GAMETE
INTERACTION

Prospects for
Immunocontraception

CONRAD WORKSHOP SERIES EDITORS

Henry L. Gabelnick, Ph.D.
Director
CONRAD Program

Gary D. Hodgen, Ph.D.
Principal Investigator
CONRAD Program

Nancy J. Alexander, Ph.D.
Director, Applied Fundamental Research
CONRAD Program

David F. Archer, M.D.
Clinical Investigator
CONRAD Program

Anibal A. Acosta, M.D.
Director, Fellowships and Andrology
CONRAD Program

Jeffrey M. Spieler, M.Sc.
Senior Biomedical Research Advisor
Research Division, Office of Population
Agency for International Development

GAMETE INTERACTION

Prospects for Immunocontraception

Proceedings of the Third Contraceptive Research and Development
(CONRAD) Program International Workshop, Cosponsored by the World
Health Organization, Held in San Carlos de Bariloche, Argentina,
November 26–29, 1989

EDITORS

NANCY J. ALEXANDER
Contraceptive Research and Development Program
Eastern Virginia Medical School
Norfolk, Virginia

DAVID GRIFFIN
World Health Organization
Geneva, Switzerland

JEFFREY M. SPIELER
Office of Population
Agency for International Development
Washington, D.C.

GEOFFREY M.H. WAITES
World Health Organization
Geneva, Switzerland

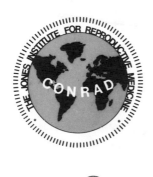
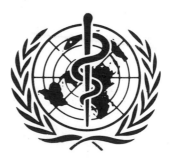

⊛ WILEY-LISS

A JOHN WILEY & SONS, INC., PUBLICATION
New York • Chichester • Brisbane • Toronto • Singapore

Address all Inquiries to the Publisher
Wiley-Liss, Inc., 41 East 11th Street, New York, NY 10003

Library of Congress Cataloging-in-Publication Data

CONRAD-WHO International Workshop (1989 : San Carlos de Bariloche, Argentina)
    Gamete interaction : prospects for immunocontraception :
proceedings of a CONRAD-WHO International Workshop, held in San
Carlos de Bariloche, Argentina, November 27–29, 1989 / editors,
Nancy J. Alexander . . . [et al.].
       p.   cm.
  Includes bibliographical references.
  Includes index.
  ISBN 0-471-56847-3
    1. Contraception, Immunological—Congresses. 2. Sperm-ovum
interactions—Congresses. I. Alexander, Nancy J.
II. Contraceptive Research and Development Program. III. World
Health Health Organization. IV. Title.
    [DNLM: 1. Contraception—congresses. 2. Sperm-Ovum Interactions—
congresses. WP 630 C754g 1989]
RG136.8.C66 1989
613.9'432—dc20
DNLM/DLC
for Library of Congress   90-12737
                                       CIP

Contents

PART I: SPERM ANTIGENS

PART II: EPIDIDYMAL AND SEMINAL PLASMA-RELATED LEADS

PART III: SPERM–ZONA INTERACTION

PART IV: ZONA PELLUCIDA ANTIGENS

Contributors

ANIBAL A. ACOSTA, Jones Institute for Reproductive Medicine, Department of Obstetrics and Gynecology, Eastern Virginia Medical School, Norfolk, VA 23510 **[471]**

G.L. ADA, Department of Immunology and Infectious Diseases, Johns Hopkins School of Hygiene and Public Health, Baltimore, MD 21205 **[565]**

KAMAL K. AHUJA, Fertility and IVF Centre, Cromwell Hospital, London SW5 0TU, and MRC Experimental Embryology and Teratology Unit, St. George's Hospital Medical School, London SW17, England **[239]**

R.J. AITKEN, MRC Reproductive Biology Unit, Centre for Reproductive Biology, Edinburgh EH3 9EW, Scotland **[293]**

NANCY J. ALEXANDER, Contraceptive Research and Development Program, Eastern Virginia Medical School, Norfolk, VA 23510; present address: Contraceptive Development Branch, National Institute of Child Health and Diseases, National Institutes of Health, Rockville, MD 20892 **[345,471]**

D.W. ANDERSON, Department of Immunopharmacology, R.W. Johnson Pharmaceutical Research Institute, Raritan, NJ 08869 **[523]**

DEBORAH J. ANDERSON, Fearing Research Laboratory, Department of Obstetrics, Gynecology, and Reproductive Biology, Harvard Medical School, Boston, MA 02115 **[103,175]**

K. ARUNAN, National Institute of Immunology, New Delhi 110067, India **[579]**

C.S. BAMBRA, Department of Reproduction, Institute of Primate Research, National Museums of Kenya, Karen, Nairobi, Kenya **[487]**

C. BARROS, Laboratorio de Embriologia, Departamento de Ciencias Fisiologicas, Facultad de Ciencias Biologicas, Pontifica Universidad Catolica de Chile, Santiago, Chile **[185]**

IGLIKA BATOVA, Institute of Biology & Immunology of Reproduction & Development of Organisms, Bulgarian Academy of Sciences, Sofia 1143, Bulgaria **[359]**

M.I. BECKER, Unidad de Immunologia, Departamento de Biologia Celular, Facultad de Ciencias Biologicas, Pontifica Universidad Catolica de Chile, Santiago, Chile **[185]**

JORGE A. BLAQUIER, FERTILAB, 1121 Buenos Aires, Argentina, and Instituto de Biologia y Medicina Experimental, 1428 Buenos Aires, Argentina **[129]**

P. BRAUDE, Department of Obstetrics and Gynecology, St. Thomas' Hospital, London, England **[293]**

D. BUNCH, Department of Cell Biology, Duke University Medical Center, Durham, NC 27710 **[225]**

The numbers in brackets are the opening page numbers of the contributors' articles.

xi

LANI J. BURKMAN, Jones Institute for Reproductive Medicine, Department of Obstetrics and Gynecology, Eastern Virginia Medical School, Norfolk, VA 23510 [471]

MÓNICA S. CAMEO, FERTILAB, 1121 Buenos Aires, Argentina [129]

R.J. CAPETOLA, Department of Experimental Therapeutics, R.W. Johnson Pharmaceutical Research Institute, Raritan, NJ 08869 [523]

C. CAPOTE, Laboratorio de Embriologia, Departamento de Ciencias Fisiologicas, Facultad de Ciencias Biologicas, Pontifica Universidad Catolica de Chile, Santiago, Chile [185]

CHRISTOPHER P. CARRON, Division of Reproductive Biology, Department of Obstetrics and Gynecology, Duke University Medical Center, Durham, NC 27710; present address: Monsanto Corporate Research, Monsanto Company, Chesterfield, MO 63198 [401]

D. CECHOVA, Institute of Molecular Genetics, Czechoslovak Academy of Sciences, Prague, Czechoslovakia [197]

C. CHEVRIER, Laboratoire de Physiologie de la Reproduction, INRA, UA-CNRS 1291, 37380 Nouzilly, France, and Laboratoire de Physiologie Comparée, Faculté des Sciences, Tours, France [111]

WILLIAM W. CHIN, Division of Genetics, Department of Medicine, Brigham and Women's Hospital, and Howard Hughes Medical Institute, Harvard Medical School, Boston, MA 02115 [419]

CHARLES C. CODDINGTON, Jones Institute for Reproductive Medicine, Department of Obstetrics and Gynecology, Eastern Virginia Medical School, Norfolk, VA 23510 [471]

DANIELA CONESA, Instituto de Biologia y Medicina Experimental, 1428 Buenos Aires, Argentina [143]

PATRICIA S. CUASNICÚ, Instituto de Biologia y Medicina Experimental, 1428 Buenos Aires, Argentina [143]

F. DACHEUX, Laboratoire de Physiologie de la Reproduction, INRA, UA-CNRS 1291, 37380 Nouzilly, France, and Laboratoire de Physiologie Comparée, Faculté des Sciences, Tours, France [111]

J.L. DACHEUX, Laboratoire de Physiologie de la Reproduction, INRA, UA-CNRS 1291, 37380 Nouzilly, France, and Laboratoire de Physiologie Comparée, Faculté des Sciences, Tours, France [111]

ADRIANA DAWIDOWSKI, Instituto de Biologia y Medicina Experimental, 1428 Buenos Aires, Argentina [129]

JURRIEN DEAN, Laboratory of Cellular and Developmental Biology, NIDDK, National Institutes of Health, Bethesda, MD 20894 [313]

A.E. DE IOANNES, Unidad de Immunologia, Departamento de Biologia Celular, Facultad de Ciencias Biologicas, Pontifica Universidad Catolica de Chile, Santiago, Chile [185]

BONNIE S. DUNBAR, Department of Cell Biology, Baylor College of Medicine, Houston, TX 77030 [277]

CHARLES J. FLICKINGER, Department of Anatomy and Cell Biology, University of Virginia, Charlottesville, VA 22908 [13]

JAMES FOSTER, Department of Anatomy and Cell Biology, University of Virginia, Charlottesville, VA 22908 [13]

DANIEL R. FRANKEN, Infertility Clinic, Tygerberg Hospital, Tygerberg 7505, South Africa [471]

A.E. FRIESS, Institute of Veterinary Anatomy, University of Bern, 3001 Bern, Switzerland [197]

J.L. GATTI, Laboratoire de Physiologie de la Reproduction, INRA, UA-CNRS 1291, 37380 Nouzilly, France [111]

ERWIN GOLDBERG, Department of Biochemistry, Molecular Biology and Cell Biology, Northwestern University, Evanston, IL 60208 [63]

FERNANDA GONZALEZ ECHE-VERRIA, FERTILAB, 1121 Buenos Aires, Argentina [129]

DAVID GRIFFIN, Special Programme of Research, Development and Research Training in Human Reproduction, World Health Organization, 1211 Geneva 27, Switzerland [501]

SATISH K. GUPTA, Gamete Antigen Laboratory, National Institute of Immunology, New Delhi 110067, India [345]

SEN-ITIROH HAKOMORI, The Biomembrane Institute, Seattle, WA 98119 [155]

A. HENSCHEN, Max Planck Institute for Biochemistry, Martinsried, Federal Republic of Germany; present address: Department of Molecular Biology & Biochemistry, University of California, Irvine, California 92717 [197]

JOHN C. HERR, Department of Anatomy and Cell Biology, University of Virginia, Charlottesville, VA 22908 [13]

TAGE HJORT, Institute of Medical Microbiology, University of Aarhus, DK-8000 Aarhus C, Denmark [333]

GARY D. HODGEN, Jones Institute for Reproductive Medicine, Department of Obstetrics and Gynecology, Eastern Virginia Medical School, Norfolk, VA 23510 [471]

MONA HOMYK, Department of Anatomy and Cell Biology, University of Virginia, Charlottesville, VA 22908 [13]

A.M. HUNDAL, Department of Genetics, University of Glasgow, Glasgow G11 5JS, Scotland [435]

M.A. ISAHAKIA, Department of Reproduction, Institute of Primate Research, National Museums of Kenya, Karen, Nairobi, Kenya [487]

SHINZO ISOJIMA, Department of Obstetrics and Gynecology, Hyogo Medical College, Nishinomiya 663, Japan [155,359]

C. JEULIN, Laboratoire de Biologie de la Reproduction et du Development, CHU Bicêtre, Kremlin Bicêtre, France [111]

EDWARD JOHN, Department of Anatomy and Cell Biology, University of Virginia, Charlottesville, VA 22908 [13]

WARREN R. JONES, Department of Obstetrics and Gynecology, Flinders Medical Centre, University of South Australia, Bedford Park SA 5042, Australia [459,595]

KINU KAMEDA, Department of Obstetrics and Gynecology, Hyogo Medical College, Nishinomiya 663, Japan [155,359]

KENNETH KLOTZ, Department of Anatomy and Cell Biology, University of Virginia, Charlottesville, VA 22908 [13]

P. THILLAI KOOTHAN, MRC Reproductive Biology Unit, Centre for Reproductive Biology, Edinburgh EH3 9EW, Scotland [293]

DENNIS E. KOPPEL, Department of Biochemistry, University of Connecticut Health Center, Farmington, CT 06030 [1]

KOJI KOYAMA, Department of Obstetrics and Gynecology, Hyogo Medical College, Nishinomiya 663, Japan [359]

THINUS F. KRUGER, Infertility Clinic, Tygerberg Hospital, Tygerberg 7505, South Africa [471]

MACIEJ KURPISŻ, Department of Immunogenetics, Institute of Human Genetics, Polish Academy of Sciences, 60-479 Poznan, Poland **[377]**

ARTHUR C. LEE, Department of Obstetrics and Gynecology, Ohio State University, Columbus, OH 43210 **[549]**

CHI-YU GREGORY LEE, Acute Care Unit, Department of Obstetrics and Gynecology, University of British Columbia, Vancouver, British Columbia V6T 2B5, Canada **[37]**

P. LE GUEN, Department of Obstetrics and Gynecology, Duke University Medical Center, Durham, NC 27710 **[225]**

D.H. LEWIS, Department of New Product Development, Stolle Research and Development Corporation, Decatur, AL 35601 **[549]**

L. LEYTON, Department of Obstetrics and Gynecology, Duke University Medical Center, Durham, NC 27710 **[225]**

MING-SUN LIU, Acute Care Unit, Department of Obstetrics and Gynecology, University of British Columbia, Vancouver, British Columbia V6T 2B5, Canada **[37]**

M. McBRIDE, Department of Genetics, University of Glasgow, Glasgow G11 5JS, Scotland **[435]**

SARAH E. MILLAR, Laboratory of Cellular and Developmental Biology, NIDDK, National Institutes of Health, Bethesda, MD 20894 **[313]**

N.A. MITCHISON, Imperial Cancer Research Fund Immunology Unit, Biology Department, University College London, London WC1E 6BT, England **[607]**

ALISON MOORE, Gamete Biology Unit, MRC/AFRC Comparative Physiology Research Group, Institute of Zooology, Zoological Society of London, Regent's Park, London NW1 4RY, England **[53]**

HARRY D.M. MOORE, Gamete Biology Unit, MRC/AFRC Comparative Physiology Research Group, Institute of Zoology, Zoological Society of London, Regent's Park, London NW1 4RY, England **[53]**

DIANA G. MYLES, Department of Physiology, University of Connecticut Health Center, Farmington, CT 06030 **[1,89]**

D.A. NICKSON, Department of Genetics, University of Glasgow, Glasgow G11 5JS, Scotland **[435]**

B.S. NIKOLAJCZYK, Laboratories for Cell Biology, Department of Cell Biology and Anatomy, University of North Carolina, Chapel Hill, NC 27599 **[213]**

SERGIO OEHNINGER, Jones Institute for Reproductive Medicine, Department of Obstetrics and Gynecology, Eastern Virginia Medical School, Norfolk, VA 23510 **[471]**

M.G. O'RAND, Laboratories for Cell Biology, Department of Cell Biology and Anatomy, University of North Carolina, Chapel Hill, NC 27599 **[213]**

R. PAL, National Institute of Immunology, New Delhi 110067, India **[579]**

M. PAQUIGNON, Laboratoire de Physiologie de la Reproduction, INRA-CNRS 1291, 37380 Nouzilly, France **[111]**

C. PARISET, UER Biomedicale des Saint Peres, Paris, France **[111]**

M. PATERSON, MRC Reproductive Biology Unit, Centre for Reproductive Biology, Edinburgh EH3 9EW, Scotland **[293]**

C. PERÉZ, Laboratorio de Embriologia, Departamento de Ciencias Fisiologicas, Facultad de Ciencias Biologicas, Pontifica Universidad Catolica de
Chile, Santiago, Chile [185]

JOHN E. POWELL, Department of
Obstetrics and Gynecology, Ohio
State University, Columbus, OH 43210
[549]

PAUL PRIMAKOFF, Department
of Physiology, University of Connecticut Health Center, Farmington, CT
06030 [1,89]

R.T. RICHARDSON, Laboratories
for Cell Biology, Department of Cell
Biology and Anatomy, University of
North Carolina, Chapel Hill, NC 27599
[213]

MICHAEL RICKEY, Depaertment
of Research and Development, Stolle
Research and Development Corporation, Cincinnati, OH 45242 [549]

LEONORA ROCHWERGER, In-
stituto de Biologia y Medicina Experimental, 1428 Buenos Aires, Argentina
[143]

ANTHONY G. SACCO, Depart-
ment of Obstetrics and Gynecology,
Wayne State University School of
Medicine, Detroit, MI 48201 [259]

P. SALING, Departments of Obstet-
rics & Gynecology and Cell Biology,
Duke University Medical Center,
Durham, NC 27710 [225]

CLAUDIA SANJURJO, FERTILAB,
1121 Buenos Aires, Argentina [129]

M. SELUB, Department of Obstetrics
and Gynecology, Duke University
Medical Center, Durham, NC 27710
[225]

R.B. SHABANOWITZ, Division of
Reproductive Endocrinology, Depart-
ment of Obstetrics and Gynecology,
University of North Carolina, Chapel
Hill, NC 27599 [213]

CHANDRIMA SHAHA, Sperm
Biotechnology Laboratory, National
Institute of Immunology, New Delhi
110067, India [75]

T. SHESHADRI, Sperm Biotechnology Laboratory, National Institute of
Immunology, New Delhi 110067, India
[75]

MINORU SHIGETA, Department
of Obstetrics and Gynecology, Hyogo
Medical College, Nishinomiya 663, Japan [155]

O. SINGH, National Institute of Immunology, New Delhi 110067, India
[579]

SHERI M. SKINNER, Department
of Cell Biology, Baylor College of Medicine, Houston, TX 77030 [277]

CAROLINE A. SMITH, Gamete Biology Unit, MRC/AFRC Comparative
Physiology Research Group, Institute
of Zoology, Zoological Society of London, Regent's Park, London NW1
4RY, England [53]

M. STEINBERGER, Andrology
Unit, Department of Dermatology,
University of Munich, D-8000 Munich
2, Federal Republic of Germany [197]

V.C. STEVENS, Department of Obstetrics and Gynecology, Ohio State
University, Columbus, OH 43210 [549]

MING-WAN SU, Andrology Laboratory, Department of Obstetrics and
Gynecology, University of British Columbia, Vancouver, British Columbia
V6T 2B5, Canada [37]

ANIL SURI, Sperm Biotechnology
Laboratory, National Institute of Immunology, New Delhi 11067, India
[75]

R.G. SUTCLIFFE, Department of
Genetics, University of Glasgow, Glasgow G11 5JS, Scotland [435]

G.P. TALWAR, Sperm Biotechnology Laboratory, National Institute of
Immunology, New Delhi 110067, India
[75,579]

THERESE M. TIMMONS, Department of Cell Biology, Baylor College of Medicine, Houston, TX 77030 **[277]**

E. TÖPFER-PETERSEN, Andrology Unit, Department of Derma- tology, University of Munich, D-8000 Munich 2, Federal Republic of Germany **[197]**

YOSHIYUKI TSUJI, Department of Obstetrics and Gynecology, Hyogo Medical College, Nishinomiya 663, Japan **[155,359]**

S.-L. WANG, Department of Genetics, University of Glasgow, Glasgow G11 5JS, Scotland **[435]**

E.E. WIDGREN, Laboratories for Cell Biology, Department of Cell Biology and Anatomy, University of North Carolina, Chapel Hill, NC 27599 **[213]**

RICHARD M. WRIGHT, Department of Anatomy and Cell Biology, University of Virginia, Charlottesville, VA 22908 **[13]**

S. ZEINALI, Department of Genetics, University of Glasgow, Glasgow G11 5JS, Scotland **[435]**

JIA-BEI ZHU, Andrology Laboratory, Department of Obstetrics and Gynecology, University of British Columbia, Vancouver, British Columbia V6T 2B5, Canada **[37]**

Preface

In cooperation with the United States Agency for International Development (USAID), the Contraceptive Research and Development (CONRAD) Program, Eastern Virginia Medical School, Norfolk, Virginia, has as its primary mission the development of new, safe, effective, and acceptable methods of fertility regulation suitable for use in developing countries. The WHO Special Programme of Research, Development and Research Training in Human Reproduction, which co-sponsored the workshop, has a similar mission within its broader overall mandate. Both programs recognize the need for international workshops that bring together leading scientists from developed and developing countries to present their work and to exchange ideas on research related to specific areas of contraception and fertility regulation.

The purpose of this workshop was to:

— Describe sperm and ovum-specific antigens and sperm-zona interaction
— Review the use of antibodies to define gamete-specific antigens
— Discuss the role of molecular biology for antigen production
— Describe methods and models for defining and evaluating gamete antigens
— Identify the steps in immunocontraceptive development
— Review the status of clinical trials of vaccines for fertility regulation
— Establish research priorities in immunocontraception

From 27 countries, the workshop attracted 43 speakers, moderators, and participants comprising many of the world's authorities in this field. Through the publication of these proceedings, we are pleased to be sharing the information presented in papers, posters, and discussions with a broader audience than was fortunate enough to have participated directly.

Nancy J. Alexander
David Griffin
Jeffrey M. Spieler
Geoffrey M.H. Waites

xvii

Defining Sperm Surface Domains

Diana G. Myles, Dennis E. Koppel,
and Paul Primakoff

For some time it has been known that the mammalian sperm surface is heterogeneous. With a variety of probes this heterogeneity can be detected in the form of an uneven distribution of surface charge, lectin-binding groups, antibody-binding sites, and intramembane particles (IMPs) as revealed by freeze fracture [reviewed by Eddy, 1988].

There are two aspects of membrane heterogeneity. First is the heterogeneity of sites on the sperm surface that can be identified by probes that recognize specific sites. Most information we have about surface heterogeneity comes from this type of information. It does not tell us the ultimate location of molecules on the surface, but it does tell us the distribution of sites recognized by a particular probe, and this information can be most relevant in terms of surface function. For example, because galactosyltransferase activity is required for binding mouse sperm to the zona pellucida [Lopez et al., 1985], the distribution of substrate-binding activity is more important in terms of the localization of this function than is the absolute distribution of the enzyme itself [Scully et al., 1987]. If the substrate-binding site were covered or occupied in all regions of the sperm surface except for one surface domain, then, for functional purposes, the enzyme activity would be localized to that specific region. The second aspect of membrane heterogeneity lies in the ultimate distribution of the molecule itself as either an integral or peripheral part of the membrane. The actual distribution of surface molecules (as opposed to surface sites) may be more difficult to determine, but is ultimately useful for understanding the mechanisms responsible for

Gamete Interaction: Prospects for Immunocontraception, pages 1–11

maintenance and dynamics of sperm surface domains. In many cases the distribution of specific surface sites may reflect the distribution of surface molecules, but the distribution of the molecules may be actually broader than the distribution of a particular accessible site on the molecule. A surface probe may not have access to a particular site if it is covert due either to conformation of the molecule or to the interaction with another molecule.

DYNAMICS OF THE SPERM SURFACE

In addition to defining molecular surface domains, there are questions of how these surface domains are maintained, created, and altered.

Maintenance

The mechanism that maintains the heterogeneity of the cell surface is probably a complex set of molecular interactions. Membrane asymmetry could result from 1) the restriction of molecular diffusion so that molecules are tethered in a particular region (through either external or internal interactions); 2) thermodynamic partitioning in which the molecule is restricted by its preference for the environment in one region over another; or 3) a barrier in the membrane that does not allow freely diffusing molecules to move from one surface domain to another. In examples 1 and 2 an initial asymmetry of membrane molecules or associated structures is implied. The third possibility, a membrane barrier, indicates a specialized membrane structure exists at the junctions of surface domains.

Creation and Alteration of Membrane Domains

The creation of specific domains occurs when the sperm is being formed in the testis and continues during passage through the male reproductive tract, when the sperm contacts reproductive tract fluids. In addition, the localization of surface molecules established at one stage is not necessarily final but can be altered until the time of fertilization.

Potential mechanisms for the creation of surface domains include 1) a new molecule being inserted into or associated with a specific region or 2) an initial whole cell distribution of a molecule becoming secondarily restricted to a specific domain. Localized insertion would require a targeting message in the molecule that directs it to a specific region of the cell. This could occur for proteins synthesized by the sperm in the testis during sperm formation, or it could theoretically occur after sperm leave the testis by the external insertion of a protein from the fluid of the male reproductive tract. Alternatively, targeting of a peripheral protein to a specific domain from an external source could be through the binding of a ligand to a previously localized receptor. Secondary restriction of a molecule could reflect elimination from the cell surface in some regions while the molecule is retained in other regions. It could also result from the movement of molecules from regions where it is to be eliminated into the specific domain where it becomes localized. If, instead of the entire molecule becoming localized, there is a localization of only the access of a probe to a specific site, then the creation of a domain can occur by the limiting of access to that site by a change in the conformation of the protein in that region or its association with another molecule that blocks access.

The alteration of existing domains may have many similarities to their initial creation. Molecules may be either eliminated from specific regions or moved from one region to another. Also, the acrosome reaction results in a major rearrangement of the plasma membrane, including the loss of the plasma membrane over the anterior head domain and the insertion of a new membrane (inner acrosomal membrane) in the anterior part of the head. This means that molecules in the anterior head domain are shed from the cell, and a new membrane, potentially with a very different set of molecules, is incorporated into the surface.

GUINEA PIG SPERM SURFACE

The surface of guinea pig sperm has been investigated by a variety of methods, including freeze fracture, lectins, lipid probes, and antibodies [Friend, 1982]. We have used monoclonal antibodies (mAbs) raised against sperm membranes to define surface domains on the sperm at various stages of sperm maturation and to investigate questions of how the domains are established, altered, and maintained.

On testicular sperm we have observed patterns of antibody binding to whole cell, whole head, anterior tail, and posterior tail [Myles and Primakoff, 1983; Phelps and Myles, 1987] (also Phelps et al., 1990; Cowan and Myles, unpublished results). Therefore, even sperm in the testis have some localized antigenic sites. On sperm taken from the epididymis, we observed patterns of antibody binding that were restricted to anterior, posterior, or whole head and anterior, posterior, or whole tail (Fig. 1). After the acrosome reaction, additional patterns included the limitation of epitopes to either the

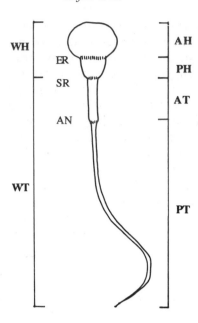

Fig. 1.   Surface domains defined by monoclonal antibodies on acrosome-intact guinea pig sperm: AH, anterior head; PH, posterior head; WH, whole head; AT, anterior tail; PT, posterior tail; and WT, whole tail. The anterior head domain extends to the bottom of the underlying acrosomal membrane. The anterior tail domain coincides with the region of the midpiece. Junctions of surface domains are marked by the following regions of plasma membrane specialization: ER, equatorial region; SR, striated ring; AN, annulus.

inner acrosomal membrane or equatorial region only. These observed distribution patterns of antigenic determinants on the guinea pig sperm surface may not be the only ones; other patterns may exist.

Maintenance of Surface Domains

One of the first questions we asked was how could these antigens be maintained in their polarized distribution. To determine if the antigens were tethered within a restricted region, we measured the lateral diffusion of two of the antigens at different stages in sperm maturation (Table 1). With the technique of fluorescence redistribution after photobleaching (FRAP), two different parameters were measured: the diffusion coefficient, D, which is the rate at which diffusion occurs in cm^2/sec, and the percent recovery, R, which is the percent mobile fraction [Koppel, 1979]. Diffusion coefficients of proteins range from about 10^{-12} cm^2/sec, which is the limit of resolution

TABLE 1. Diffusion Coefficients and Percent Recovery of PH-20
and PT-1 Proteins

Antibody	Sperm type	Localization	$D \times 10^9$ (cm^2/sec)	Percent recovery
PH-20	Testicular	Whole cell	0.019	72
	Cauda, acrosome intact	Posterior head	0.18	73
	Cauda, acrosome reacted	Inner acrosomal membrane	4.9	78
PT-1	Cauda, fresh	Posterior tail	2.5	90
	Cauda, after capacitation	Whole tail (measured in the anterior tail)	1.0	~30

for most measurements and is considered to be immobile, and 2–5 ×
10^{-9} cm^2/sec, which is at the theoretical limit of a protein in a lipid
bilayer and is considered to be freely diffusing. PH-20 protein on
testicular sperm and on acrosome-intact sperm from the cauda
showed restricted diffusion; on testicular sperm diffusion was very
restricted, and on acrosome-intact sperm it was typical of membrane
proteins that show some restriction in their diffusion. Therefore, on
testicular sperm, restriction of the lateral diffusion of the PH-20 protein prevents its movement from one region to another, but in this
case it shows a whole cell distribution. This restriction may result
from interactions with an external coat or matrix but cannot result in
a direct interaction of all the PH-20 molecules with a cytoplasmic
structure, since PH-20 is anchored in the membrane via a lipid anchor, glycosyl phosphatidylinositol (GPI), and is therefore only inserted into the outer half of the lipid bilayer [Phelps et al., 1988]. On
acrosome-intact sperm from the cauda, PH-20 may also have some
transient interactions in the outer half of the membrane that maintain
it in the posterior head region [Cowan et al., 1987]. However, PH-20,
localized to the inner acrosomal membrane of acrosome-reacted
cells, and PT-1, restricted either to the posterior tail of sperm taken
fresh from the cauda or on the whole tail after capacitation, are both
freely diffusing in the membrane (Table 1) [Cowan et al., 1987; Myles
et al., 1984]. This lack of constraint indicates that there must be a
mechanism other than restriction of diffusion that prevents these
antigens from diffusing out of their domains into new regions of the
cell surface. We have suggested that there are barriers in the membrane that prevent diffusion between domains and that these barri-

crs occur at the equatorial region, the posterior ring (the junction between the head and the tail), and the annulus (the junction between the anterior and posterior tail regions) [Myles and Primakoff, 1986; Myles et al., 1987]. In all three of these regions, specialized structures associated with the membrane have been described with freeze fracture techniques [Friend and Fawcett, 1974]. The maintenance of specific molecular domains of the guinea pig sperm surface may involve a combination of mechanisms, but, for the surface distributions that we have described, the existence of three such membrane barriers could be invoked to explain any of the described distribution patterns.

Creation and Alteration of Domains

Specific antibody-binding patterns were detected in testicular sperm, but we do not yet have any information about how they were created. We have, however, studied the mechanism(s) of how domains are created and altered during epididymal passage, capacitation, and the acrosome reaction.

During epididymal maturation there are some antibody-binding patterns that are left unaltered, some antibody-binding patterns that become restricted in their distribution, and some epitopes that first appear during passage through the epididymis. One example of an antibody-binding pattern that becomes restricted is that of the three mAbs PH-20, PH-21, and PH-22, which bind to the PH-20 protein. All three antibodies bind to the entire surface of testicular sperm, but are restricted in their binding to the posterior head of sperm taken from the cauda (Fig. 2) [Phelps and Myles, 1987]. We have recently made measurements of antibody bound in the posterior head region of sperm populations that were prelabeled with antibody and then induced to restrict their distribution in an in vitro system that mimics epididymal passage. These experiments indicate that the change in distribution of PH-20 during epidiymal maturation involves the migration of the protein from other region(s) into the posterior head region. Some loss or covering of the epitope (or molecule) may also be involved (Phelps et al., 1990). PH-30 monoclonal antibody represents an antibody in which binding does not occur on testicular sperm; binding of this mAb is first observed on cauda sperm, where it is restricted to the posterior head region (Fig. 2) [Primakoff et al., 1987]. In this case, the epitope recognized by the PH-30 mAb is not available on testicular sperm even though the PH-30 protein is present. The PH-30 protein has been detected on the whole head of testicular sperm with several different polyclonal antibodies raised

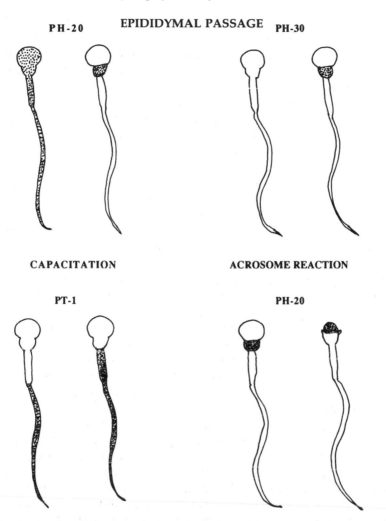

Fig. 2. Examples of alterations of monoclonal antibody (mAb)–binding patterns that occur during sperm maturation. After epididymal passage, PH-20 mAb binding is restricted to the posterior head region and PH-30 mAb is able to bind newly to the sperm. Even though the PH-30 protein is present on the testicular sperm, the epitope recognized by the PH-30 mAb is covert or missing on testicular sperm. During capacitation, PT-1 mAb-binding pattern increases to include the whole tail. After the acrosome reaction, the binding pattern of PH-20 mAb is changed from a posterior head pattern to inner acrosomal membrane only.

against purified PH-30 protein, and it can be either immunoprecip-itated (Phelps et al., 1990) or immunoblotted (Blobel et al., 1990) by polyclonal antibodies. The epitope recognized by the PH-30 mAb must be either created or uncovered during epididymal passage. The

changes in surface domains that we have observed during epididymal passage can be mimicked in vitro by brief trypsin treatment
(Phelps et al., 1990). This indicates that one of the factors active in
creating and altering domains during epididymal passage could be
limited proteolysis.

We have also explored the mechanisms(s) that could be responsible
for the alterations in membrane domains that occur during capacitation and the acrosome reaction. During capacitation there is a change
in the binding of the PT-1 mAb from posterior tail only to whole tail
(Fig. 2). Prelabeling experiments demonstrated that this change results from the migration of a part of the population of the PT-1 protein
from the posterior tail region to the anterior tail [Myles and Primakoff,
1984]. A substantial population of the PT-1–labeled protein on the
anterior tail is immobilized, whereas the posterior tail region has a
high mobile fraction (Table 1). Furthermore, photobleaching experiments indicated that there was no systematic flow or drift of PT-
1–labeled protein in the direction of the anterior tail. Rather, the
comparison of data simulations to actual experiments indicate that
there is a partially permeable barrier at the anterior tail–posterior tail
junction during migration [Koppel et al., 1986]. These data are consistent with the migration being the result of protein diffusion from
the posterior tail to a trap in the anterior tail region.

Similarly, there is a migration of prelabeled PH-20 protein from the
posterior head domain to the inner acrosomal membrane after the
acrosome reaction (Fig. 2) [Myles and Primakoff, 1984]. However,
video analysis of PH-20 protein during migration indicates that there
may be an entirely different mechanism involved. Early in the migration process, an intensity gradient is observed for fluorescently
labeled PH-20 protein on acrosome reacted sperm. The gradient increases in the direction of PH-20 migration; if PH-20 were diffusing
from the posterior head region and being trapped in the region of the
inner acrosomal membrane, no such gradient should be formed.
These results indicate that migration of PH-20 does not result from
diffusion to a trap but that there is an active mechanism that moves
PH-20 from the posterior head domain into the newly inserted inner
acrosomal membrane [Cowan et al., 1986a; manuscript submitted].

SUMMARY AND CONCLUSIONS

Segregation of surface sites and molecules into defined surface
domains on the sperm surface is complex. It occurs at different times
and perhaps via different mechanisms. These arrangements are not
static but can be altered at different stages in sperm maturation.

Rearrangements of surface molecules can occur as the result of external signals and includes the creation or uncovering of new epitopes on preexisting surface molecules.

Potentially the dynamics of these surface domains could regulate surface functions. They provide a mechanism for bringing together regulatory molecules with catalytic sites and also for concentrating molecules on the surface that could be a prerequisite for both cell adhesion [Norment et al., 1988] and cell–cell fusion [Ellens et al., 1989].

ACKNOWLEDGMENTS

This work was supported by National Institutes of Health grants HD16580 (to D.G.M.) and GM-23585 (to D.E.K.). D.G.M. was supported by an American Cancer Society Faculty Research Award. The authors thank Ms. Diane Malena for preparation of the manuscript.

REFERENCES

Blobel CP, Myles DG, Primakoff P, White JM (1990): Proteolytic processing of a protein involved in sperm-egg fusion correlates with acquisition of fertilization competence. J Cell Biol 111:69–78.

Cowan AE, Myles DG, Koppel DE (1986a): Migration of the PH-20 plasma membrane protein on individual guinea pig sperm analyzed by computer-enhanced video microscopy. J Cell Biol 103:468a.

Cowan AE, Myles DG, Koppel DE (1987): Lateral diffusion of the PH-20 protein on guinea pig sperm: Evidence that barriers to diffusion maintain plasma membrane domains in mammalian sperm. J Cell Biol 104:917–923.

Cowan AE, Myles DG, Koppel DE: Migration of the guinea pig sperm membrane protein PH-20 from one localized domain to another involves active translocation (manuscript submitted).

Cowan AE, Primakoff P, Myles DG (1986b): Sperm exocytosis increases the amount of PH-20 antigen on the surface of guinea pig sperm. J Cell Biol 103:1289–1297.

Eddy EM (1988): The Spermatozoon. In Knobil E, Neill JD (eds): The Physiology of Reproduction. New York: Raven Press, pp 27–68.

Ellens H, Bentz J, Mason D, White JM (1989): The fusion site of influenza HA-expressing fibroblasts requires more than one HA trimer. J Cell Biol 109:159a.

Friend DS (1982): Plasma-membrane diversity in a highly polarized cell. J Cell Biol 93:243–249.

Friend, DS, Fawcett DW (1974): Membrane differentiations in freeze-fracture mammalian sperm. J Cell Biol 93:243–249.

Koppel DE (1979): Fluorescence redistribution after photobleaching. Biophys J 28:281–292.

10   *Myles et al.*

Koppel DE, Primakoff P, Myles DG (1986): Fluorescence photobleaching analysis of cell surface regionalization. In Taylor DL, Waggoner AS, Murphy RF, Lanni F, Birge RR (eds): Applications of Fluorescence in the Biolmedical Sciences. New York: Alan R. Liss, pp 477–497.

Lopez LC, Bayna EM, Litoff D, Shaper NL, Shaper JH, Shur BD (1985): Receptor function of mouse sperm surface galactosyltransferase during fertilization. J Cell Biol 101:1501–1510.

Myles DG, Koppel DE, Cowan AE, Phelps BM, Primakoff P (1987): Rearrangement of sperm surface antigens prior to fertilization. Cell Biol Testis Epidid 513:262–273.

Myles DG, Primakoff P (1983): Establishment of sperm surface topography during development analyzed with monoclonal antibodies. In Andre J (ed): The Sperm Cell. The Hague: Martinus Nijhoff, pp 127–130.

Myles DG, Primakoff P (1984): Localized surface antigens of guinea pig sperm migrate to new regions prior to fertilization. J Cell Biol 99:1634–1641.

Myles DG, Primakoff P (1986): Topographic distribution of sperm surface proteins and sperm–egg interaction. J Electron Microsc (Suppl) 35:1889–1982.

Myles DG, Primakoff P, Koppel DE (1984): A localized surface protein of guinea pig sperm exhibits free diffusion in its domain. J Cell Biol 98:1905–1909.

Norment AM, Salter RD, Parham P, Engelhard VH, Littman DR (1988): Cell–cell adhesion mediated by CD8 and MDC class I molecules. Nature 336:79–81.

Phelps B, Myles DG (1987): The guinea pig sperm surface protein, PH-20, reaches the surface via two transport pathways and becomes localized to a domain after an initial uniform distribution. Dev Biol 123:63–72.

Phelps BM, Koppel DE, Primakoff P, Myles DG (1990): Evidence that proteolysis of the surface is an initial step in the mechanism of formation of sperm cell surface domains. J Cell Biol (in press).

Phelps BM, Primakoff P, Koppel DE, Low MR, Myles DG (1988): Restricted lateral diffusion of PH-20, a PI-anchored sperm membrane protein. Science 240:1780–1782.

Primakoff P, Hyatt H, Tredick-Kline J (1987): Identification and purification of a sperm surface protein with a potential role in sperm–egg membrane fusion. J Cell Biol 104:141–149.

Scully NF, Shaper JH, Shur BD (1987): Spatial and temporal expression of cell surface galactosyltransferase during mouse spermatogenesis and epididymal maturation. Dev Biol 124:111–124.

DISCUSSION

DR. BURGOS: My question is related to the appearance of the epitope recognized by the PH-30 monoclonal antibody in the caudal region of the epididymis. In fact, it's more than a question, it's an addition to your presentation. Our research has indicated that sperm become gradually positive for this epitope as they reach the proximal caudal epididymis. If we apply trypsin to epididymal sperm, all become positive. So, perhaps there is an unmasking of the PH-30 protein in a particular portion of the epididymis.

DR. MYLES: We have now analyzed the location of the appearance of the epitope recognized by PH-30 MAb in guinea pigs, looking at epididymal sections. And, it's exactly where you suggest—right where you move into the proximal portion of the epididymis. It's a very distinct line. No staining occurs proximally, but at that region the sperm become positive.

DR. HAMILTON: After seeing your abstract at the Cell Biology meetings in San Francisco concerning your studies with guinea pigs, we went home and repeated your studies with rats using our monoclonal antibodies. I have to say that there must be species variations or antigen variations, because none of our antibodies that we had behaved the way your antibodies did. This is merely an observation and a caution that the finding can't be generalized.

DR. MYLES: You treated testicular sperm with trypsin and you saw no change?

DR. HAMILTON: Correct.

DR. GROOTEGOED: You showed the presence of PH-20 and two subunits of PH-30 on spermatogenic cells. Can you tell us at what stage of spermatogenesis these proteins are first expressed? At the spermatocyte or spermatid stage?

DR. MYLES: We first detected PH-20 on round spermatids, at the earliest stages when the acrosome is forming. For PH-30, I'm not sure, because most of our localization studies we have done have employed the monoclonal antibody that doesn't recognize antigen until the cauda.

DR. HECHT: With PH-20 there was a slight change in the electrophoretic mobility before it was clipped. Is that essential for the processing event?

DR. MYLES: It is not essential when the proteolytic clip is mimicked by trypsin treatment. It may, of course, be essential in order to allow PH-20 to function, but I don't know for sure.

DR. HECHT: Do you know what that change is?

DR. MYLES: No, but as you saw in the nonreducing gel, the decrease that is happening is in the 41,000 to 48,000 fragment and not in the 26,000 fragment.

DR. DACHEUX: After treatment with trypsin, do all spermatozoa react similarily?

DR. MYLES: Yes. The population after treatment with trypsin is generally around 90%.

2

Monoclonal Antibody MHS-10 and Its Cognate Intra-Acrosomal Antigen SP-10

John C. Herr, Richard M. Wright, Edward John, Kenneth Klotz, Mona Homyk, James Foster, and Charles J. Flickinger

The World Health Organization Task Force on Contraceptive Vaccines, which met in June 1986 at the time of the 3rd International Congress of Reproductive Immunology, designated the human sperm protein SP-10 as a "primary vaccine candidate" [Anderson et al., 1987]. This designation was based on three criteria that were apparently fulfilled by a monoclonal antibody to SP-10 (termed *mAb MHS-10*, or *S20* in WHO nomenclature): "1) reactivity with human testicular germ cells and abundant surface antigens on mature spermatozoa; 2) no, or minimal, cross reactivity with somatic cells; and 3) inhibition of at least one sperm function assay." The goals of this paper are 1) to review our major findings [Herr et al., 1990 a–c; Homyk et al., 1990; Wright et al., 1990] regarding the biochemical and morphological characterization of the SP-10 protein and the coding region of the SP-10 gene, 2) to indicate where our recent data clarify or modify the conclusions of the WHO Task Force, and 3) to discuss the relevance of our basic biochemical and morphological data to the potential of SP-10 as a vaccine immunogen.

Gamete Interaction: Prospects for Immunocontraception, pages 13–36
© 1990 Wiley-Liss, Inc.

MORPHOLOGY

SP-10 is a differentiation antigen that arises during spermiogenesis and appears to be testis specific [Anderson et al., 1987; Herr et al., 1990]. Figure 1 illustrates the immunohistochemical staining pattern with the MHS-10 monoclonal antibody on paraffin-embedded human testis sections. The reaction product is first detected in round spermatids as ovoid granules (Fig. 1B, arrowheads) and in later germ cell stages as crescent-shaped structures (arrows) associated with the sperm head. Complementary results employing electron microscopic immunocytochemistry on human testis sections with the MHS-10 mAb and colloidal gold coated with antimouse antibody (Fig. 2) showed a concentration of gold particles located over electron-dense material contained within the nascent acrosomal granule. Together, the light and electron microscopic observations indicate that SP-10 is expressed in round spermatids at the Golgi phase of spermatogenesis and is detectable at appreciable levels in the acrosomal granule. Specificity for round spermatids and subsequent stages of spermatogenesis is shown by the lack of reactivity with spermatogonia or Sertoli or Leydig cells in testis sections (Fig. 1). The WHO workshop concluded that the MHS-10 antibody did not react with any tissues other than testis.

Electron microscopic (EM) immunolocalizations of SP-10 in baboon testes have shown a colloidal gold pattern similar to that in human testes. SP-10 was detected in nascent acrosomal granules in round spermatids and within the developing acrosome in subsequent stages (Fig. 2C).

Using immunofluorescence microscopy on fresh ejaculated sperm, greater than 90% of sperm routinely fluoresced with MHS-10 in a cap-shaped pattern on the anterior portion of the sperm head, a pattern similar in shape to the known morphology of the acrosome (Fig. 3). However, this cap-shaped pattern was not obtained unless sperm were permeabilized with detergent, ethanol, or methanol treatments—a finding that indicated that SP-10 is not localized on the plasma membrane of intact sperm.

This conclusion was supported by electron microscopic localizations on mature, acrosome-intact sperm with colloidal gold techniques and the MHS-10 antibody (Fig. 4), which localized the SP-10 antigen within the acrosomal compartment. In many specimens, a bilaminar array of gold particles was observed in areas in which the acrosomal membranes were sectioned obliquely (Fig. 4, arrowheads). This finding suggested that SP-10 is nonuniformly disposed in some sperm within the acrosomal matrix, possibly in association

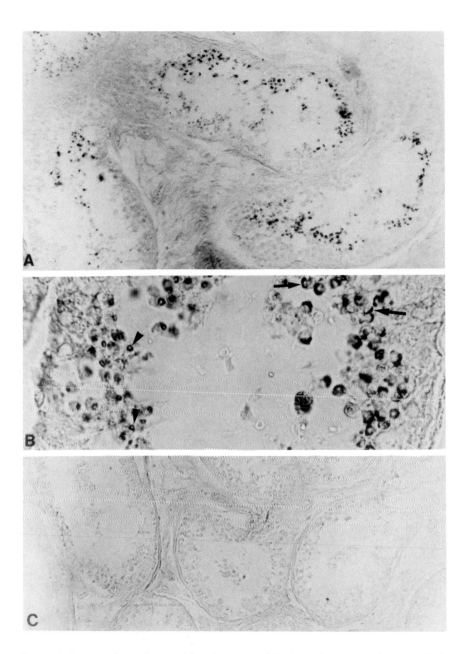

Fig. 1. Immunohistochemical localization of SP-10 within seminiferous tubules of the human testis. **A:** Cross sections of seminiferous tubules reacted with the MHS-10 monoclonal antibody (1:1,000) demonstrate dark reaction product in the adluminal compartment. ×180. **B:** At higher magnification, both crescent-shaped and smaller granular reaction product (arrowheads) are observed in cohorts of similar-stage germ cells within a single seminiferous tubule. ×720 **C:** Tissue section treated with the control murine IgG$_1$ shows no staining. ×180.

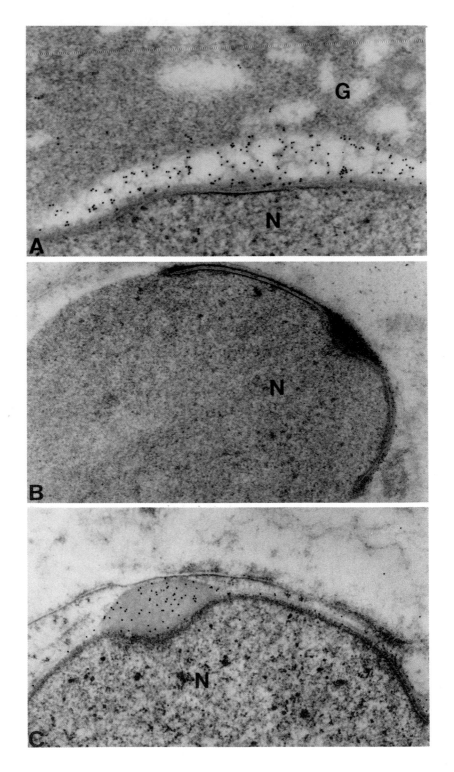

with the inner aspect of the outer acrosomal membrane and the outer aspect of the inner acrosomal membrane.

The observation that SP-10 is an intra-acrosomal protein in acrosome-intact sperm may, to some, diminish its potential as a vaccine immunogen. Molecules exposed on the surface plasma membrane are often regarded as the best target immunogens for immobilizing or agglutinating actions of immune effectors. However, our data indicate that SP-10 remains associated with the sperm head following the acrosome reaction (Fig. 5). It is well known that following the acrosome reaction the outer acrosomal membrane fuses with the plasma membrane and the inner acrosomal membrane becomes the limiting membrane of the anterior portion of the sperm head. Furthermore, in many sperm, both inner and outer acrosomal membranes remain intact beneath the equatorial segment [Nagae et al., 1986; Sathananthan et al., 1986; Yudin et al., 1988]. Figure 5 shows immunofluorescent images of a population of human sperm acrosome reacted with the calcium ionophore A23187. Following ionophore treatment, the incidence of sperm showing faint caps and belt-like bars (Fig. 5, curved arrows) or bars alone (Fig. 5, arrowheads) increased. We interpret the faint cap to indicate that SP-10 is associated, following the acrosome reaction, with the inner acrosomal membrane and the belt-like bar to indicate association of SP-10 with the equatorial segment. These findings thus indicate retention of SP-10 on the sperm head following the acrosome reaction. It is possible that the inhibition by MHS-10 mAb of sperm–egg interaction in the hamster egg penetration test, reported in the WHO study, may be due to an interaction of antibody with its target antigen exposed following the acrosome reaction.

BIOCHEMICAL CHARACTERIZATION

A molecular characterization of SP-10 has been obtained by Western blots [Towbin et al., 1979] of one- and two-dimensional gels on which sperm homogenates were electrophoresed. Western blots of a

Fig. 2. **A:** Electron micrograph of round human spermatid showing immunogold localization of SP-10 within the nascent acrosomal vesicle adjacent to the nucleus. ×55,000. **B:** Cap phase human spermatid showing SP-10 immunogold localization in the acrosomal matrix. ×25,300. **C:** Cap phase spermatid of *Papio papio* (baboon) showing similar distribution of SP-10 in the acrosome as in human spermatids. ×31,250. All sections were reacted with MHS-10 mAb and 10 nm colloidal gold coated with goat antimouse IgG. Tissue is unosmicated. N, nucleus; G, Golgi region.

Herr et al.

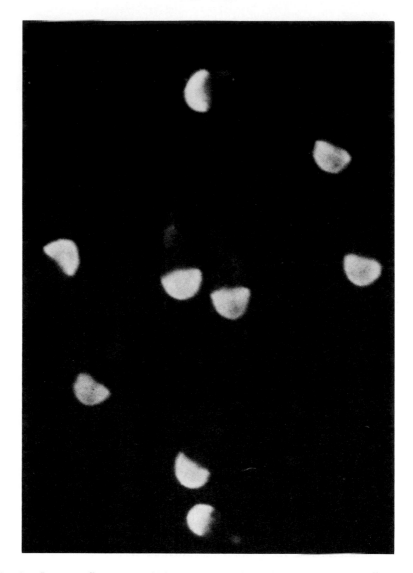

Fig. 3.   Immunofluorescent light micrograph localizing SP-10 in ejaculated human sperm. The image demonstrates cap-shaped fluorescence over the anterior portion of the sperm head. ×3220.

10% acrylamide, one-dimensional SDS-PAGE gel [Laemmli, 1970] allowed resolution of at least 14 distinct immunoreactive sperm peptide bands (Fig. 6B), which ranged from 18 to 34 kd. Sperm homogenates treated with SDS and the disulfide bond–reducing agent B-mercaptoethanol were compared with homogenates that were not

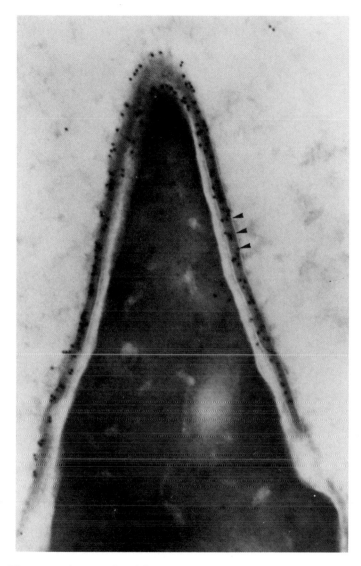

Fig. 4. Electron micrograph of human sperm head following reaction with monoclonal antibody MHS-10 and protein-A gold. Gold particles are observed over the acrosomal compartment. In regions where the acrosome was sectioned obliquely, as at the sperm apex, the gold particles follow a bilaminar distribution. Arrowheads indicate location of acrosomal membranes that are electron lucent in this unosmicated material. × 42,000.

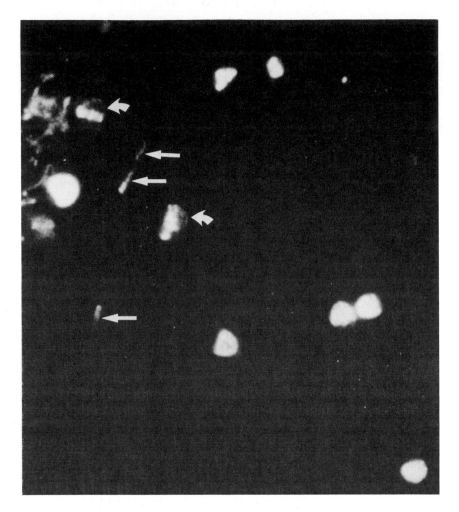

Fig. 5.   Sperm following artificial induction of the acrosome reaction with the calcium ionophore A23187. In the experiment from which this photo was taken, 47.5% of sperm showed full fluorescent caps (unreacted); 20.3%, faint fluorescent caps (curved arrows [acrosome reacted]); 22.4%, equatorial bars (straight arrows [acrosome reacted]); and 9.9%, unstained. ×2,550.

exposed to the reducing agent (Fig. 6B). The pattern of immunoreactive peptides was identical whether or not B-mercaptoethanol was present, indicating that reduction of disulfide bonds did not alter the apparent molecular weights of the immunoreactive peptides.

Figure 6B shows that immunoreactive SP-10 from different individuals were very similar. The relative intensity of antibody reactivity with any one peptide band was similar in different individuals, as

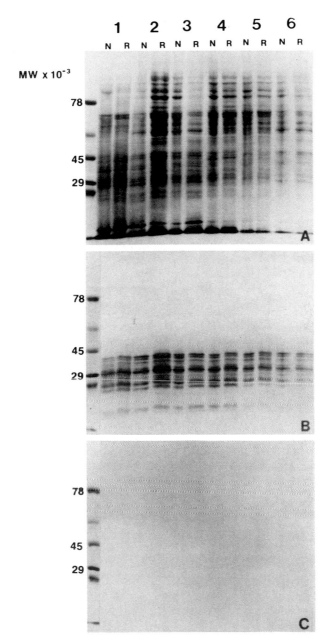

Fig. 6.   One-dimensional SDS-PAGE gel (10% acrylamide) nitrocellulose elec-
troblot stained with amido black (**A**) and identical nitrocellulose sheet reacted
with the MHS-10 mAb (**B**) or control IgG$_1$ (**C**). Sperm extracts from six donors
(1–6) contained B-mercaptoethanol (lanes marked R, reduced) or lacked this
agent (N, nonreduced). Twenty-five micrograms of protein was run per lane.
The pattern of SP-10 immunoreactive peptides (B) is identical both between
persons and in reduced and nonreduced extracts.

was the presence in each sperm homogenate of the full complement of 14 distinct immunoreactive peptide bands (Fig. 6B). To date, no sperm sample tested, with either immunofluorescence or Western blots (N = 60), has failed to react with the MHS-10 monoclonal antibody, indicating that SP-10 is highly conserved in the human population.

Silver stain of a sperm homogenate that was electrophoresed on a two-dimensional gel [O'Farrell, 1975] showed many protein spots possessing isoelectric points over the pH range 4.3–6.5 (Fig. 7A). The MHS-10 monoclonal antibody immunoreacted (Fig. 7B) with a series of peptide spots that ranged in apparent molecular weight from 18 to 34 kd. Immunoreactive peptides with apparent molecular weights from 24 to 34 kd had isoelectric points of approximately 4.9, while the immunoreactive peptides in the 18 kd range were slightly more basic, with pIs from 5.1 to 5.4.

WESTERN BLOTS OF SP-10 IN OTHER PRIMATES

The presence of SP-10 was studied in sperm from baboons and rhesus monkeys [Herr et al., 1990c]. Sperm were obtained from the cauda epididymides of *Macaca mulatta, Macaca fascicularis,* and *Papio cynocephalus anubis* at sacrifice and were extracted in 4× Laemmli buffer with mercaptoethanol for SDS-PAGE. Peptides immunoreactive with the MHS-10 monoclonal antibody were detected on Western blots containing these sperm extracts (Fig. 8). Sperm from each of these primates showed a polymorphic pattern of immunoreactivity similar to that observed on extracts of human sperm; however, the primate sperm extracts showed immunoreactive peptides of lower apparent mass than those in the human sperm extracts and including a band at approximately 14 kd. On the Western blot, sperm extracts from each primate showed immunoreactive bands at approximately 29 kd in the upper range of the pattern. These bands are of approximately the mass predicted from the nucleotide sequence for SP-10 (see below). Like the human sperm extracts, multiple immunoreactive forms below 29 kd were observed. This similarity in polymorphism between human, baboon, and macaque SP-10 suggests that the mechanisms responsible for generation of the polymorphism of SP-10, be it proteolysis or multiple gene products or a combination of these, are operating in baboon and macaque sperm as well as in human sperm.

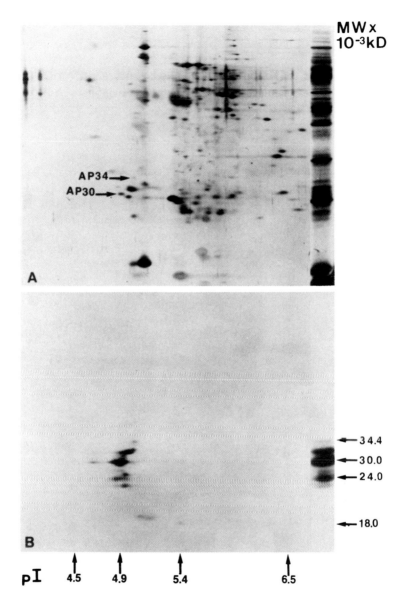

Fig. 7. Silver-stained two-dimensional gel (**A**) and immunoblot (**B**) with MHS-10 mAb on proteins extracted from human sperm. A one-dimensional lane showing the silver stain and immunoblot pattern of the sperm extract lies at the right of each part. Molecular weights (MW) and isoelectric points (pI) are indicated on the right and bottom margins, respectively. Arrows on the silver stain in A indicate the locations of SP-10 proteins (AP) at 34 and 30 kd, which can be compared with bands and spots of similar mass on the immunoblot below in B. Two- and one-dimensional gels were loaded with 75 and 15 μg of sperm protein, respectively. Immunoreactive SP-10 peptides from 24 to 34 kd have a pI of 4.9, the 18 kd spots range in pI from 5.1 to 5.4.

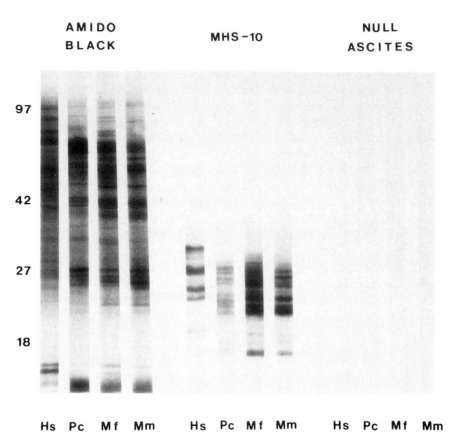

Fig. 8.   Immunoblot of human (Hs), *Papio cynochephalus* (Pc), *Macaca mulatta* (Mm), and *Macaca fascicularis* (Mf) sperm extracted with 1% SDS. Each lane was loaded with 10 μg of protein that had been separated by SDS-PAGE and transferred to nitrocellulose. Lanes were stained with amido black, a 1:2,000 dilution of MHS-10 ascites, or a 1:2,000 dilution of null ascites as indicated. Lanes incubated with ascites were subsequently incubated with horseradish peroxidase (HRP)-labeled goat antimouse IgG secondary antibody followed by 0.05% diaminobenzidine (DAB) and hydrogen peroxide. The sperm extracts of baboon and rhesus react with the MHS 10 mAb in a polymorphic pattern similar to the human.

THE OPEN READING FRAME AND THE PREDICTED AMINO ACID SEQUENCE FOR SP-10

The MHS-10 monoclonal antibody was used to probe a gt11 expression library from human testis [Wright et al., 1990]. This library was constructed by Jose Millan and coworkers [1987] and is commercially available from CLONTECH (Palo Alto, CA). The library was plated at a density of 5×10^3 plaque-forming units (pfu) per 150 mm petri dish with *Escherichia coli* Y1090 as host bacteria. After growth at 42°C and induction with isopropyl-B D-thiogalactoside, the nitrocellulose filters were screened with a 1:1,000 dilution of MHS-10 monoclonal antibody (isotype IgGl), with another IgGl monoclonal antibody as a control. Bound monoclonal antibody was detected by use of a goat antimouse IgG coupled to horseradish peroxidase (Jackson Immuno-Research Laboratories). A putative clone was identified upon screening 50,000 pfu from the expression library. This clone was isolated and was subsequently plaque purified through two additional rounds of screening with the monoclonal antibody until uniform plaque reactivity with the antibody was obtained. This clone contained an insert of 0.214 kilobase pairs (kbp).

The 0.214 kbp fragment was nick translated (Bethesda Research Labs) with ^{32}PdCTP (ICN) and used to reprobe the gtll library to identify additional clones according to the procedure of Benton and Davis [1977]. Five additional clones were identified.

Three plaques homologous to the 0.214 kbp clone were purified, and the cDNA inserts were isolated and subcloned into pGEM3Zf (ProMega). These three subcloned cDNAs were designated pGEM-SP-10-5, pGEM-SP-10-8, and pGEM-SP-10-10. Nested deletions were made in pGEM-SP-5 and pGEM-SP-10 with the Erase-a-Base System (ProMega). Both strands of the inserts were then sequenced with a Sequenase sequencing kit (U.S. Biochemicals).

Based on assembling overlapping sequences from the two cDNAs, we determined that the open reading frame for SP-10 consists of 795 nucleotides encoding a protein of 265 amino acids (Fig. 9). The predicted molecular weight of this protein is 28,156 daltons. The polyadenylation consensus sequence AATAAA begins 236 base residues 3' from the termination codon. A single mRNA decay consensus motif [Shaw and Kamen, 1986; Caput et al., 1986] ATTTA begins 71 base residues 3' to the termination codon. A consensus sequence for eukaryotic initiation sites [Kozak, 1984] is present 5' to the ATG start codon. The open reading frame for SP-10 contains a single internal EcoR1 site (Fig. 9, arrowhead).

The predicted amino acid sequence for SP-10 contains two canonical Asp-X-Ser (Thr) sequences for N-linked glycosylation. These potential sites for N-ether–linked glycosylation exist at asparagine residues located at amino acids 48 and 258.

Perhaps the most interesting feature in the amino acid sequence for SP-10 is a repeat motif consisting of Ser-Gly-Glu-Gln-Pro, which occurs five times (single underlines in Fig. 9). Three additional variants of this motif are present in the same region of the protein. Each

```
                                                                GGTTTCTCTTGCTAATGAGTCTT
AATTCCCGGCTATGAAGAACCTGTGTCCCACACTGGGGTCCCCTCTTTTCCTAAATCCAGATGAACAGGTTTCTCTTGCTAATGAGTCTT      90
      TER                                                  TER ~~~~  M  N  R  F  L  L  L  M  S  L    10

TATCTCCTTGGATCTGCCAGAGGAACATCAAGTCAGCCTAATGAGCTTTCTGGCTCCATAGATCATCAAACTTCAGTTCAGCAACTTCCA      180
TATCTCCTTGGATCTGCCAGAGGAACATCAAGTCAGCCTAATGAGCTTTCTGGCTCCATAGATCATCAAACTTCAGTTCAGCAACTTCCA
  Y  L  L  G  S  A  R  G  T  S  S  Q  P  N  E  L  S  G  S  I  D  H  Q  T  S  V  Q  Q  L  P      40

GGTGAGTTCTTTTCACTTGAAAACCCTTCTGATGCTGAGGCTTTATATGAGACTTCTTCAGGCCTGAACACTTTAAGTGAGCATGGTTCC      270
GGTGAGTTCTTTTCACTTGAAAACCCTTCTGATGCTGAGGCTTTATATGAGACTTCTTCAGGCCTGAACACTTTAAGTGAGCATGGTTCC
  G  E  F  F  S  L  E  N  P  S  D  A  E  A  L  Y  E  T  S  S  G  L  N  T  L  S  E  H  G  S      70
                                                                         -cho-

AGTGAGCATGGTTCAAGCAAGCCACACTGTGGGGGAGCACACTTCTGGAGAACATGCTGAGAGTGAGCATGCTTCAGGTGAGCCCGCTGGG      360
AGTGAGCATGGTTCAAGCAAGCCACACTGTGGGGGAGCACACTTCTGGAGAACATGCTGAGAGTGAGCATGCTTCAGGTGAGCCCGCTGGG
  S  E  H  G  S  S  K  H  T  V  A  E  H  T  S  G  E  H  A  E  S  E  H  A  S  G  E  P  A  A      100

ACTGAACATGCTGAAGGTGAGCCATACTGTAGGGTGAGCCAGCCTTCAGGAGAACAGCCTTCAGGTGAACACCTCTCGGGAGAACAGCCTTTG      450
ACTGAACATGCTGAAGGTGAGCCATACTGTAGGGTGAGCCAGCCTTCAGGAGAACAGCCTTCAGGTGAACACCTCTCGGGAGAACAGCCTTTG
  T  E  H  A  E  G  E  H  T  V  G  E  Q  P  S  G  E  Q  P  S  G  E  H  L  S  G  E  Q  P  L      130

AGTGAGCTTGAGTCAGGTGAACAGCCTTCAGATGAACAGCCTTCAGGTGAACATGGCTCGGGTGAACAGCCTTCTGGTGAGCAGGCCTCG      540
AGTGAGCTTGAGTCAGGTGAACAGCCTTCAGATGAACAGCCTTCAGGTGAACATGGCTCGGGTGAACAGCCTTCTGGTGAGCAGGCCTCG
  S  E  L  E  S  G  E  Q  P  S  D  E  Q  P  S  G  E  H  G  S  G  E  Q  P  S  G  E  Q  A  S      160
                    + + + + +

GGTGAACAGCCTTCAGGTGAGCAGCCTTCAGGGGAACAGCCTTCAGGTGCACCAAATTTCAAGCACATCTACAGGCACAATATTAAAATTGC      630
GGTGAACAGCCTT---------------------------------------------------------CAGGCACAATATTAAAATTGC
  G  E  Q  P  S  G  E  H  A  S  G  E  Q  A  S  G  A  P  I  S  S  T  S  T  G  T  I  L  N  C      190
              + + + +

TACACATGTGCTTATATGAATGATCAAGGAAAATGTCTTCGTGGAGAGGGAACCTGCATCACTCAGAATTCCCAGCCAGTGCATGTTAAAG      720
TACACATGTGCTTATATGAATGATCAAGGAAAATGTCTTCGTGGAGAGGGAACCTGCATCACTCAGAATTCCCAGCCAGTGCATGTTAAAG
  Y  T  C  A  Y  M  N  D  Q  G  K  C  L  R  G  E  G  T  C  I  T  Q  N  S  Q  Q  C  M  L  K      220

AAGATCTTTGAAGGTGGAAAACTCCAATTCATGGTTCAAGGGTGTGAGAACATGTGCCCATCTATGAACCTCTTCTCCCATGGAACGAGG      810
AAGATCTTTGAAGGTGGAAAACTCCAATTCATGGTTCAAGGGTGTGAGAACATGTGCCCATCTATGAACCTCTTCTCCCATGGAACGAGG
  K  I  F  E  G  G  K  L  Q  F  M  V  Q  G  C  E  N  M  C  P  S  M  N  L  F  S  H  G  T  R      250

ATGCAAATTATATGCTGTCGAAATCAATCTTTCTCGCAATAAGATCTAGAAGCCTGGGCCCTTGCTTGTTTTGACTCAGGCAGTAAAAAGC      900
ATGCAAATTATATGCTGTCGAAATCAATCTTTCTCGCAATAAGATCTAGAAGCCTGGGCCCTTGCTTGTTTTGACTCAGGCAGTAAAAAGC
  M  Q  I  I  C  C  R  N  Q  S  F  C  N  K  I TER                                               265
                                            -cho-

CTCCATCACTCTATTTGGCTCATTTTATATTTAGTTCCTTCCCCAGTCAACAACTGACCACATCTGCCTCTGCCTGAGCATTAGGATGCT      990
CTCCATCACTCTATTTGGCTCATTTTATATTTAGTTCCTTCCCCAGTCAACAACTGACCACATCTGCCTCTGCCTGAGCATTAGGATGCT
                                                         *****

CAAACATCCTATCTTTCTTCTTCTATTCATGCTTTTATCCATTCTTCTCGTGTCCGTCTTCCCTGCCTCCAACTCTTTCTCTCAATATTCC      1080
CAAACATCCTATCTTTCTTCTTCTATTCATGCTTTTATCCATTCTTCTCGTGTCCGTCTTCCCTGCCTCCAACTCTTTCTCTCAATATTCC

TGATTTTTTTTTCAATAAATTTCACATGCCCGAATTC    3'                                                    1117
TGATTTTTTTTT  ^^^^^^
```

Fig. 9. Complete nucleotide and predicted protein sequences derived from overlapping SP-10-5 and SP-10-10 cDNAs. The single letter amino acid code for the protein sequence is indicated below the nucleotide sequence. The top line in each pair of sequences was derived from the SP-10-5 cDNA and the bottom line from the SP-10-10 cDNA as indicated. The numbering to the right indicates the nucleotide and amino acid positions. The solid line in the SP-10-10 sequence spanning nucleotides 554–610 represents the putative alternatively spliced region of SP-10-10. Repeated motifs one, two, and three are designated by single, double, and triple underlined sequences, respectively. Sites of potential N-linked glycosylation are denoted by the symbol -cho-, and sites of potential O-linked glycosylation are underscored with the symbol (+ + +). The 5' consensus nucleotide sequence flanking eukaryotic ATG start codons is underscored with the symbol (~~), a poly A addition signal is underscored with the symbol (^^^), and an mRNA consensus degradation sequence is underscored with the symbol (***). The two in-frame termination codons 5' of the ATG are designated by TER. An internal EcoR1 site is indicated at the arrowhead.

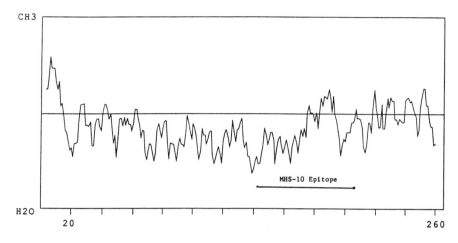

Fig. 10. A hydrophobicity/hydrophilicity plot, deduced from the predicted amino acid sequence for SP-10. The amino terminus contains a region typical of a secretory signal sequence. The central portion of the protein, in the region containing the repeat motifs, contains a considerable stretch of hydrophilic residues. The region adjacent to the carboxy terminus is decidedly hydrophobic. The region containing the MHS-10 epitope is indicated.

variant contains a single amino acid substitution of the five amino acid sequence indicated above. These motifs are underlined in Figure 9. This area of sixteen repeat motifs occurs in the central hydrophilic portion of the protein.

HYDROPHOBICITY/HYDROPHILICITY

A hydrophobicity/hydrophilicity plot, deduced from the predicted amino acid sequence for SP-10, is presented in Figure 10. The amino terminus contains a region typical of a secretory signal sequence [von Heijne, 1986]. The central portion of the protein, in the region containing the repeat motifs, contains a considerable stretch of hydrophilic residues. The region adjacent to the carboxy terminus is decidedly hydrophobic. The region containing the MHS-10 epitope lies within amino acid residues 143–213.

SEQUENCE ANALYSIS

Homology searches of the Genbank, National Biomedical Research Foundation protein and Swiss Protein Library databases were performed with the Pearson and Lipman FASTA and tFASTA programs

[Pearson and Lipman, 1988]. Comparisons were run with ktups of 1 and 2. Local similarity analyses were performed with the LFASTA program. No significant protein or nucleic acid homologies to SP-10 were observed in these banks. These findings indicate that SP-10 is a novel acrosomal protein.

NORTHERN BLOTS/THE mRNA FOR SP-10

Human testes were obtained from patients undergoing surgical orchiectomy for prostate cancer; and baboon (*Papio papio* and *P. cynocephalus anubis*) and rhesus (M. mulatta) testes were received frozen from the University of Washington Regional Primate Research Center. PolyA$^+$ RNA was isolated from these tissues with Oligo(dT)-Cellulose Type 3 (Collaborative Research, Inc., Bedford, MA). One microgram of human testis polyA$^+$ RNA, 2 µg of human placental and liver polyA$^+$ RNA, and 10 µg of primate, dog, and cat polyA$^+$ RNA were electrophoresed on a 1% formaldehyde-agarose gel according to published procedures [Lehrach et al., 1977; Goldberg, 1980]. The RNA was blotted to a Biotrace membrane (Gelman) and probed with a ^{32}P labeled 634 bp fragment containing part of the coding region from the SP-10-5 cDNA. This fragment results from an internal EcoR1 site within the SP-10 open reading frame. Figure 11 shows that the 634 bp fragment hybridizes to a 1.35 kb mRNA in the human testis RNA preparation. RNA isolated from testes of several individuals showed an identical 1.35 kb mRNA. No hybridization was observed on polyA$^+$ RNA isolated from human liver or placenta at high stringency.

It should be noted (Fig. 9) that we have obtained cDNA sequence data on 1,117 residues; thus about 200 bases in the mRNA remain to be elucidated 3' or 5' to the open reading frame. PolyA$^+$ RNA from human placenta and liver gave no evidence of hybridization with the 634 bp probe, indicating these tissues do not express SP-10 mRNA. Although we have not studied all tissues, we have not detected MHS-10 reactivity in any tissue other than testis, confirming the WHO workshop's conclusion regarding testis specificity. Thus all evidence to data continues to indicate that SP-10 is expressed specifically in the testis.

Northern blots (Fig. 11) that were loaded with polyA$^+$ RNA purified from testes of *P. papio*, *P. cynocephalus anubis*, and *M. mulatta* demonstrated that these species testes contained a 1.35 kb mRNA that hybridized with the 634 bp SP-10 probe. This 1.35 kb mRNA was of similar size to human testicular mRNA (Fig. 11). PolyA$^+$ RNA from dog and cat testes did not hybridize with the probe.

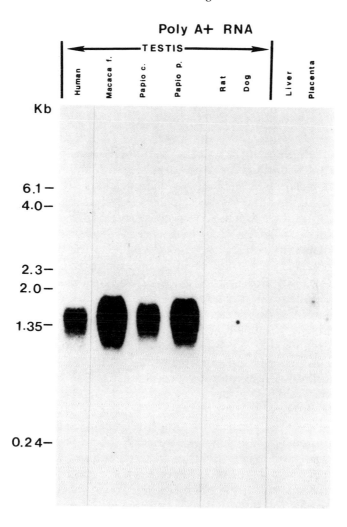

Fig. 11.   Northern blot of polyA$^+$ RNA isolated from testes of human, baboon (*Papio papio, Papio cynocephalus anubis*), *Macaca fascicularis*, dog, and cat as well as human placenta and liver. The blot was hybridized with a ^{32}P-labeled probe spanning 634 bp of the open reading frame for human SP-10. A 1.35 kb mRNA is observed in lanes containing human, baboon, and monkey polyA$^+$ testis RNA. Lanes were loaded with 1 μg human testis RNA, 2 μg human liver or placental RNA, and 10 μg primate testis RNA.

The observation that a 1.35 kb mRNA for SP-10 is common to baboons, macaques, and humans provides additional evidence supporting the homologies demonstrated in immunoreactive SP-10 on Western blots. Together these data indicate that macaques and baboons may be appropriate primate models for testing the antifertility potential of a recombinant SP-10 vaccine.

CONCLUSIONS

The observations that the MHS-10 monoclonal antibody reacts with only round spermatids and subsequent stages of spermiogenesis on testis sections and localizes within the acrosome at the EM level, coupled with the report that somatic tissues were nonreactive with the MHS-10 monoclonal antibody [Anderson et al., 1987], together indicate that SP-10 may be classified as a "differentiation antigen" [Bennett et al., 1972], i.e., a tissue-specific molecule expressed at a precise stage of human spermatogenesis. MHS-10 immunoreaction product on light micrographs was evident in the seminiferous epithelium as small ovoid granules adjacent to the nucleus of round spermatids, and at the EM level within acrosomal granules. Now that cDNA probes are available for SP-10, we are initiating in situ hybridization studies to determine when during spermatogenesis the SP-10 mRNA is first detectable.

The absence of cross-reactivity of MHS-10 with somatic tissues, coupled with its stage-specific expression during germ cell differentiation, is germane to the possible utility of SP-10 as a contraceptive vaccine immunogen. Potential problems of autoimmunity, which would be anticipated if common somatic antigens were utilized as vaccine immunogens, may not be found with SP-10.

Our immunofluorescence evidence indicated that in acrosome-intact, membrane-permeabilized sperm, SP-10 localized in a cap-shaped immunofluorescent pattern that appeared to encompass the entire extent of the acrosome. There was no evidence that the MHS-10 antibody recognized its cognate antigen on the plasmalemma of living sperm. This is at variance with the report of the WHO workshop [Anderson et al., 1987, p 249], which concluded that the MHS-10 antibody (S20) showed "reactivity . . . with abundant surface antigens on mature sperm." It should be emphasized that our more recent results do not agree with the workshop's conclusion for acrosome-intact, nonpermeabilized sperm.

Our results show that after ionophore-induced acrosome reaction, there was an increase in the number of sperm displaying fluorescent bars or fluorescent bars together with fainter fluorescent caps. We interpret the reduced immunofluorescence of the cap (faint cap) to indicate that following the acrosome reaction SP-10 is displayed on the sperm surface, most likely in association with the inner acrosomal membrane. The retention of immunofluorescence after the acrosome reaction in a belt-like bar likely represents retention of SP-10 within the equatorial segment. The equatorial bar immunofluorescence, although covering a much smaller region than the fluorescent cap, appeared to be of varying intensity, indicating that the amount of SP-10 remaining after ionophore induction within the equatorial segment is different from one sperm to another.

The WHO-sponsored multicenter study presented evidence that the MHS-10 monoclonal antibody inhibited sperm egg interactions in the hamster egg penetration test [Anderson et al., 1987]. Our model to explain this result postulates that, although the SP-10 antigen is sequestered within the limits of the acrosomal membranes in intact, nonacrosome-reacted sperm, it is accessible to the actions of the MHS-10 antibody following the acrosome reaction. Current concepts regarding key events of fertilization are relevant to this model. During fertilization, human sperm must undergo the acrosome reaction in order to penetrate the zona pellucida [Singer et al., 1985] and fuse with the egg plasma membrane [Sathananthan and Chen, 1986]. After the acrosome reaction, the acrosomal contents are externalized and the inner acrosomal membrane becomes the limiting membrane of the anterior sperm head [Nagae et al., 1986; Yudin et al., 1988; Cross et al., 1986]. Most sperm observed on the human zona after 1 min of binding in vitro have intact acrosomes [Cross et al., 1988]. The numbers of acrosome-reacted sperm on the zona then rapidly increase with time, as the zona acts as a potent inducer of the acrosome reaction [Cross et al., 1988]. After penetration of the zona, the site of initiation of fusion between sperm and egg in man, as in other eutherian animals, is thought to occur between the plasma membrane over the equatorial segment and the egg plasma membrane [Bedford et al., 1979; Sathananthan and Chen, 1986]. Important questions remain to be elucidated regarding immunocontraception based on SP-10 or other intra-acrosomal immunogens. Are the sperm of humans or other primates acrosome reacted *prior to* or *during* zona binding during in vivo fertilization in the oviduct? Can antibodies in oviductal fluids be induced by vaccination to reach sufficient levels to agglutinate, immobilize, or lyse acrosome-reacted sperm? Can such antibodies in secretions of the female tract can gain access in vivo to antigens on the inner acrosomal membrane or equatorial segment to block either sperm penetration of the zona or fusion with the egg membrane? Some of these questions will be addressed when trials of an SP-10–based vaccine are undertaken in primates.

A common assumption regarding selection of appropriate sperm immunogens for contraceptive vaccine development is that the target molecules should be surface components accessible to humoral or cellular immune effectors [Anderson and Alexander, 1983]. Although the intra-acrosomal localization of the SP-10 peptides in the mature, nonacrosome-reacted sperm appears at first glance not to fulfill this caveat, the remodeling of the sperm head membranes that accompany the acrosome reaction opens the possibility that constituents of the acrosome, although sequestered from the immune system in intact sperm, should not be dismissed as candidates for contraceptive vaccines without examination of their fate following the acrosome reaction.

Mitigating against the idea of SP-10 as a vaccine immunogen are data on immunization with acrosin and hyaluronidase. Like SP-10, acrosin is retained on the inner acrosomal membrane and equatorial segment following the acrosome reaction [Tesarik et al., 1988]. In rabbits, antibodies formed in response to systematic immunization with acrosin were found only in low amounts in oviductal fluid [Syner et al., 1979]. Immunization with hyaluronidase has also not resulted in significant reductions in fertility [Morton and McAnulty, 1979]. On the other hand, studies with guinea pig sperm have provided remarkable evidence that full but reversible contraception can be achieved by immunizing female animals with the purified sperm protein PH-20 [Primakoff et al., 1988]. This molecule of 64,000 daltons is present on both the plasma membrane and, following the acrosome reaction, the inner acrosomal membrane [Primakoff et al., 1985, 1988a; Myles and Primakoff, 1984; Cowan et al., 1986] of guinea pig sperm. Although SP-10 and PH-20 appear to be different molecules based on consideration of apparent molecular weight and immunoreactivity, they share the property of persistence on the sperm head following the acrosome reaction. The remarkable effectiveness of PH-20 in eliciting a contraceptive effect in guinea pigs [Primakoff et al., 1988b] suggests certain antigens associated with acrosome-reacted sperm are effective targets for immunocontraception. SP-10 appears to be a model molecule in humans for this type of intra-acrosomal immunogen.

The observation of a high degree of similarity between individuals in the immunoreactive forms of SP-10 on Western blots and consistent immunofluorescent localizations on each individual's sperm indicate that SP-10 is conserved in the human population. This knowledge is essential in choosing a contraceptive vaccine molecule, because it must be present on most, if not all, sperm in order for a vaccine to achieve the widest possible effectiveness. The multiple forms of SP-10 peptides identified by Western blotting may represent post-translational modifications, proteolytic processing of the protein within the acrosome, multiple gene products, or several of these possibilities combined. However, the high degree of similarity between individuals on Western blots suggests that the mechanism(s) producing polymorphism in antigenic peptides operate similarly in different individuals. The fact that reduction did not alter the pattern of immunoreactive SP-10 peptides suggests a lack of interchain and few or no intrachain disulfide bonds in SP-10.

The MHS-10 monoclonal antibody was successfully used to isolate cDNA clones from a λgt11 library of human testis, suggesting that the antibody recognizes a proteinaceous rather than a carbohydrate epitope. The open reading frame for the cDNAs that we have identified and sequenced predicts that SP-10 has a molecular weight of 28.15 kd. When comparing this predicted molecular weight to the immunoblot results, it can be appreciated that a protein of 28.15 kd would lie centrally within the 24–34 kd cluster of immunoreactive peptides, possibly corresponding to the strongly immunoreactive band at approximately 29 kd. We speculate that N-linked glycosylation occurs to a varying degree at both potential N-linked sites, resulting in the peptide bands observed above 29 kd. Our current speculation regarding the immunoreactive peptides below 29 kd posits proteolytic mechanisms for their generation.

Given the arguments presented above both for and against the premise that an intra-acrosomal sperm immunogen such as SP-10 might serve as an effective contraceptive vaccine immunogen, we conclude that the potential of SP-10 must be tested in fertility trials. The evidence presented above demonstrates the presence of SP-10 mRNA in baboons and macaques and shows that the distribution of SP-10 in spermatids is similar in humans and baboons, providing ideal primate models in which to proceed.

REFERENCES

Anderson DJ, Alexander NJ (1983): A new look at antifertility vaccines. Fertil Steril 40: 557–571.

Anderson DJ, Johnson PM, Alexander NJ, Jones WR, Griffin PD (1987): Monoclonal antibodies to human trophoblast and sperm antigens: Report of two WHO-sponsored workshops, June 30, 1986—Toronto, Canada. J Reprod Immunol 10:231–257.

Bedford JM, Moore HDM, Franklin LE (1979): Significance of the equatorial segments of the acrosome of the spermatozoa in eutherian mammals. Exp Cell Res 119:119–126.

Bennett D, Goldberg E, Dunn LC, Boyse EA (1972): Serological detection of a cell-surface antigen specified by the T (brachyury) mutant gene in the house mouse. Proc Natl Acad Sci USA 69:2076–2080.

Benton WD, Davis RW (1977): Screening λ g+ recombinant clones by hybridization to single plaques in situ. Science 196:180–182.

34 *Herr et al.*

Caput D, Beutler B, Hartog K, Thayer R, Brown-Shimer S, Cerami A (1986): Identification of a common nucleotide sequence in the 3' untranslated region of mRNA molecules specifying inflammatory mediators. Proc Natl Acad Sci USA 83:1670–1674.

Cowan AE, Primakoff P, Myles DG (1986): Sperm exocytosis increases the amount of PH-20 antigen on the surface of guinea pig sperm. J Cell Biol 103:1289–1297.

Cross NL, Morales P, Overstreet JW, Hanson FW (1986): Two simple methods for detecting acrosome-reacted human sperm. Gamete Res 15:213–244.

Cross NL, Morales P, Overstreet JW, Hanson FW (1988): Induction of acrosome reactions by the human zona pellucida. Biol Reprod 38:235–244.

Goldberg DA (1980): Isolation and partial characterization of the *Drosophila* alcohol dehydrogenase gene. Proc Natl Acad Sci USA 77:5794–5798.

Herr JC, Flickinger CJ, Homyk M, Klotz K, John E (1990a): Biochemical and morphological characterization of the intra-acrosomal antigen SP-10 from human sperm. Biol Reprod 42:181–193.

Herr JC, Wright RM, Flickinger CJ (1990b): Biochemical, ultrastructural and genetic characterization of human acrosomal antigen SP-10. In Mettler L, Billington WD (eds): Proceedings of the 4th International Congress of Reproductive Immunology. Amsterdam: Elsevier, pp 51–59.

Herr JC, Wright RM, John E, Foster J, Flickinger CJ (1990c): Identification of human acrosomal antigen SP-10 in primates and pigs. Biol Reprod 42:377–382.

Homyk M, Anderson DJ, Wolff H, Herr JC (1990): Differential diagnosis of immature germ cells in semen utilizing monoclonal antibody MHS-10 to the intra-acrosomal antigen SP-10. Fertil Steril 53:323–329.

Kozak M (1984): Compilation and analysis of sequences upstream from the translational start site in eukaryotic mRNAs. Nucleic Acids Res 12:857–873.

Laemmli UK (1970): Cleavage of structural proteins during the assembly of the head of bacteriophase T4. Nature 227:680–685.

Lehrach H, Diamond D, Wozney JM, Doedtker H (1977): RNA molecular weight determinations by gel electrophoresis under denaturing conditions: A critical reexamination. Biochemistry 16:4743–4751.

Millan JL, Driscoll CE, LeVan KM, Goldberg E (1987): Epitopes of human testis-specific lactate dehydrogenase deduced from a cDNA sequence. Proc Natl Acad Sci USA 84:5311–5315.

Morton DB, McAnulty PA (1979): The effect on fertility of immunizing female sheep with ram sperm acroson and hyaluronidase. J Reprod Immunol 1:61–73.

Myles DG, Primakoff P (1984): Localized surface antigens of guinea pig sperm migrate to new regions prior to fertilization. J Cell Biol 99:1634–1641.

Nagae T, Yanagimachi R, Srivastava P, Yanagimachi H (1986): Acrosome reaction in human spermatozoa. Fertil Steril 45:701–707.

O'Farrell PH (1975): High resolution two-dimensional electrophoresis of membrane proteins. J Biol Chem 250:4007–4021.

Pearson WR, Lipman DJ (1988): Improved tools for biological sequence camparison. Proc Natl Acad Sci USA 85:2444–2448.

Primakoff P, Cowan A, Hyatt H, Tredick-Kline J, Myles DG (1988a): Purification of the guinea pig sperm PH-20 antigen and detection of a site-specific endoproteolytic activity in sperm preparations that cleaves PH-20 into two disulfide-linked fragments. Biol Reprod 38:921–934.

Primakoff P, Hyatt H, Myles DG (1985): A role for the mitgrating sperm surface antigen PH-20 in guinea pig sperm binding to the egg zona pellucida. J Cell Biol 101:2239–2244.

Primakoff P, Lathrop W, Woolman L, Cowan A, Myles D (1988b): Fully effective contraception in male and female guinea pigs immunized with the sperm protein PH-20. Nature 335:543–546.

Sathananthan AH, Chen C (1986): Sperm–oocyte fusion in the human during monospermic fertilization. Gamete Res 15:177–186.

Sathananthan AH, Ng SC, Edirisinghe R, Ratnam SS, Wong PC (1986): Human sperm–egg interaction in vitro. Gamete Res 15:317–326.

Shaw G, Kamen R (1986): A conserved AU sequence from the 3' untranslated region of GM-CSF mRNA mediates selective mRNA degradation. Cell 46:659–667.

Singer SL, Lambert H, Overstreet JW, Hanson FW, Yanagimachi R (1985): The kinetics of human sperm binding to the human zona pellucida and zona-free hamster oocyte in vitro. Gamete Res 12:29–39.

Syner FN, Kuras R, Moghissi KS (1979): Active immunization of female rabbits with purified rabbit acrosin and effect on fertility. Fertil Steril 32:468–473.

Tesarik J, Drahorad J, Peknicova J (1988): Subcellular immunochemical localization of acrosin in human spermatozoa during the acrosome reaction and zona pellucida penetration. Fertil Steril 50:133–141.

Towbin H, Staehelin T, Gordon G (1979): Electrophoretic transfer of proteins from polyacrylamide gels to nitrocellulose sheets: Procedures and some applications. Proc Natl Acad Sci USA 76:4350–4354.

von Heijne G (1986): A new method for predicting signal sequence cleavage sites. Nucleic Acids Res 14:4683–4691.

Wright RM, John E, Flickinger CJ, Herr JC (1990): Cloning and sequencing of cDNAs coding for the human intra-acrosomal antigen SP-10. Biol Reprod 42:693–701.

Yudin AI, Gottlieb W, Meizel S (1988): Ultrastructural studies of the early events of the human sperm acrosome reaction as initiated by human follicular fluid. Gamete Res 20: 11–24.

DISCUSSION

DR. ANDERSON: You mentioned in your introduction that you don't find surface expression of this antigen, yet you are going ahead to use it for a contraceptive vaccine candidate in animal models. Could you clarify this issue?

DR. HERR: There is evidence from the WHO Sperm Antigen Workshop that, in the hamster test, the monoclonal antibody inhibited sperm–egg interactions. The model of this is the obvious existence of the protein in association with the inner acrosomal membrane in the equatorial segment, following the acrosome reaction. The monoclonal antibody may thus be able to interdict the events of fertilization by binding in those regions. Our hope is to take polyclonal antisera from injected baboons and demonstrate in acrosomal-reactive baboon sperm that this exists. This is the model that we have in mind for the potential mechanism of action.

MR. SPIELER: You described a model in which you took the 207 amino acid sequence combined with beta-galactosidase, and injected it into rabbits. Are you going to evaluate the fertility of the immunized animals?

DR. HERR: No plans at present. After combining the monoclonal antibody with rabbit sperm, we found no cross-reactivity. So, the MHS-10 epitope is not there. And on high stringency studies with RNA extracted from rabbits, we do not get hybridization with the SP-10 cDNA probe. Nonetheless, since we have not completed a whole set of zoo blots at low stringency, we are not certain whether there is a rabbit homologue that shows partial SP-10 sequence identity.

3

Studies of Sperm Antigens Reactive to HS-11 and HS-63 Monoclonal Antibodies

Chi-Yu Gregory Lee, Ming-Sun Liu,
Ming-Wan Su, and Jia-Bei Zhu

It has been known for decades that certain sperm antigens are auto- or isoimmunogenic [Menge et al., 1979; Tung, 1980]. Clinically, the presence of naturally occurring antisperm antibodies, especially those secreted locally in the reproductive tract, has been implicated in 10–15% of unexplained human infertility [Ingerslev, 1981; Menge, 1980; Shulman, 1982]. Generally speaking, the presence of antisperm antibodies in the reproductive tract can result in agglutination or immobilization of sperm in the presence of complements and interfere with sperm–egg interaction, fertilization, or implantation of early embryos [Isojima et al., 1968; Shulman, 1982]. Logically, if sperm-specific antigens that elicit naturally occurring sperm antibodies are associated with human infertility, immunization with well-characterized antigens in the form of a vaccine could also serve the purpose of fertility control [Anderson and Alexander, 1983; D'Almeida et al., 1981; Lee et al., 1982; Tung, 1976].

Therefore, the development of immunocontraceptive vaccines using sperm antigens for human application is justified. For practical purposes, there is also a need to expand contraception technology for the control of global population. With the advances of biotechnology, the immunologic means of fertility control are just beginning to evolve.

In view of the known effects of sperm antibodies on sperm functions and their association with human infertility, sperm antigen-based immunocontraceptive vaccines appear to be an ideal choice for

Gamete Interaction: Prospects for Immunocontraception, pages 37–51
© 1990 Wiley-Liss, Inc.

prefertilization contraception in humans and animals. Furthermore, the fact that those individuals who suffer from sperm antibody-related infertility have no more health problems than any normal individual provides supportive safety data.

Since 1981, we have been involved in the generation of monoclonal antibodies against sperm surface antigens, assessment of their effects on sperm function and fertilization, and purification and biochemical/immunologic characterizations of specific sperm antigens for contraceptive vaccine development [Lee et al., 1982, 1984a–c, 1986, 1987; Liu et al., 1989a,b, 1990; Menge et al., 1987]. Among the monoclonal antibodies that we produced, HS-11 and HS-63 were found to react specifically with the sperm acrosome of several mammalian species, but not with any other somatic tissues.

In 1986, a workshop was held by the World Health Organization to conduct interlaboratory evaluations of all monoclonal antibodies against sperm and trophoblast antigens submitted worldwide [Anderson et al., 1987]. In view of their high specificity and significant antifertility effects, both HS-11 and HS-63 were selected for further consideration. Hence, a research project was undertaken in our laboratory in 1987 under the support of the CONRAD program to purify and characterize the relevant sperm antigens for subsequent development of contraceptive vaccines [Liu et al., 1990]. The progress of this research work is herein summarized.

PURIFICATION OF SPERM ANTIGENS REACTIVE TO HS-11 AND HS-63 MONOCLONAL ANTIBODIES

Mouse Sperm Antigens Reactive to HS-63 (MSA-63)

In testis homogenate, the antigen reactive to HS-63 monoclonal antibody was found to be present predominantly in the supernatant of detergent-free testis homogenate. Therefore, a conventional protein purification procedure, including ammonium sulfate fractionation and DEAE ion exchange chromatography, was adopted for the initial stages of antigen purification from the mouse testis homogenate. Immunoaffinity chromatography with purified HS-63 as the affinity ligand was employed as the last step of antigen purification. During purification, the immunoactivity of the target antigen was followed by an established indirect immunofluorescent inhibition assay [Liu et al., 1989b].

As shown in Table 1, about 1,000-fold protein purification was required to obtain a homogeneous antigen preparation from the

TABLE 1. Purification of Sperm Antigens Reactive to HS-11 and HS-63 Monoclonal Antibodies From Mouse Testis Homogenate

Sperm antigens	Purification steps	Fold of protein purification
MSA-63	1. Crude extract	1.0[a]
	2. Ammonium sulfate fractionation	1.4
	3. DEAE ion exchange chromatography	9.0
	4. HS-63 immunoaffinity chromatography	1,100
MSA-11	1. Crude extract	1.0[b]
	2. HS-11 Immunoaffinity chromatography	912

[a]Determined by indirect immunofluorescent inhibition assay [Liu et al., 1989b].
[b]Determined by dot blot immunobinding assay.

crude testis homogenate. The purified MSA-63 was shown to be comprised of three major soluble glycoproteins with molecular weight of 50, 43, and 42 kd, respectively, on SDS-PAGE (Fig. 1). The immunospecificity of purified MSA-63 to HS-63 was determined by established immunoassay procedures such as enzyme-linked immunosorbent assay (ELISA) with sperm or purified MSA-63 coated on microwells and a radioimmunosorbent inhibition assay (RISA). Similarly, the rabbit sperm antigen (RSA-63) reactive to HS-63 was also purified by the same purification scheme and was shown to have molecular sizes similar to those of MSA-63.

Mouse Sperm Antigen Reactive to HS-11 (MSA-11)

In contrast, the antigenic epitope specific to HS-11 is relatively unstable and sensitive to irreversible inactivation during routine laboratory manipulations. Furthermore, the presence of mild nonionic detergents such as Tween-20 and Triton X-100 greatly enhanced the stability and recovery of relevant sperm antigens during protein purification. The purification of MSA-11 was best achieved by a single-step immunoaffinity chromatographic procedure from detergent-solubilized mouse testis homogenate. A dot radioimmunobinding assay was used to follow the immunoactivity of MSA-11 before and after immunoaffinity chromatography. When analyzed by SDS-PAGE (Fig. 1), the purified MSA-11 was shown to be a group of seven glycoproteins with molecular weight ranging from 35 to 50 kd. The isoelectric points of these glycoproteins ranged from 4.4 to 4.7 as determined by two-dimensional gel electrophoresis. This also represented a 1,000-fold protein purification from the crude mouse testis homogenate (Table 1).

The HS-11–related immunoactivity was found to decrease with

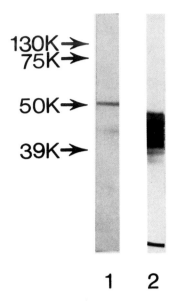

130K→
75K→

50K→

39K→

1 2

Fig. 1. Sodium dodecylsulfate polyacrylamide gel electrophoresis (10% acrylamide gels) of purified MSA-63 (**lane 1**) and MSA-11 (**lane 2**) sperm antigens. Molecular weight standards are (from top to bottom) 130, 75, 50, and 39 kd. [Liu et al., 1989b].

time and storage conditions. To investigate the microheterogeneity of the purified sperm antigen, the purified MSA-11 was subjected to analysis for molecular size distribution of the purified native antigen by a Sephacryl S-300 gel filtration chromatography. It was subsequently observed that MSA-11 appeared to be a wide molecular range of undefined aggregates in the native state (100–2,000 kd). Unexpectedly, fractions with peak immunoactivity to HS-11 did not coincide with those of the high protein concentration. Much higher immunoactivity to HS-11 was found in the early fractions of high-molecular-weight regions, which had relatively low protein concentration. The existence of high-molecular-weight aggregates appeared to be essential for the antigenic epitope to be recognized by HS-11 monoclonal antibody. The protein and activity profiles of a typical gel filtration column are presented in Figure 2. Furthermore, when the protein fractions eluted from Sephacryl S-300 gel filtration columns were grouped according to three different molecular weight ranges and analyzed by SDS-PAGE, the patterns of protein bands in each group were not significantly different from those initially purified from the immunoaffinity column. Judging from these observations, it is therefore suggested that MSA-11 is a protein complex

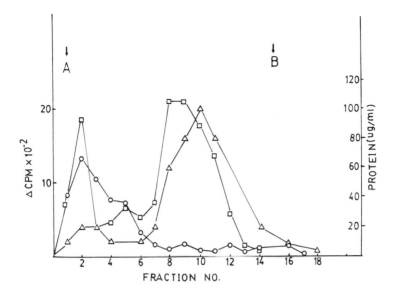

Fig. 2. Sephacryl S-300 gel filtration chromatography to reveal the molecular size distribution and HS-11 and HS-63 immunoactivities of the purified MSA-11 antigen: △, protein concentration in μmg/ml; □, ○, immunoactivities to HS-11 and HS-63 in each eluted fraction, respectively. Arrows A and B indicate the position of the void volume and the column volume, respectively.

localized on the sperm acrosome held together by noncovalent hydrophobic/hydrophilic interactions.

IMMUNOLOGIC AND ANTIFERTILITY STUDIES OF MSA-63 AND MSA-11 SPERM ANTIGENS

Both purified MSA-63 and MSA-11 are auto- and isoimmunogenic in mice and immunogenic in rabbits. This was clearly demonstrated by active immunization with the purified sperm antigens. In the case of MSA-63, the titer of mouse antisera can be as high as 1:20,000 serum dilution when analyzed by the indirect immunofluorescent assay, whereas those of rabbits could reach a titer of 1:200,000. Both mouse and rabbit antisera were highly specific to antigens in sperm and testis and did not cross-react with any other somatic tissues when examined by quantitative tissue adsorption experiments and/ or tissue sections. Similar to the original HS-63 monoclonal antibody, anti-MSA-63 sera cross-react with the sperm acrosome of several mammalian species, including human, mouse, and rabbit.

Similarly, MSA-11 is also highly immunogenic in rabbits and mice, and high titers of antisera were raised. By Western blot assay, the

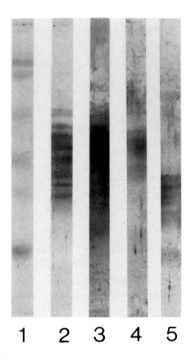

1   2   3   4   5

Fig. 3. The Western blot assay to reveal the proteins bands recognized by mouse or rabbit antisera against purified MSA-11: **Lane 1,** molecular weight standards (from top to bottom) are the same those described in Figure 1; **lane 2,** purified MSA-11 on the nitrocellulose strip detected by mouse anti-MSA-11 sera; **lane 3,** purified MSA-11 detected by rabbit anti-MSA-11 sera; **lane 4,** mouse sperm homogenate detected by rabbit anti-MSA-11 sera; **lane 5,** human sperm homogenate detected by rabbit anti-MSA-11 sera.

protein patterns recognized by mouse or rabbit antisera on nitrocellulose strips to which mouse sperm proteins were transferred were not significantly different from those of the purified MSA-11 (Fig. 3). Unexpectedly, the molecular weights of the protein bands detected on the strips of human sperm extract appeared to be lower than those on mouse sperm (molecular weights 20–35 kd in human vs. 35–50 kd in mouse).

Through active immunization with the purified MSA-63 or MSA-11 in mice, the raised isoimmune sera were shown to exhibit strong antifertility effects as determined by mouse in vitro fertilization and by the sperm penetration assay using zona-free hamster ova. As shown in Tables 2 and 3, the degree of antifertility effects with isoimmune sera seemed to be stronger than those by the original HS-11 and HS-63 monoclonal antibodies.

TABLE 2. Effect of HS-63, HS-11, and Antisera Against MSA-63 and MSA-11 on the In Vitro Fertilization of Mouse Oocytes[a]

Antibodies	No. of assays	Ova examined (No.)	Ova fertilized (No.)	Fertilization rate (%)
HS-63	5	118	28	24
Control	*8*	*116*	*63*	*54*
HS-11	2	39	13	33
Control	*3*	*68*	*27*	*65*
Mouse Anti-MSA-63	7	181	8	4.4
Control	*8*	*116*	*63*	*54*
Rabbit Anti-MSA-63	6	123	6	4.8
Control	*4*	*53*	*33*	*62*
Mouse Anti-MSA-11	4	95	11	11.6
Control	*3*	*68*	*27*	*65*
Rabbit Anti-MSA-11	2	30	1	3.3
Control	*4*	*43*	*32*	*74.4*

[a]Details of experimental conditions are presented elsewhere [Liu et al., 1989b].

TABLE 3. Effect of HS-63 and Antisera Against MSA-63 on the Sperm Penetration Assay Using Zona-Free Hamster Ova[a]

Antibodies	No. of assays	Ova examined (No.)	Ova fertilized (No.)	Fertilization rate (%)
HS-63	4	63	7	11.1
Control	*4*	*74*	*40*	*54.1*
Mouse Anti-MSA-63	4	75	7	9.0
Rabbit Anti-MSA-63	4	73	7	9.5
Control	*2*	*43*	*25*	*58.1*

[a]Details of experimental conditions are presented elsewhere [Liu et al., 1989b].

The mechanism by which HS-11 and HS-63 monoclonal antibodies and relevant polyclonal antisera inhibit fertilization was elucidated. As shown in Figure 4, both HS-11 and HS-63 inhibit A23187-induced as well as zona-induced sperm acrosome reaction in a time- and dose-dependent manner. These observations may explain why both HS-11 and HS-63 and relevant polyclonal antisera inhibit fertilization of mouse oocytes in vitro [Liu et al., 1989b].

MOLECULAR CLONING OF SPERM ANTIGEN GENE

Our preliminary experiments have demonstrated that two purified sperm antigens, MSA-11 and MSA-63, are isoimmunogenic. The

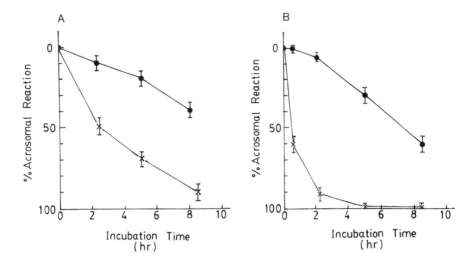

Fig. 4. Time-dependent inhibition of A23187-induced human sperm (**A**) and mouse sperm (**B**) acrosome reaction by HS-63 monoclonal antibody (●). Phosphate-buffered saline was used as the negative control (×) [Liu et al., 1989a].

raised antisera exhibit a strong antifertility effect in vitro. It is essential to mass produce these sperm antigens for animal studies to assess the feasibility of contraceptive vaccine development. Therefore, subsequent research and development requires the application of recombinant DNA technology to isolate genes encoding desirable sperm antigens.

In collaboration with Dr. Chris Lau at the University of California, San Francisco, we have successfully isolated the mouse gene coding for MSA-63 protein. Initially, specific rabbit antisera were raised against the purified MSA-63. These polyclonal antibodies were then used to immunoscreen a mouse testis cDNA library constructed with a λgt11 expression vector. Out of 5×10^5 cDNA clones that have been screened, four express a recombinant fusion protein that could be recognized by rabbit anti-MSA-63 sera. Following a cross-hybridization experiment, cDNA probes for the MSA-63 gene were isolated and subjected to DNA sequencing analysis, which was then used to deduce the corresponding protein amino acid sequence. The results of this analysis together with the restriction map are presented in Figure 5. By using Northern analysis, it was clearly demonstrated that the isolated cDNA probe could only hybridize with a single 1.5 kb mRNA strand from the adult mouse testis, but not with any other mouse tissues such as brain, liver, ovary, or fetal testis [Liu et al., 1990]. The results of this analysis are demonstrated in Figure 6.

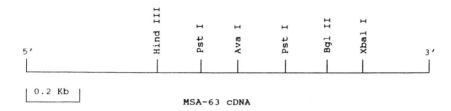

MSA-63 cDNA

DNA/PROTEIN SEQUENCE OF pMSA-12

```
  1 GTTA ATC TTA CTG GGT CTT TAT CTG CTT GGA TCT GCC CAA GGA
    Leu Ile Leu Leu Gly Leu Tyr Leu Leu Gly Ser Ala Gln Gly
 44 GCA CCA CCA GGT CAG CCT GAG GAG CTT CTT GAC TCT GTA GAC
    Ala Pro Pro Gly Gln Pro Glu Glu Leu Leu Asp Ser Val Asp
 86 CAA CAA GCT TCG GTT CAG CAA CTT TCA AGC GAG TAT CTC TCA
    Gln Gln Ala Ser Val Gln Gln Leu Ser Ser Glu Tyr Leu Ser
128 CTC GCA AAC CCT TCA GAT GCC GAG GCT TTA TAT GAA ACT CCT
    Leu Ala Asn Pro Ser Asp Ala Glu Ala Leu Tyr Glu Thr Pro
170 TTA GAT GAG AAG ACT CTG AGT GGT CAT AGT TCA AGT GAA CAG
    Leu Asp Glu Lys Thr Leu Ser Gly His Ser Ser Ser Glu Gln
212 GAA TCA AGT GAG CAT GCT GTA GCT GAA CAT TCT GCA GGT GAG
    Glu Ser Ser Glu His Ala Val Ala Glu His Ser Ala Gly Glu
254 CAC TCT TCA GGA GAA CAG TCT TCA CAA CAC ATG TCA GGT GAC
    His Ser Ser Gly Glu Gln Ser Ser Glu His MET Ser Gly Asp
296 CAC ATG TCA GGA CAG CAC TTG TCA GAA CAC ACT TCA GAG GAG
    His MET Ser Gly Gln His Leu Ser Glu His Thr Ser Glu Glu
338 CAC TCC TCG GGC GAG CAC ACT TGC ACC GAG CAC ACT TCA GGT
    His Ser Ser Gly Glu His Thr Cys Thr Glu His Thr Ser Gly
380 GAA CAA CCT GCA ACT GAA CAG TCC TCA AGT GAC CAG CCC TCC
    Glu Gln Pro Ala Thr Glu Gln Ser Ser Ser Asp Gln Pro Ser
422 GAA GCA TCT TCA CGT GAA GTT TCG GGT GAC GAA GCA GGT GAA
    Glu Ala Ser Ser Gly Glu Val Ser Gly Asp Glu Ala Gly Glu
464 CAG GTG TCT AGC GAG ACA AAT GAC AAA GAA AAT GAT GCT ATG
    Gln Val Ser Ser Glu Thr Asn Asp Lys Glu Asn Asp Ala MET
506 AGT ACA CCA CTT CCA AGC ACA TCT GCA GCC ATA ACA ATA AAT
    Ser Thr Pro Leu Pro Ser Thr Ser Ala Ala Ile Thr Ile Asn
548 TGC CAC ACA TGT GCT TAT ATG AAT GAT GAT GCA AAA TGT CTC
    Cys His Thr Cys Ala Tyr MET Asn Asp Asp Ala Lys Cys Leu
590 CGT GGA GAA GGA GTA TGC ACC ACT CAA AAC TCC CAG CAG TGC
    Arg Gly Glu Gly Val Cys Thr Thr Gln Asn Ser Gln Gln Cys
632 ATG TTA AAG AAG ATC TTT GAA GGT GGA AAC TCC AGT TCA TGG
    MET Leu Lys Lys Ile Phe Glu Gly Gly Asn Ser Ser Ser Trp
674 TTC AAG GGT GTG AGA ACA TGT GCC CAT CTA TGA ACCTCTTC
    Phe Lys Gly Val Arg Thr Cys Ala His Leu TER
715 TCT CAT GGA ACA AGA ATG CAA ATT ATG TGC TGT CGG AAT GAA
757 CCT CTC TGC AAC AAG GTC TAG ATG CCC GTG CCC TAC TTC TTG
799 CTC TGA CTT AGG CAG GTT CAC CAC TCT ACT TGG CTC AAT TTA
841 TGT TCA ACT TCA ACA ACT AAT CAC ATC GGC TCT GCC TGA TCA
883 CCA GAT AAG AAG CTC AAA CCT TGT CTT TAT TGA TAC CCC ATT
925 GCC TAT GTC CTC TGC CTT ACT TTG CTC CCA TCC TTC GCG CAG
967 ATG TTC TTT TTT GCA ATA AAT TGC TAT TAA AGA 25 polyA tail
```

Fig. 5. The restriction map (restriction enzymes at the top) and the partial nucleotide as well as the corresponding amino acid sequence of the MSA-63 gene (bottom) through the initial immunoscreening of the mouse testis cDNA library. A cDNA clone (pMSA-12) was used for the sequencing analysis [Liu et al., 1990].

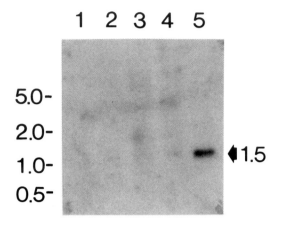

Fig. 6.   Northern analysis to reveal the hybridization of a single 1.5 kb mRNA strand from the adult mouse testis (**lane 5**), but not with any other mouse tissues, including brain (**lane 1**), liver (**lane 2**), ovary (**lane 3**), and fetal testis (**lane 4**). The mRNA size markers are shown on the left [Liu et al., 1990].

CHARACTERIZATION OF RECOMBINANT FUSION PROTEIN

The specificity of the recombinant fusion protein produced by lysogenic bacteria that carried the desirable recombinant cDNA insert was determined by radioimmunosorbent inhibition assay with the sperm extract or purified MSA-63 coated on microwells. The Western blot assay with the bacteria extract transferred to nitrocellulose strips was also used to detect the expression of 150 kd recombinant fusion protein. The selected results of such immunologic analysis are given in Figure 7.

By using Sephacryl S-300 gel filtration chromatography, the recombinant fusion protein, partially purified from bacteria extract, was used to immunize mice and rabbits actively. Similar to HS-63 and to the corresponding polyclonal antisera raised against MSA-63, antisera against the fusion protein also reacted with the sperm acrosome. The specific binding between the raised antisera and MSA-63 coated on microwells was also demonstrated by ELISA. In summary, these experimental results have helped us to establish the basic strategy and protocol from which specific sperm antigen-based immunocontraceptive vaccines can be developed in the near future.

Recently, the cDNA of human SA-63 protein (HSA-63) was successfully isolated from a human testis cDNA library by with ^{32}P-labeled MSA-63 cDNA fragment as the probe [Maniatis et al., 1982]. The longest cDNA fragment was shown to have a size of 1.5 kb and

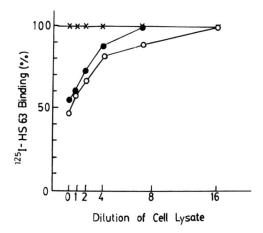

Fig. 7. Radioimmunosorbent assays to reveal dose-dependent percent inhibition of the binding between ^{125}I-labeled HS-63 and mouse sperm coated on microwells in the presence of lysates from the recombinant bacteria containing pMSA-6 insert (●), pMSA-12 insert (○), and those from the original bacteria host Y1089 (X). The initial protein concentrations of the cell lysates were adjusted to be 5 mg/ml, and 1×10^5 cpm/well was used for each assay [Liu et al., 1990].

was subcloned to a plasmid vector for DNA sequence analysis. In the near future, the full-length cDNA of HSA-63 will be constructed to a suitable vector and will be expressed in a mammalian cell system for recombinant protein production. It is expected that suitable immunocontraceptive vaccines for humans may be mass produced by recombinant DNA technology.

BIOCHEMICAL/IMMUNOLOGIC RELATIONSHIPS OF SPERM ANTIGENS REACTIVE TO HS-11 AND HS-63

Both HS-11 and HS-63 monoclonal antibodies recognized conserved antigens that were localized on the sperm acrosome of several mammalian species. Both were able to inhibit in vitro fertilization of mouse oocytes by blocking sperm acrosome reaction [Liu et al., 1989a]. Judging from the relative stability of their respective antigenic epitopes, it was suspected that HS-11 and HS-63 react with two different types of antigenic epitopes. The corresponding sperm antigens MSA-11 and MSA-63 were purified by completely different protocols [Liu et al., 1989a,b, 1990]. MSA-63 was shown to consist of three soluble proteins with molecular weights of 40–50 kd on SDS gel, whereas MSA-11 appeared to be a group of membrane-associated proteins with sizes ranging from 35 to 50 kd. The HS-11–specific

Lee et al.

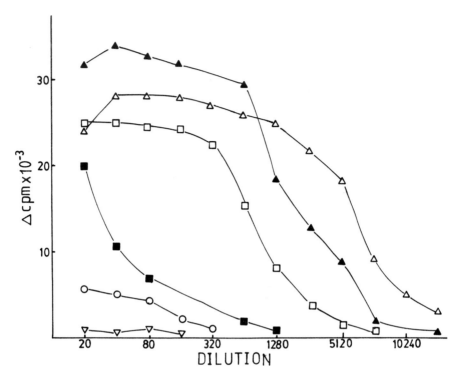

Fig. 8. Radioimmunobinding assays to reveal the binding and the mutual cross-reactivity between ^{125}I-labeled MSA-11 or MSA-63 and relevant monoclonal antibodies or polyclonal antisera in different dilutions (in log scale). △, ^{125}I-MSA-11 and rabbit anti-MSA-11; □, ^{125}I-MSA-11 and rabbit anti-MSA-63; ○, ^{125}I-MSA-11 and HS-63 monoclonal antibody; ▽, ^{125}I-MSA-11 and HS-11 monoclonal antibody; ▲, ^{125}I-MSA-63 and rabbit anti-MSA-11; ■, ^{125}I-MSA-63 and rabbit anti-MSA-63. To each binding assay, 1×10^5 cpm of ^{125}I-labeled MSA-11 or MSA-63 was used and incubated with antibodies of different dilutions according to the procedures described elsewhere [Chow et al., 1985].

epitope of MSA-11 proteins require a certain organized structure for immunoactivity and nonionic detergent for stability.

Immunologically, rabbit antisera against MSA-63 cross-react with MSA-11. Similarly, cross-reactivity was observed between rabbit anti-MSA-11 and MSA-63 when analyzed with radioimmunobinding assay with ^{125}I-labeled purified sperm antigens as respective tracers. The results of this analysis are presented in Figure 8.

Following gel filtration chromatography of the purified MSA-11, the protein in the molecular weight range of 50–100 kd appeared to be recognized only by HS-63 (Fig. 2). This observation indicates that certain immunologic cross-reactivities exist between the purified

MSA-11 and MSA-63 antigens. Rabbit antisera against fusion protein did not cross react with MSA-11 proteins by immunoblot. On the other hand, rabbit antisera against MSA-63 only recognized part of the protein bands displayed by purified MSA-11 on nitrocellulose strips.

Since epitope-specific monoclonal antibodies were used as affinity ligands for antigen purification, immunologic cross-reactivity of the raised polyclonal antisera implies that the epitopes recognized by HS-11 and HS-63 are shared by both purified MSA-11 and MSA-63 antigens. HS-11 monoclonal antibody only recognized protein aggregates of certain molecular size and appeared to be specific to a certain conformational determinant of an acrosome–protein complex. On the other hand, HS-63 reacts specifically with an epitope of peptide determinant. However, both HS-11 and HS-63 failed to recognize determinants on the renatured antigens that had been previously denatured during SDS- PAGE. This was clearly demonstrated by the Western blot assay (unpublished observations). Finally, it is HS-63, not HS-11, that reacts with a protein determinant derived from the recombinant fusion protein expressed by cDNA clones initially immunoscreened with anti-MSA-63 sera.

Because of these observations, it is reasonable to suggest that HS-11 and HS-63 recognize different epitopes of proteins in an acrosome–protein complex. The monoclonal and polyclonal antibodies specific to certain auto- and isoimmunogenic epitopes of this protein complex may be capable of inhibiting the sperm acrosome reaction and the subsequent fertilization processes. Therefore, the auto- and isoimmunogenic properties of this acrosome complex could be the basis for the design of potential immunocontraceptive vaccines.

ACKNOWLEDGMENTS

Support for this project was provided by the Contraceptive Research and Development Program (CONRAD 009), Eastern Virginia Medical School, under a Cooperative Agreement with the United States Agency for International Development (A.I.D.; DEP-3044-A-00-6063-00) and by the Medical Research Council of Canada (5-99802). The views expressed by the authors do not necessarily reflect the views of A.I.D. and CONRAD.

REFERENCES

Anderson DJ, Alexander NJ (1983): A new look at antifertility vaccines. Fertil Steril 40:557.

Anderson DJ, Johnson PM, Alexander NJ, Jones WR, Griffin PD (1987): Monoclonal antibodies to human trophoblast and sperm antigens. J Reprod Immunol 10:231.

Chow SN, Ouyang PC, Lee CL, Lee CYG (1985): Studies of monoclonal antibodies against human chorionic gonadotropin. I. Characterization of monoclonal antibodies specific to beta subunit of human chorionic gonadotropin. J Chin Biochem Soc 14:1.

D'Almeida M, Lefroit-Jolig M, Voisin GA (1981): Studies on human spermatozoa autoantigens. Clin Exp Immunol 44:359.

Ingerslev HJ (1981): Antibodies against spermatozoal surface-membrane antigens in female infertility. Acta Obstet Gynecol Scand (Suppl) 100:1.

Isojima S, Li TS, Ashitaka Y (1968): Immunologic analysis of sperm-immobilizing factor found in sera of women with unexplained sterility. Am J Obstet Gynecol 101:677.

Lee CYG, Lum V, Wong E, Memge AC, Huang YS (1982): Identification of human sperm antigens to antisperm antibodies. Am J Reprod Immunol 3:183.

Lee CYG, Wong E, Menge AC (1984a): Monoclonal antibodies to rabbit sperm autoantigens. Fertil Steril 41:131.

Lee CYG, Wong E, Richter DE, Menge AC (1984b): Monoclonal antibodies to human sperm antigens, II. J Reprod Immunol 6:227.

Lee CYG, Wong E, Teh CZ (1984c): Analysis of sperm isoantigens using monoclonal antibodies. Am J Reprod Immunol 6:27.

Lee CYG, Wong E, Zhang JH (1986): Inhibitory effects of monoclonal sperm antibodies on the fertilization of mouse oocytes in vitro and in vivo. J Reprod Immunol 9:261.

Lee CYG, Zhang JH, Wong E, Chow SN, Yang Y, Sun P, Leung HY (1987): Sex difference of antifertility effect by passively immunized monoclonal sperm antibodies. Am J Reprod Immunol Microbiol 13:9.

Liu MS, Chan K, Lau YF, Lee CYG (1990): Molecular cloning of an acrosomal sperm antigen gene and the production of its recombinant protein for immunocontraceptive vaccine. Mol Reprod Develop 25:302.

Liu MS, Yang Y, Lee CYG (1989a): Inhibition of acrosome reaction by monoclonal antibodies reactive to sperm acrosome. Mol Androl 1:358.

Liu MS, Yang Y, Pan J, Liu HW, Menge AC, Lee CYG (1989b): Purification of acrosomal antigen recognized by a monoclonal antibody and antifertility effects of isoimmune sera. Int J Androl 12:451.

Maniatis T, Fritsch ET, Sambrook J (1982): Molecular Cloning: A Laboratory Manual. New York: Cold Spring Harbor.

Menge AC (1980): Clinical immunological infertility. In Dhinsda D, Schumacher GFB (eds): Immunologic Aspects of Infertility and Fertility Regulation. Amsterdam: Elsevier-North Holland, p 205.

Menge AC, Peegal H, Riolo ML (1979): Sperm fractions responsible for immunologic induction of pre- and postfertilization infertility in rabbits. Biol Reprod 20:931.

Menge AC, Shoultz GK, Kelsey DE, Lee CYG (1987): Characterization of monoclonal antibodies against human sperm antigens by immunoassays including sperm function assays and epitope evaluation. Am J Reprod Immunol 13:108.

Shulman S (1982): Immunological Factors in Human Reproduction. Serono Symposium, Vol 45. New York: Academic Press, p 5.

Tung KSK (1976): Antifertility vaccines: Considerations of their potential immunopathologic complications. Int J Fertil 21:197.

Tung KSK (1980): Autoimmunity of the testis. In Dhinsda DS, Schumacher GFB (eds): Immunologic Aspects of Infertility and Fertility Regulation. Amsterdam: Elsevier-North Holland, p 33.

DISCUSSION

DR. ANDERSON: What is the mechanism of acrosome reaction inhibition?

DR. LEE: We use chlorotetracycline as a probe to study inhibition of the monclonal antibodies on the sperm acrosome reaction. We found that the acrosome reaction is arrested at the S phase. Apparently it may have something to do with the involvement of the acrosome component in fusion with other acrosomal membranes to form vesicles. This hypothesis requires further testing.

DR. SURI: You had immunoaffinity-purified the HS623 antigen. When you raised the polyclonal sera against that, in your blot you showed a group of identifying bands. Can you explain that result against a specific antigen?

DR. LEE: If this antigen has autolytic activity, or it has proteolytic activity in testes or sperm preparations, this antigen can easily be broken down into many bands. This is commonly observed in many sperm antigen preparations. They are recognized by one single monoclonal antibody or polyclonal antibody.

DR. SURI: With respect to your antigen, is it tissue specific?

DR. LEE: Yes, it is tissue specific.

DR.HECHT: In your Northern blot data, which tissues did you examine and how much RNA were you running on each gel?

DR. LEE: In high-stringency conditions, we run fetal testes, fetal brain, adult liver, and many different tissues compared with adult mouse testes. This is in collaboration with Dr. Chris Lau from San Francisco.

4

Morphological Development and Function of the Mammalian Sperm Acrosome Explored With 18.6 Monoclonal Antibody

Harry D.M. Moore, Caroline A. Smith, and Alison Moore

The first contact of the mammalian spermatozoon with the egg anchors and orientates the sperm head so that it can begin to penetrate the zona pellucida [see Moore and Bedford, 1983; Yanagimachi, 1988]. Because this initial interaction between sperm and ovum is vital for fertilization and appears to be mediated by gamete-specific receptors on the sperm plasmalemma and zona surface, it is an obvious target for immunocontraceptive action. The acrosome and its membranes play a critical role during sperm–egg binding. Only spermatozoa that have lost their apical membranes and acrosomal contents (as a result of an acrosome reaction) can penetrate the zona matrix and undergo fusion with the oolemma. The question that remains to be answered unequivocally is: What is the state of the acrosome of the fertilizing sperm at the moment of contact with the zona surface? In rodent species, such as the mouse and hamster, and also in the human, the consensus view is that it is the plasma membrane overlying the apical surface of an intact or partially reacted acrosome that initially binds the *fertilizing* sperm to the zona [Wassarman, 1987; Yanagimachi, 1988; Cross et al., 1988]. In the mouse, there is good evidence to suggest that in vitro, at least, the zona protein ZP3 can trigger the acrosome reaction at sperm–egg contact

Gamete Interaction: Prospects for Immunocontraception, pages 53–61

[Bleil and Wassarman, 1983; Leyton and Saling, 1989]. More information about the role of the acrosome is clearly required for other laboratory species and man for effective contraception to be devised.

Monoclonal antibodies (mAbs) generated against acrosome components can be used to explore the morphological development of the acrosome and its role during fertilization. Furthermore, in conjunction with appropriate fertilization assays in vivo and in vitro, these mAbs can be used to identify pertinent antigens involved in sperm–egg interactions. One such monoclonal antibody, designated 18.6, has proved particularly valuable as a specific marker of the acrosome. This paper summarizes the results of several investigations [Ellis et al., 1985; Moore et al., 1985, 1987a,b] and of more recent unpublished studies.

MATERIALS AND METHODS

Production of Monoclonal Antibodies

Monoclonal antibody 18.6 was produced as described previously [Moore and Hartman, 1984]. Briefly, Balb/C mice were immunized intraperitoneally with intact hamster spermatozoa (10^7) recovered from the cauda epididymis. After 6 weeks, the mice were given a booster injection and then sacrificed 4 days later for the fusion and cloning procedures, as outlined elsewhere [Ellis et al., 1985]. Characterization of secreted immunoglobulin was carried out by affinity chromatography on a 5 ml protein-A Sepharose column (Pharmacia) as described by Trincheri [1979].

Solid Phase Immunoassay (ELISA) With Purified Acrosomal Membranes

An ELISA assay was developed with purified acrosomal material dried and fixed on 96 well microtiter plates [Moore et al., 1987b]. Assays were performed with 100 µl aliquots (in triplicate) of cultured supernatant and three reference-negative controls (preimmune serum, saline, and myeloma cell culture supernatant). The second antibody was rabbit antimouse IgG conjugated to alkaline phosphatase.

Immunocytochemistry

Immunofluorescent localization was carried out as described previously [see Moore et al., 1987b]. Ultrastructural observation of antibody binding was carried out using an immunoperoxidase technique [Smith et al., 1986].

Fertilization Assays

The inhibition of fertilization by antibody was tested in a hamster in vitro fertilization assay [Moore and Hartman, 1984; Ellis et al., 1985] with intact and zona-free oocytes and in a human in vitro zona-binding assay with salt-stored oocytes [Moore et al., 1987a].

RESULTS

ELISA and Characterization of Antigen

Enzyme-linked immunosorbent assays with purified acrosomes as a solid-phase antigen indicated that culture supernatant exhibited high titers of antibody (Fig. 1). Assays with brain, liver, heart, and lung tissue demonstrated no cross-reactivity. Immunoglobulin was of the class IgG_2.

Under very mild denaturing conditions, 18.6 mAb recognized a large antigen of apparent molecular weight of more than 500 kd [Ellis et al., 1985], but this value was probably due to incomplete dissociation from membrane. Investigations with dot blots showed that the antigen was sensitive to detergent and heat treatment.

Expression and Localization of Antigen

On fixed sections of hamster testis 18.6 antibody recognized an antigen on specific sections of the seminiferous tubule corresponding with late spermatids (stages 14–17). This localization was shown at higher magnification to be specific to the acrosome. In cell suspensions of seminiferous tubules antigen was expressed at all stages of spermatid development (Fig. 2), suggesting that antibody access to antigen was restricted in sections possibly by overlying Sertoli cells. The antibody was acrosome specific (Fig. 2) but cross-reacted strongly with spermatozoa from most eutherian mammals thus far tested (only faint fluorescence on Giant Panda sperm).

At the ultrastructural level, antigen was associated with developing inner and outer acrosomal membranes and, in fully mature spermatozoa, with acrosomal matrix material (Fig. 3). This intracellular localization of antigen is consistent with the absence of immunofluorescence with intact live spermatozoa. During capacitation in capacitating medium, the proportion of motile spermatozoa exhibiting

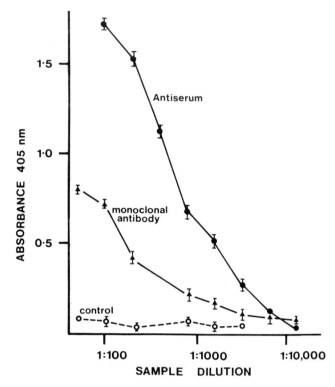

Fig. 1. Enzyme-linked immunosorbent assay with purified acrosomes as solid-phase antigen. A graph of optical density at 405 nm against titers of antihamster sperm antiserum (●), culture supernatant containing 18.6 antibody (▲), and control supernatant (○).

fluorescence in the presence of FITC-conjugated antibody was correlated with the proportion of acrosome-reacted spermatozoa in a time-dependent manner (Fig. 4).

Fertilization Assays

The ability of antibody to inhibit fertilization was assessed in vitro in the hamster and human. mAb 18.6 failed to inhibit fertilization of intact or zona-free hamster eggs or the binding of human sperm to salt-stored oocytes, whereas, for comparison, mAb 97.25 (specific to a 90/95 kd antigen of the acrosome) specifically blocked fertilization and human sperm/zona binding (Tables 1 and 2).

DISCUSSION

mAb 18.6 failed to block fertilization events in either the hamster or human; therefore, it is unlikely that it identifies an antigen that

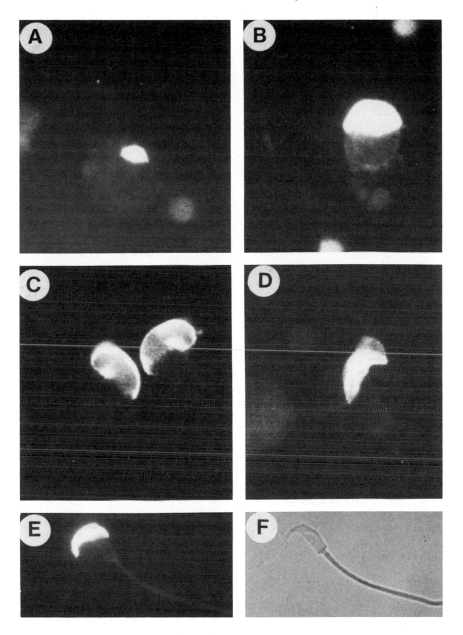

Fig. 2. Immunofluorescent localization of binding of 18.6 antibody to various stages of spermatid development. ×1,050. **A:** Fluorescence on an acrosomal granule of a round spermatid. **B:** Spreading of fluorescence with the lateral movement of the acrosome over the anterior acrosome. **C,D:** Pattern of fluorescence during spermatid elongation. **E,F:** Immunofluorescent localization of 18.6 antibody and corresponding light micrograph on a cauda epididymal spermatozoon.

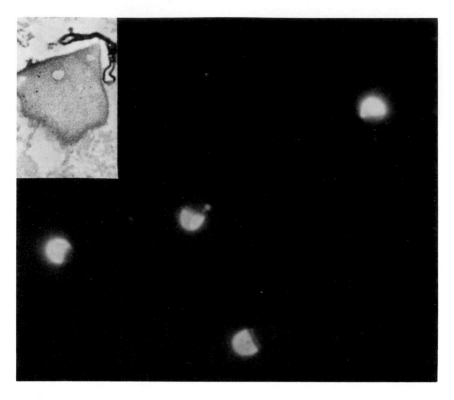

Fig. 3. A micrograph of immunofluorescent localization of monoclonal antibody binding to human spermatozoa. **Inset:** Ultrastructural localization over acrosome membranes of developing spermatid.

could be used in an antifertility vaccine. Nevertheless, investigations with this antibody have shown it to be an extremely useful marker of the acrosome during its development and function and also have established approaches that may yield antigens that are potential candidates for vaccine development [Moore et al., 1987a]. In this respect, the most important feature of any antibody is its specificity for spermatozoa and, in particular, postmeiotic stages of development. By using hamster spermatozoa as immunogen and screening hybridoma supernatants for cross-reactivity with human spermatozoa or acrosome fragments, it is clear that antibodies can be selected that are sperm specific. It is also more likely that they recognize antigens that have been conserved during evolution and therefore may be important for fertilization processes. That 18.6 cross-reacts with all eutherian spermatozoa thus far tested but does not react with marsupial or other vertebrate spermatozoa is interesting. From

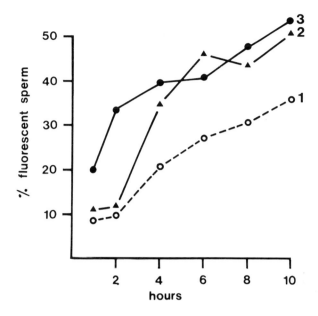

Fig. 4.   A graph of the proportion of live spermatozoa in three samples exhibiting immunofluorescence against the length of incubation in BWW (Biggers, Whitten and Whittingham) capacitating medium.

TABLE 1. In Vitro Sperm Penetration of Intact and Zona-Free Hamster Oocytes in the Presence of Monoclonal Antibodies

Monoclonal antibody	Proportion of oocytes penetrated		Titer of supernatant
	Intact	Zona free	
18.6	54/60	38/38	1:10
	52/58	24/25	1:50
97.5	0/42	26/30	1:10
	7/32	25/25	1:50
	12/47	22/22	1:100
	31/34	28/31	1:500

a practical point of view, broad cross-species reactivity is an advantage because screening assays of sperm function can first be undertaken in a laboratory species.

The most important use of 18.6 is as a marker (at the light microscopic level) of the acrosome in human spermatozoa [Moore et al., 1987b]. Its use has enabled us to determine the proportion of sperm undergoing the acrosome reaction and to therefore identify poten-

TABLE 2. In Vitrò Sperm Attachment of Human Spermatozoa to Salt-Stored Human Oocytes in the Presence of Monoclonal Antibodies

Monoclonal antibody	No. of zona examined	Mean No. of sperm bound	Titer of antibody
18.6	23	32.3 + 8.1	1:50
97.5	20	2.3 + 3.3*	1:50

*$P < 0.005$.

tially subfertile semen samples in the human and other species. It has also been used to demonstrate that usually only acrosome-reacted spermatozoa can bind to the egg membrane.

ACKNOWLEDGMENTS

These studies were supported by a program grant from the Medical Research Council and the Agricultural and Food Research Council and by a grant from the Wellcome Trust.

REFERENCES

Bleil JD, Wassarman PM (1983): Sperm–egg interactions in the mouse: Sequence of events and induction of the acrosome reaction by a zona pellucida glycoprotein. Dev Biol 95: 317–324.

Cross NL, Morales P, Overstreet JW, Hanson FW (1988): Induction of acrosome reactions by the human zona pellucida. Biol Reprod 38:235–244.

Ellis DH, Hartman TD, Moore HDM (1985): Maturation and function of the hamster spermatzoon probed with monoclonal antibodies. J Reprod Immunol 7:299–314.

Leyton L, Saling P (1989): 95 Kd sperm proteins bind ZP3 and serve as tyrosine kinase substrates in response to zona binding. Cell 57:1123–1130.

Moore HDM, Bedford JM (1983): The interaction of mammalian gametes in the female. In Hartman JF (ed): Mechanism and Control of Animal Fertilization. New York: Academic Press, pp 453–497.

Moore HDM, Hartman TD (1984): Localization by monoclonal antibodies of various surface antigens of hamster spermatozoa and the effect of antibody on fertilization in vitro. J Reprod Fertil 70:175–183.

Moore HDM, Hartman TD, Brown AC, Smith CA, Ellis DA (1985): Expression of sperm antigens during spermatogenesis and maturation detected with monoclonal antibodies. Exp Clin Immunogenet 2:84–96.

Moore HDM, Hartman TD, Bye AP, Lutjen P, De Witt M, Trouson AO (1987a): Monoclonal antibodies against a sperm antigen Mr 95,000 inhibits attachment of human spermatozoa to the zona pellucida. J Reprod Immunol 11:157–166.

Moore HDM, Smith CA, Hartman TD, Bye AP (1987b): Visualization and characterization of the acrosome reaction of human spermatozoa by immunolocalization with monoclonal antibodies. Gamete Res 17:245–259.

Smith CA, Hartman TD, Moore HDM (1986): A determinant of Mr 34000 expressed by hamster epididymal epithelium binds specifically to spermatozoa in co-culture. J Reprod Fertil 78:337–345.

Trincheri G (1979): Purification of immunoglobulins produced by the hybrid cells. In Hybridoma Technology With Special Reference to Parasitic Diseases. Geneva: UNDO/World Bank/WHO, pp 67–69.

Wassarman PM (1987): The biology and chemistry of fertilization. Science 235:553–554.

Yanagimachi R (1988): Mammalian fertilization. In Knobil E, et al. (eds): The Physiology of Reproduction. New York: Raven Press, pp 135–185.

DISCUSSION

DR. ISOJIMA: By using monoclonal 97 and by means of the fluorescence stain, do you see staining of the ejaculated living human sperm?

DR. MOORE: Yes. The stain is localized over the head and in the equatorial region.

DR. ISOJIMA: Have you tried staining other human tissues using the sensitive ABC stain?

DR. MOORE: Yes. We have stained human testes and ovary and find that we get staining only on germ cells.

DR. HERR: I am intrigued with the idea of using the bacterial lysates in the bioassay. Are you working with an expression system that gives you the soluble protein?

DR. MOORE: No. It is a problem to evaluate how the bioassay really is going to be affected. We can do it by just comparing different clones, and, with some, we definitely get an inhibition that can be reversed by pulling it out with an antibody. Eventually, it may offer a means of screening the library for potentially important clones at an early stage.

5

Lactate Dehydrogenase C_4 as an Immunocontraceptive Model

Erwin Goldberg

Lactate dehydrogenase (LDH) is a glycolytic enzyme that exists in multiple molecular forms or isozymes consisting of subunit types A, B, and C. These subunits, each a distinct gene product, combine as homo- or heterotetrameric proteins with distinct tissue and functional specificities [Markert, 1962]. The most rigid specificity is seen with the LDH-C_4 isozyme of mammalian testes and spermatozoa, which was first described by Goldberg [1963] and by Blanco and Zinkham [1963]. This isozyme appears with the onset of puberty during prophase of the first meiotic division of the primary spermatocyte [Hintz and Goldberg, 1977] and is found on and in the mature spermatozoan [Goldberg, 1977]. While the functional role of LDH-C_4 (mC_4) within the germinal epithelium, or as a sperm enzyme, has never been clearly elucidated [Wheat and Goldberg, 1983], its association with the sperm cell and its dissimilarity to the somatic LDH isozymes suggested its potential in development of a contraceptive vaccine [Goldberg et al., 1983; Wheat and Goldberg, 1983].

The prospect of developing a vaccine for contraception using sperm antigens has been pursued vigorously since the turn of the century. Promising, but often confusing, results have been obtained, primarily because of the undefined nature of the antigenic preparations, how they might be manipulated to gain maximum antifertility effectiveness, and lack of understanding of the specific immune responses that result in infertility. Availability of well-characterized antigens is required to overcome these problems.

With only a few exceptions, it has been almost impossible to iso-

Gamete Interaction: Prospects for Immunocontraception, pages 63–73
© 1990 Wiley-Liss, Inc.

late, characterize, and produce in quantity individual sperm antigens for use in a monospecific vaccine. Recent advances in recombinant DNA technology may provide new impetus for immunocontraceptive studies. Molecular probes can be used to screen cDNA libraries prepared from testes to identify a gene or genes encoding sperm antigens. Genetic engineering can then be used to obtain the gene product from bacterial or viral expression systems.

PROPERTIES OF LDH-C$_4$

LDH-C$_4$ satisfies an essential requirement of a sperm antigen: It provokes antibodies that are absolutely cell specific and do not cross-react with the somatic LDH isozymes [Wheat and Goldberg, 1983; Liang et al., 1986]. LDH-C$_4$ is never synthesized by females and is sequestered from the immune system of the male by the blood–testis barrier. Therefore, immunization of both males and females with purified LDH-C$_4$ provokes an immune response. Antibodies to LDH-C$_4$ suppress fertility in female mice, rabbits, and baboons [Goldberg, 1975; Wheat and Goldberg, 1983]. More important than this, however, is the fact that LDH-C$_4$ was the first antigenic component of spermatozoa that has been obtained in relative abundance for structural and immunological characterization. Isolation of gram quantities of LDH-C$_4$ from mouse testes is relatively routine [Lee et al., 1982], and antibodies to this isozyme not only bind to LDH-C$_4$ from other species but also agglutinate spermatozoa from rabbit, mouse, and man. Inhibition of fertility presumably involves transudation of circulating antibody to reproductive tract fluids, where binding to spermatozoa in vaginal, uterine, and oviducal secretions would occur [Kille and Goldberg, 1979, 1980]. According to this scenario, sperm would be impeded in movement through the female reproductive tract and rendered nonfunctional. The contraceptive action would, therefore, prevent fertilization.

CONTRACEPTIVE VACCINE DEVELOPMENT

Antigenic Determinants

Our initial strategy for developing an immunocontraceptive vaccine based on LDH-C$_4$ was to study the antigenic structure of the protein [Wheat and Goldberg, 1985]. As noted above, immunization of female animals with LDH-C$_4$ purified from mouse testes results in the production of highly specific antisera and in the suppression of fertility [Goldberg, 1973; Goldberg et al., 1981]. We felt that replacement of the natural product LDH-C_4 with a synthetic antigen would ensure availability and homogeneity of vaccine preparations, as well as guarantee antigenic specificity for the spermatozoal LDH isozyme [Goldberg et al., 1981]. With the refined structure of LDH-C_4 available [Hogrefe et al., 1987] and the amino acid sequence of the C subunit known, it was possible to map the antigenic determinants of LDH-C_4 by synthesizing a panel of peptides chosen according to a number of criteria such as surface accessibility, segmental flexibility, and evolutionary variability [Hogrefe et al., 1989].

Synthetic Peptides

Nine peptides encompassing the most flexible and accessible segments of the LDH-C_4 tetramer, and therefore the most likely to be immunogenic, were synthesized. These peptides were assembled from 10–15 amino acids each and, in total, represent greater than 50% of the solvent-accessible surface of the tetramer [Hogrefe et al., 1989]. In addition, topographic epitopes were designed to yield peptides that assumed a predetermined secondary structure (α-helix; helical bundle) in solution [Kaumaya et al., 1989]. Each of the linear peptides were conjugated to diphtheria toxoid for immunization, and each provoked antibodies in rabbits and mice that recognized the native protein [Wheat and Goldberg, 1985; Wheat et al., 1985; Hogrefe et al., 1989]. The relative titers of antisera to the peptides were lower, by 1 order of magnitude, than anti-LDH-C_4, and the peptides differed from each other in their immunogenicity primarily according to their evolutionary divergence from the homologous sequences in the somatic isozymes [Hogrefe et al., 1989]. The topographic determinants were immunogenic without conjugation to carrier (Goldberg, unpublished data, 1989).

Our studies with LDH-C_4 from the mouse indicate the feasibility of using synthetic peptides corresponding to epitopes of proteins to elicit a specific immune response to the intact native protein. Furthermore, one of these synthetic "vaccines," mC5–16 (previously designated mC5–15 [Wheat and Goldberg, 1985]), conjugated to diphtheria toxoid (DT) did induce protective immunity against pregnancy. In a recently completed fertility trial, only three pregnancies occurred among 14 female baboons immunized with a synthetic peptide representing amino acid residues 5–16 of mouse LDH-C_4. In the control group (injected with DT), 10 of 14 animals conceived. All of the immunized animals were mated at least four times, and they all developed circulating antibodies that recognized both mouse and baboon LDH-C_4. Furthermore, five of eight immunized animals subsequently conceived within 2–4 months of the final booster immunization, indicating that fertility suppression was reversible. Because of these results, and our previously published studies [Wheat and Goldberg, 1983; Goldberg and Shelton, 1986], LDH-C_4 continues to serve as a useful model sperm antigen for contraceptive vaccine development utilizing synthetic peptides containing epitopes of the native protein. A next step is to establish whether immunosuppression of fertility in primates can be enhanced with, for example, an epitope of human LDH-C_4 (hC_4) or with genetically engineered human LDH-C_4. Efficacy in a homologous system may be reflected in the results of Primakoff and coworkers [1988], who observed 100% suppression of fertility in guinea pigs immunized with PH-20, an antigen isolated from guinea pig sperm. Since human LDH-C_4 is not easily available, a genetic engineering approach was used to obtain this isozyme.

MOLECULAR BIOLOGY OF HUMAN LDH-C_4

A human testes cDNA expression library packaged in λgt11 was screened with polyclonal and monoclonal antibodies to murine LDH-C_4 [Millan et al., 1987]. We were able to clone and sequence the entire open reading frame for the Ldh-c gene and from this deduce the amino acid sequence of the human LDH-C_4 isozyme. Comparison with mouse LDH-C_4 revealed 74% sequence similarity and a number of amino acid substitutions in those sequences that contained epitopes [Millan et al., 1987; Hogrefe et al., 1989]. For example, the sequence encompassing residues 5–16 is as follows:

mC5–16 –Glu–**Gln**–Leu–Ile–**Gln**–**Asn**–Leu–**Val**–**Pro**–Asp–**Glu**–**Lys**
hC5–16 –Glu–Glu–Leu–Ile–Glu–Lys–Leu–Ile–Glu–Asp–Asp–Gly
       5   10   15

Amino acid differences between mouse and human LDH-C_4 at positions 10 (Asn→Lys) and 13 (Pro→Glu) could significantly influence immunogenicity of these peptides. It is probable that Pro 13 affects the conformation of the peptide and extent of cross-reaction between αmC_4 and hC_4. On the basis of these results and other differences observed in amino acid sequences of epitopes, we decided to engineer the cDNA for expression in *Escherichia coli*. Catalytically active human LDH-C_4 was expressed in this microbial system. With hC_4 available, antisera to mC5–16 and hC5–16 were compared for specificities. These results, presented in Figure 1, confirm that αmC_4 has a titer at least 1 order of magnitude higher with

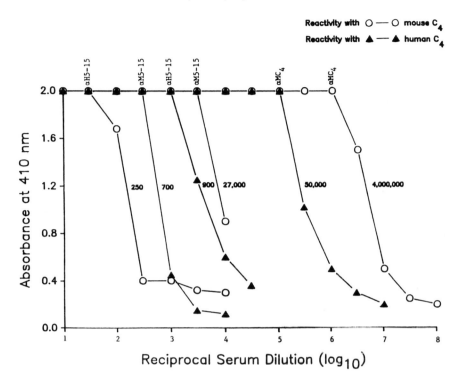

Fig. 1. Binding of antisera to mouse and human LDH-C_4. ELISA titers shown on each curve were calculated as the serum dilution giving an A_{410nm} of 0.4 units above background. The sera tested were raised against mouse LDH-C_4 (αmC_4) and synthetic peptides 5–16 of the mouse sequence ($\alpha m5$–15) or human sequence ($\alpha h5$–15). See text for further explanation.

mC_4 than with hC_4. Similarly, the antipeptide antibodies had higher titers to the cogent peptides than to the heterologous peptide. These findings suggest the need to test the antigen in as nearly homologous a system as possible for biological efficacy. The availability of a microbial system to yield large quantities of the recombinant human isozyme by a relatively routine purification scheme not only makes such studies possible, but also has obvious advantages to obtaining the protein from natural sources.

VACCINIA EXPRESSING hC_4

Mammalian proteins are relatively poor antigens and require adjuvants to provoke a robust immune response. As an alternative, recombinant viruses may be constructed that will express foreign DNA. The expression of foreign genes in vaccinia virus provides a

generic approach for using these genetically engineered vectors as
live recombinant vaccines directed against a variety of antigens
[Mackett et al., 1982; Panicali and Paoletti, 1982]. Experimental animals infected with vaccinia virus recombinants containing genes
coding for hepatitis B [Smith et al., 1983], rabies [Kieny et al., 1984],
and malaria [Smith et al., 1984] have been shown to be protected
against challenge infection with the corresponding infectious agent.
Expression of the AIDS virus envelope gene in a recombinant vaccinia has been accomplished [Chakrabarti et al., 1986; Hu et al.,
1986]. Additional examples of success and popularity of inserting
foreign genes into vaccinia include genes that encode biochemical
markers such as the herpes simplex virus thymidine kinase [Panicali
and Paoletti, 1982], chloramphenicol acetyltransferase [Mackett et
al., 1984], β-galactosidase [Chakrabarti et al., 1985], and neomycin
resistance [Franke et al., 1985]. These inserts have enabled vaccinia
to be used as a cloning vector with the advantage of assayable biochemical markers. Plasmid vectors that facilitate the insertion and
expression of foreign genes in vaccinia virus as well as the selection
of recombinants have been described [Mackett et al., 1984; Chakrabarti et al., 1985].

Using these principles, we have successfully engineered the human Ldh-c cDNA to produce a recombinant vaccinia that expresses
LDH-C_4. The strategy employed is described in Figure 2. Preliminary
results have been obtained and demonstrate that vaccinated rabbits
produce antibodies to human LDH-C_4.

Observations thus far involve only small numbers of laboratory
animals, but the potential attraction of such recombinant vaccines
include not only their low cost and ease of production (once suitable
recombinants are established) but also ease of administration and a
high degree of stability that would put them within reach of populations in developing countries. It must be noted, however, that
adverse reactions to vaccinia virus can occur and were documented
[Fenner, 1984] during the smallpox eradication program. Studies are
in progress [Piccini and Paoletti, 1986] aimed at generating a virus
with only the genetic material for replication, deleting those parts of
the genome responsible for pathogenesis.

ANIMAL MODEL FOR FERTILITY TRIALS

The obvious next stage for the development of human LDH-C_4 as
a contraceptive vaccine is to select an appropriate animal model for
fertility trials. No species has yet been identified that accurately mimics both the human immune system and the human reproductive

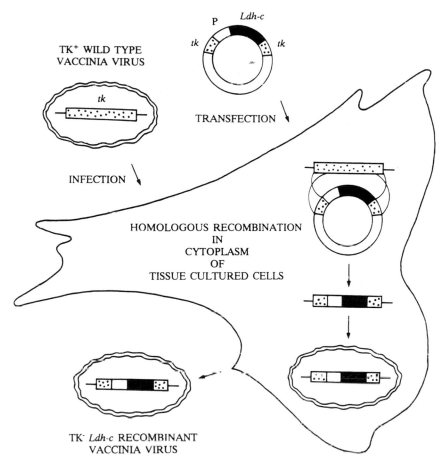

RECOMBINANT PLASMID

TK⁺ WILD TYPE
VACCINIA VIRUS

TRANSFECTION

INFECTION

HOMOLOGOUS RECOMBINATION
IN
CYTOPLASM
OF
TISSUE CULTURED CELLS

TK⁻ *Ldh-c* RECOMBINANT
VACCINIA VIRUS

Fig. 2. The strategy employed to engineer recombinant virus with the Ldh-c cDNA for immunization.

system. Immunocontraceptive antigens that are safe and effective in nonhuman primates, such as baboons, may prove to be less effective or produce unacceptable side effects in humans. Alternatively, a sperm-specific antigen like human LDH-C_4 may prove to be more effective in the homologous species than in any heterologous species. Ultimately, human clinical trials will be necessary to begin to accumulate a body of data to enable researchers to predict success and to bring the field of immunocontraception from the laboratory to the public.

CONCLUSIONS

The application of current techniques of immunochemistry, peptide synthesis, and molecular biology should lead to the development of contraceptive vaccines. LDH-C_4 has served as a useful model protein for designing such studies on sperm antigens in vaccine development. The need for vaccines to supplement the other contraceptive technologies is apparent. The failure of conventional prophylactic measures to control population growth in many parts of the developing world has focused attention on the great benefits that would accrue from the availability of effective birth control vaccines.

ACKNOWLEDGMENTS

I thank the following colleagues and students for their major contributions to the research described here: Dr. J. Curl, Dr. P.T.P. Kaumaya, Dr. P.A. O'Hern, Ms. C.D. Brooke, Ms. K. LeVan, Ms. C. Moses, Ms. R. Tekula, and Ms. M. Benoit. This work was supported by grants from NIH.

REFERENCES

Blanco A, Zinkham WH (1963): Lactate dehydrogenases in human testes. Science 139:601–602.

Chakrabarti S, Brechling K, Moss B (1985): Vaccinia virus expression vector: Coexpression of β-galactosidase provides visual screening of recombinant virus plaques. Mol Cell Biol 5:3403–3409.

Chakrabarti S, Robert-Guroff M, Wong-Stall F, Gallo RC, Moss B (1986): Expression of the HTLV-III envelope gene by a recombinant vaccinia virus. Nature 320:535–537.

Fenner F (1984): Viral vectors for vaccines. In Bell R, Torrigiani G (eds): New Approaches to Vaccine Development. Basel: Schwabe & Co. AG, pp 187–196.

Franke CA, Rice CM, Strauss JH, Hruby DE (1985): Neomycin resistance as a dominant selectable marker for selection and isolation of vaccinia virus recombinants. Mol Cell Biol 5:1918–1924.

Goldberg E (1963): Lactic and malic dehydrogenases in human spermatozoa. Science 139:602–603.

Goldberg E (1973): Infertility in female rabbits immunized with lactate dehydrogenase X. Science 181:458–459.

Goldberg E (1975): Lactate dehydrogenase-X (crystalline) from mouse testes. In Wood WA (ed): Methods in Enzymology Vol. XLI: Carbohydrate Metabolism, Part B. New York: Academic Press, pp 318–322.

Goldberg E (1977): Isozymes in testes and spermatozoa. In Rattazzi MC, Scandalios JG, Whitt GS (eds): Isozymes: Current Topics in Biological and Medical Research, Volume 1. New York: Alan R. Liss, Inc., pp 79–124.

Goldberg E, Gonzales-Prevatt V, Wheat TE (1981): Immunosuppression of fertility in females by injection of sperm-specific LDH-C_4 (LDH-X): Prospects for development of a contraceptive vaccine. In Semm K, Mettler L (eds): Proceedings of III World Congress of Human Reproduction. Amsterdam: Excerpta Medica, pp 360–364.

Goldberg E, Shelton JA (1986): Control of fertilization by immunization with peptide fragments of sperm-specific LDH-C_4. Adv Exp Med Biol 207:395–406.

Goldberg E, Wheat TE, Shelton JA (1983): Sperm-specific LDH and development of a synthetic contraceptive vaccine. In Isojima S, Billington WD (eds): Reproductive Immunology, 1983. Amsterdam: Elsevier Biomedical, pp 215–223.

Hintz M, Goldberg E (1977): Immunohistochemical localization of LDH-X during spermatogenesis in mouse testes. Dev Biol 57:375–384.

Hogrefe HH, Griffith JP, Rossmann MG, Goldberg E (1987): Characterization of antigenic sites on the refined 3Å structure of mouse testicular lactate dehydrogenase-C_4. J Biol Chem 262:13155–13162.

Hogrefe HH, Kaumaya PTP, Goldberg E (1989): Immunogenicity of synthetic peptides corresponding to flexible and antibody-accessible segments of mouse lactate dehydrogenase (LDH)-C_4. J Biol Chem 264:10513–10519.

Hu SL, Kosowski SG, Dalrymple JM (1986): Expression of AIDS virus envelope gene in recombinant vaccinia viruses. Nature 320:537–540.

Kaumaya PTP, Berndt KD, Heidorn DB, Trewhella J, Kezdy FJ, Goldberg E (1989): Synthesis and biophysical characterization of engineered topographic immunogenic determinants with αα topology. Biochemistry 29:13–23.

Kieny MP, Lathe R, Drillien R, Spehner D, Skory S, Schmitt D, Witkor T, Koprowski H, Lecocq JP (1984): Expression of rabies virus glycoprotein from a recombinant vaccinia virus. Nature 312:163–166.

Kille JW, Goldberg E (1979): Female reproductive tract immunoglobulin responses to a purified sperm specific antigen (LDH-C_4). Biol Reprod 28:863–871.

Kille JW, Goldberg E (1980): Inhibition of oviductal sperm transport in rabbits immunized against sperm-specific lactate dehydrogenase (LDH-C_4). J Reprod Immunol 2:15–21.

Lee CY, Yuan JH, Goldberg E (1982): Lactate dehydrogenase from the mouse. Methods Enzymol 89:351–362.

Liang ZG, Shelton JA, Goldberg E (1986): Non-crossreactivity of antibodies to murine LDH-C_4 with LDH-A_4 and LDH-$_4$. J Exp Zool 240:377–384.

Mackett M, Smith GL, Moss B (1982): Vaccinia virus: A selectable eukaryotic cloning and expression vector. Proc Natl Acad Sci USA 79:7415–7419.

Mackett M, Smith GL, Moss B (1984): General method for production and selection of infectious vaccinia virus recombinants expressing foreign genes. J Virol 49:857–864.

Markert CL (1962): Isozymes in kidney development. In Metcoff J (ed): Hereditary Developmental and Immunologic Aspects of Kidney Disease. Chicago: Northwestern University Press, pp 54–64.

Millan JL, Driscoll CE, LeVan KM, Goldberg E (1987): Epitopes of human testis-specific lactate dehydrogenase deduced from a cDNA sequence. Proc Natl Acad Sci USA 84: 5311–5315.

Panicali D, Paoletti E (1982): Construction of poxviruses as cloning vectors: Insertion of the thymidine kinase gene from herpes simplex virus into the DNA of infectious vaccinia virus. Proc Natl Acad Sci USA 79:4927–4931.

Piccini A, Paoletti E (1986): The use of vaccinia virus for the construction of recombinant vaccines. Bioessays 5:248–252.

Primakoff P, Lathrop W, Woolman L, Cowan A, Myles D (1988): Fully effective contraception in male and female guinea pigs immunized with the sperm protein PH-20. Nature 335:543–546.

Smith GL, Godson GN, Nussenzweig V, Nussenzweig RS, Barnwell J, Moss B (1984): *Plasmodium knowlesi* sporozoite antigen: Expression by infectious recombinant vaccinia virus. Science 224:397–399.

Smith GL, Mackett M, Moss B (1983): Infectious vaccinia virus recombinants that express hepatitis B virus surface antigen. Nature 302:490–495.

Wheat TE, Goldberg E (1983): Sperm-specific lactate dehydrogenase C_4: Antigenic structure and immuno-suppression of fertility. In Rattazzi MC, Scandalios JG, Whitt GS (eds): Isozymes: Current Topics in Biological and Medical Research, Volume 7: Molecular Structure and Regulation. New York: Alan R. Liss, Inc., pp 113–130.

Wheat TE, Goldberg E (1985): Antigenic domains of the sperm-specific lactate dehydrogenase C_4 isozyme. Mol Immunol 22:643–649.

Wheat TE, Shelton JA, Gonzales-Prevatt V, Goldberg E (1985): The antigenicity of synthetic peptide fragments of LDH-C_4. Mol Immunol 22:1195–1199.

DISCUSSION

DR. ALEXANDER: Based on your former studies in baboons, which demonstrated a reduction in infertility, and your current studies, which do not, are you still of the opinion that LDH-C_4 would be a perfect vaccine candidate?

DR. GOLDBERG: I feel it is as "perfect" as any other at this time. There is no evidence to rule it out.

DR. TALWAR: Your previous work testing these antigens in a variety of animal species did not show 100% reduction of fertility, but rather 50, 70, or 80% reduction in rodents and primates. The puzzling part of your presentation is that even though the ELISA titers, with either the peptides or the vaccinia, expressed total protein, or an equal amount of expressed total protein, you don't have a complete fertility block, which may require having the antibodies in the genital tract, rather than only in the serum. I wonder whether you would comment on this?

DR. GOLDBERG: I agree that one of the observations that we have made over the years in the fertility trials that we have conducted is that there is no correlation between circulating antibodies and fertility. I think that is because measuring the antibody levels in the serum doesn't get to the heart of the matter. That is, the antibody in the reproductive tract is doing the job. I think that this is one of the problems with fertility trials in rodents in comparison with some primates where the female reproductive tract is open to aspiration of peritoneal fluid that contains antibodies. This would be common in the human situation, which is why baboons were chosen as a model for some of our experiments. So, I think it is true that one needs to stimulate a local immune response.

DR. SEHGAL: I understand that Dr. Gupta worked in your lab some time ago and learned how to isolate enzymes. He then returned to Punjab University, repeated the experiments with mice, and was not able to show any block of fertility in mice.

DR. GOLDBERG: I am aware of this. In fact, I saw Dr. Gupta in Germany earlier this year, and he presented some data where he found an enhancement or protection of pregnancy by immunization with LDH-C_4.

DR. JONES: I believe you published information on local immunization with one of your preparations?

DR. GOLDBERG: Actually, we are just starting collaboration with Roy Curtiss at Washington University in St. Louis in which the plasmid will be cloned to make recombinant *Salmonella* that is attenuated. This would presumably stimulate a local immune response. So we may eventually have some answers to that question.

6

Sperm Antigens Defined From Polyclonal Antisera

Chandrima Shaha, T. Sheshadri, G.P. Talwar, and Anil Suri

The presence of antisperm antibodies can result in infertility in both men and women [Isojima, 1969; Hjort and Hansen, 1971; Boettcher, 1974]. This finding suggests that sperm antigens could be used as a basis for antifertility vaccines. Both monoclonal and polyclonal antibodies have been used to identify antigens on spermatozoa that are important in the process of fertilization. Identification of these antigens may allow manipulation of reproduction. Monoclonal antibodies have been used extensively to identify and characterize sperm antigens [Anderson et al., 1987] but polyclonal antibodies have been used only sparingly for the same purpose [Shaha et al., 1988; O'Rand, 1981; Benet-Rubinat et al., 1989; Wang et al., 1989]. Both systems of detection have their advantages and disadvantages. Monoclonal antibodies involve a great deal of work for mere production, and, in addition, in some circumstances their extreme monospecificity may be a disadvantage. Whereas monoclonal antibodies are indispensable tools in some facets of work, polyclonal antibodies can be extremely useful. Here we describe the possibility of identifying sperm antigens using polyclonal antibodies as probes.

USE OF HYPERIMMUNIZED RABBIT SERA

In our laboratory, we have produced polyclonal antisera from rabbits hyperimmunized against sperm and then used these antisera to locate antigens relevant to fertility. We describe the use of one such polyclonal antiserum to identify an interesting sperm antigen.

Antiserum was raised against washed human spermatozoa. The

Gamete Interaction: Prospects for Immunocontraception, pages 75–88
© 1990 Wiley-Liss, Inc.

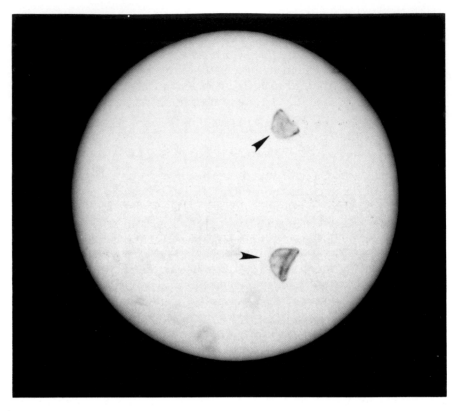

Fig. 1. Human sperm acrosome reacted with antiserum I as revealed by indirect immunoperoxidase technique. Arrowheads indicate position of the acrosomes. ×1,000.

serum obtained was subsequently adsorbed with tissue powders from liver, lungs, and muscle of rabbit.

Indirect Immunofluorescence

By indirect immunofluorescence, the antiserum recognized the acrosomal region of sperm from many species. Human (Fig. 1), monkey, rabbit, hamster, rat, and mice sperm reacted with the serum in the same acrosome region [Shaha et al., 1988]. This specific acrosomal localization indicated that the antigen recognized by antiserum I was conserved through evolution. This was a convenient characteristic, because the serum could be used for efficacy studies as well as for defining mechanism(s) of action.

Ultrastructural Localization

For an antigen to be a vaccine candidate, it must be accessible so that antibodies targetted against it bind easily. Immunolocalization studies at the ultrastructural level were carried out on rat spermatozoa. The antibody bound to antigens on the plasma membrane of rat sperm acrosome as evidenced by immunogold localization [Shaha et al., 1988].

Functional Studies

Functional studies with the antiserum using human spermatozoa revealed strong agglutination but no immobilization. We next did passive immunization studies with mice. Superovulated BALB/c outbred female mice were injected with globulins from antiserum I (partially purified by 50% ammonium sulfate cut) and then mated. When oviducts were flushed for embryos 48 hr after the appearance of vaginal plugs, embryos were recovered from five of 25 animals in the experimental group (passively injected with antiserum I), whereas in the control group (passively immunized with normal rabbit serum) embryos were recovered from 21 of 27 animals. Oocytes obtained from superovulated mice were incubated with mouse sperm treated with the antiserum for a period of 30 min. Binding of sperm to oocytes were reduced to 1.2% in experimentals compared with 100% of controls (sperm were treated with normal rabbit serum). Hence, the antiserum was able to prevent the binding of sperm to oocytes both in vivo and in vitro.

Western Blots

Western blots with human sperm extracts were used to determine molecular weight. A distinct dark band at 40 kd (Fig. 2a) and some minor ones at 42 and 72 kd were observed. Western blots with a monkey sperm extract showed a band around 69 kd. To look for a plentiful antigen source, immunoblots were done with rat testicular cytosol; the antiserum recognized a heavy protein band around 24 kd (Fig. 2b). Western blots of cytosol from rat spleen, kidney, liver, and lungs did not show any reaction with antiserum I (Fig. 3), indicating that this antigen was specific to spermatozoa. Western blots with human testicular cytosol also showed a band at around 24 kd.

Ontogeny

Rat testis sections were immunostained with antiserum I in order to trace the origin and localization of the testicular antigen. The

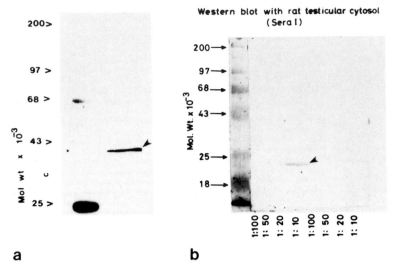

a   b

Fig. 2.   Western blot with human sperm extract (**a**) and rat testicular cytosol (**b**) using antiserum I. Rat testicular cytosol was loaded at a concentration of 1 mg/ml. Arrowheads indicate position of the bands.

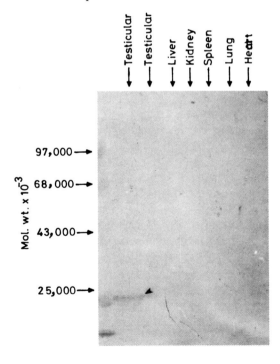

Fig. 3.   Antigen–antibody reaction on immunoblot with cytosol preparations from various rat tissues using antiserum I. Arrowhead indicates position of the 24 kd band with rat testicular cytosol.

antiserum first recognized spermatozoa at the spermatid stage. The pattern of immunostaining changed as the developing acrosome shifted in shape from the spermatid stage to the mature spermatozoon. This finding demonstrates that this acrosomal antigen is located inside the blood–testis barrier in rat testis and develops from the spermatid stage onward [Shaha et al., 1988].

Active Immunization Studies

After it was established that the antiserum recognized an important antigen, the next logical step was to conduct active immunization of animals for efficacy studies. These studies were initiated with rat testicular cytosol as the antigen source. Gel bands at 24 kd were isolated from the SDS gels and chopped into fine pieces, and the protein was eluted out by electroelution [Shaha et al., 1989b].

Active immunization studies were conducted using two different routes of immunization. One was an oral route and the other an intramuscular route.

Oral immunization. Oral immunizations by feeding the animals with the 24 kd antigens by gavage were done. Adjuvants used were SPLPS (a thyalated derivative of lipopolysaccharide) and alum in one group and MDP (muramyl dipeptide) in another group. Both groups showed significant inhibition of fertility. It was interesting that the antibody titers increased (Fig. 4) with mating in the immunized groups. In the group with SPLPS and alum, serum IgG titers were higher as compared with serum IgA titers in all animals, whereas in vaginal washings the IgA titers tended to be higher. In the second group, with MDP as an adjuvant, serum IgA did not differ significantly from IgA in the vaginal washings, and serum IgG titers were significantly higher than vaginal washing IgG titers. One animal with vaginal washing IgA titers below 0.3 O.D. became pregnant. This finding indicates the importance of IgA titers in the vaginal washings.

Intramuscular immunizations. Animals were injected with the 24 kd antigen along with SPLPS and alum as adjuvants in one group and with MDP as adjuvant in another group. Both groups had normal fertility rates. Animals with high serum titers, which were manifested in agglutination and by indirect immunofluorescence, did not become pregnant for 17–18 cycles, whereas animals with lower titers became pregnant within 1–2 cycles (Fig. 5). Unfortunately, the titers of antibody in the vaginal washings were not monitored in this group; therefore, a direct comparison with the animals in the oral immunization group could not be made. These two studies showed

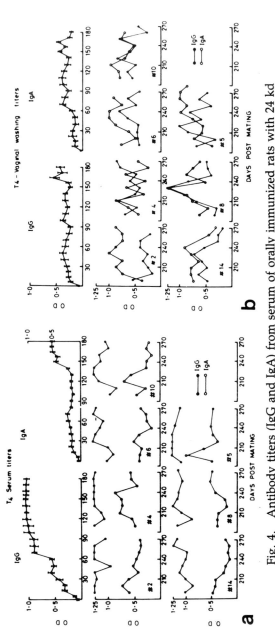

Fig. 4. Antibody titers (IgG and IgA) from serum of orally immunized rats with 24 kd antigens (a) and titers of the same in vaginal washings (b) as measured by enzyme-linked immunoadsorbant assay. The upper panels represent average titers; the lower two panels depict titers of IgA and IgG in individual animals after mating.

that antibodies against the 24 kd antigen in the circulation were able to block pregnancy.

Studies were conducted using the same antigens in mice of different strains (BALB/c inbred, BALB/c outbred, Swiss outbred, CBA, and nude). There was no marked difference in the build-up of titers in different strains except that nude mice did not respond at all, a finding indicating that this is a T-dependent antigen. The normal fertility rate was affected in all strains, but there was no difference in terms of efficacy of the antigen to inhibit fertility between the strains.

Mechanisms of Action

From the oral immunization studies it was seen that IgA-secreting antibodies were present in the vaginal washings of the immunized animals in higher amounts after mating as compared with serum IgA (unpublished data). An immunohistological study showed that IgA immunocytes were higher in number on day 1 (Fig. 6b) and day 3 postmating and were located nearer to the luminal border as compared with mated controls (Fig. 6a) on the same days. This supports the concept that IgA is secreted into the lumen in a larger quantity than is IgG (IgG immunocytes were found in lesser numbers than those of IgA and were the same in both control and experimental groups). The local response to IgA noted in these animals is probably because of the deposition of sperm during coitus toward which an immune reaction was mounted by the memory lymphocytes to IgA immunocytes present in the genital tract.

In a separate study using both oral and intramuscular routes of administration in mice with semipurified rat testicular cytosol, we found that animals that showed a higher titer of IgA in serum had less embryos (Figs. 7, 8). With this method, the ability of a spermatozoa to fertilize oocytes could be related directly to the titers of IgA levels in the reproductive tract. The titers generated in the intramuscularly immunized group were higher than those of the orally immunized group. Five of six animals remained infertile in the oral group, whereas four of six remained infertile in the intramuscular group. The ratio between IgG and IgA may be an important factor in the success of fertility.

A monoclonal antibody raised against this antigen [Shaha et al., 1989a] also inhibited binding of hamster and mice sperm to respective oocytes. Most of the sperm show agglutination; however, the ones that remained free were unable to bind to the oocytes. This experiment indicated that the level of blockade was at the stage of sperm oocyte attachment.

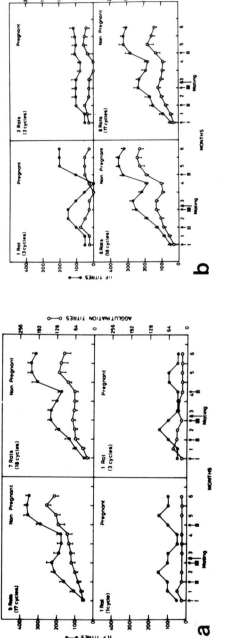

Fig. 5. Serum IgG titers in rats immunized systemically with 24 kd antigens. **a**: Titers of the animals immunized with SPLPS and alum as adjuvants. **b**: Titers of animals immunized using nor-MDP as an adjuvant. The antibody titers were measured in terms of indirect immunofluorescence and agglutination.

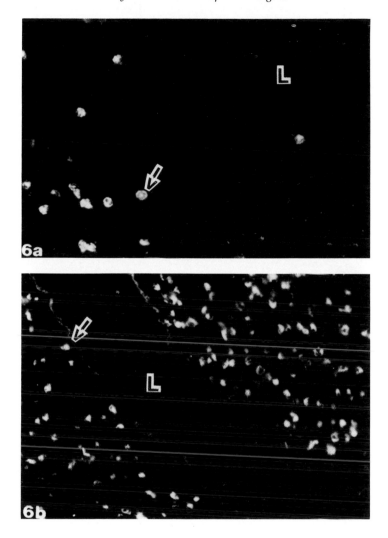

Fig. 6.   Immunohistochemistry with anti-IgA antibody using tissues from orally immunized rats from control and experimental groups on day 1 of mating. IgA immunocytes were further from the lumen in tissue of a mated control rats (**a**) as compared with the increased number of immunocytes, which are closer to the lumen in tissue from the mated immunized animal (**b**). L, lumen; arrows indicate immunocytes.

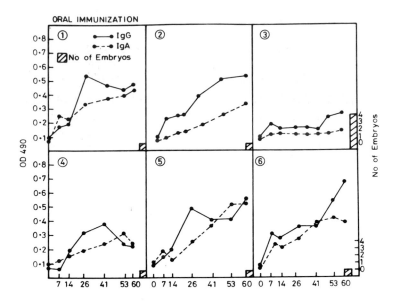

Fig. 7.   Serum IgA and IgG titers in orally immunized mice with semipurified rat testicular cytosol. Numbers of embryos are also depicted on the right-hand side of each panel.

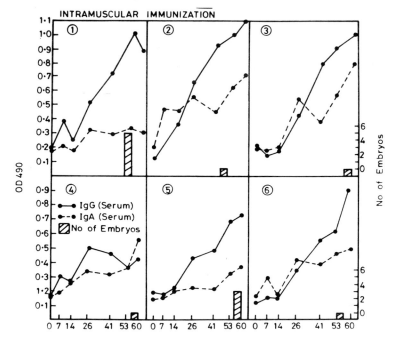

Fig. 8.   Serum IgG and IgA titers in mice immunized intramuscularly using Leiras basic adjuvant. Numbers of embryos are depicted on the right-hand side of each panel.

USE OF HUMAN INFERTILE SERA

General Characters of the serum

Serum (IF-10) from a male subject having high titers of agglutinating antisperm antibodies with a 2 year history of primary infertility was used to characterize antigens on human sperm that could regulate fertility. This subject was normal in all respects, free from any autoimmune disorders, and had 80% immobilized sperm in his semen in free or agglutinated form. His sera caused sperm agglutination at dilutions of 1:252 and also had immobilizing properties.

Localization on Sperm

Immunofluorescence. The serum IF-10 recognized antigens on the main tail piece of human and monkey spermatozoa. It was found to be cross-reactive with sperm of many species. It identified the acrosome of rabbit and hamster spermatozoa, whereas the guinea pig sperm acrosome was faintly stained with two distinct spots on the midpiece. In hamster sperm a similar pattern was noted.

Western blots. Serum immunoblots with sperm extracts of different species reacted with IF-10 to several molecular sizes of antigens. A 80 kd band on the human spermatozoa (Fig. 9) and a similar band on rabbit spermatozoa along with a 56 kd band were found. Four bands were recognized with hamster sperm extracts (Fig. 10).

Monospecific Antisera Against the Relevant Antigens

Monospecific antisera were raised against the 80 and 56 kd antigen bands of gels made of rabbit sperm antigen; an antiserum was also produced to a nonrelevant band of 96 kd. The sera against the 80 and 56 kd bands agglutinated human sperm as strongly as was originally observed with the infertile sera. A similar pattern of immunofluorescence was detected by both of the sera. They were also able to prevent binding of hamster sperm to hamster oocytes. However, the serum against 96 kd neither agglutinated sperm nor reduced hamster sperm to oocyte binding.

The characterization of target sperm antigens for a contraceptive vaccine involves not only cell specificity and their distribution but also whether the antigens are membrane bound or subsurface, because only the former are accessible to immunological attack. The biological functions of sperm antigens are important whether they are structural, protective, or concerned with sperm selection or with

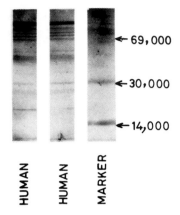

Fig. 9. Western blot of human sperm extract with antiserum IF-10, showing a prominent band around 80 kd.

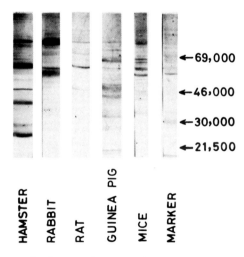

Fig. 10. Antigen–antibody reactions on the immunoblot with sperm extracts from various species using IF-10. Note four strong bands with hamster sperm extract and two strong bands with rabbit sperm extract.

fertilizing capacity. All of these properties bear on selectivity and effectiveness of immunization regimes. Our studies show how it is possible to identify sperm antigens by using polyclonal sera from various sources. Monospecific rabbit sera are important tools for this purpose. Although in most cases one will encounter antibodies against multiple antigens in the same molecular weight, the polyclonal serum is by no means an inferior reagent. With the advent of two-dimensional gel technology and the feasibility of producing antibodies to polypeptides from two-dimensional gels, the idea of using polyclonal antisera has become more attractive.

REFERENCES

Anderson DJ, Johnson PM, Alexander NJ, Jones WR, Griffin PO (1987): Monoclonal antibodies to human trophoblast and sperm antigens: Report of the WHO sponsored workshop, June 30, 1986, Toronto, Canada. J Reprod Immunol 10:231–257.

Benet-Rubinat JM, Martinez P, Andolz P, Garcia-Fram's V, Bielsa MA, Egozcue J (1989): Analysis of human sperm antigens obtained by affinity chromatography with polyclonal antsperm antibodies. J Reprod Immunol Suppl p 38.

Boettcher B (1974): The molecular nature of sperm agglutinins and sperm antibodies in human sera. J Reprod Fetil Suppl 21:151.

Hjort T, Hansen KB (1971): Immunofluorescent studies on human spermatozoa. 1. The detection of different spermatozoal antibodies and their occurrence in normal and infertile women. Clin Exp Immunol 1:9–23.

Isojima S (1969): Relationship between antibodies to spermatozoa and sterility in females In Edwards RG (ed): Immunology and Reproduction. London: IPPG, pp 267–277.

O'Rand MG (1981): Inhibition of fertility and sperm zona binding by antiserum to the rabbit sperm membrane autoantigen RSA-1. Biol Reprod 25:621–628.

Schulman S (1975): Sperm antibodies in serum of men and women in cervical mucus. In Proceedings of the 8th World Congress on Fertility and Sterility, Buenos Aires, 1974. Amsterdam: Excerpta Medica, pp 3–9.

Shaha C, Sheshadri T, Talwar GP, Suri A (1989a): Characterization of a monoclonal antibody against a 24KD antigen from rat testis important for fertility regulation. Hybridoma 8:647–660.

Shaha C, Suri A, Talwar GP (1988): Identification of sperm antigens that regulate fertility. Int J Androl 11:479–491.

Shaha C, Suri A, Talwar GP (1990): Induction of infertility in female rats after active immunization with 24KD antigens from rat testes. Int J Androl 13:17–25.

Tyler A (1961): Approaches to the control of fertility based on immunological phenomena. J Reprod Fertil 2:473.

Wang LF, Miao SY, Liu QY, Bai Y, Xu C, Chen F, Yan YC, Koide S (1989): Antisperm antibodies in sera of Chinese infertile subjects and identification of cDNA coding for a specific antigen. J Reprod Immunol Suppl 16:50.

DISCUSSION

DR. THAU: In your comparative studies, did boosters suggest an irreversible immunization?

DR. SHAHA: We don't know that. We have separated the rats for a long time, and when they mated, they were fertile.

DR. MITCHISON: Concerning your strategy of using polyclonal antisera, it seemed that your aim was to move rapidly from polyvalent antiserum to picking up a single strong antigen. What I do not understand is that this approach seems to overlook the fact that these polyvalent antisera are valuable reagents for picking up as broad a range of antigens as possible. Would it not be worth taking a second look at what the polyvalent antisera identify? For example, when you use a polyvalent antiserum, can you pick up two antigens? Twenty antigens? Two hundred antigens?

DR. SHAHA: Well, what we have here are 24 kd antigens, because the single band in two-dimensional gels gives us six spots. What we are doing is observing what each of the spots is responsible for.

DR. MITCHISON: Have you considered looking at the numbers to see how many different antigens you can pick up, for instance, by screening a library?

DR. SHAHA: Yes, we are in the process of doing this now.

7

Progress Toward a Birth Control Vaccine That Blocks Sperm Function

Paul Primakoff and Diana G. Myles

"The development of a fundamentally new birth control procedure, usable by millions of people over prolonged periods of time, is one of the most difficult problems in biomedical research" [Djerassi, 1979, p xix]. Research on development of a birth control vaccine is in its infancy and faces a number of formidable problems. These include the political and economic problems surveyed by Djerassi [1979, 1989] and scientific manpower problems. As an example of the latter, there are only a very small number of basic researchers studying mammalian sperm surface antigens. Even fewer researchers are defining human sperm surface antigens, the antigens that must be used for an anti-sperm vaccine. To our knowledge, less than five human sperm plasma membrane proteins have been identified, none have been purified, and no genes for these antigens have been cloned. In contrast, at the 4th International Workshop on Human Leukocyte Differentiation Antigens in February 1989, workers from 525 laboratories submitted and/or jointly evaluated about 1,100 different monoclonal antibodies to surface proteins. More than 70 human leukocyte surface antigens were identified. Many of these leukocyte surface proteins have been purified and the corresponding genes cloned [Knapp et al., 1989].

Despite the dearth of basic research on human sperm surface antigens, there is a clear conceptual basis for anti-sperm and other modes of immunological birth control. Figure 1 contrasts this immune approach with contraception that targets the endocrine system. The endocrine system supports ovarian/testicular function and

Gamete Interaction: Prospects for Immunocontraception, pages 89–102
© 1990 Wiley-Liss, Inc.

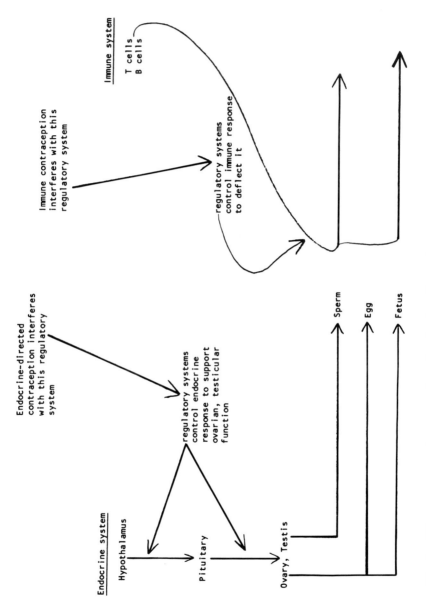

Fig. 1. Diagram comparing strategies of endocrine-directed contraception to immune contraception.

gestation through a variety of hormones whose production is regulated via feedback loops. Endocrine-directed contraception interferes with the endocrine regulatory systems. In the normal physiological situation, the immune system does not respond to sperm, egg, or fetus. Specific regulatory systems control immunocompetent cells to eliminate effectively the responses to gametes and fetus. Immune contraception is designed to interfere with these immune regulatory systems (Fig. 1). One of the difficulties in doing this, in the case of sperm, is that the nature of the immune regulatory systems is largely unknown. Thus, in designing an anti-sperm vaccine, we must overcome immune mechanisms that normally block responses to sperm (in the male and/or female), but we have little information as to what these mechanisms are.

Compared with anti-egg or anti-fetus immune contraception, an anti-sperm vaccine has two theoretical advantages. First, it might work in both males and females; second, it would not raise problems of autoimmunity in the female if a sperm-specific protein is used. A variety of scientific questions face a real-life anti-sperm vaccine; some of the major ones are listed in Table 1 and discussed below.

QUESTION 1: WHAT SPERM SURFACE PROTEIN(S) TO USE AS ANTIGEN?

This is the major research focus at the moment and has been the primary concern in our laboratory. We will discuss it in detail below. Very few mammalian sperm surface proteins have been purified (about six, if all reports of purification and location on the cell surface are reliable). Even among these, an essential function in fertilization remains to be rigorously established for most of them. Thus, the choice of good candidate sperm antigens is quite limited.

QUESTION 2: WHAT ADJUVANT TO USE IN HUMANS FOR AN ANTI-SPERM VACCINE?

This is a problem for all new vaccines, because, for human use, alum, a relatively ineffective adjuvant, is the only one currently approved. Until the other questions in Table 1 are resolved, the adjuvant question will probably remain in the background.

QUESTION 3: HOW TO MAINTAIN HIGH TITER?

A birth control vaccine is different from almost all other vaccines in that it will require the long-term presence of a sufficiently high an-

TABLE 1. Some Questions Facing an Anti-Sperm Contraceptive Vaccine

1. What sperm protein(s) to use as antigen?
2. What adjuvant to use in humans?
3. How will sufficiently high titer be maintained?
4. How will the contraceptive effect be terminated?
    a. By normal decline in antibody titer?
       i. Will person-to-person variation in the rate of this decline make the period of induced infertility unacceptably variable?
       ii. Will presence of sperm (from intercourse) in female reproductive tract boost titers, making the duration of infertility depend on the frequency of intercourse?
    b. By providing in female tract large amounts of soluble form of the sperm surface antigen used in the vaccine (this soluble antigen would have to be introduced in the female tract at sufficiently high levels to bind up the anti-sperm antibody and in a relatively nonimmunogenic form that did not boost the immune response)?
5. What are potential side effects?
    a. Autoimmune reactions to cross-reactive components of female tissues and autoimmune damage to the testis in males?
    b. Hypersensitivity reactions to the presence of sperm in the female reproductive tract—including IgE-mediated allergic reactions and immune complex-mediated inflammation and tissue injury?

tibody titer to give protection. (Drastic declines in titers are generally tolerable with other vaccines against infectious agents that can rely on the memory response to the agent.) A sufficiently high titer to give conveniently long infertile periods may be achievable by initial immunization or might require a method for long-term administration of the antigen (e.g., subdermal implant that would slowly release a protein antigen).

QUESTION 4: HOW WILL THE CONTRACEPTIVE EFFECT BE TERMINATED?

This is an infrequently discussed difficulty facing any birth control vaccine, including an anti-sperm vaccine. It is often assumed that return to fertility will be readily obtained by decline in antibody titers, and a small amount of evidence supports this. However, two factors could make the rate of antibody titer decline variable and thus

TABLE 2. Contraceptive Effect of PH-20 Immunization[a]

	Amount of PH-20 injected (μg)	No. of animals	No. with litters (% with litters)	No. of progeny	Average No. progeny in control
Group 1 females	50	1	0	0	
	30	1	0	0	
	20	1	0	0	
	10	1	0	0	
	0 (control)	13	12 (92)	46	3.5
Group 2 females	20	14	0	0	
	10	4	0	0	
	5	3	0	0	
	0 (control)	23	22 (96)	74	3.2
Total PH-20– immunized females		25	0 (0)	0	
Total control females		36	34 (94)	120	3.3
			Females with fetuses mated females		
Group 3 Males	50	1	0/2	0	
	30	1	0/2	0	
	20	1	0/2	0	
	10	1	0/2	0	
	5	1	0/2	0	
	2.5	1	0/2	0	
	0 (control)	7	14/14	62	4.4
Total PH-20– immunized males		6	0/12 (0)		
Total control males		7	14/14 (100)		

[a]Female or male Hartley guinea pigs (about 300 gm at the time of the first injection) received two injections containing PH-20 in the stated amount. PH-20, purified from sperm by mAb affinity chromatography, showed no detectable contaminants using silver staining of high loads (5 μg) of proteins on SDS gels. Purity of each PH-20 preparation used for immunization of females or males was verified by SDS-PAGE and silver staining. The affinity-purified PH-20, in 0.375 ml phosphate-buffered saline (PBS) containing 3 mM octylglucoside (OG), was emulsified with 0.375 ml complete Freund's adjuvant (CFA). Each animal received 0.5 ml of the emulsion subcutaneously in the back and 0.25 ml intramuscularly in a rear leg. About 1 month later the same amount of PH-20 in PBS and 3 mM OG, emulsified with incomplete Freund's adjuvant (IFA), was injected into the same sites in each animal. (A single exception was that the male that received 30 μg PH-20 had only the primary injection.) Control females and males received the same injections on the same schedule containing PBS and 3 mM OG and CFA or IFA but lacking PH-20. To allow the injected females to mate, about 2 months after the initial injection they were housed with males for 3 weeks. Each cage contained one male (575–600 gm), two or three PH-20–immunized females, and two to four control-injected females. After 3 weeks, the females were separated from the males, pregnant females proceeded to have litters, and progeny were counted. Control-injected females that failed to become pregnant had been in cages where the other controls did become pregnant, indicating all males, mated with immunized females, were fertile. To allow the injected males to mate, about 2 months after the initial injection each injected male was housed with two females (about 600 gm) for 3 weeks. The females and males were then separated, and, after an additional 5 weeks, females were sacrificed and fetuses counted. Reproduced from Primakoff et al. [1988], with permission of the publisher.

TABLE 3. Antisera Binding in Radioimmune Assay[a]

Antiserum from animals injected with PH-20 (μg)	Antiserum dilutions						
	10^{-2}	10^{-3}	10^{-4}	10^{-5}	10^{-6}	10^{-7}	10^{-8}
0 (control)	27[b]	5	2	1	1	1	1
5	156	152	120	44	14	5	2
10	150	149	130	66	21	8	4
20	150	147	128	66	24	10	5
30	155	148	113	43	13	4	2
50	142	140	130	64	18	6	2

[a]Binding of antisera, obtained 1 week before the first mating and diluted as indicated, was measured in a radioactive solid-phase (microtiter plate) assay using an octylglucoside extract of live sperm as antigen and ^{125}I-protein A as the second reagent. Nonspecific binding was blocked with 3% nonfat dry milk in PBS. Values shown were determined in duplicate in one experiment and were from one immunized female (50 and 30 μg) or the averages of four females (0 μg), two females (5 μg), one group 1 and two group 2 females (10 μg), and one group 1 and three group 2 females (20 μg). Group 2 females, immunized with 10 or 20 μg, had somewhat higher titers than group 1 females immunized with 10 or 20 μg. Reproduced from Primakoff et al. [1988], with permission of the publisher.
[b]^{125}I cpm bound in microtiter well ($\times$ 10^{-2}).

make the period of induced infertility unacceptably variable. First, there may be person-to-person variations in the rate of titer decline below the threshold necessary to restore fertility to that individual. The threshold titer may also show variability. Second, in women it is possible that sperm in the reproductive tract (after intercourse) would boost the effective antibody titers, and thus duration of infertility would depend on frequency of intercourse. Regardless of these possibilities of individual variation, in any one person there may well be a period of infertility, followed by a period of subfertility, then fertility. The subfertile period may be unacceptable to some potential users. An alternative approach to terminate the contraception would be to place soluble antigen in the female reproductive tract. (By "soluble antigen" we mean a genetically engineered form of the vaccine's sperm membrane antigen that would lack the membrane anchor and thus not aggregate/precipitate). This soluble antigen (presented in a nonimmunogenic form) might bind up sufficient anti-sperm antibody to leave the sperm effectively antibody free. This is a theoretical possibility for females and potentially for males, if in the males the antibody is present only in seminal fluid and thus contacts the sperm only in the vagina after ejaculation. Certain anti-sperm antibodies responsible for spontaneous immune infertility in men apparently have these properties [Bronson et al., 1984].

QUESTION 5: WHAT SIDE EFFECTS CAN BE EXPECTED?

A variety of potential side effects must be considered, the most obvious and serious being the possibility of autoimmune problems (question 5, Table 1).

DISCUSSION

All of the questions in Table 1 can be answered through research, and their number and complexity indicate the scope of research required. It is premature to begin extensive investigation of questions 2–5 (about adjuvants, titer maintenance, termination, and side effects) until sperm antigens, fully effective in inducing infertility, are identified. Thus our energies have been directed toward identifying effective sperm antigens. We have succeeded in finding a sperm surface protein, the PH-20 protein of guinea pig sperm, which is a fully effective contraceptive immunogen.

The PH-20 protein has a required function in sperm–zona binding [Primakoff et al., 1985]. When either male or female guinea pigs are immunized with purified PH-20, 100% effective contraception is obtained. In our initial study [Primakoff et al., 1988], 25 females and 6 males were immunized, and all became infertile (Table 2). Subsequently, an additional 22 males were immunized with PH-20 and all have become infertile, while all additional control-injected males were fertile (Primakoff, Woolman and Tung, unpublished results).

In the first study we found that the immunized females had very high anti-PH-20 antibody titers. These titers could be measured either by RIA or by testing the ability of immunized female sera to inhibit a sperm–zona binding assay (Tables 3 and 4). Sera from females, immunized with 5–50 μg PH-20, inhibited sperm binding to the guinea pig zona 90% or greater at a dilution of 10^{-3} and continued to inhibit substantially even at a dilution of 10^{-5} (Table 4). Titers taken at the time of the first infertile mating (2 months after the initial injection) were compared with those at second mating (6 months). About a fourfold drop in titer (see legend, Table 5) was found for individual females immunized with 10, 20, or 30 μg PH-20. The 10 and 20 μg immunized females were fertile at 6 months, but the 30 μg immunized female with an identical titer remained infertile (Table 5). This suggests that when serum titers have declined fourfold, an individual female has a certain chance of being either fertile or infertile.

The contraceptive effect is reversible in both males [Primakoff et al., 1988; Primakoff, Woolman and Tung, unpublished results] and

TABLE 4. Percent Inhibition of Sperm–Zona Binding[a]

Antiserum from animals injected with PH-20 (µg)	Antiserum dilutions			
	10^{-2}	10^{-3}	10^{-4}	10^{-5}
0 (control)	0[b]	0		
5	92	94	84	58
10	94	91	63	48
20	94	94	67	26
30	92	92	57	50
50	92	90	72	37

[a]The ability of antisera, diluted as indicated, to inhibit sperm binding to the zona pellucida of guinea pig eggs was measured as previously described for anti-PH-20 mAbs. Sperm, capacitated and allowed to acrosome react in modified Tyrode's medium, were preincubated with the diluted antiserum for 15–20 min and then added to eggs in the continuing presence of diluted antiserum. After 30 min, eggs with bound sperm were washed into sperm-free drops, fixed, and the number of sperm bound to the zona counted in one plane of focus. The mean number of sperm/egg was 16.4 ± 3.3 in the absence of antiserum in 13 experiments compiled in the table. Percent inhibition is (1.0 − the number of sperm bound in the presence of antiserum/number of sperm bound in the absence of antiserum in the same experiment) × 100%. Antiserum from one female injected with each stated amount of PH-20 was tested one time at each dilution to determine percent inhibition. Antiserum from the control-injected female was tested twice at 10^{-2} dilution. Reproduced from Primakoff et al. [1988], with permission of the publisher.
[b]Percent inhibition.

females (Table 6). Group 1 females (Table 2) had slightly lower titers (see legend, Table 3) than group 2 females (Table 2). Group 1 females' return to fertility was somewhat more rapid than that in group 2 (Table 6). By 15–18 months, 4/4 (100%) of group 1 and 16/20 (80%) of group 2 females had returned to fertility. We have insufficient data to say whether some or all of the remaining four immunized, infertile females were infertile before immunization, became infertile because of their age (almost 2 years), or remained infertile as a result of immunization. The data indicate there was a considerable spread in the time that different females receiving the same dose (10 or 20 µg PH-20) returned to fertility (6–18 months). This suggests the need for careful study of factors that determine (and may make variable) the time period of induced infertility. One of these factors in our study may have been the use of Freund's adjuvant, which may lead to antigen remaining in the animals for variable, prolonged periods.

Antisera, from females immunized with 5–50 µg PH-20, detected only PH-20 in Western blots of total extracts of intact sperm cells. Antiserum from the female receiving the highest PH-20 dose (50 µg) bound to sperm extracts in an RIA but showed no binding to a range of tissue types from female guinea pigs. This suggests that PH-20 is

TABLE 5. Antisera Binding Before First Mating Compared With Second Mating[a]

Antiserum from animals injected with PH-20 (μg)	Mating	Antiserum dilutions						
		10^{-2}	10^{-3}	10^{-4}	10^{-5}	10^{-6}	10^{-7}	10^{-8}
0 (control)	1st	26[b]	6	2	1	1	1	1
	2nd	25	5	2	1	1	1	1
10	1st Infertile	144	145	110	40	9	5	3
	2nd Fertile	139	128	59	13	4	4	2
20	1st Infertile	142	139	105	33	10	6	3
	2nd Fertile	144	129	59	16	6	4	3
30	1st Infertile	155	144	109	42	14	6	3
	2nd Infertile	152	132	60	14	5	4	2
50	1st Infertile	142	144	125	59	18	8	3
	2nd Infertile	145	139	104	37	12	8	3

[a]Binding of antisera, obtained 1 week before the first mating or 1 week before the second mating, diluted as indicated, was measured as in Table 3. Values shown are averages determined in duplicate in two experiments. Cpm bound specifically at 10^{-2} dilution is maximal binding. Antiserum titer is defined as the dilution at which cpm bound = half maximal binding. Reproduced from Primakoff et al., [1988], with permission of the publisher.
[b]^{125}I cpm bound in microtiter well ($\times 10^{-2}$).

TABLE 6. Reversibility of Contraceptive Effect in Females

Months after initial injection	Group	No. with litters/total[a]
6	1	2/4 (50)
	2	2/19 (11)
9–11	1	3/4 (75)
	2	8/20 (40)
15–18	1	4/4 (100)
	2	16/20 (80)

[a]Values in parentheses are percentages.

a sperm-specific antigen, and the immune response to it may not include significant levels of antibodies cross-reactive with female tissues. Thus PH-20 may have one of the theoretical advantages of a sperm immunogen: that it will not lead to problems of autoimmunity in females [Primakoff et al., 1988].

One of the questions that remains concerning PH-20 is whether it is present on sperm of mammalian species other than guinea pig. Particularly critical from the contraceptive point of view is the pos-

TABLE 7. Binding of Antiguinea Pig PH-20 Antibodies to Human Sperm

Antibody	Indirect immunofluorescence on swim-up sperm	RIA on detergent extract of sperm
Mouse monoclonal	0/3	0/3
Rabbit polyclonal	2/2	2/2
Guinea pig polyclonal	2/3	15/20

sible presence of a PH-20 homologue on human sperm. Whereas the three monoclonal antibodies we have to PH-20 do not bind to human sperm in indirect immunofluorescence or RIA, a variety of anti-PH-20 polyclonal antibodies do bind to human sperm in these two assays (Table 7). Recently, we completed cloning and sequencing DNA for guinea pig PH-20 [Lathrop et al., 1989]. We are currently doing cross-species Southern blots to test for a PH-20–related gene in other mammals, including human.

ACKNOWLEDGMENTS

This work was supported by NIH grant HD21989 to P.P.

REFERENCES

Bronson RA, Cooper GW, Rosenfeld DL (1984): Sperm antibodies: Their role in infertility. Fertil Steril 42:171–183.

Djerassi C (1979): The Politics of Contraception. San Francisco: W.H. Freeman and Co.

Djerassi C (1989): The bitter pill. Science 245:356–361.

Knapp W, Rieber P, Dorken B, Schmidt RE, Stein H, Borne AEGKUD (1989): Towards a better definition of human leucocyte surface molecules. Immunol Today 10:253–257.

Lathrop W, Carmichael E, Myles DG, Primakoff P (1989): Cloning and sequencing of the gene for the PH-20 protein of guinea pig sperm. J Cell Biol Abstr 109:125a.

Primakoff P, Hyatt H, Myles DG (1985): A role for the migrating antigen PH-20 in guinea pig sperm binding to the egg zona pellucida. J Cell Biol 101:2239–2244.

Primakoff P, Lathrop W, Woolman L, Cowan A, Myles DG (1988): Fully effective contraception in male and female guine pigs immunized with the sperm protein PH-20. Nature 335:543–546.

DISCUSSION

DR. ALEXANDER: You showed that after immunization with PH-20 there were no sperm in the cauda epididymis. Was this due to an immune response? Were there many macrophages in the caput epididymidis?

DR. PRIMAKOFF: No. I neglected to mention that. Ken Tung told me that there was no sign of epididymitis. There were no macrophages, lymphocytes, or anything unusual around the epididymis. And he also feels the sperm are absent from the caput and the cauda, and there is, for some unknown reason, a small reservoir of some sperm in the corpus. It may be that there is complement-mediated lysis and phagocytosis by the epithelial cells in the epididymis.

DR. SWERLOFF: You were able to demonstrate that, after a certain period of active immunization, there was reversibility. Yet you then demonstrated that there was, in fact, evidence of orchitis. However, if you applied these techniques to humans, undoubtedly you would need additional immunization. Have you attempted to reimmunize the animals, or boost them, to see to what degree damage occurred and whether reversibility was still possible?

DR. PRIMAKOFF: No. We have not done that. That is a very important experiment. As far as the reversibility of the orchitis goes, by itself, the initial orchitis is an unacceptable side effect.

DR. SURI: When you were speaking about the mechanism of infertility in males, you said you could not locate macrophages in the epididymis. Did you find any blockage of sperm production in your testicular sections, or was there normal spermatogenesis? And, did you check for PH-20 antibodies in the seminal fluid?

DR. PRIMAKOFF: In terms of the orchitis causing a block to spermatogenesis, that may well have occurred in local areas. The extent of the orchitis was variable from animal to animal, so certainly in some animals the orchitis had some impact on spermatogenesis per se. Concerning your second question, we have only looked for antibody in these animals in the serum; we have not looked at any reproductive tract fluids.

DR. SURI: When you mated the animals, did you check for ovulation?

DR. PRIMAKOFF: No.

DR. ISOJIMA: You said the mouse monoclonal antibody against the PH-20 did not cross-react with human spermatozoa, but rabbit polyclonal antibody against PH-20 cross-reacted with human sperm. Does that mean that the PH-20 is not a pure component? Also, what component do you use for the analysis of the amino acid sequence?

DR. PRIMAKOFF: In answer to your first question, it is a common finding that, because monoclonals look at a single epitope, they will not bind in a cross-species or cross-tissue reactivity test, whereas a polyclonal, because it surveys many epitopes, will bind. So, I think that it is reasonable to find that the monoclonals don't bind and the polyclonals do. As to your second question, we determined the amino acid sequence of six tryptic peptides by the standard methods of purifying the PH-20 protein and fragmenting with trypsin.

DR. ISOJIMA: Did you use the 64 kd component?

DR. PRIMAKOFF: Yes. That is all there is.

DR. ISOJIMA: Do you think there may be some contamination molecules included?

DR. PRIMAKOFF: No. Purified PH-20 protein is unusually pure. We tested this by silver staining on SDS-PAGE gels and found that contaminants were present at less than one part per 2,000, which is actually unusual.

DR. ISOJIMA: You mentioned using the absorption test for specificity, but I doubt that the absorption procedure is possible. One usually uses some more specific staining method to evaluate cross-reactivity in other tissues.

DR. PRIMAKOFF: I agree with you. The question of whether other tissues contain the PH-20 protein or are cross-reactive is very difficult to answer. We should probably use an RIA kind of assay, tissue fluorescence, and Northern blots and, after you do all those things, examine a large number of tissues.

DR. DONCEL: Did you immunize other species besides the guinea pig? It is well known that the guinea pig easily develops autoimmune orchitis, which is not the case in humans.

DR. PRIMAKOFF: No. In experiments in which whole testis homogenates were injected, guinea pigs were more sensitive to development of autoimmune orchitis than other species. That is something that we are quite interested in.

DR. DONCEL: Did you check the histology of the vas deferens in order to detect vasitis? Vasitis or abscesses are often present, initially, in autoimmune orchitis in guinea pigs.

DR. PRIMAKOFF: Ken Tung said that he saw no epididymitis and no vasitis.

DR. TALWAR: In the males, did you have to use an adjuvant like Freund's complete adjuvant?

DR. PRIMAKOFF: Yes, in both males and females, we used Freund's adjuvant. We used complete Freund's in the first injection, and, if they received a second injection, it was with incomplete Freund's.

DR. TALWAR: Does it work without Freund's adjuvant or with any other adjuvants?

DR. PRIMAKOFF: We have not yet tried any other adjuvants.

DR. TALWAR: I think that that is very important, because, as you know, there is a barrier between the immune system and the testis.

If one has to use an adjuvant like Freund's complete adjuvant, then obviously we have a restriction, a systemic immunization.

DR. SHAHA: Did I understand that your rabbit polyclonal did not reveal high titers in immunofluorescence?

DR. PRIMAKOFF: Yes.

DR. SHAHA: How about RIA?

DR. PRIMAKOFF: It was positive in RIA. In fact, both rabbit polyclonals were positive in RIA.

DR. SHAHA: Positive, but not like the guinea pig?

DR. PRIMAKOFF: No. Some of the guinea pig polyclonals were not positive. I think that is a sign that the expected cross-reactivity to human sperm is obviously low. But, that experiment is really inconclusive, because, if we take those same sera that are positive in those assays and use them in immunoblot or immunoprecipitation, we don't detect a human sperm antigen.

DR. DACHEUX: You said that there was a sperm pocket in the corpus region of the epididymis? Was sperm transport from the epididymis stopped?

DR. PRIMAKOFF: We are not really evaluating sperm transport. The testes were fixed at the time that the animal was sacrificed, so it is really a static picture.

DR. BURGOS: Are you affecting the inhibition of the sperm released or spermiation?

DR. PRIMAKOFF: There is no evidence for that from the histology. Apparently, most of the seminiferous tubules appear to contain a normal number of sperm in the lumen. Thus release after spermiation appears to be normal, except where the tubules are inflamed.

DR. BURGOS: How do you explain the empty epididymal regions?

DR. PRIMAKOFF: We don't have an explanation for that.

DR. BURGOS: One point would be to detect that no spermatozoa are in the rete testes; a lowering of the number of spermatozoa in the rete testes or caput of the epididymis can point to diminution of the sperm released.

DR. PRIMAKOFF: But that does not appear to be what is occurring. The sperm released look normal, and the number of sperm in the rete testis looks normal. What is abnormal is that the sperm are absent in most regions of the epididymis.

DR. JOHNSON: PH-20 is a glycosylphosphatidylinositol (GPI)-linked membrane protein. Also, within the male reproductive tract, there is believed to be quite a significant amount of phosphatidylinositol-specific phospholipase, so one might expect release of PH-20 protein from the surface of sperm within its natural environment. Could you comment on this?

DR. PRIMAKOFF: I don't think anyone has shown that the enzymes in the epididymis can actually release GPI-anchored membrane proteins. But there may be a loss of PH-20 antibody-binding sites when PH-20 goes through the epididymis. PH-20's change from whole surface distribution to posterior head distribution involves migration of some of the molecules and possibly a loss of some others. Thus it could be through an effect like that.

DR. JOHNSON: Do you know what the effect of treating sperm with a GPI-specific enzyme is on sperm–zona binding?

DR. PRIMAKOFF: Yes. We have conducted that experiment. In fact, the point is that when the membrane anchor is glycosylphosphatidylinositol, the membrane protein can be released by an enzyme that cuts at the phosphate so that the whole protein is released into the medium. We found in looking at the acrosome-reacted sperm in our sperm–zona binding assay, PH-20 appears to be the only surface protein (on acrosome-reacted sperm) that is anchored this way. When you release it you inhibit sperm–zona binding substantially, between 55 and 60% inhibition.

8

World Health Organization Sperm Antigen Workshops and Sperm Antigen Nomenclature Project

Deborah J. Anderson

SPERM ANTIGEN WORKSHOP I: TORONTO, CANADA, JULY 1986.

The β-hCG peptide vaccine has been the focus of the World Health Organization Task Force on Vaccines for Fertility Regulation for the past 10 years. However, in 1985, the Task Force broadened the scope of its program to include research on sperm, trophoblast, and zona pellucida antigens as antifertility vaccine candidates. It was recognized that rapid advances in the field of genetic engineering now make the production of such cell-associated antigens for vaccines feasible. To evaluate the status of the sperm antigen field, a workshop was held in 1986. A literature search was performed to identify investigators who had produced antisperm monoclonal antibodies, and these individuals were requested to submit sperm-specific monoclonal antibodies to the workshop. A total of 66 mouse monoclonal antibodies reacting with human sperm were submitted by 16 laboratories. The antibodies were aliquotted and coded in a central laboratory and then distributed to 42 independent evaluating laboratories. The major objectives of the first workshop were:

1   To assess the quality and abundance of sperm-specific monoclonal antibodies for identification and characterization of sperm surface antigens

Gamete Interaction: Prospects for Immunocontraception, pages 103–106
© 1990 Wiley-Liss, Inc.

2   To establish criteria for the identification and development
    of sperm vaccine candidates
3   To identify sperm-specific antigens that might be pursued
    as contraceptive vaccine candidates
4   To assess the reproducibility of current antisperm antibody
    assays.

The results of the 1986 workshop were published [Anderson et al., 1987]. The following criteria were established for initial selection of monoclonal antibodies with which to identify sperm antigen candidates: 1) reactivity with human testicular germ cells and abundant surface antigens on mature spermatozoa, 2) no detectable cross-reactivity with somatic cells, and 3) inhibition of at least one sperm function assay. Three monoclonal antibodies, S20 (Chapter 2, this volume), S37 (Chapter 3, this volume), and S61 (Chapter 4, this volume), met these criteria. It is of interest that all of these antibodies have subsequently been shown to react with acrosomal antigens that are expressed during or following the acrosome reaction. These antigens are currently being cloned by the originating laboratories, and are planned to be used as sperm antigen vaccine prototypes. An unexpected finding was the extensive cross-reactivity of most antisperm monoclonal antibodies with human somatic tissues. Sixty-three of the 66 antibodies submitted to the sperm antigen workshop cross-reacted with antigens present in other human tissues. It was concluded that immunization of mice with washed human sperm (or washed semen cells) is not an efficient approach for the production of sperm-specific monoclonal antibodies, as it most often results in the production of heterophilic (human-specific but not tissue-specific) monoclonal antibodies. Alternate approaches to identifying human sperm-specific determinants such as production of human monoclonal antibodies from lymphocytes of infertility patients or the use of difference cDNA libraries may be possibilities.

Only 31 of the workshop monoclonal antibodies reacted with antigens expressed on the sperm surface, and these antibodies did not begin to map the surface of the human spermatozoon. Furthermore, several laboratories reported that many of the antibodies reacted with a subpopulation of sperm in any given preparation. This focused attention on differences in antigen expression that accompany changes in the sperm surface during sperm processing in the female reproductive tract, including capacitation, and the acrosome reaction. The fact that few of these antibodies reacted with all sperm in a preparation introduced the concept that a multideterminant sperm vaccine might be required for contraceptive purposes.

A number of operational problems were encountered in the first workshop: 1) laboratory protocols differed widely and contributed to a lack of reproducibility of data, 2) there were in many cases a lack of accordance of workshop data with information published by the source laboratory (most frequently concerning the issue of sperm specificity), and 3) definitive biochemical data (i.e., molecular weight, isoelectric point, molecular composition of epitope) was not obtained for most of the antigens. It was proposed that subsequent workshops in this area might focus on 1) the standardization of functional, biochemical, and immunohistological tests for the characterization of antisperm monoclonal antibodies and their antigenic targets and 2) use of more rigorous techniques to obtain definitive molecular information.

SPERM ANTIGEN WORKSHOP 2: BARILOCHE, ARGENTINA, NOVEMBER 1989.

Ten new monoclonal antibodies were submitted to Workshop 2. Six of the antibodies reacted with testicular germ cells and abundantly expressed sperm surface antigens. Five of these antibodies were reactive with acrosomal/equatorial region antigens, and three of these have demonstrated lack of cross-reactivity against a limited panel of somatic tissues; however, most showed a curious cross-reactivity with trophoblast cells in placenta sections.

The following recommendations were made: 1) a third sperm antigen workshop should be held to focus on biochemical and molecular techniques and data (this workshop should be held in Rome, Italy, in 1992 in conjunction with the International Reproductive Immunology Congress), 2) a committee should be appointed to standardize protocols for the various antisperm antibody assays, and 3) a sperm antigen nomenclature committee should be established and a sperm antigen nomenclature system be published following the 1992 workshop.

WHO SPERM ANTIGEN NOMENCLATURE PROGRAM

A sperm antigen nomenclature committee was appointed by the Task Force. Members were selected on the basis of experience, expertise, and geographical considerations: D. Anderson (Chairman), N. Alexander (U.S.A.), J. Herr (U.S.A.), G. Lee (Canada), M. Isahakia (Kenya), A. De Ioannes (Chile), H. Moore (U.K.), D. Griffin (Switzerland, WHO Secretariat), C. Shaha (India), S. Isojima (Japan),

X. Chong (China), M. Kurpisz (Poland), and P. Johnson (U.K.; Trophoblast Antigen Nomenclature Liaison). The first committee meeting was held in Bariloche, Argentina, in November 1989, and the committee proposed that the following information concerning each sperm antigen be obtained to served as a basis for the nomenclature system: 1) sperm surface localization, 2) PI and molecular weight, 3) peptide sequence (when known), and 4) DNA sequence (when known). It was concluded that the Third Sperm Antigen Workshop be a concerted effort to obtain definitive data on as many human sperm surface antigens as possible, that a computerized database be established containing all available data on human sperm surface antigens from the workshops and the literature, and that the WHO sperm antigen nomenclature be published in 1993, in conjunction with corresponding information generated in the WHO human trophoblast antigen nomenclature program.

REFERENCES

Anderson DJ, Johnson PM, Alexander NJ, Jones WR, Griffin PD (1987): Monoclonal antibodies to human trophoblast and sperm antigens: Report of two WHO-sponsored workshops, June 30, 1986—Toronto, Canada. J Reprod Immunol 10:231.

General Discussion

DR. ANDERSON: At this point in the workshop, we will have a general discussion on which antigens appear to be the best candidates for a contraceptive vaccine. The majority of the vaccine candidates that have been identified, thus far, have been acrosomal matrix or acrosomal membrane antigens. My question is: Why haven't more reagents been generated to human sperm-specific antigens that are expressed on the plasma membrane? And is there a strategy to pursue such antigens specifically for contraceptive vaccine development programs?

DR. HERR: It is clear, in working with human coating antigens from the human seminal vesicle, that certain seminal vesicle proteins coat the entire surface of the human sperm very effectively. The use of ejaculated sperm as targets may not be as effective as taking epididymal sperm that can be obtained from a urologist at vasectomy.

DR. PRIMAKOFF: I agree. Our experience has been that when we make monoclonal antibodies to ejaculated human sperm, the large majority of antibodies are to seminal fluid proteins. Certain seminal fluid proteins may be looked at as vaccine candidates. But, because everyone is focusing on proteins made in the testes, to get them you either have to get a source of human epididymal sperm, which is rare, or immunosuppress mice against seminal fluid proteins. Then you can do the fusions against the human sperm and raise a number of relevant antibodies to integral sperm membrane proteins. But, concerning what occurred in the first WHO Sperm Antigen Workshop, a number of the antibodies that turned out to be to intracellular components were identified as being to surface antigens. I think we have to be careful to make that distinction and ensure that the antibodies do, in fact, belong to live, swim-up sperm.

DR. HERR: But the surface has to be extended to include the inner acrosomal membrane exposed on the head of the sperm following the acrosome reaction. The surface is fine as long as we don't restrict it to the plasma membrane but also account for the postacrosomal events.

DR. JONES: Traditionally, looking at the prospects of the sperm vaccine in the female by observing the natural model of infertility, we always assume that it has to operate on some of the aspects of sperm transport, although it would have to be a locally mediated IgA effect.

Gamete Interaction: Prospects for Immunocontraception, pages 107–109
© 1990 Wiley-Liss, Inc.

There have been concerns about how this can be effective in relation to the large sperm load. I have two comments about this issue. First, with the advent of sperm–egg in vitro tests and IVF in humans, we have begun to realize that many of the antibodies in human infertility probably operate at that level. We have also heard that the large proportion of the monoclonal antibodies presented are directed against events of sperm–oocyte interaction, that is, with notable exceptions such as Dr. Shaha's work with a polyclonal antibody that acted at two levels. But, in most cases, they are biologically active or have implications for biological activity at that level. Thus it raises the possibility that we may be overemphasizing the need for local immunity. The most important issue relates to getting a reasonable level of trasudated IgG antibodies into the follicular fluid or in the fallopian tubes.

DR. ISAHAKIA: In terms of selecting epididymal sperm as a source of initial antigen, appropriate animal models, in particular primates, are necessary. We have found that, by using epididymal sperm, 90% of antibodies that we generated cross-reacted with human sperm. Recently, we worked with chimpanzee epididymal sperm and found that 100% of antibodies raised against chimp sperm essentially cross react with human sperm. This was true not only in terms of cross-reactivity but also in terms of localization. In fact, the domains were exactly the same as those of the human. If we continue to utilize animals, particularly primates, as a source of antigen, we should be able to generate antibodies that are specific to our human sperm antigens.

DR. HJORT: I think we should be very careful in going from in vitro to in vivo studies. There are several experiments, for example, those concerning the sperm and its relationship to humans, where you have good impact of IgG antibodies in the in vitro experiments, but when it comes to observing the patient, there is very little evidence that the IgG antibodies have an effect in vivo.

DR. FICHOROVA: We have data that sera from infertile patients react more strongly with epididymal sperm than with ejaculated sperm. This is another reason to pay more attention to epididymal sperm, although it is very difficult to isolate epididymal sperm from men. But, if you have high cross-reactivity between human and baboon epididymal sperm, we can use more epididymal sperm to raise monoclonal antibodies that are more important in infertility.

DR. ANDERSON: Clearly, we all agree that we should try harder to look for antigens expressed on epididymal sperm. This is why the animal work has progressed further along the lines of identifying sperm plasma membrane antigens than the human work. I would also urge those researchers working on animal sperm to try to use cross-reactivity of their clones to pull out equivalent antigens from human DNA libraries.

9

Sperm Biochemical Changes During Epididymal Maturation

J.L. Dacheux, C. Chevrier, F. Dacheux,
C. Jeulin, J.L. Gatti, C. Pariset, and
M. Paquignon

In all mammals, including man, the spermatozoa that leave the testis are infertile. To be able to meet, recognize, and fertilize an oocyte, the sperm must undergo several successive biochemical transformations during their transit in the male and female genital tracts. This postgonadal maturation represents the last step of cellular differentiation that transforms a gonocyte into several fertile spermatozoa. In the testis, the genome of the germ cell controls the successive cellular transformations. However, in the last stages of spermatogenesis, the sperm modifications are mainly influenced by the surrounding somatic cells.

In the male genital tract the principal post-testicular sperm biochemical modifications occur during epididymal transit. The major postgonadal modifications studied are 1) changes in metabolic pathways mostly linked to the energy supply of the gamete and to its survival during epididymal storage, 2) intracellular modifications of the axonema and the molecular system related to flagellar movement, and 3) the nature of external signals and their effects on the plasma membrane and transduction by eventual second intracellular messengers.

The importance of each sperm modification of fertilizing ability is difficult to establish for several reasons: 1) the modifications may be assessed for each gamete, but the fertilizing ability can be estimated only with a sperm population (several thousands) that is always

Gamete Interaction: Prospects for Immunocontraception, pages 111–128
© 1990 Wiley-Liss, Inc.

heterogeneous; and 2) the fertilization of the oocyte requires a succession of several events on the spermatozoa, but the final result is expressed as a "yes" or "no" answer: fertilized or not fertilized.

However, as acquisition of fertilizing ability by the spermatozoa in the epididymis is progressive, studies of sequential sperm modifications during epididymal maturation, using different species, may be able to give good correlations between biochemical modifications and fertilizing power.

BIOCHEMICAL CHANGES ASSOCIATED WITH THE DEVELOPMENT OF SPERM MOTILITY

The most visible result of biochemical changes during epididymal transit is the appearance of cellular movement. The biochemistry involved in the mature spermatozoa motility is composed of highly complex and integrated enzymatic reactions that are far from being known. However, analysis of the flagellar movement during epididymal initiation of sperm motility may contribute to the understanding of the sequential biochemical changes necessary for the gametes to be fully motile.

Mechanochemical Mechanism of Sperm Motility

Mammalian sperm movement is the result of flagellar beating. The flagellum is a highly complex structure containing a "9 + 2" microtubule axonema, nine outer dense fibers, and an envelope of fibrous sheath. The flagellar movement results from transient interactions between dynein ATPases and tubulin molecules that generate local sliding of the axonemal microtubules. The specific structures of the axonema, such as nexin links and radial spokes, and the presence of outer dense fibers create resistance to this active sliding, inducing shear forces that result in the curvature of the flagellum. The characteristics of the mobility of the spermatozoa can be described by 1) the form of the curvature or bend (which is an equilibrium between active and resistant forces); 2) the velocity at which these curvatures propagate along the flagellum (which is dependent on the activities of the mechanochemical enzymes); and 3) the rapidity with which these curvatures are generated alternatively on each side of the axonema (which may be related to the energetic possibility of the gametes).

In mammalian sperm, the length of the flagellum that is curved (the bend) increases as this bend propagates over the proximal half of the flagellum. For the same wave (a propagated bend), the cur-

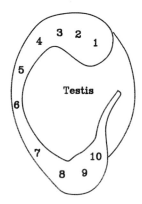

Fig. 1. Schematic representation of the mammalian epididymis. Regions 1 to 4 represent the caput, 5 to 7 the corpus, and 8 to 10 the cauda.

vature differs according to the position of the wave on the flagellum. The bend angle value is dependent on the proximity of the immediately preceding bend [Chevrier and Dacheux 1987]. These characteristics of the mammalian flagellar movement are linked to the elastic resistance property of their flagellum. This elastic resistance is largely influenced by the presence of changing periaxonemal structures such as the dense fibers and the fibrous sheath and/or by changes inherent in the axonemal force-generating machinery.

Evolution of Flagellar Movement During the Epididymal Transit

In mammals, the ultimate structure of the sperm flagella is already established when spermatozoa leave the testis; however, motility of the gametes appears only during their transit in the epididymal duct. For all mammals studied, the percentage of motile spermatozoa (all flagellar movement included) increases throughout the anterior region and is maximal in the corpus of the epididymis (Figs. 1–3) [Paquignon et al., 1983].

The maturation of flagellar movement is characterized by an increase in the flagellar beat frequency and by the appearance of symmetrical bending, which induces forward motility and rotation when the spermatozoa reach the last part of the epididymis [Chevrier and Dacheux, 1989; Bork et al., 1988].

In the ram, the flagellar movement of distal caput epididymal sperm is characterized by the presence of a great static bending in the first part of the flagellum and oscillations of the flagellum without

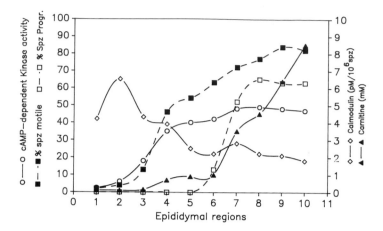

Fig. 2. Biochemical modifications in ram sperm during epididymal transit. Sperm are sampled from the 10 regions in Figure 1. The values shown are according to Besançon et al. [1985] for carnitine, Chevrier and Dacheux [1989] for motility, and Pariset et al. [1985] for calmodulin and protein kinase.

apparent propagating waves (Fig. 4) [Chevrier and Dacheux, 1989]. This static curvature is not observed with testicular or anterior caput epididymal spermatozoa.

In the corpus of the epididymis, most of the spermatozoa have a circular motion and erratic displacements because of transitory flagellar movements between simple oscillations and symmetric and synchronous beats. The flagellar movement of these spermatozoa is characterized by highly asymmetrical bends and several sites of initiation of waves.

Regulatory Factors of the Intrinsic Dynein–Tubulin Interactions

Microtubule sliding. Epididymal sperm mobility is controlled by a regulatory pathway involving cAMP. Numerous investigations have shown that motility increases in the presence of phosphodiesterase inhibitors (such as caffeine) or in the presence of dibutyryl cAMP. The requirement for cAMP to activate flagellar sperm movement decreases as sperm mature [Garbers et al., 1971; Dacheux and Paquignon, 1980; Amann et al., 1982]. The lack of a regulatory subunit of sperm adenylate cyclase makes the regulation of cAMP very unusual. In vivo, only bicarbonate has been found to stimulate sperm adenylate cyclase of several species [Okamura et al., 1985].

Activity of cAMP-dependent protein kinases rises dramatically

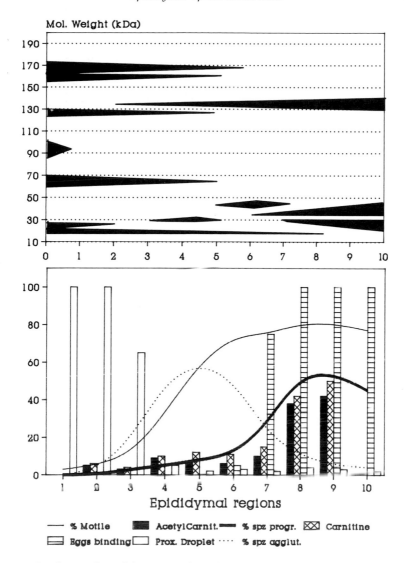

Fig. 3. Biochemical modifications of epididymal boar sperm. **Top:** Changes in the major sperm surface membrane as a function of epididymal transit as described by Dacheux et al. [1989]. **Bottom:** Changes in the percentage of motile and progressive sperm, intracellular concentrations of carnitine and acetylcarnitine (nM/10^8 spermatozoa [spz]) [Jeulin et al., 1987], zona-free hamster egg binding ability (percentage of eggs totally covered with spermatozoa from Dacheux and Voglmayr [1983]), percentage of sperm with proximal cytoplasmic droplets, and percentage of sperm agglutinated after dilution [Dacheux and Voglmayr, 1983].

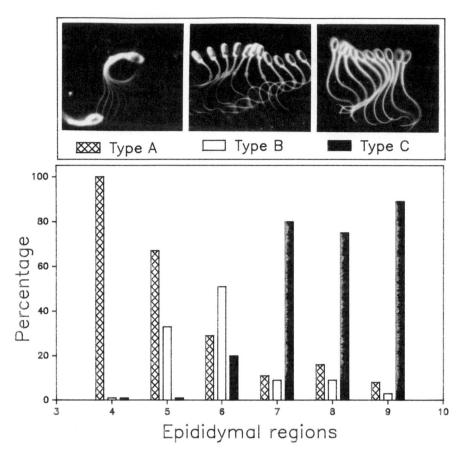

Fig. 4.   Distribution of the different types of motility patterns of motile ram spermatozoa during epididymal transit. **Type A:** Spermatozoa that only show flagella oscillations. **Type B:** "Erratic" movement with circular displacement. **Type C:** Forward progressive spermatozoa. The micrographs corresponding to the motility types are obtained with the stroboscopic techniques described by Chevrier and Dacheux [1987].

during epididymal transit (Fig. 2). In the ram, cAMP-dependent protein kinase subunits RIIa and C have been localized within the sperm motility apparatus as soon as the gametes leave the testis, and in the corpus and cauda epididymal sperm, RIIa also appeared localized between coarse fibers and mitochondria [Pariset et al., 1985, 1989].

   The correlation between cAMP-dependent protein kinase activity and flagellar beats provides evidence that cAMP-dependent protein phosphorylations are involved in the motility process. Actually, only one or two proteins of 56 kd (axokinin and RIIa subunit) have been described to be phosphorylated in a cAMP-dependent manner [Tash et al., 1984; Horowitz et al., 1989]. However, the increased catalytic subunit activity is associated only with the increased percentage of motile spermatozoa, and not with the appearance of forward progression, which occurs later in the epididymis (Fig. 2) [Pariset et al., 1985].

Bending of the flagella. Study of the sequential changes of flagellar bending pattern during epididymal maturation suggests that two types of mechanochemical interactions may be involved. The first one is the generation of the static curvature of the flagellum observed in immature sperm, and the second is the induction of propagating asymmetrical then symmetrical waves on the flagellum when the spermatozoa are mature [Chevrier and Dacheux, 1989].

The waves' propagation on each side of the axonema are associated with the presence of reversible dynein–tubulin binding between microtubule doublets. The angulation of the flagella is related to the rate of sliding and to the length of the axonema involved in this sliding [Gibbons, 1981]. All of these parameters are dependent on the time of attachment of the dynein arms to the microtubules. The in vivo regulation of the kinetics of the enzymatic mechanisms involved in attachment–detachment is still unknown.

Various observations on both invertebrate and mammalian sperm have demonstrated that calcium regulates the curvature of the axonema [Brokaw, 1979; Okuno and Brokaw, 1981; Eshel and Brokaw, 1987]. The Ca^{2+} effect may be mediated by its binding to calmodulin present in sperm flagella [Lindemann and Kanous, 1989]. The role of this ion in the modification of bending during epididymal transit is uncertain because no significant variations in external Ca^{2+} concentration or Ca^{2+} sperm membrane permeability can be found during epididymal transit. However, the abrupt and large decrease in calmodulin activity observed in rams during sperm transit can modulate Ca^{2+} action [Pariset et al., 1985]. Interactions between calcium and cAMP have also been described in rat spermatozoa in which decrease in intracellular Ca^{2+} is accompanied by an increase in cAMP, motility, and curvature of the flagella [Lindemann et al., 1987].

Changes in the bending of the flagellum have also been induced with various phosphodiesterase inhibitors. The effects of such inhibitors are variable according to the maturation step of the gametes. For caput epididymal spermatozoa, hairpin-curved forms of flagella can be produced [Dacheux and Paquignon, 1980]. The role of cAMP in this flagellar bending is unknown.

General Factors Involved in Motility Regulation

Intracellular pH. Intracellular pH controls the activity of several enzymes of metabolism, adenylate cyclase, and Ca^{2+}-binding protein. Increases in internal pH (pHi) stimulate the motility and metabolism of ejaculated bull sperm [Vijarayagavhan et al., 1985; Babcock et al., 1983; Wong and Lee, 1983], and it has also been proposed that, during epididymal transit, the motility of the sperm of several mammalian species is controlled by internal pH [Carr et al., 1985]. In eukaryotic cells, pHi can be regulated by sodium–proton exchange and/or bicarbonate-transport systems, proton permeability of the plasma membrane, buffering power of the cell, and plasma membrane potential.

In mammalian sperm, pHi is strongly dependent on the external pH (pHe); immediately after sperm dilution, the internal pH equilibrates toward the value of external pH. Regulation of the internal pH appears to be species specific [Carr et al., 1985]. In boar and ram, pHi is unaffected by the external concentration of sodium or potassium, ruling out mechanisms such as sodium–proton or potassium–proton exchange as the pHi regulatory mechanism (unpublished data). In the rat, the pHi of sperm from the cauda epididymis is controlled by a sodium–proton exchange similar to the one found in sea urchin sperm [Wong and Lee, 1983]. In the bull, the pHi can be raised to some extent by the addition of external potassium [Babcock et al., 1983].

In ram and boar, the regulatory system of the pHi is already in place when the sperm leave the gonad and remains unchanged during epididymal maturation (Fig. 5). However, in the boar it has been demonstrated that a membrane anion (HCO_3^- and SO_4^{--}) transport exists, and its activity decreases as the sperm travel through the anterior part of the epididymis [Okamura et al., 1988].

Motility of epididymal sperm depends strongly on the pH of the dilution medium and less on its ionic composition [Pholpramool and Chaturapanich, 1979]. For boar sperm, an acidic pH strongly inhibits motility, which is observed only at neutral or alkaline pH (Fig. 6). Motility can be affected by an internal pH shift either by a direct effect on dynein ATPase, which is fully active at pH 7.8–8.0, or on adenylate kinase present in the sperm flagella [Schoff et al., 1989]. However, motility and metabolism have zones of pHe optima that are directly affected by the cations, anions, and metabolic substrates present in the media. Motile ram sperm can be observed even when pHe reaches extreme values such as pH 6 or 9 in the presence of sodium and potassium, and even pH 10 in choline media (Fig. 6).

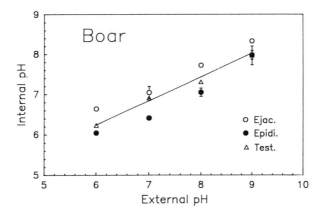

Fig. 5. Internal changes in pH of testicular (test.), epididymal (Epidi.), and ejaculated (Ejac.) boar spermatozoa as a function of the external values. The results were obtained after a 30 min incubation.

The presence of a significant percentage of motile spermatozoa at these extremes of pH indicate that the pH control of motility is only a part of a more complex regulation system.

Carnitine and acetylcarnitine. A relationship between the carnitine concentration in epididymal fluid and sperm motility has been suggested [Hinton and Hernandez, 1985; Johansen and Bohmer, 1979]. Carnitine is present in the epididymis at higher concentrations than in other body tissues in all species studied. In spermatozoa, carnitine is rapidly acetylated and thus can be indirectly involved in energy supply to the gametes. During epididymal transit, the concentration of carnitine increases in the fluid and in the spermatozoa from the corpus to the distal region (Fig. 2) [Hinton et al., 1979; Besançon et al., 1985]. The gametes do not appear to concentrate carnitine, as its concentrations outside and inside the mature spermatozoa are very similar [Jeulin et al., 1987]. Sperm membrane permeability to carnitine is unchanged during epididymal transit; however, in some animals the uptake increases for caudal epididymal spermatozoa (Jeulin and Dacheux, unpublished data). The value of the acetylcarnitine:carnitine ratio does not change throughout sperm maturation, and the carnitine acetyltransferase is already functional in immature spermatozoa [Brooks, 1979; Jeulin et al., 1987].

During epididymal transit, the rise in the percentage of motile spermatozoa occurs before the concentration of carnitine increases. However, the evolution of the percentage of progressive spermatozoa is always associated with their internal carnitine and acetylcarnitine concentrations (Fig. 3). These observations suggest that car-

Dacheux et al.

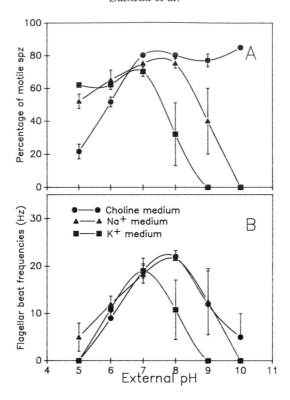

Fig. 6.   Influence of the external ionic conditions on the motility and flagellar beat frequency of the ram epididymal spermatozoa. Sperm were diluted (final concentration, 10^8 sperm/ml) in media containing either sodium, potassium, or choline as the main cation and buffered at the different pHs indicated. The percent of motile sperm **(A)** and their average flagellar beat frequency **(B)** were measured 60 min after dilution. Sperm from four animals were used; the bars indicate standard errors of the mean.

nitine is not directly involved in the initiation of sperm motility but may be an important metabolic factor in the high energy requirement of progressive spermatozoa.

SPERM PLASMA MEMBRANE CHANGES DURING EPIDIDYMAL TRANSIT

Maturation-associated membrane changes have been described in several species with various techniques. All of these investigations showed extensive and sequential surface modifications characterized by large surface renovations in the caput epididymis and the acquisition of new compounds at the surface membrane as the sperm travel through the terminal part of this organ. Because sperm possess a limited biosynthetic capability, it would appear that the interactions of the spermatozoa with the surrounding fluid play a major role in these changes in the surface membrane.

Evolution of the Sperm Surface Membrane Compounds

Testicular sperm surface membrane is characterized by the presence of major species-specific high-molecular-weight proteins [105–115 kd in the boar, Dacheux et al., 1989; 95–119 kd in the ram, Dacheux and Voglmayr, 1983; 110–130 kd in the rat, Jones et al., 1981; 110 kd in man, Dacheux et al., 1987]. Most of these testicular surface proteins gradually disappear in the first part of the epididymis. Some other compounds are removed very soon, such as 75–97 kd compound in boar [Dacheux et al., 1989] (Fig. 3) and a 78–88 kd compound in the ram [Dacheux and Voglmayr, 1983]. Several mechanisms have been postulated to induce these changes on the sperm surface. Among these are enzymatic activities (either intra- or extracellular-like proteinases, glycosidases, and galactosyl-transferases) and the association of new exogenous compounds able to mask other surface polypeptides such as the 105–115 kd sperm surface glycoproteins in the boar [Dacheux et al., 1989]. However, most of the sperm membrane polypeptides that disappear from the surface are never found in the epididymal surrounding plasma and are probably degraded during their surface release.

The disappearance of these sperm surface proteins is sometimes associated with the appearance of new proteins. In the boar, the progressive decrease in the 170 and 160 kd compounds during epididymal transit is always associated with a progressive appearance of a new 135 kd surface compound characterized by a similar pI (7.2, Fig. 3) [Dacheux et al., 1989]. In the ram, a similar association has been described for two major 97 kd testicular sperm surface compounds (97a and 97b) for which the progressive disappearance is also linked to the appearance of a more glycosylated 97 kd surface polypeptide [Dacheux and Voglmayr, 1983]. A direct relationship between these compounds has not been established, but their association may be linked to structural modifications of the sugar residues.

New Major Glycoproteins and Sialoproteins on the Sperm Surface

Among the new membrane surface compounds of the sperm appearing during epididymal transit, most are characterized by a low molecular weight (range, 14–36 kd) and a high glycosylation level. Such events have been described in the rat [Brown et al., 1983; Brooks and Tiver, 1984], the ram [Voglmayr et al., 1982, 1985], the hamster [Moore and Hartman, 1986], the chimpanzee [Gould et al., 1984], and the human [Dacheux et al., 1987] sperm. In the boar, detailed two-dimensional gel electrophoresis studies of the sperm surface proteins reveals that numerous compounds are present in these molecular weight ranges. Most of these low-molecular-weight proteins appear to be species specific, as no cross-reactivity has been obtained with antibodies.

For those surface proteins that have been characterized, their features on the sperm surface are variable. Some bind to the membrane only during epididymal transit and disappear in the female tract [Gould et al., 1984] but others, like a 28 kd compound in the surface membrane of boar sperm (Fig. 7), are still present in the membrane during oocyte fertilization (Dacheux, unpublished data).

Relationships Between the Epididymal Fluid and the Sperm Surface

In several species (mice, rat, ram, rabbit, boar, chimpanzee, human), a similarity between the protein composition of the sperm membrane and epididymal fluid has been assessed by comparison of electrophoretic characteristics. With this method, several major epididymal proteins and surface membrane compounds were noted as related proteins [Tezon et al., 1985; Iusem et al., 1989; Hall and Killian, 1989; Russell et al., 1984; Young et al., 1985]. The number of associated compounds is variable according to the species and the authors. In the boar, three membrane proteins in the sperm from caput and two from corpus and cauda were associated with epididymal compounds. However, complete identification of proteins cannot be assumed only on electrophoretic criteria, because comparisons become very hazardous with high polymorphic compounds. The epididymal origin of several membrane proteins has been confirmed with immunological techniques by concomitant localization of compounds both in the epithelium cell and on the sperm surface. Nevertheless, some compounds that are electrophoretically similar appear to be immunologically different, such as the major 135 kd compound present both on the sperm surface and in the fluid in the boar (Okamura and Dacheux, unpublished data).

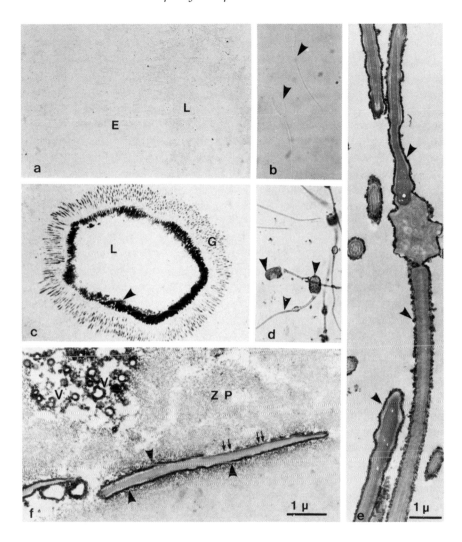

Fig. 7. Immunolocalization with a monoclonal antibody and immunoperoxidase staining of a 28 kd protein in the boar epididymal tissue and of sperm
during epididymal maturation and fertilization. **a,b:** The 28 kd protein is not
present in the epithelium tissue (E), lumen (L) or spermatozoa (arrowheads) of
the epididymal caput. **c:** In the corpus region, the 28 kd compound is localized
in the Golgi complex (G) of the epithelial cells and in the lumen (L) and is
essentially associated with the adluminal border of the epithelium (arrowhead).
d,e: The protein appears on the sperm (head and flagellum) from the corpus of
the epididymis and is associated with the plasma membrane (arrowheads). **f:**
After in vivo fertilization, the 28 kd protein is localized on/in the plasma membrane of sperm (arrowheads) inside the zona pellucida (ZP), except for the
portions of membrane (arrows) associated with the acrosomal reaction that are
found as positive vesicles (V) at the periphery of the oocyte.

Relationship Between Sperm Surface Changes and Sperm Activities

The relationship between the changes in sperm surface and the motility and fertilizing abilities of the sperm is still obscure. However, comparisons between different sequential sperm transformations and physiological sperm properties suggest some associations such as appearance of new surface glycopeptides and the forward progressive motility or the fertilizing ability of the gametes (Fig. 3) [Dacheux et al., 1983]. However, the simultaneity of several membrane modifications makes correlations very hazardous. No clear relationship has been established between these membrane changes and variations of an internal second messenger (cAMP or Ca^{2+}) that may be involved in the control of the flagella motility.

CONCLUSION

Epididymal maturation represents the last stages in the spermatozoa for acquisition of the ability to fertilize an oocyte. Following the dramatic cellular changes that characterize spermiogenesis, these postgonadal cellular differentiations are composed of a series of fine biochemical modifications that result in the activation or the control of enzymatic mechanisms already present in the immature gametes. The regulation of flagellar movement is one of the more important steps for the spermatozoa. Flagellar movement mechanisms are a complex and highly integrated process. Our knowledge of the sliding tubule mechanism is very limited, and its regulation is far from being understood. Links between cAMP or Ca^{2+} signals and sliding tubules are as yet unknown. External influences on sperm maturation are now fully evident, but the origin and the nature of the signals for the sperm changes are still uncertain. Analysis of the compositions of the epididymal fluid and sperm surface proteins provides numerous candidates that may mediate the control of the biochemical changes of the sperm. However, further experiments are needed to clarify the exact mechanisms by which the epididymal spermatozoa become motile and fertile.

REFERENCES

Amann R, Hay S, Hammersted S (1982): Yield, characteristics, motility and cAMP content of sperm isolated from seven regions of ram epididymis. Biol Reprod 27:723–733.

Babcock DF, Rufo GA, Lardy HA (1983): Potassium-dependent increases in cytosolic pH stimulate metabolism and motility of mammalian sperm. Proc Natl Acad Sci USA 50:1327–1331.

Besançon J, Dacheux JL, Paquin R, Tremblay RR (1985): Major contribution of epididymis to glucosidase content of ram seminal plasma. Biol Reprod 33:296–301.

Bork K, Chevrier C, Paquignon M, Jouannet P, Dacheux JL (1988): Analyse de la motilité et du mouvement flagellaire des spermatozoïdes de verrat au cours du transit épididymaire. Reprod Nutr Dev 28:1307–1315.

Brokaw CJ (1979): Calcium-induced asymmetrical beating of Triton-demembranated sea-urchin sperm flagella. J Cell Biol 82:401–411.

Brooks DE, (1979): Carnitine, acetylcarnitine and the activity of carnitine acyltransferase in seminal plasma and spermatozoa of men, rams and rats. J Reprod Fertil 56:667–673.

Brooks DE, Tiver K, (1984): Analysis of surface proteins of rat spermatozoa during epididymal transit and identification of antigens common to spermatozoa, rete testis fluid and cauda epididymal plasma. J Reprod Fertil 71:249–257.

Brown CR, Von Glos KI, Jones R (1983): Changes in plasma membrane glycoproteins of rat spermatozoa during maturation in the epididymis. J Cell Biol 96:256–226.

Carr DW, Usselman MC, Acott S (1985): Effects of pH, lactate and viscoelastic drag on sperm motility: A species comparison. Biol Reprod 33:588–595.

Chevrier C, Dacheux JL (1987): Analysis of the flagellar bending waves of ejaculated ram sperm. Cell Motil Cytoskeleton 8:261–273.

Chevrier C, Dacheux JL (1989): Analysis of the flagellar bending waves during the maturation of ram sperm in the epididymis. Cell Motil Cytoskeleton (submitted).

Dacheux JL, Chevrier C, Lanson Y (1987): Motility and surface transformations of human spermatozoa during epididymal transit. Ann NY Acad Sci 513:560–563.

Dacheux JL, Dacheux F, Paquignon M (1989): Changes in sperm surface membrane and luminal protein fluid content during epididymal transit in the boar. Biol Reprod 40:635–651.

Dacheux JL, Paquignon M (1980): The effects of caffeine on ram and boar spermatozoa: Influence of their stage of maturation and the medium; initiation of progressive motility of testicular spermatozoa. In Steinberger E, Steinberger A (eds): Testicular Development: Structure and Function. New York: Raven Press, pp 513–522.

Dacheux JL, Paquignon M, Combarnous Y (1983): Head-to-head agglutination of ram and boar epididymal spermatozoa and evidence for an epididymal antagglutinin. J Reprod Fertil 67:181–189.

Dacheux JL, Voglmayr JK (1983): Sequence of sperm cell surface differentiation and its relationship to exogenous fluid proteins in the ram epididymis. Biol Reprod 29:1033–1046.

Eshel D, Brokaw CJ (1987): New evidence for a "biased baseline" mechanism for calcium-regulated asymmetry of flagellar bending. Chem Motil Cytoskeleton 7:160–168.

Garbers DL, Lust WD, First NL, Lardy HA (1971): Effects of phosphodiesterase inhibitors and cyclic nucleotides on sperm respiration and motility. Biochemistry 19:1825–1831.

Gibbons IR (1981): Transient flagellar waveforms during intermittent swimming in sea urchin sperm. II. Analysis of tubule sliding. J Musc Res Cell Motil 2:83–130.

Gould KG, Young LG, Hinton BT (1984): Alteration in surface charge of chimpanzee sperm during epididymal transit and at ejaculation. Arch Androl 6:20–24.

Hall JC, Killian GJ (1989): 2-Dimensional gel electrophoretic analysis of rat sperm membrane: Interaction with cauda epididymal fluid. J Androl 10:64–76.

Hinton BT, Hernandez H (1985): Selective luminal absorption of l-carnitine from the proximal regions of the rat epididymis. possible relationships to development of sperm motility. J Androl 6:300–305.

Hinton BT, Snoswell AM, Setchell BP (1979): The concentration of carnitine in the luminal fluid of the testis and epididymis of the rat and some other mammals. J Reprod Fertil 61:59–64.

Horowitz JA, Voulalas P, Wasco W, Macleod J, Paupard MC, Orr GA (1989): Biochemical and immunological characterization of the flagellar-associated regulatory subunit of a type-II cyclic adenosine 5'-monophosphate-dependent protein kinase. Arch Biochem Biophys 270:411–418.

Iusem ND, Pineiro L, Blaquier JA, Belocopitow E (1989): Identification of a major secretory glycoprotein from rat epididymis—Interaction with spermatozoa. Biol Reprod 40: 307–316.

Jeulin C, Soufir JC, Marson J, Paquignon M, Dacheux JL (1987): The distribution of carnitine and acetylcarnitine in the epididymis and epididymal spermatozoa of the boar. J Reprod Fertil 79:523–529.

Johansen L, Bohmer T (1979): Motility related to the presence of carnitine/acetyl-carnitine in human spermatozoa. Int J Androl 2:202–210.

Jones R, Brown CR, Von Glos KI, Gaunt SJ (1981): Development of a maturation antigen on the plasma membrane of rat spermatozoa in the epididymis and its fate during fertilization. Exp Cell Res 156:31–44.

Lindemann CB, Goltz JS, Kanous KS (1987): Regulation of activation state and flagellar wave form in epididymal rat sperm: Evidence for the involvement of both Ca^{2+} and cAMP. Cell Motil Cytoskeleton 8:324–332.

Lindemann CB, Kanous KS (1989): Regulation of mammalian sperm motility. Arch Androl 23:1–22.

Moore HDM, Hartmann TD (1986): In vitro development of the fertility ability of hamster epididymal spermatozoa after co-culture with epithelium from the proximal cauda epididymis. J Fertil Reprod 78:347–352.

Okamura N, Tajima Y, Soejima A, Masuda H, Sugita Y, (1985): Sodium bicarbonate in seminal plasma stimulates the motility of mammalian spermatozoa through direct activation of adenylate cyclase. J Biol Chem 260:9699–9705.

Okamura N, Talima Y, Sugita Y (1988): Decrease in bicarbonate transport activities during epididymal maturation of porcine sperm. Biochem Biophys Res Commun 157:1280–1287.

Okuno M, Brokaw CJ (1981): Calcium-induced change in form of demembranated sea-urchin sperm flagella immobilized by vanadate. Cell Motil 3:349–362.

Paquignon M, Dacheux JL, Jeulin C, Fauquenot A (1983): Laser light scattering study of spermatozoa motility of domestic animals. In André J (ed): The Sperm Cell. The Netherland: Martinus Nijhoff, pp 332–335.

Pariset C, Feinberg J, Dacheux JL, Oyen O, Jahnsen T, Weinman S (1989): Differential expression and subcellular localization for subunits of cAMP-dependent kinase during ram spermatogenesis. J Cell Biol 109:1195–1205.

Pariset CC, Feinberg J, Dacheux JL, Weinman S (1985): Changes in calmodulin level and cAMP-dependent protein kinase activity during epididymal maturation of ram spermatozoa. J Reprod Fertil 74:105–112.

Pholpramool C, Chaturapanich G (1979): Effect of sodium and potassium concentrations and ph on the maintenance of motility of rabbit and rat epididymal spermatozoa. J Reprod Fert 57:245–251.

Russell LD, Peterson RN, Hunt W, Strack LE (1984): Posttesticular surface modifications and contributions of reproductive tract fluids to the surface polypeptide composition of boar spermatozoa. Biol Reprod 30:959–978.

Schoff PK, Cheetham J, Lardy HA (1989): Adenylate kinase activity in ejaculated bovine sperm flagella. J Biol Chem 264:6086–6091.

Tash JS, Kadar SS, Means AR (1984): Flagellar motility requires the cAMP-dependent phosphorylation of a heat-stable NP-40-soluble 56 kd protein, axokinin. Cell 38:551–559.

Tezon JG, Ramella F, Cameo MS, Vazquez MH, Blaquier JA (1985): Immunochemical localization of secretory antigens in the human epididymis and their association with spermatozoa. Biol Reprod 32:591–597.

Vijarayagavhan S, Critchlow LM, Hoskins DD (1985): Evidence for a role for cellular alkalinization in the cyclic adenosine 3',5'-monophosphate-mediated initiation of motility in bovine caput spermatozoa. Biol Reprod 32:489–500.

Voglmayr JK, Fairbanks G, Vespa DB, Collela JR (1982): Studies on the surface modifications in the ram spermatozoa during the final stages of differentiation. Biol Reprod 26:483–500.

Voglmayr JK, Sawyer RF, Dacheux JL (1985): Glycoproteins: A variable factor in the surface transformation of ram spermatozoa during epididymal transit. Biol Reprod 33:165–176.

Wong PYD, Lee WM (1983): Potassium movement during sodium-induced motility initiation in the rat caudal epididymal spermatozoa. Biol Reprod 28:206–212.

Young LG, Hinton BT, Gould KG (1985): Surface change in chimpanzee sperm during epididymal transit. Biol Reprod 32:399–412.

DISCUSSION

DR. MOORE: It has been known for some time that if you ligate the epididymis it is possible to bring about an increase in the progressive motility of sperm in the more distal region. I have always thought this indicated the intrinsic development of progressive motility. However, when we try to bring about this progressive motility by in vitro cocultures with epithelium, we have always failed. In your opinion, is this an intrinsic change in the flagellum, or is it dependent on secretions from the epididymis?

DR. DACHEUX: In the presence of epididymal proteins, testicular and anterior caput epididymal spermatozoa never developed motility in vitro. When an intracellular increase of cAMP was induced in these cells, flagellar movements appeared. Such observations suggested that the motility apparatus is functional very soon. An external signal has to be present to induce directly or indirectly an intracellular trigger of the motility.

10

Changes in Sperm-Specific Antigens During Epididymal Maturation

Mónica S. Cameo, Adriana Dawidowski, Claudia Sanjurjo, Fernanda Gonzalez Echeverria, and Jorge A. Blaquier

Mammalian spermatozoa develop the capacity to fertilize oocytes as they pass through the epididymis [reviewed by Cooper, 1986]. One expression of this maturation phenomenon are the changes in antigenic properties accorded the spermatozoa during epididymal transit as a result of the addition, subtraction, and modification of antigens on the cell surface. The epididymis actively participates in this maturation process and does not simply provide an adequate millieu for the expression of a potential capacity of the spermatozoon. However, the nature of the maturation mediators is still the subject of investigation, and the mechanisms involved in the production of the functional changes are poorly understood.

Substantial progress has been achieved in recent years with the demonstration that androgen-induced glycoproteins secreted by the epididymis become associated with the surface of spermatozoa during maturation. Synchronous with this interaction, the cells develop the fertilizing ability characteristic of mature sperm. Based on these observations, a possible biological role for these substances as mediators of maturation is reasonable.

The direct action of androgen-induced epididymal glycoproteins in maturation has been an important advance. Immature spermatozoa from the proximal epididymal segments gain the ability to bind the zona pellucida and fertilize ova after incubation with preparations of secreted epididymal glycoproteins [hamster, Cuasnicú et al.,

Gamete Interaction: Prospects for Immunocontraception, pages 129–141

TABLE I. Relationship Between Purification of Hamster
Epididymal Proteins EP2-EP3 and Their Biological Activity[a]

Purification step	EP2-EP3 (%)[b]	Biological activity[c]
Starting material	6	1
I	16	35
II	60	245

[a]Reproduced from Blaquier et al. [1986], with permission of the publisher.
[b]Percent EP2-EP3 in total protein.
[c]Calculated from the dose required to double the fertilizing capacity of distal corpus spermatozoa.

1984b; Gonzalez Echeverria et al., 1984; Moore and Hartman, 1986; rat, Orgebin-Crist and Fournier-Delpech, 1982].

Most preparations used for these experiments were not purified to homogeneity, but the biological activity of the preparations (induction of fertilizing capacity), copurified with epididymal secretory proteins in the hamster through several purification steps (Table 1), reduces the possibility that contaminants are responsible for the effect observed [Blaquier et al., 1986].

Supporting evidence for a biological role of epididymal glycoproteins in maturation was obtained using the alternative approach of blocking the biological activity of these antigens with specific antibodies. Such an effect was obtained by Fournier-Delpech et al. [1985] in rats immunized in vivo with an epididymal antigen and also by directly reacting mature spermatozoa with antisera directed against epididymal proteins [Cuasnicú, et al., 1984a].

From these data a hypothesis evolved suggesting the participation of epididymal proteins, incorporated onto the surface of spermatozoa, in the development of sperm-oocyte recognition sites. Most of the following data summarize the results obtained during the course of our investigations aimed at extending this kind of knowledge.

SPERM MATURATION IN THE HUMAN EPIDIDYMIS

Earlier studies in animals have only recently been supported by data demonstrating the occurrence of analogous phenomena to human spermatozoa during epididymal transit. Hinrichsen and Blaquier [1980] and Moore et al. [1983] were able to demonstrate the capacity to penetrate zona-free hamster ova as spermatozoa passed through the successive segments of the human epididymis (Fig. 1). These observations were interpreted as indicative of the existence of

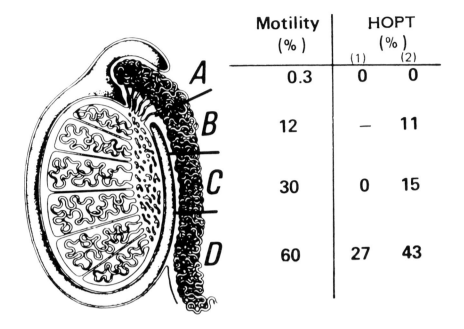

	Motility (%)	HOPT (%)	
		(1)	(2)
A	0.3	0	0
B	12	—	11
C	30	0	15
D	60	27	43

Fig. 1. Spermatozoa maturation in the human epididymis. HOPT: Percent penetration in the zona-free hamster oocyte penetration test. Data are from 1: Hinrichsen and Blaquier [1980] and 2: Moore et al. [1983].

a process of maturation (acquisition of fertilizing capacity) in the human epididymis.

This idea, however, has been recently challenged by publications reporting the fertilizing capacity of spermatozoa recovered from the most proximal segments of the epididymis (even fron rete testis) in patients undergoing surgical treatment for epididymal obstruction [Silber, 1988; Silber et al., 1988]. The authors speculated that human sperm may be fertile as they leave the testis.

In this respect, we raise a cautionary note about the validity of drawing physiological conclusions from a pathological model. Indeed, we suggest it is appropriate to study sperm maturation in a situation in which the flow of sperm through the epididymis is unimpaired, such as that found in samples from patients undergoing orchiectomy as treatment for prostatic carcinoma. Samples obtained from obstructed patients, an abnormal condition that usually has a long evolution that may provoke adaptive functional changes in the organ, are not appropriate material in which to study maturation.

Data discussed below indicate that the antigens secreted by the proximal segments of the epididymis tend to accumulate in the epi-

TABLE II. Some Characteristics of Androgen-Induced Proteins From the Human Epididymis[a]

	Relative mobility R (albumin)				
	0.31	0.43	0.68	0.81	1.01
Molecular mass (kd) (native form)	38	21	69	13.9	29
Isoelectric point	5.8	6.2	5.1	6.8	6.8
Binding of concanavalin A	+	+	+	+	−
Present in sperm	+	+	−	−	+

[a]Reproduced from Tezón et al. [1985b], with permission of the publisher.

didymal plasma and on spermatozoa as they pass through the organ, suggesting a gradual incorporation of antigen from the surrounding millieu into the cells. In cases of obstruction, the reduced velocity of transit may permit completion of the association between sperm and antigen at a site proximal to where it is normally completed.

Because of the nature of the tissues used in our investigation, an organ culture technique permitting an adequate survival of cells was adapted for the human epididymis in our laboratory [Tezón and Blaquier, 1981]. Samples were obtained from patients undergoing orchiectomy for a valid medical reason who gave free, informed, written consent for the use of specimens.

When this preparation was stimulated with androgens, the response closely paralleled that obtained in androgen-stimulated castrated rats with respect to protein and nuclei acid synthesis [Tezón et al., 1982], trophic parameters [Vazquez et al., 1989], and preservation of androgen receptor number [Vazquez et al., 1986]. Faced with a remarkable lack of information about the physiology of the human epididymis, these results suggested that the data obtained with this preparation resembled the physiological effects of androgens.

Application of this procedure to 20 different human epididymides resulted in the identification of a group of proteins whose synthesis and secretion were consistently stimulated by the addition of physiological amounts of androgen to the cultures [Tezón et al., 1985b]. Some characteristics of these proteins in their native state are listed in Table 2.

These proteins were produced mainly in the proximal segments of the organ, and some became associated with spermatozoa [Tezón et al., 1985a]. Based on this observation, antigens were extracted from the surface of ejaculated spermatozoa, and a fraction corresponding to proteins of epididymal origin was used to raise a polyclonal antiserum (anti-KCl) in rabbits, the characteristics of which are given in Table 3. This antiserum localized the antigens mainly on the acroso-

TABLE III. Partial Characterization of Anti-KCl

1. Specific for the human epididymis: negative for human testis and prostate and for epididymides from other species
2. Specific for epididymal sperm: recognizes epididymal but not testicular spermatozoa
3. Species specific: negative for ejaculated sperm from eight other mammals
4. Recognizes epididymal antigens 17.6 and 18.7 kd

mal cap region of the ejaculated spermatozoon, with minor localizations on the midpiece and flagellum as revealed by indirect immunofluorescence.

POSSIBLE ROLE OF EPIDIDYMAL ANTIGENS ON SPERM–OOCYTE INTERACTION

The antiserum was applied to the study of the biological role of the antigens. In a first approach we compared the amount of antigens and their localization in spermatozoa isolated from semen samples from fertile donors and patients with unexplained infertility. Results indicated that, among the latter population, a subgroup could be identified in which the antigens were abnormally localized on spermatozoa, and the total antigen content of spermatozoa was significantly decreased [Blaquier et al., 1986], suggesting a relationship between infertility and defective antigen content or localization.

Recently we tested the effect of the antiserum on several aspects of sperm function. For this purpose we used ejaculates from normal fertile donors from which spermatozoa were selected by swim-up. This population was capacitated by overnight incubation in medium BWW supplemented with 3.5% human serum albumin (BWW-HSA) at room temperature. This was followed by incubation for 2 hr at 37°C in the same medium, to complete capacitation, prior to functional testing of spermatozoa. Unless noted otherwise, it was during this incubation period (2 hr at 37°C) that different aliquots of the swim-up were exposed to anti-KCl or to a control preparation of the immunoglobulin fraction of preimmune normal rabbit serum (NRS).

The most relevant initial finding was obtained with the zona-free hamster oocyte penetration test. Exposure of spermatozoa to anti-KCl, at a dilution of 0.098 mg protein/ml, significantly decreased (34% inhibition with respect to control) their ability to penetrate denuded hamster oocytes (Table 4). The inhibitory effect of the antiserum became maximal at a dilution containing 0.39 mg protein/ml

TABLE IV. Effect of Pretreatment of Capacitated Human
Spermatozoa With Anti-KCl or Normal Rabbit Serum (NRS)
Upon Their Ability to Penetrate Zona-Free Hamster Oocytes

Treatment		N	Oocytes (penetrated/total)	Percent penetration (mean + SD)	Inhibition (%)
Control		14	102/246	41.5 + 26.8	
NRS	1:6	8	54/160	33.8 + 20.8[a]	19
Anti-KCl	1:6	14	46/316	14.7 + 11.7[*,†]	65
	1:12	3	13/59	22.2 + 7.1[‡]	47
	1:24	3	15/56	26.8 + 8.7[‡]	34

[a]Not significantly different from control.
*$P < 0.005$ vs. control.
†$P < 0.005$ vs. NRS.
‡$P < 0.05$ vs. control.

(1:6, 65% inhibition) beyond which testing became unreliable because of agglutination of spermatozoa. The blocking effect was not reproduced by the control preparation of NRS used at the same dilutions.

Investigation of the mechanism by which the antiserum produced this effect led to the conclusion that motility parameters, both percent motile cells and linear velocity, were not altered by anti-KCl and that agglutination caused by the antiserum involved only 7% of the motile cells at the highest concentration used (while penetration was inhibited by 65%).

From these data it was concluded that inhibition of hamster ova penetration was not due to a decrease in the probability of sperm–ova interactions because of decreased sperm motility.

We proceeded to examine whether anti-KCl diminished the number of acrosome-reacted spermatozoa at the completion of the incubation period or caused a premature acrosome reaction, because both conditions may decrease ova penetration. The triple-stain technique of Talbot and Chacon [1981] was used for these experiments.

The rate of spontaneous acrosome reactions was found to be equal in control (8.9%), anti-KCl–exposed (9.7%), and NRS-exposed (9.4%) cells. Furthermore, anti-KCl did not modify the effect of human follicular fluid (hFF) as inducer of the acrosome reaction [Suarez et al., 1986]. In our conditions, exposure of capacitated spermatozoa to 25% hFF (in BWW-HSA) for 30 min at 37°C results in 22% of spermatozoa being acrosome reacted. Preincubation of aliquots of spermatozoa with anti-KCl did not change the rate of hFF-induced acrosome reactions.

These data led to the conclusion that inhibition of penetration of

TABLE V. Effect of Exposure of Human Sperm to Anti-KCl and
NRS Upon Their Ability to Bind Tightly to Zona-Free
Hamster Ova

Group	N	No. oocytes	Percent ova with bound sperm		
			<5	5–10	>10
Control	8	122	53	19	28
Anti-KCl	8	168	70	20	10*
NRS	5	107	26*	19	55*

*$P < 0.05$ vs. control.

denuded hamster oocytes by anti-KCl was not mediated by modifications of the proportion of acrosome-reacted cells during sperm–
ova coincubation.

In our standard procedure, hamster ova are subjected to three
wash steps after incubation with spermatozoa and prior to fixation.
Each step involves pipetting through a finely drawn glass Pasteur
pipette with the aim of dislodging loosely bound spermatozoa. Thus
the number of spermatozoa attached to the oolemma after fixation is
an indication of the tightness of binding between sperm and oocyte.

Table 5 shows a frequency distribution of oocytes with different
numbers (low, medium, high) of bound spermatozoa after incubation with aliquots of the same sperm sample treated with anti-KCl or
NRS. Treatment with NRS significantly increased the binding of
spermatozoa to oocytes while exposure to anti-KCl, at the same protein concentration and under identical conditions, significantly reduced the proportion of oocytes with large numbers of bound
sperm. In summary, the data presented suggest that binding of anti-
KCl to antigens on the sperm surface interferes with the attachment
of sperm to the oolemma, and, as a consequence, the number of
penetrated ova is decreased.

Exploring one step further, we began investigations on the effect
of treatment with anti-KCl on the ability of normal ejaculated spermatozoa to bind to the human zona pellucida. Human zonae are
collected from noninseminated spare oocytes obtained from in vitro
fertilization (IVF), gamete intrafallopian transfer (GIFT), or other assisted reproduction procedures. In our practice, no more than four
oocytes are fertilized or transferred, and requests for freezing of the
remaining gametes are rare. Therefore, many patients have excess
oocytes. After obtaining informed consent, oocytes are kept in culture for 24–48 hr in medium Ham-F-10 supplemented with 10%
serum from the patient to allow extrusion of the first polar body, the

TABLE VI. Effect of Preincubation of Capacitated Spermatozoa With Anti-KCl Upon Their Ability to Bind Tightly to the Human Zona Pellucida

Exp. No.	Sperm bound per zona		Percent inhibition
	Control	Anti-KCl	
1	15	1	93
2	10	3	70
3	42	16	62
4	11	2	82
Mean	19.5	5.5	77
SD	13	6	12

cumulus cells are removed by incubation with hyaluronidase, and the oocytes are stored in a solution of 1 M $MgCl_2$, 0.5 M $(NH_4)_2 SO_4$, 0.1% dextran, and 0.02% sodium azide at 4°C under a layer of mineral oil. This treatment is known to preserve the characteristics of the zona pellucida for several months and to render the oocytes nonviable [Yanagimachi et al., 1979]. Prior to use, oocytes are transferred to 2 ml BWW and left overnight at 4°C. Next morning, the cells are passed through two changes of fresh BWW for 30 min each, the last one containing 3.5% human serum albumin, and used for the binding assay.

For the binding assay, one to three oocytes are placed in 0.3 ml BWW-HSA containing $3-5 \times 10^5$ sperm/ml and incubated for 4–5 hr at 37°C in an atmosphere of 5% CO_2. At the end of this period oocytes are transferred to fresh BWW-HSA and repeatedly pipetted in and out of a finely drawn pipette to dislodge loosely bound spermatozoa. The oocytes are then mounted on a slide and slightly flattened with a coverslip to permit counting of firmly attached spermatozoa.

Table 6 depicts preliminary data (N = 4) showing a 77% inhibition in zona pellucida binding in aliquots of spermatozoa treated with anti-KCl. In spite of the error introduced by high individual variations in sperm binding among zonae, even when derived from the same patient, the results obviously indicate a tendency toward substantial inhibition of sperm–zona binding.

DISCUSSION

Data generated in our laboratory and by others demonstrate the existence of functional changes in human spermatozoa during epididymal transit, analogous to the process of maturation recognized in other mammals. During this journey the spermatozoon is changed by addition, removal, and modification of molecules onto its surface. By analogy to what is known in laboratory animals, we postulate that incorporation of epididymal secretory proteins onto sperm is a crucial step of maturation leading to the development of the ability to recognize and bind to the homologous oocyte.

Taken collectively, the results presented in the previous section support this postulate and suggest that the antigens recognized by anti-KCl have a substantial participation in the events immediately preceeding fertilization of the oocyte. Further experimentation is required to improve these initial data, which are mostly indirect and derived from determinations made using a polyclonal antiserum that may recognize other antigens. In spite of these shortcomings, the data also suggest that the antigens under study have the potential to become suitable candidates for an immunological approach to contraception. Furthermore, these molecules could also serve as markers of epididymal function and of sperm maturation.

REFERENCES

Blaquier J, Cameo M, Stephany D, Piazza A, Tezón J, Sherins R (1986): Abnormal distribution of epididymal antigens on spermatozoa from infertile men. Fertil Steril 47: 302–309.

Blaquier J, Piñeiro L, Dawidowski A, Echeverria FG (1986): The role of epididymal proteins in spermatozoa maturation in the hamster. Proceedings of the 12th World Congress on Fertility and Sterility, Singapore, p 912.

Cooper TG (1986): The Epididymis, Sperm Maturation and Fertilisation. Berlin: Springer Verlag, pp 1–8.

Cuasnicú P, Gonzalez Echeverria F, Piazza A, Cameo M, Blaquier J (1984a): Antibodies against epididymal glycoproteins block fertilizing ability in rat. J Reprod Fertil 72:467–471.

Cuasnicú P, Gonzalez Echeverria F, Piazza A, Piñeiro L, Blaquier J (1984b): Epididymal proteins mimic the androgenic effect on zona pellucida recognition by immature spermatozoa. J Reprod Fertil 71:427–431.

Fournier-Delpech S, Courot M, Dubois MP (1985): Decreased fertility and motility of spermatozoa from rats immunized with a pre-albumin, epididymis-specific glycoprotein. J Androl 6:246–250.

Gonzalez Echeverria F, Cuasnicú P, Piazza A, Piñeiro L, Blaquier J (1984): Addition of an androgen-free epididymal protein extract increases the ability of immature hamster spermatozoa to fertilize in vivo and in vitro. J Reprod Fertil 71:433–437.

Hinrichsen MJ, Blaquier JA (1980): Evidence supporting the existence of sperm maturation in the human epididymis. J Reprod Fertil 60:291–294.

Moore H, Hartman T (1986): In vitro development of the fertilizing ability of hamster epididymal spermatozoa after co-culture with epithelium from the proximal cauda epididymis. J Reprod Fertil 78:347–352.

Moore H, Hartman T, Pryor J (1983): Development of the oocyte penetrating capacity of spermatozoa in the human epididymis. Int J Androl 6:310–318.

Orgebin-Crist MC, Fournier-Delpech S (1982): Sperm-egg interaction: Evidence for maturational changes during epididymal transit. J Androl 3:429–433.

Silber S (1988): Pregnancy caused by sperm from vasa efferentia. Fertil Steril 49:373–375.

Silber S, Balmaceda J, Ord T, Zuluago C, du Plessis Y, Borrero C, Asch R (1988): Fertilizing capacity of epididymal sperm in the human. Abstract 017: Proceedings of the 44th Annual Meeting of the American Fertility Society.

Suarez S, Wolf DP, Meizel S (1986): Induction of the acrosome reaction in human spermatozoa by a fraction of human follicular fluid. Gamete Res 14:107–121.

Talbot P, Chacon R (1981): A triple stain technique for evaluating normal acrosome reactions of human sperm. J Exp Zool 215:201–208.

Tezón J, Blaquier J (1981): The organ culture of human epididymal tubules and their response to androgens. Mol Cell Endocrinol 21:233–242.

Tezón J, Cuasnicú PS, Scorticati C, Blaquier JA (1982): Development and characterization of a model system for the study of epididymal physiology in man. In: De Nicola AF, Blaquier JA, Soto RJ (eds): Physiopathology of Hypophysial Disturbances and Diseases of Reproduction. New York: Alan R Liss, Inc., pp 251–275.

Tezón J, Ramella E, Cameo M, Vazquez M, Blaquier J (1985a): Immunochemical localization of secretory antigens in the human epididymis and their association with spermatozoa. Biol Reprod 32:591–597.

Tezón J, Vazquez M, Piñeiro L, de Larminat M, Blaquier J (1985b): Identification of androgen-induced proteins in human epididymis. Biol Reprod 32:584–590.

Vazquez M, de Larminat M, Blaquier J (1986): Effect of androgens on androgen receptors in cultured human epididymis. J Endocrinol 111:343–348.

Vazquez M, de Larminat M, Blaquier J (1989): The effect of in vitro androgen stimulation upon androgen metabolism and trophic parameters in cultured human epididymis. Andrologia 21:9–17.

Yanagimachi R, Lopata A, Odom C, Bronson R, Mahi C, Nicolson G (1979): Retention of biologic characteristics of zona pellucida in highly concentrated salt solution: The use of salt-stored eggs for assessing the fertilizing capacity of spermatozoa. Fertil Steril 31:562–574.

DISCUSSION

DR. ALEXANDER: How do your findings compare with those of Dr. Silber and Dr. Asch, who have collected sperm from the epididymis for in vitro fertilization?

DR. BLAQUIER: I think that Dr. Silber and Dr. Asch are working with infertile men, which could be considered an abnormal model. They are working with obstructed epididymides in which the capability of the epididymal epithelium to produce antigens or proteins may be altered. As you, yourself, have observed, the caput epididymis produces very little antigen. Thus I think it is unfair to draw physiological conclusions, saying that the epididymis is not necessary in man for sperm maturation, from a pathological model. I still believe that, under normal physiological conditions, sperm maturation occurs in man.

DR. O'RAND: I think that you have presented very interesting results. When you extract sperm with 0.6 M KCl, do you know whether any membrane proteins actually extracted? In other words, is the membrane disrupted? Are these two epididymal antigens an integral part of the plasma membrane, or do they merely adhere to the surface?

DR. BLAQUIER: We have compared the KCl extracts with detergent or SDS extracts and found that they were entirely different. As a matter of fact, if we put KCl plus sperm in the cold for only a half an hour, it extracts very little protein. I think that that treatment with 0.6 M KCl is not strong enough to extract integral proteins from the membrane, although I cannot be sure.

DR. O'RAND: I am also curious to know if you have any information on whether patients with antisperm antibodies have antibodies to these epididymal antigens.

DR. BLAQUIER: This is one of our research projects, but at present but we do not have any information.

DR. ISOJIMA: Most humans have immobilizing antibodies against a carbohydrate portion. It is very rare to raise the antibody against the peptide portion. What is your interpretation regarding the reaction to carbohydrate in your extract?

DR. BLAQUIER: I believe that the antibody is raised against the peptide portion, although I am not entirely sure. Nonetheless, it is not a monoclonal antibody, so it is not monospecific. Thus, because it recognizes at least two different antigens, I am unable to answer your questions.

DR. ISOJIMA: You showed an in vitro fertilization case. We have several cases in which the oocyte is the problem; oocytes are not always normal, so sperm may never be able to fertilize them.

DR. BLAQUIER: That was controlled for, Dr. Isojima. In two of the previous in vitro fertilization attempts, oocytes after failing to fertilize with the husband's semen were exposed to donor semen and fertilized, although they did not give rise to a pregnancy.

DR. VASQUEZ: Can you say something about the modification or inhibition of binding to the oolema and the redistribution of the antigen in the membrane after this antibody application?

DR. BLAQUIER: The only information that we have on the behavior of the antibody during capacitation is on sperm recovered after IVF attempts that are supposedly fully capacitated, or as capacitated as possible under seminatural conditions. We find a very marked decrease in the amount of antigen on the surface of sperm, although the antigen does not disappear entirely.

DR. VASQUEZ: With respect to the specific IVF case presented, did you not expect that the presence of this extract of protein from these extra sperm would be having some latent affects on antigen binding as previously shown in detail in your positive results?

DR. BLAQUIER: That is an interesting point. We had other aliquots of the sperm incubated with different fluids—human follicular fluid, donor semen, seminal plasma—and apparently there were no obvious stimulatory effects of this incubation scheme. The sperm sample incubated with the KCl extract was exactly the same in terms of motility, a factor that we can appreciate readily. We are running zona pellucida–binding assays using sperm treated or not with the extract.

DR. VASQUEZ: The antigens that are present on the surface of the sperm remain intact because of the presence of epididymal secretions, whereas those seminal secretions don't. Maybe other proteins produced in the male tract or even in the female tract can be modified and therefore are not intact at the time of presentation, and perhaps your extract is preventing this?

DR. BLAQUIER: Acting as a decapacitation factor of sorts?

DR. VASQUEZ: Well, yes.

DR. MAZZOLLI: What about your antigen after the acrosomal reaction? Does it disappear or remain on the surface?

DR. BLAQUIER: That's what we discussed one moment ago. A large proportion of the antigen goes, but some remains on the sperm surface.

DR. MAZZOLLI: I thought you suggested, some years ago, that these antigens disappeared.

DR. BLAQUIER: Well, fortunately, with better methods, we have found that there is indeed antigen on the sperm surface.

MR. ADOYO: In your method of KCl antigen extraction, how did you establish the surface nature of these antigens?

DR. BLAQUIER: Essentially, there are several methods of extraction of surface proteins. We selected the mildest method, one that does not destroy the cell. The membrane is not in too good a shape after extracting with KCl, but it is not destroyed. And the organelles are intact. As such, we presume that we are not extracting anything from inside of the cell. I think that the most obvious evidence is evaluation of the biological activity of the antibody on swim-up sperm, which are inhibited in penetrating hamster eggs or the zona pellucida. It must be a surface protein, because antibodies will not get into the cells.

MR. ADOYO: Did you carry out any procedure, for example, EM, to check whether these sperms were not in any way damaged and that the membrane was still intact postextraction?

DR. BLAQUIER: We have planned to carry on EM localization studies, but, thus far, we have not.

11

Potential Contraceptive Use of an Epididymal Protein That Participates in Fertilizaton

Patricia S. Cuasnicú, Daniela Conesa, and
Leonora Rochwerger

A growing body of evidence supports the concept that epididymal secretory glycoproteins in the sperm surface are modified during epididymal maturation [Lea et al., 1978; Olson and Hamilton, 1978; Kohane et al., 1980b; Moore, 1980, 1981; Gonzalez Echeverria et al., 1982; Tezon et al., 1985]. The role of epididymal factors as mediators of sperm maturation has been supported by data showing that the addition of these proteins to immature rat and hamster spermatozoa is accompanied by an increase in their ability to recognize the zona pellucida [Orgebin Crist and Fournier-Delpech, 1982; Cuasnicu et al., 1984a,c] and to fertilize [Gonzalez Echeverria et al., 1984; Moore and Hartmann, 1986] and by the antifertility effect of specific antibodies against them [Moore, 1981; Cuasnicu et al., 1984b].

Because epididymal proteins become associated with maturing spermatozoa, they may possess the requisite specificity for a true block to male fertility. Moreover, immunologic approaches might well be translated to the female tract, because immunity to epididymal sperm surface glycoproteins could perhaps even more readily suppress some aspect of sperm function in the female, preventing fertilization.

The main component of the secreted epididymal glycoproteins that associates with sperm in the rat has been highly purified and characterized in our laboratory [Garberi et al., 1979]. Protein DE,

Gamete Interaction: Prospects for Immunocontraception, pages 143–153

with a molecular weight (MW) of 37,000, is synthetized and secreted in an androgen-dependent manner by the epithelium of the proximal segments of the epididymis [Kohane et al., 1980a]. Indirect immunofluorescence (IIF) experiments with a specific antibody against DE raised in rabbits (anti-DE) revealed the localization of this protein over the head of the sperm [Garberi et al., 1979] and demonstrated that rat sperm first become coated with DE as they leave the initial segment and then remain coated throughout epididymal transit [Kohane et al., 1980b]. Further ultrastructural studies by SEM demonstrated that DE is localized on the external surface of the sperm plasma membrane covering the acrosomal region of the sperm head [Cameo et al., 1986]. Although the partial loss of DE obtained under capacitating conditions first suggested that DE might act as a decapacitation factor [Kohane et al., 1980b], the reduction of fertilization obtained by exposure of sperm to anti-DE prior to uterine insemination [Cuasnicu et al., 1984b], together with the permanence of a remnant of DE on the acrosome-reacted sperm [Cameo et al., 1986], opened the possibility of a different role for this protein in the process of fertilization itself. Furthermore, recent results indicating that protein DE redistributes to the equatorial segment of the sperm head during capacitation (Cuasnicú and Rochwerger, in press) suggest the possible involvement of this protein in a more specific event such as interaction of sperm with the oolema, since sperm–egg fusion occurs through this region of the sperm head [Yanagimachi, 1981]. The aims of the present work, therefore, have been to examine the specific participation of protein DE in fertilization and to explore whether this epididymal protein might be of use in contraceptive vaccine development.

RESULTS

Participation of Protein DE in Fertilization

Although the reduction of fertilizing ability obtained in vivo by preincubation of sperm with anti-DE before insemination suggests that DE may play a role in fertilization, we cannot answer the question as to whether the antibody has interfered with capacitation or with fertilization itself. To investigate the participation of DE in the process of fertilization and, more specifically, in sperm–egg fusion, we conducted a series of experiments in vitro in which mature cauda spermatozoa were capacitated in vitro during 5 hr and then incubated with either normal rabbit IgG (NRIgG) or anti-DE during 15 min before the addition of zona-free eggs. Table 1 shows the results obtained using 2–5×10^5 sperm/ml and three different concentrations

TABLE 1. Effects of Anti-DE on Penetration of Zona-Free Eggs[a]

Antibody (mg/ml)	No. of eggs tested	Percent of zona-free eggs with			mean ratio spz/egg	Percent inhibition
		1 spz	2–7 spz	>7 spz		
Normal IgG	56	0	12	88	11.8	
0.25	45	0	87	13	4.9	58
0.50	33	9	82	9	3.9	67
0.75	41	7	93	0	2.9	75

[a]Mean ratio sperm/egg: number of incorporated sperm/number of eggs tested. Spz, spermatozoa.

of antibody (0.25, 0.50, and 1 mg/ml). We observed that under these conditions there was a significant reduction (75%) in the number of sperm incorporated per egg compared with control (2.9 vs. 11.8). When sperm concentration was reduced to 2–5 $\times$ 10^4 sperm/ml, conditions under which we obtained monospermia, an important inhibition (70%) in the percentage of penetrated eggs was obtained with the lowest anti-DE concentration (0.25 mg/ml) whereas complete inhibition (100%) was obtained with 1 mg/ml of the antibody (Fig. 1).

This inhibitory effect of anti-DE on sperm–egg fusion was not caused by an effect of the antibody on sperm motility, because no major change in motility or evidence of agglutination was observed in these preparations. Finally, when zona-free eggs were incubated with anti-DE for 45 min, washed, and then exposed to untreated sperm, no reduction in the number of incorporated sperm per egg or in the percentage of fertilized zona-free eggs was observed, indicating that the inhibition was not due to a direct effect of the antibody on the eggs.

Potential Contraceptive Use of DE

The results described above suggest that epididymal protein DE might play an important role in fertilization and, more specifically, in fusion events. However, two questions arise in considering whether this may have a potential use in efforts to develop new contraceptive approaches in the male or female and concern 1) the accessibility of epididymal spermatozoa to specific antibodies raised in males or of inseminated spermatozoa to antibodies produced by females and 2) the potential auto- or alloantigenicity of epididymal secretions.

With regard to the first point, both the oviduct and uterine cavity of the female tract are readily accessible to circulating antibodies [McAnulty and Morton, 1978; Saling and Waibel, 1985]. Therefore, passive or active immunization of females might effectively interfere

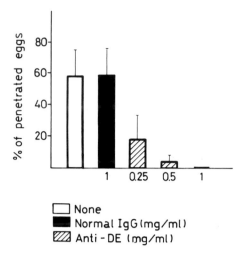

Fig. 1. Effect of anti-DE on the percentage of penetration of zona-free eggs. Mature cauda spermatozoa were capacitated in vitro during 5 hr and then incubated during 15 min at a concentration of 2–5 10⁴ sperm/ml in medium alone or medium containing either 1 mg/ml of normal rabbit IgG or different concentrations of the specific antibody against DE (anti-DE). Zona-free eggs were then added to the sperm suspensions and the percentage of penetrated eggs determined.

with sperm–egg interaction, subsequent embryo development, or implantation. The entry of immunoglobulins into the epididymal lumen, however, remains controversial. A blood epididymal barrier does exist for large molecules [Alexander and Fulgham, 1978], including those given by passive immunization [Wong et al., 1983]. Nevertheless, the level of specific IgG in epididymal fluid detected after active immunization with a potent antigen was significantly greater than that reported in testicular fluid (reaching a calculated ratio of 40,000 molecules IgG/spermatozoa) and perhaps great enough to affect spermatozoa if directed against some related component [Weininger et al., 1982]. If a similar phenomenon occurred in the rat, the concentration of IgG would be enough to neutralize the estimated 400–600 molecules of rat epididymal 32K protein bound per spermatozoa [Wong and Tsang, 1982].

The second issue, the isoantigenicity of epididymal components, is also controversial. Fournier-Delpech et al. [1985] reported the presence of antibodies in the sera of 90% of the male rats actively immunized against an acidic epididymal glycoprotein and a concomitant reduction in their fertility. Esponda and Bedford [1985], on the other hand, reported that macromolecules secreted by the epididymis, including those that associate with spermatozoa, do not act as auto- or alloantigens, indicating the lack of promise of this approach as a contraceptive measure.

To investigate whether an in vivo immunologic interference with protein DE can suppress sperm function in either sex and prevent fertilization, male and female rats of different strains (Sprague-Dawley, Wistar, and Lewis) were immunized (subcutaneously and intramuscularly) with purified DE (50 or 100 μg) four times (initially with complete Freund's adjuvant) at intervals of 3 weeks. Two weeks after the last injection, the animals were bled to obtain the sera, and the presence of anti-DE was determined by immunodiffusion. To test fertility, control and immunized animals were mated at intervals with animals of proven fertility over a period of 6 months.

The results obtained are presented in Figure 2 and indicate that while none of the sera from Sprague-Dawley rats (not even those from animals injected with higher doses of DE: 250 μg) caused immunodiffusion bands (0/14), 92% (11 of 12) of the sera from Wistar and 93% (14 of 15) of those from Lewis immunized animals caused a positive reaction. The period elapsed until detection of the bands was dependent on the strain and on the amount of protein injected. While 5–11 and 1–2 days were needed for detection of reactions in Wistar animals injected with 50 and 100 μg of DE, respectively, the presence of antibodies was detected after only 1–2 days in the sera of Lewis animals injected with either 50 or 100 μg of the protein. We did not detect antibodies in any of the sera (0/18) of control animals.

The fertility of immunized animals was also different depending on the strain and dose employed. While all Sprague-Dawley animals were 100% fertile over a period of 6 months, Wistar animals reached a minimum fertility of 40% and 33% for males and females, respectively, and male and female Lewis rats were completely infertile 3–4 months after initial immunization. The reduction in fertility also correlates with the period required for detection of immunodifusion bands.

When analyzed for reversal of the contraceptive effect, results indicated that 70% of male Wistar and 60% of male Lewis rats had recovered their fertility 6 months after the initial injection. While 70% of the female Wistar rats had recovered their fertility after 6 months, none of the Lewis rats were yet fertile at the end of this period.

With the established procedures for in vitro fertilization of zona-free rat eggs, the inhibitory effects of sera from the infertile male and female Lewis rats (100 μg) were studied and evaluated. The results of the experiments indicate that, like anti-DE raised in rabbits, these sera (1/50) significantly decreased the percentage of fertilization com-

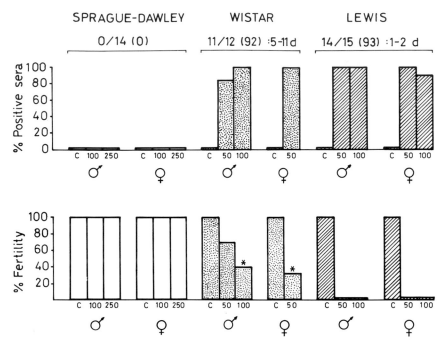

Fig. 2. Immunologic response and subsequent fertility of male and female rats of different strains after immunization against epididymal protein DE. Young adult male and female Sprague-Dawley, Wistar, and Lewis rats were immunized with 50 and 100 µg of purified protein DE subcutaneously and intramuscularly, four times at intervals of 3 weeks. Two weeks after the last injection, the immunized animals were mated with fertile animals and the presence of antibodies in their sera determined by immunodiffusion. The percentage of fertility was calculated as number of pregnant females/total number of mated females for males and as number of pregnant females/total number of matings for females at the time of minimum fertility (3–4 months after initial injection).

pared with that obtained with sera from control immunized animals (37% male and 38% female vs. 73% control, $P < 0.05$). In no instance did we detect evidence of immobilization or agglutination in these samples.

DISCUSSION

The overall aims of our work were to examine the participation of protein DE in fertilization and to explore its potential use as a contraceptive agent. Our results on the effect of anti-DE on penetration of zona-free eggs in vitro suggest that DE might play a specific role in the interaction of sperm with the oolema, because, depending on the concentration of sperm employed, the antibody was able either to significantly reduce the number of sperm incorporated per egg or to completely inhibit the zona-free egg penetration. However, because our assay detects the occurrence of fusion by observation of a subsequent event such as decondensation of sperm nucleus or pronucleus formation in the ooplasma, we cannot exclude the possibility that DE is involved in another event that occurs between fusion and sperm head swelling.

The participation of DE in fertilization together with previous evidence in favor of the possible entry of immunoglobulins into the epididymis encouraged us to explore whether this protein could be of use in contraceptive vaccine development. The present study indicates that epididymal protein DE is auto- and alloantigenic, because reactive antibody was detected in about 90% of the sera from male and female Wistar and Lewis rats. Moreover, immunization with DE resulted in a reduction of fertility dependent on the strain of rat and dose of DE injected, reaching values of 100% for male and female Lewis rats injected with the highest dose.

Our results indicating differences in the immune response to DE in different rat strains are consistent with the work of Bigazzi et al. [1977], who reported that antibodies to rat spermatozoa could be detected after vasectomy in the sera of some strains (Lewis, Wistar, Buffalo) but not others (Sprague-Dawley, Fisher), Lewis rats being the highest responders to sperm antigens. Furthermore, maximum incidence of sperm autoantibodies was detected 3 to 4 months after vasectomy, at which time maximum reduction of fertility was found in our immunized animals.

The mechanisms by which immunization with DE affected fertility in these animals remain to be elucidated. In females, antibodies may have interacted with inseminated sperm in the uterus or oviduct, preventing fertilization. In males, the reduction of fertility may have resulted from the interaction of immunoglobulins with epididymal spermatozoa or, alternatively, from an effect of the antibodies on the synthesis and/or secretory function of epididymal epithelial cells. We cannot exclude, however, the interaction of immunoglobulins with spermatozoa, after their release from the epididymis, at the moment of ejaculation. Further immunologic and histologic data must be obtained to answer these questions.

CONCLUSIONS AND PERSPECTIVES

The described experiments have to be considered in the context of developing a sperm immunologic contraceptive vaccine for humans, to be used as a reversible mode of contraception. Many sperm proteins have been previously tested as contraceptive immunogens with variable effects on fertility [Morton and McAnulty, 1979; Goldberg et al., 1981; Mettler et al., 1983; Primakoff et al., 1988]. While immunization of females with sperm antigens will probably only interfere with some aspect of sperm function, immunization of males with sperm proteins might compromise testicular function. In this regard, the use of specific epididymal antigens involved in the acquisition of sperm fertilizing ability represents a promising area for antisperm vaccine development in man. Finally, it is interesting to note that human functional analogs to DE have already been identified and are therefore likely candidates for use as contraceptive agents.

ACKNOWLEDGMENTS

This investigation was partially supported by OMS grant 87094.

REFERENCES

Alexander NJ, Fulgham DL (1978): Antibodies to spermatozoa in male monkeys: Mode of action. Fertil Steril 30:334–342.

Bigazzi PE, Kosuda L, Harnick L (1977): Sperm autoantibodies in vasectomized rats of different inbred strains. Science 197:1282–1283.

Cameo MS, Gonzalez Echeverria F, Blaquier JA, Burgos M (1986): Immunochemical localization of epididymal protein DE on rat spermatozoa: Its face after induced acrosome reaction. Gamete Res 15:247–257.

Cuasnicú PS, Gonzalez Echeverria MF, Piazza AD, Blaquier JA (1984a): Addition of androgens to cultured hamster epididymis increases zona recognition by immature spermatozoa. J Reprod Fertil 70:541–547.

Cuasnicú PS, Gonzalez Echeverria MF, Piazza AD, Cameo MS, Blaquier JA (1984b): Antibodies against epididymal glycoproteins block fertilizing ability in the rat. J Reprod Fertil 72:467–471.

Cuasnicú PS, Gonzalez Echeverria MF, Piazza AD, Pineiro L, Blaquier JA (1984c): Epididymal proteins mimic the androgenic affect on zona pellucida recognition by immature hamster spermatozoa. J Reprod Fertil 71:427–431.

Cuasnicú PS, Rochwerger L: Redistribution of sperm epididymal protein after capacitation and its participation in sperm–egg interaction. Proceedings of the VI International Symposium of Spermatology, Siena, Italy, 1990 (in press).

Esponda P, Bedford JM (1985): Epididymal fluid macromolecules do not act as auto or allo antigens. J Androl 6:359–364.

Fournier-Delpech S, Courot M, Dubois P (1985): Decreased fertility and motility of spermatozoa from rats immunized with a prealbumin epididymal specific glycoprotein. J Androl 4:246–250.

Garberi JC, Kohane AC, Cameo MS, Blaquier JA (1979): Isolation and characterization of specific rat epididymal proteins. Mol Cell Endocrinol 13:73–82.

Goldberg E, Wheat TE, Powell JE, Stevens VC (1981): Reduction of fertility in female baboons immunized with lactate dehydrogenase C$_4$. Fertil Steril 35:214–217.

Gonzalez Echeverria MF, Cuasnicú PS, Piazza AD, Pineiro L, Blaquier JA (1984): Addition of an androgen-free epididymal protein extract increases the ability of immature hamster spermatozoa to fertilize in vivo and in vitro. J Reprod Fertil 71:433–437.

Kohane AC, Cameo MS, Pineiro L, Blaquier JA (1980a): Distribution and site of production of specific proteins in the rat epididymis. Biol Reprod 23:181–187.

Kohane AC, Gonzalez Echeverria MF, Pineiro L, Blaquier JA (1980b): Interaction of proteins of epididymal origin with spermatozoa. Biol Reprod 23:737–742.

Lea OA, Petrusz P, French FS (1978): Purification and localization of acidic epididymal protein (AEG): A sperm coating protein secreted by the rat epididymis. J Androl Suppl 2:592–605.

McAnulty PA, Morton DB (1978): The immune response of the genital tract of the female rabbit following systemic and local immunization. J Clin Lab Immunol 1:255–260.

Mettler L, Czuppon AB, Tinneberg HR (1983): Immunization with spermatozoal peptide antigens resulting in immuno-suppression of fertility rates in female rats. Andrologia 15(6):670–675.

Moore HDM (1980): Localization of specific glycoproteins secreted by the rabbit and hamster epididymis. Biol Reprod 22:705–718.

Moore HDM (1981): Glycoprotein secretion of the epididymis in the rabbit and hamster: Localization on epididymal spermatozoa and the effect of specific antibodies on fertilization in vivo. J Exp Zool 2:77–85.

Moore HDM, Hartmann TD (1986): In vitro development of the fertilizing ability of hamster epididymal spermatozoa following co-culture with epithelium from proximal cauda epididymis. J Reprod Fertil 78:347–352.

Morton DB, McAnulty PA (1979): The effect on fertility of immunizing female sheep with ram sperm acrosin and hyaluronidase. J Reprod Immunol 1:61–72.

Olson GE, Hamilton DW (1978): Characterization of the surface glycoproteins of rat spermatozoa. Biol Reprod 19:26–35.

Orgebin Crist MC, Fournier-Delpech S (1982): Sperm-egg interaction: Evidence for maturational changes during epididymal transit. J Androl 3:429–433.

Primakoff P, Lathrop W, Woolman L, Cowan A, Myles D (1988): Fully effective contraception in male and female guinea pigs immunized with the sperm protein PH-20. Nature 335:543–546.

Saling PM, Waibel R (1985): Mouse sperm antigens that participate in fertilization III. Passive immunization with a single monoclonal antisperm antibody inhibits pregnancy and fertilization in vivo. Biol Reprod 33:537–544.

Tezon JG, Ramella E, Cameo MS, Vazquez MH, Blaquier JA (1985): Immunochemical localization of secretory antigens in the human epididymis and their association with spermatozoa. Biol Reprod 32:591–597.

Weininger RB, Fisher S, Rifkin J, Bedford JM (1982): Experimental studies on the passage of specific IgG to the lumen of the rabbit epididymis. J Reprod Fertil 66:251–258.

Wong PYD, Tsang AYF (1982): Studies on the binding of a 32K rat epididymal protein to rat epididymal spermatozoa. Biol Reprod 27:1239–1246.

Wong PYD, Tsang AYF, Fu WO, Lau HK (1983): Restricted entry of an anti-rat epididymal protein IgG into the rat epididymis. Int J Androl 6:275–282.

Yanagimachi R (1981): Mechanism of fertilization in mammals. In Mastroiani L, Biggers JB (eds): Fertilization and Embryonic Development In Vitro. New York: Plenum Press, pp 81–182.

DISCUSSION

DR. MITCHISON: One striking aspect of these data was that the male and the female rats seemed to have the same titer of antibodies. Is that correct?

DR. CUASNICÚ: The figures show the number of animals with the percentage of positive responses. The antibody titer was not given. What is similar is the number of positive animals in the male and female groups. But I don't know about the titer, because we did not make strict measurements of antibodies by ELISA or by any another specific assay.

DR. MITCHISON: If it is true that males and females are responding at the same rate, it would be nice to have quantitative information on the amount of antibodies. But, even if they are responding at the same rate, that tells us something very interesting about the compartmentalization of this protein. It seems as if the protein can't possibly be reaching the immune system, even in concentrations as low as 10^9 M or so—concentrations known to cause tolerization and that are expected to produce a difference between males and females. Also, you referred to earlier studies in which immunization to epididymal proteins did not cause an immune response. Was there any difference in the responses of males and females in that report?

DR. CUASNICÚ: Neither developed antibodies.

DR. DACHEUX: What is the key after the immunization if the initial suppression occurred after immunization?

DR. CUASNICÚ: These are very recent results. What I can say is that no rats showed signs of orchitis or epididymitis, and control animals behaved the same as immunized animals. We only have three animals at this time, so I cannot say anything else.

DR. ALEXANDER: It is very disturbing to see such variations between different strains of animals. It makes us cognizant of the necessity of using multiple antigens when developing a vaccine.

DR. CUASNICÚ: In the case of the Sprague-Dawley rats, which did not develop antibodies, it appeared that they never developed antibodies against anything, even after vasectomy. Thus it seems to be a problem of this strain and not of the antigen.

DR. ALEXANDER: Sprague-Dawley rats can respond to certain antigens. Furthermore, after vasectomy, they don't develop as many granulomas as some of the other strains of rats. Also, it could be variability in the total amount of sperm that are produced daily and thus in the amount of antigen available to activate the immune system.

12

Coating Antigens of Human Seminal Plasma Involved in Fertilization

Shinzo Isojima, Yoshiyuki Tsuji, Kinu Kameda,
Minoru Shigeta, and Sen-itiroh Hakomori

By 1950, Weil et al. had already reported that antihuman seminal plasma (HSP) antibodies (Abs) were generated when rabbits were immunized with washed sperm. They insisted that the ejaculated sperm were firmly coated with HSP components that were difficult to remove even by repeated washings.

In our studies of sperm immobilizing (SI) Abs in the sera of sterile women, we found that the majority of SI-positive patients' sera could be absorbed with HSP components (azoospermic semen), and a few patients' sera required washed sperm to remove SI activity [Isojima et al., 1968, 1972]. Many researchers have studied the membrane antigens of human sperm, but the HSP components firmly bound to sperm membrane should not be neglected. Our research group has been concerned with HSP antigens relevant to SI Abs; many women raised SI Abs to HSP as sperm-coating antigens (SCA), and we can easily obtain enough material for purification.

To obtain the sperm membrane antigen, a detergent must be used [Mettler and Shrabei, 1979], but a small amount of detergent contaminating the extract could be harmful for delicate SI tests. For these reasons, we studied HSP components by analyzing and purifying sperm antigens relevant to SI Abs.

Gamete Interaction: Prospects for Immunocontraception, pages 155–174
© 1990 Wiley-Liss, Inc.

CHARACTERISTICS OF SPERM ANTIGENS RELEVANT TO SPERM-IMMOBILIZING ANTIBODIES PRESENT IN STERILE WOMEN WITH UNKNOWN CAUSE

Twenty-five SI-positive sera samples (1 ml each) were absorbed with lyophylized azoospermic semen (50 mg). SI activites in all sera were found to be absorbed with azoospermic semen.

To analyze the chemical components of the corresponding antigen, the HSP was precipitated by saturation with $(NH_4)_2SO_4$, dialyzed against water, and the dialyzate then treated with trifluoromethane sulfonic acid (TFMS) according to the method of Edge et al. [1981]. Surprisingly, all 25 sera whose SI activities were absorbed with HSP retained their SI activities after absorption with TFMS-treated HSP (Table 1). To examine whether the peptide moiety of HSP might be damaged by treatment with TFMS, an antibody was generated in rabbits, and the antibody to TFMS-treated HSP reacted to the TFMS-treated HSP. From these results, we speculate that most sterile women having SI Abs generated Abs to the carbohydrate moiety of HSP. However, when the SI-positive patients' sera that could be absorbed with ejaculated sperm were used for absorption experiments with sperm treated with periodic acid [Kubota, 1987], only approximately half the sera retained their SI activity. This finding suggests, because periodic acid is effective only on type 1 neolactosamine, that the majority of SI-positive sera were raised to the sperm antigen composed of type 2 neolactosamine structure, and, among them, half of the SI-positive sera might be raised to the HSP antigen composed of both types 1 and 2 neolactosamines [Table 2].

ANALYSIS OF HSP BY IMMUNOELECTROPHORESIS

Shulman and Bronson [1969] studied the antigenic components of HSP. By utilizing immunoelectrophoresis, they defined several antigenic components using rabbit anti-HSP as a probe. We also analyzed antigens of HSP by immunoelectrophoresis of HSP protein using rabbit anti-HSP after absorption with human serum protein, extracts of human liver, and kidney tissues [Isojima et al., 1974]. In immunoelectrophoresis, six HSP-specific precipitation lines (HSP Nos. 3, 4, 6, 7, 9, and 10) were found. HSP No. 3 Ag proved to be lactoferrin [Heckman and Rümke, 1969], and the novel HSP No. 7 Ag, discovered by our group, was named *Ferrisplan* [Koyama et al., 1983]; it contained iron and shared antigenicity with human milk protein.

Previously, we found that the antibodies to sperm in women's sera

TABLE 1. Effect of TFMS Treatment of HSP on the Absorbing Activity of Sperm-Immobilizing Antibodies

No. of patients	Dilution of serum	Sperm motility (%) after absorption with		
		None	HSP	TFMS-HSP
1	1:2	8	50	15
2	1:2	27	64	25
3	1:2	16	51	11
4	1:2	15	50	13
5	1:2	17	50	17
6	1:4	23	43	21
7	1:4	11	63	22
8	1:4	6	30	8
9	1:4	13	45	19
10	1:4	21	47	18
11	1:4	18	47	19
12	1:4	18	57	16
13	1:8	10	59	15
14	1:8	21	56	17
15	1:8	4	51	10
16	1:8	12	37	12
17	1:8	10	47	17
18	1:16	7	48	12
19	1:16	18	58	26
20	1:16	15	35	21
21	1:64	40	71	48
22	1:64	3	72	4
23	1:64	21	49	29
24	1:64	7	43	15
25	1:64	12	40	10

were heterogeneous. Some only bound to sperm [Husted, 1975; Mathur et al., 1979; Moyes, 1969; Lynch et al., 1986; Bronson et al., 1984], and others were biologically relevant to SI and sperm agglutinating (SA) activities and also blocked sperm binding to the zona pellucida. The purification of HSP antigens therefore, could be very difficult, because sperm antibodies in patients and experimental animals are polyclonal. For these reasons, monoclonal antibodies (mAbs) to HSP were essential to analyze and to purify HSP antigens.

TABLE 2. Effect of Periodic Acid Treatment of Ejaculated Sperm on the Absorbing Activity of Sperm-Immobilizing Antibodies[a]

No. of patients	Dilution of serum	Sperm motility (%) after absorption with		
		None	Sperm	PA sperm
1	1:6	11	77	71
2	1:10	16	60	52
3	1:1	12	68	56
4	1:2	11	69	56
5	1:10	8	67	48
6	1:1.5	1	55	32
7	1:10	13	62	37
8	1:4	11	66	20
9	1:10	17	68	23
10	1:3	6	61	4

[a]PA, periodic acid. Washed sperm (20 × 10^6/ml) were treated in 10 mM PA for 10 min and then washed three times with PBS.

FIRST SUCCESS IN PRODUCING mAb TO HSP THAT POSSESSED A STRONG SI ACTIVITY

In 1980, we first succeeded in establishing rat–mouse heterohybridoma 1C4 against HSP, which secreted a strong SI mAb [Shigeta et al., 1980]. In 1979, Bechtol et al. produced a mouse mAb that recognized differentiation antigens of spermatogenesis in the mouse, but this was to mouse sperm, and no biological relevancy was demonstrated. Before creation of this mAb 1C4 (IgM), the relationship of anti-HSP to SI activity had not been accepted.

The mAb made a precipitin line with HSP protein and human milk protein by immunodiffusion, and both precipitin lines completely fused. By immunoelectrophoresis, the antigen corresponding to mAb 1C4 was defined as HSP No. 7 antigen (Ferrisplan), which contains iron in the molecule and is common with human milk. The purification of the antigen was performed by immunoaffinity chromatography on bound mAb 1C4, and it was purified 196 times. The purified antigen was fractionated in a 15 kd molecule by SDS-PAGE. However, this antigen is not a good candidate for immunological contraception, because the antigenicity is shared with human milk protein [Isojima et al., 1982].

TABLE 3. Characteristics of mAbs to HSP[a]

mAB	Ig subclass	Ag specificity	Ab to sperm	Purification of corresponding Ag (SIA/protein)	Nature corresponding Ag
1C4	IgM	HSP HM	Immobil. (+ + +) Aggl. (+)	196	Glycoprotein
2C6	IgM	HSP	Immobil. (+ + +) Aggl. (+ +) Fertil. block (+)	29	Glycoprotein
2E5	IgG3	HSP	Immobil. (+ +) Aggl. (+)	N.D.	Glycoprotein
2B6	IgG3	HSP	Immobil. (+ +) Aggl. (+)	N.D.	Glycoprotein

[a]HSP, human seminal plasma; mAb, monoclonal antibody; HM, human milk; Immobil., immobilization; Ag, antigen; Aggl., agglutination; N.D., not determined; SIA, sperm-immobilizing activity.

After production of mAb 1C4, mouse mAbs 2C6 (IgM), 2E5 (IgG3), and 2B6 (IgG3) were produced in our laboratory [Isojima, 1989]. The summarized characteristics of these mAbs are given in Table 3. All mAbs were HSP specific and possessed strong SI and SA activities. mAb 2C6 also blocked sperm binding to human zona pellucida. The binding of all mAbs to sperm were not inhibited by SI-positive patients' sera. One possibility is that the binding affinity of mouse mAbs is higher than that of human antibodies, and another is that the mouse recognizes a xenogenic epitope of HSP but humans recognize other isogenic epitopes of HSP. For these reasons, we attempted to produce a human mAb to HSP that had biological effects on sperm. In 1986, Kyurkchiev et al. succeeded in producing human mAbs to HSP possessing SA or SI activities, and Herr et al. [1985] studied the human mAbs to sperm that had binding activity to sperm by fusing lymphocytes of vasectomized men with mouse myeloma cells. Later Isojima et al. [1987] succeeded in establishing a stable human hybridoma that secreted human mAb H6-3C4, IgM(λ). This mAb expressed extremely high titers of SI (5,000 SI_{50}) [Isojima and Koyama, 1976] and SA (1:1,600 dilutions) activities. The SI activity of mAb H6-3C4 was absorbed only with HSP, ejaculated sperm, and fluid of seminal vesicle and epididymal tissue extracts, and the absorption of antibody with sperm was species specific except for boar sperm. The summarized characteristics of human mAb H6-3C4 are given in Table 4.

TABLE 4. Summary of Characteristic Properties
of Human mAb H6-3C4[a]

Immunoglobulin class	Human IgM(λ)
Sperm immobilization	+ + (SI_{50} unit = 5,000)
Sperm agglutination	+ + (1:1,600 dilution)
Antigen localization	Antibody absorption test
Genital organ	
Testis	−
Epididymis	+
Seminal vesicle	+
Prostate	−
Somatic organ	
Liver	−
Kidney	−
Spleen	−
Brain	−
Cells	
Ejaculated spermatozoa	+
Red blood cells	−
White blood cells	−
Body fluid	
Seminal plasma	+
Milk	−
Saliva	−
Serum	−

[a]+, positive; −, negative.

ANALYSES OF SPERM-COATING ANTIGENS CORRESPONDING TO mAbs PRODUCED AGAINST HSP

Binding Experiments With Lectins

HSP was treated with trypsin and passed through Sephacryl S-300. The fraction obtained (partially purified HSP [P-HSP]) was used for absorption with RCA-120 Agarose columns. The absorption capability of P-HSP in SI activities of mAbs H6-3C4, 2C6, 2E5, and 2B6 disappeared after passing through the column, but the eluted fraction from the column with 0.1 M lactose resumed the antigenic properties for these mAbs. Therefore, we assumed that the antigenic epitopes corresponding to these mAbs might have a Gal–GlcNAc structure. When the effects of lectins on antibody binding to coated sperm were examined by ELISA, lectins of RCA and wheat germ agglutinin (WGA) inhibited the binding of mAb H6-3C4 to sperm;

thus the involvement of Gal–GlcNAc, galactose, and sialic acid in the antigenic epitope to mAb H6-3C4 was presumed. The binding of mAb 2C6 to sperm was also blocked with RCA; thus the antigenic eiptope to mAb 2C6 was also assumed to have a Gal–GlcNAc structure. From these inhibition experiments with lectins, the antigenic epitopes corresponding to all mAbs that expressed SI and SA activities seemed to have a carbohydrate structure.

Destruction of Carbohydrate Components on Sperm Surface Antigens and Its Effect on Binding of mAbs to Sperm (by ELISA)

Washed sperm were treated with TFMS according to the method of Omer-Ali et al. [1986]. Washed sperm were also treated with periodic acid [Shapiro and Erickson, 1981]. Fifty microliters per well of treated sperm suspension (6 × 10^{6}ml of PBS) was put in Falcon assay plate-3912 and dried. The ELISA assays were performed by the usual procedures, and the damage of carbohydrate antigen on binding mAbs was examined. The antigenicities to mAbs H6-3C4, 2B6, and 2E5 were almost completely destroyed by treating sperm with either TFMS or periodate, but the antigenicity to mAb 2C6 was retained to some degree compared with that to other mAbs. These results indicate that the antigenic epitope to mAb H6-3C4 may be glycolipid, but that to mAb 2C6 may be composed of carbohydrate as the major moiety and peptide as the minor moiety.

Effect of Treating HSP With TFMS on Absorption Capability for SI Activities of mAbs H6-3C4 and 2C6

HSP was precipitated by saturating it with $(NH_4)_2SO_4$ and was completely dialyzed against water. Then 10 mg/ml of dialysate was treated with TFMS at 4°C for 2 hr, according to the method of Edge et al. [1981]. After TFMS treatment, the absorption capability of HSP for SI activity of mAb H6-3C4 was completely destroyed, but that of mAb 2C6 was somewhat retained. These results confirmed the previous results that the antigenic epitope in HSP corresponding to mAb H6-3C4 may be glycolipid but that to mAb 2C6 may be composed of carbohydrate as the major moiety and peptide as the minor moiety.

Molecular Weight of HSP Components That Contain Antigenic Epitopes Corresponding to These mAbs

When HSP was fractionated by Sephacryl S-300, a macromolecule 670 kd fraction possessed the absorption capability for SI activity of

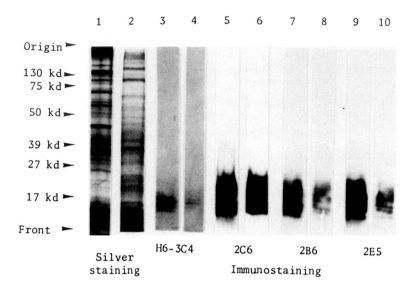

Fig. 1.   SDS-PAGE and Western blot analysis. **Lanes 1, 3, 5, 7, 9,** sperm membrane extract with 0.5% NP-40; **Lanes 2, 4, 6, 8, 10,** partially purified HSP.

mAb H6-3C4. When the 670 kd fraction was fractionated further by SDS-PAGE, the ~20 kd band showed antigenicity to mAb H6-3C4 by Western blot. Not only human mAb H6-3C4 reacted to the 20 kd band of HSP, but also mAbs 2C6, 2E5, and 2B6 reacted to the 20 kd fraction of HSP. Fig. 1 indicates the 20 kd band reacted to various mAbs. Therefore, the important carbohydrate moiety or glycoprotein relevant to raise SI Abs might be contained in the 20 kd molecule in HSP.

INTERFERENCE OF MOUSE mAbs AGAINST HUMAN SPERM OR HSP ON SPERM BINDING OF HUMAN mAb H6-3C4

As shown in Table 5, mouse mAbs 2C6, 2E5, and 2B6 produced in our laboratory reduced sperm binding of mAb H6-3C4. These experiments were performed by using ^{125}I antihuman IgM as a second antibody, after applying various mouse mAbs and mAb H6-3C4 to fixed sperm in wells of a Falcon plate. mAbs 2C6, 2E5, and 2B6 seemed to recognize a carbohydrate epitope similar to that of mAb H6-3C4, or the location of the carbohydrate epitope to these mouse mAbs may be very close to the epitope corresponding to mAb H6-3C4. The several WHO mouse mAbs to human sperm that showed

TABLE 5. Results of Competitive Binding Inhibition Assay With
[125]I-Labeled mAb H6-3C4 to Human Spermatozoa by Different
Monoclonal Antisperm Antibodies[a]

Mabs	Percent binding inhibition	Mabs	Percent binding inhibition	Mabs	Percent binding inhibition
S01[b]	−7.6	S19[b]	69.8	S37	21.4
S02[b]	−15.9	S20	12.8	S38[b]	74.5
S03	−6.8	S21	12.8	S39[b]	62.3
S04	0.6	S22	11.3	S40	4.8
S05[b]	59.6	S23	−3.4	S41	3.2
S06	2.3	S24	15.2	S42	13.0
S07	5.9	S25	−2.2	S43	0.5
S08	11.3	S26	12.2	S44	13.7
S09	16.1	S27	−4.4	S45	12.2
S10	17.0	S28	0.0	S46	18.4
S11	2.5	S29	−3.7	S47	−12.4
S12	6.1	S30	−5.5	S48	17.5
S13	12.4	S31	0.3	S49	7.0
S14	−1.3	S32	11.3	2C6[b]	76.0
S15	0.9	S33	−0.3	2E5[b]	96.7
S16	−1.3	S34[b]	11.1	2B6[b]	76.1
S17	−5.9	S35	7.0	1C4[b]	3.7
S18	−25.8	S36	17.2	H6-3C4[b]	97.8

[a]mAbs, monoclonal antibodies.
[b]Monoclonal antibodies that are SIT positive. mAbs S01–S49, diluted with 10% normal
human serum in PBS; mAbs 2C6, 2E5, 2B6, 1C4, H6-3C4, not diluted.

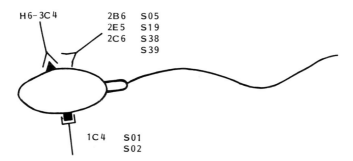

Fig. 2.   Monoclonal antibodies are as follows: H6-3C4, human–mouse hybridoma; 2B6, 2E5, 2C6, mouse hybridomas; 1C4, rat–mouse hybridoma; S01, S02,
S05, S19, S38, S39, mouse hybridomas from WHO.

strong SI activities also inhibited sperm binding of mAb H6-3C4 to some degree. This implies that the antigenic epitopes of sperm surface components relevant to producing SI Abs may have similar structures (Fig. 2).

CHEMICAL STRUCTURE OF ANTIGENIC EPITOPE CORRESPONDING TO mAb H6-3C4

In previous experiments, it was assumed that the antigen corresponding to mAb H6-3C4 might have a Gal–GlcNAc structure or galactose or sialic acid in the molecule. Recently, Tsuji et al. [1988] identified the antigenic epitope to mAb H6-3C4 by immunostaining and solid-phase RIA for glycolipids. The glycolipids were preared by extracting red blood cells and placenta by isopropanol/hexane/water 55:30:25, followed by Folch's partition repeated three times, DEAE cellulose chromatography, HPLC on porous silica gel column, and, finally, purification on high-performance thin-layer chromatography (HPTLC) as free state or as acetate. Each glycolipid preparation was homogeneous on HPTLC, and some of their structures were identified by nuclear magnetic resonance (NMR) and fast-atom bombardment mass spectrometry (FAB-MS). Thin-layer chromatography immunostaining of glycolipids was performed on HPTLC [Kannagi et al., 1982; Kannagi et al., 1982, 1983] as originated by Magnami et al. [1980]. Solid-phase RIA was performed on 96-well flexible vinyl plastic plates [Kannagi et al., 1983]. Table 6 shows the reaction of H6-3C4 to various glycolipids of which the chemical structures are well-known. mAb H6-3C4 reacted to lactonorhexaosylceramide (which is an i blood group antigen), $2\rightarrow3$ sialyl i antigen, $2\rightarrow6$ sialyl i antigen, and lactonoroctaosylceramide. It is interesting to see that this mAb could react to i Ag regardless of substitution with sialic acid at the terminal region. Such wide reactions for mAb are very unusual. Table 6 also shows the reactions of various mAbs to the glycolipids that defined their chemical structures. mAb NUH_2 (Hakomori) obtained from a hybridoma against malignant tumor cells, reacted to disialyllactoisooctaosylceramide (sialyl I Ag).

Only mAbs H6-3C4 and NUH_2 could immobilize the sperm with complement; thus the existence of antigenic epitopes composed of sialyl i Ag and sialyl I Ag was clearly proven. That sialic acid might be substituted at the terminus of the carbohydrate chain on the surface of sperm was also proven, because, after removal of sialic acid from the surface of sperm by gentle treatment with neuraminidase, mAbs 1B2, 1B9, Dench, and C6 could immobilize sperm. From this evidence, it could be assumed that sialylated neolactosamine struc-

TABLE 6. Reaction of mAb H6-3C4 to Various Glycolipids of Known Chemical Structures[a]

	mAbs						Ag on sperm
	H6-3C4	1B2	1B9	Dench	C6	NUH$_2$	
SIT using fresh sperm	+	−	−	−	−	+	
SIT using neuraminidase treated sperm	+	+	−	+	+	−	
o—•—o—©PG	−	+	−	−	−	−	−
♦—o—•—o—©2.3.SPG	−	−	−	−	−	−	+
◇—o—•—o—©2.6.SPG	−	−	+	−	−	−	−
o—•—o—•—o—©i	+	+	−	+	−	−	−
♦—o—•—o—•—o—©2.3.S-i	+	−	−	−	−	−	+
◇—o—•—o—•—o—©2.6.S-i	+	−	+	−	−	−	−
branched ©I	−	+	−	−	+	−	−
branched ©2.3.S-I	−	−	−	−	−	+	+

[a] ♦, 2.3.sialic acid; ◇, 2.6.sialic acid; o, Gal; •, GlcNac; ©, Glc; PG, paragloboside; 2.3.SPG, 2→3 sialylparagloboside; 2.6.SPG, 2→6 sialylparagloboside; i, lactonorhexaosylceramide; 2.3.S-i, 2→3 sialyl i; 2.6.S-i, 2→6 sialyl i; I, lactoisooctaosylceramide; 2.3.S-I: disialyllactoisooctaosylceramide.

tures of carbohydrate are present in the antigenic epitopes of HSP, relevant to producing SI and SA Abs in humans and mice.

EXISTENCE OF COMMON CARBOHYDRATE ANTIGEN BETWEEN HUMAN SPERM AND PLACENTAL TROPHOBLAST

The existence of a sialyl 2→3(Galβ1—4GlcNAc)n structure is clearly proved on the surface of ejaculated sperm by using human sperm-immobilizing mAb H6-3C4 in our laboratory. We recently showed a carbohydrate structure in the chorionic trophoblast similar to that in sperm and HSP. The ABC tissue staining with mAbs produced to various neolactosamine carbohydrate chains indicated very similar patterns between ejaculated sperm and chorionic trophoblast. mAb H6-3C4, which recognized i antigen regardless of substitution with sialic acid at the terminal region, reacted to both sperm and trophoblast; mAb NUH$_2$, which recognized only sialyl I antigen, also reacted to both sperm and trophoblast tissue (Table 7).

TABLE 7. Expression of Sialyllactosamine Antigen on Human Sperm and Trophoblast[a]

mAbs	Human sperm Non-treated	Human sperm Sialidase treated	Human trophoblast Non-treated	Human trophoblast Sialidase treated
○—●—○—●—○—◎i				
◆—○—●—○—●—○—◎2.3.S-i				
◇—○—●—○—●—○—◎2.6.S-i H6-3C4	+	+	+	+
◆—○—●				
○—●—○—◎2.3.S-l NUH₂	+	−	+	−
◆—○—●				
○—●—○—◎PG 1B2	−	+	−	+
○—● ╲ ╲ ○—●—○—◎l C6 ○—● ╱	−	+	−	+
◇—○—●—○—◎2.6.SPG 1B9	−	−	−	−
○—●—○—●—○—◎i Dench	−	+	−	+

[a] ◆, 2.3.sialic acid; ◇, 2.6.sialic acid; ○, Gal; ●, GlcNac; ◎, Glc; PG, paragloboside; 2.3.SPG, 2→3 sialylparagloboside; 2.6.SPG, 2→6 sialylparagloboside; i, lactonorhexaosylceramide; 2.3.S-i, 2→3 sialyl i; 2.6.S-i, 2→6 sialyl i; l, lactoisooctaosylceramide; 2.3.S-l, disialyllactoisooctaosylceramide.

TABLE 8. Raising of Sperm-Immobilizing Antibodies in BALB/c Mice Immunized by Hydatidiform Mole Trophoblasts[a]

1. Villi were injected to BALB/c mice
2. Mice were boosted three times at 1 week intervals
3. Sperm-immobilizing activity was examined using immunized and nonimmunized mice sera

[a] Immunized mice, $SI_{50} = 80$; nonimmunized mice, $SI_{50} = 1$.

Table 8 shows the SI activity of mouse antiserum immunized with hydatidiform mole cells. Mabs to chorionic trophoblast that expressed SI or SA activities were also produced. BALB/c mice were immunized with trophoblast tissue derived from chorionic tumor, and the spleen cells from the immunized mice were fused with mouse myeloma cells (NS-1); three mAbs to chorionic trophoblast were produced. Two of the three mAbs (1H-12 [IgM] and 10H-2 [IgM]) immobilized human sperm remarkably, and the other mAb, 9-12 (IgG₁), agglutinated human sperm. All three mAbs stained syn-

TABLE 9. mAbs to HSP Peptide[a]

	mAbs	
	3B2-F7	3B10
Deglycosylated HSP	+ +	+ +
SI activity	+	−
SA activity	−	−
Blocking of sperm binding to Z.P.	+	+
Molecular weights (kd) of corresponding antigen (SDS-PAGE)	37	15
ABC staining		
Testis	+	+
Epididymis	+	+
Prostate	+	+
Fresh sperm	−	−
Fixed sperm	+	+
Connective tissues	+ +	+ +
Placenta (trophoblast)	N.D.	+ +
Purification	Yes	N.D.
Identification of antigen	Kallikrein family	N.D.
	γ-Seminoprotein	N.D.

[a]N.D., not determined; SI, sperm immobilizing; SA, sperm agglutinating; +, positive; −, negative.

tiotrophoblast and cytotrophoblast of the placenta on ABC tissue staining. The 50 kd glycoprotein fraction from the extract of trophoblast on SDS-PAGE was purified as a single component by DEAE immunoaffinity chromatography followed by HPLC, and it reacted with all three mAbs by Western blot procedures. From these results, it was shown that antigenic epitopes of sialyl i antigen and sialyl I antigen existing on the surface of ejaculated sperm seem to be present in the chorionic trophoblast. This evidence may give some information in the future concerning sterility and pregnancy loss caused by antisperm antibodies.

PEPTIDE ANTIGENS IN HSP THAT ARE RELEVANT TO PRODUCE SPERM-IMMOBILIZING ANTIBODY OR BLOCKING ANTIBODY ON SPERM BINDING TO ZONA PELLUCIDA

In our laboratory, two mAbs against HSP that reacted only to deglycosylated HSP were produced. mAb 3B2-F7 was IgM(K) and showed a weak SI activity ($SI_{50} = 256$ units) and a blocking effect of sperm binding to human zona pellucida. HSP was precipitated by saturating with $(NH_4)_2SO_4$, and the obtained protein was completely dialyzed. The HSP protein was fractionated by SDS-PAGE, and the 36 kd band was proved to contain antigenic epitope corresponding to mAb 3B2-F7 by Western blot procedure. The 36 kd band was cut and collected and then further purified by HPLC. The amino acid sequence of this purified component was analyzed and proved to show Ile-Val-Gly-Gly-□-Glu-□-Glu-Lys-His-Ser-Glu-Pro-□-Gln-Val-Leu-□-Ala-□. From these results, it was assumed that this antigenic component may belong in the kallikrein family and probably the γ-seminoprotein.

However, we recognized that our speculation might be wrong from further experiments, because γ-seminoprotein was excreted from the prostate and antibody generated to γ-seminoprotein did not react with the purified antigenic component corresponding to mAb 3B2-F7. Therefore, this antigen may have an epitope different from γ-seminoprotein and may be secreted from the epididymis. Further study is now going on to identify the antigen corresponding to mAb 3B2-F7.

The ABC staining of various human tissue with this mAb indicated that the localization of the antigenic epitope to it was distributed in many tissues, especially in the connective tissue. mAb 3B-10, which also reacted to deglycosylated HSP protein, had no SI or SA activity, but had a blocking effect on sperm binding to human zona pellucida. The localization of antigenic epitope corresponding to mAb 3B-10 was also distributed widely in somatic tissues, especially in the connective tissue. The epitopes corresponding to mAbs 3B2-F7 and 3B-10 existed also in testicular germ cells. The antigenic epitope to mAb 3B-10 localized more densely in germ cells of testis; therefore, this peptide antigenic epitope is assumed to be a sperm membrane intrinsic antigen (Table 9). From these experiments, the antigenic epitopes of HSP components that are relevant to producing SI or SA Abs may have a carbohydrate structure as a major moiety. The peptide antigens in HSP could produce antibodies to block sperm binding to zona pellucida, but antigenic epitopes seem to be distributed widely in other tissues, especially in connective tissues. However, there is still a possibility that a sperm-specific peptide epitope in HSP relevant to producing SI or SA Abs or sperm-blocking antibodies to zona pellucida may exist on the surface of sperm.

ANTIBODIES AGAINST SPERM ANTIGENS, INCLUDING SEMINAL PLASMA COMPONENTS, RAISED IN WOMEN

Most women's sera containing SI Abs were absorbed with human seminal plasma components (azoospermic semen); thus the SI Abs

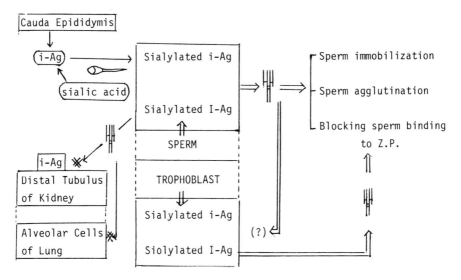

Fig. 3.   Sperm-coating carbohydrate antigens (sialylated i- and I-Ags) on sperm and trophoblast, and generation of biologically active antibodies against sperm.

seemed to be raised against sperm-coating antigens. When HSP was treated with TFMS and the carbohydrate structure of the molecule was destroyed, the antigenic capability to absorb SI Abs in all women's sera examined drastically diminished, implying that the SI Abs in women's sera might be raised against carbohydrate or carbohydrate-associated epitopes of HSP. We have succeeded in establishing the very stable human–mouse heterohybridoma H6-3C4, which secreted extremely high titers of SI and SA mAbs, and defined chemical structures of an antigenic epitope corresponding to mAb H6-3C4. The antigenic epitope was clarified as sialyllactonorhexaosylceramide (sialyl i Ag). By using another Mab (NUH$_2$), we proved that another carbohydrate epitope, disialyllactoisocaosylceramide (sialyl I Ag), was also present on the surface of sperm. The SI Abs in sterile women's sera that competitively inhibit the sperm binding of mAb H6-3D4 to sperm were very rare; therefore, carbohydrate epitopes corresponding to most women's SI Abs might not be exactly similar to that to mAb H6-3C4, though they could be closely correlated. The i Ag was secreted from epithelium of cauda epididymis and adhered firmly on the surface of sperm after sialylation at the terminal region. Ejaculated sperm were coated densely with carbohydrate (probably glycoprotein) seminal plasma components all over the surface, and probably no intrinsic membrane component was exposed in fresh ejaculated sperm. When ejaculated sperm were fixed, surface conditions of sperm membrane were changed, and some intrinsic membrane antigens could be exposed. We followed the adhered HSP antigens of ejaculated sperm until capacitation and found that sperm immobilization occurred in sperm capacitated with mAb H6-3C4.

From our experimental results, we assume that women raise SI or SA Abs against carbohydrate epitopes of sperm-coating antigens, but we cannot rule out the possibility that peptide molecules of HSP are responsible. At fertilization, antibodies to peptide antigens of sperm membrane may be relevant to block sperm binding to zona pellucida or sperm penetration. Another important fact is that a sterile woman from whom lymphocytes were drawn for establishing human hybridoma H6-3C4 was proved very healthy by repeated medical examinations even though she had a high titer of SI Ab and was sterile. In her serum, high titers of circulating SI Ab, which could be the same Ab as mAb H6-3C4, were present, and there was a common antigen in the distal tubules of kidney; however, this circulating SI Ab did not seem to impair kidney functions. Therefore, the presence of common antigens with sperm in other tissues may not necessarily induce an autoimmune disease in vivo by immunizing with sperm antigen. There may be some defense mechanism to protect somatic organs from circulating antibodies in vivo (Fig. 3).

CONCLUSIONS

1   Most sterile women, for an unknown reason, seem to raise SI Abs against carbohydrate or carbohydrate-associated epitopes of human seminal plasma antigens adhered on the surface of ejaculated sperm.

2   A stable human hybridoma mAb, H6-3C4, was established by fusing lymphocytes of a sterile women possessing a high titer of SI Ab with mouse myeloma cells. The hybridoma secreted a human Mab (IgMλ) with extremely high titers of SI and SA activities for almost 4 years.

3   The mAb H6-3C4 reacted to type 2 neolactosamines such as lactonorhexaosylceramide (i Ag), sialyl (2→3 and 2→6) lactonorhexaosylceramide (sialyl i Ag), and lactonoroctaosylceramide. On the surface of ejaculated sperm, sialyl i Ag was distributed all over the sperm. By using mAb NUH$_2$, which reacts to disialyllactoisooctaosylceramide (sialyl I Ag), the existence of sialyl I Ag on the surface of sperm was also proved.

4   The i Ag corresponding to mAb H6-3C4 was secreted from epithelium of caudal epididymis and might adhere firmly all over the surface of sperm after sialylation at the terminal region of the carbohydrate chain.

5   Besides epithelium of caudal epididymis, HSP, ejaculated sperm, the distal tubules of kidney, and placental tropho- blast indicated the presence of i or sialyl i Ag. However, a high titer of anti-i antibody in a sterile woman from whom lymphocytes were taken to establish the human hybridoma H6-3C4 proved very healthy by repeated medical examina- tions. Therefore, the existence of a certain antigen common to sperm in other somatic tissues seems to be not necessarily harmful in vivo by circulation of antibody against this anti- gen. This phenomenon is an important consideration when developing a contraceptive vaccine.

6   Peptide antigens on the surface of ejaculated sperm may not be relevant to raise SI and SA Abs, but may generate block- ing antibodies for sperm binding to zona pellucida.

ACKNOWLEDGMENTS

We thank Ms. A. Hasegawa for her help with the fertilization experiments.

REFERENCES

Bechtol KB, Brown SC, Kennett RH (1979): Recognition of differentiation antigens of spermatogenesis in the mouse by using antibodies from spleen cell–myeloma hybrids after syngeneic immunization. Proc Natl Acad Sci USA 76:363–367.

Bronson R, Cooper G, Rosenfeld D, Watkin SS (1984): Detection of spontaneously oc- curring sperm-directed antibodies in infertile couples by immunobead binding and en- zyme-linked immunosorbent assay. Ann NY Acad Sci 438:504–507.

Edge SB, Faltynek CR, Hof L, Reichert Jr LE, Weber P (1981): Deglycosylation of glyco- proteins by trifluoromethanesulfonic acid. Anal Biochem 118:131–137.

Heckman A, Rümke P (1969): The antigens of human seminal plasma, with special ref- erence to lactoferrin as a spermatozoa-coating antigen. Fertil Steril 20:312–324.

Herr JC, Flowler JE Jr, Howards SS, Sigman M, Sutherland WM, Koons DJ (1985): Human antisperm monoclonal antibodies constructed postvasectomy. Biol Reprod 32: 695–711.

Husted S (1975): Sperm antibodies in men from infertile couples: Analysis of sperm ag- glutinins and immunofluorescent antibodies in 657 men. Int J Fertil 20:113–121.

Isojima S (1989): Human sperm antigens corresponding to sperm- immobilizing antibodies in the sera of women with infertility of unknown cause: Personal review of our recent studies. Hum Reprod 4 (in press).

Isojima S, Kameda K, Tsuji Y, Shigeta M, Ikeda Y, Koyama K (1987): Establishment and characterization of a human hybridoma secreting monoclonal antibody with high titers of sperm immobilizing and agglutinating activities against human seminal plasma. J Reprod Immunol 10:67–78.

Isojima S, Koyama K (1976): Quantitative estimation of sperm immobilizing antibody in the sera of women with sterility of unknown etiology: The 50% sperm immobilization unit (SI$_{50}$). Excerpta Med Int Congr Ser 370:11–14.

Isojima S, Koyama K, Fujiwara N (1982): Purification of human seminal plasma No. 7 antigen by immunoaffinity chromatography on bound monoclonal antibody. Clin Exp Immunol 49:449–456.

Isojima S, Koyama K, Tsuchiya K (1974): The effect on fertility in women of circulating antibodies against human spermatozoa. J Reprod Fertil Suppl 21:125–150.

Isojima S, Li TS, Ashitaka Y (1968): Immunologic analysis of sperm-immobilizing factor found in sera of women with unexplained sterility. Am J Obstet Gynecol 101:677–683.

Isojima S, Tsuchiya K, Koyama K, Tanaka C, Naka O, Adachi H (1972): Further studies on sperm-immobilizing antibody found in sera of unexplained cases of sterility in women. Am J Obstet Gynecol 112:199–207.

Kannagi R, Levery SB, Ishigami F, Hakomori S, Shevinsky LH, Knowles BB, Solter D (1983a): New globoseries glycophospholipids in human teratocarcinoma reactive with the monoclonal antibody directed to a developmentally regulated antigen: Stage specific embryonic antigen 3. J Biol Chem 258:8934–8942.

Kannagi R, Nudelman E, Levery SB, Hakomori S (1982): A series of human erythrocyte glycosphingolipids reacting to the monoclonal antibody directed to a developmentally regulated antigen, SSEA-1. J Biol Chem 257:14865–14874.

Kannagi R, Stroup R, Cochran NA, Urdal DL, Young Jr WW, Hakomori S (1983b): Factors affecting expression of glycolipid tumor antigens: Influence of ceramide composition and coexisting glycolipid on the antigenicity of gliotraosylceramide in murine lymphoma cells. Cancer Res 43:4997–5005.

Koyama K, Takada Y, Takemura T, Isojima S (1983): Localization of human seminal plasma No. 7 antigen (Ferrisplan) in accessory glands of male genital tract and spermatozoa. J Reprod Immunol 5:135–143.

Kubota K (1987): Heterogeneity of sperm immobilizing antibodies in sera of sterile women. Acta Obstet Gynaecol Jpn 39:1121–1128.

Kyurkchiev SD, Shigeta M, Koyama K, Isojima S (1986): A human–mouse hybridoma producing monoclonal antibody against human sperm coating antigen. Immunology 57: 489–492.

Lynch DM, Leali BA, Howe SE (1986): A comparison of sperm agglutination and immobilization assays with a quantitative ELISA for anti-sperm antibody in serum. Fertil Steril 46:285–292.

Magnani JL, Smith DF, Ginsburg V (1980): Detection of gangliosides that bind cholera toxin: Direct binding of ^{125}I-labeled toxin to thin-layer chromatograms. Anal Biochem 109:399–402.

Mathur S, Williamson HO, Landgrebe SC, Smith CL, Fudenberg HH (1979): Application of passive hemagglutination for evaluation of antisperm antibodies and a modified Coombs' test for detecting male autoimmunity to sperm antigens. J Immunol Methods 30:381–393.

Mettler L, Shrabei H (1979): Isolation of a human spermatozoal hapten "II$_{22}$" and its reaction with naturally occurring human sperm immobilizing sera from infertile patients. J Reprod Immunol 1:173–183.

Moyes RW (1969): Antibody binding of spermatozoa. Fertil Steril 20:43–49.

Omer-Ali P, Magee AI, Kelly C, Simpson AJG (1986): A major role for carbohydrate epitopes preferentially recognized by chronically infected mice in the determination of *Schistosoma mansoni* schistosomulum surface antigenicity. J Immuol 137:3601–3607.

Shapiro M, Erickson RP (1981): Evidence that the serological determinant of H-Y antigens is carbohydrate. Nature 290:503–505.

Shigeta M, Watanabe T, Murayama S, Koyama K, Isojima S (1980): Sperm-immobilizing monoclonal antibody to human seminal plasma antigens. Clin Exp Immunol 42:458–462.

Shulman S, Bronson P (1969): Immunochemical studies on human seminal plasma. II. The major antigens and their fractionation. J Reprod Fertil 18:481–491.

Tsuji Y, Clausen H, Nudelman E, Kaizu T, Hakomori S, Isojima S (1988): Human sperm carbohydrate antigens defined by an antisperm human monoclonal antibody derived from an infertile woman bearing antisperm antibodies in her serum. J Exp Med 168:343–356.

Weil AJ, Kotsevalov O, Wilson L (1956): Antigens of human seminal plasma. Proc Soc Exp Biol Med 92:606–610.

DISCUSSION

DR. TALWAR: I believe that the incidence of immobilizing and agglutinating antibodies in Japanese women is the highest in the world. I wonder whether you have had occasion to determine whether the sera from Dr. Hjort's bank from other countries recognized the same specificity or some other.

DR. ISOJIMA: We also sent our mAb 2C6, which possessed a high sperm immobilizing (SI) titer, to the WHO antisperm bank and found that many other laboratories surprisingly reported that it was negative for SI titers. This is a problem and an important point. You mentioned the high percentage of SI and sperm agglutinating antibodies among Japanese women. The standardization of technical problems must be considered. We collaborated with Dr. Hjort's bank to examine many sera from other countries and found that there were many discrepancies between the results from our laboratory and from other laboratories.

DR. TALWAR: Did you study serum from other countries that have immobilizing properties and observe whether they recognize the same specificity?

DR. ISOJIMA: We could not examine the antigenic specificities of SI antibodies from WHO, but some mAbs from WHO recognized antigenic structures very similar to those of the epitope corresponding to our mouse mAbs 2C6, 2B6, and 2B5, which are closely related to the epitope to human mAb H6-3C4. Several other mAbs from WHO recognized a different epitope corresponding to our different mAb 1C4.

13

Immunologic Cytokines and Reproduction

Deborah J. Anderson

The reproductive tissues of both males and females contain diverse immunologic cell types, whose roles in reproductive processes are only beginning to be appreciated. Recent evidence indicates that immunologic cytokines released by activated lymphocytes, macrophages, and other accesory cells of immunologic reactions in the genital tract can benefit or adversely affect various reproductive events. The type of effect appears to depend on various factors: the types and concentrations of cells and cytokines present, the timing and duration of exposure of reproductive cells to cytokines, and possibly factors that may locally regulate cytokine production in reproductive tissues and the expression of cytokine receptors on reproductive cells. Our laboratory for the past several years has studied immunologic cell types and responses in reproductive tissues and the effects of immunologic cytokines on reproductive performance. An overview of our work is reported here.

IMMUNOLOGIC CYTOKINES AND MALE REPRODUCTION

The human testis contains numerous macrophages in the interstial tissues between seminiferous tubules. Isolated testicular cells secrete large amounts of an interleukin-1α (Il-1α)-like factor, but the origin of this factor is not yet clear. Gustafsson et al. [1988] and Syed et al. [1988] suggest that Sertoli cells may be the primary source of this factor. Recent reports have indicated that Il-1 can regulate the production of testosterone by Leydig cells [Callcino et al., 1988; Warren et al., 1989] and may be an intratesticular growth factor that

Gamete Interaction: Prospects for Immunocontraception, pages 175–184
© 1990 Wiley-Liss, Inc.

promotes spermatogenesis (Syed et al., 1988). Testicular macrophages express HLA-DR and Fc receptors, but their function has not been fully explored. Most studies on testicular macrophages have been performed on cells isolated from testes of experimental animals; it is critical to devise ways also to assess testicular macrophage function in situ, as in vitro experiments remove cells from local regulatory influences and therefore may be misleading.

In addition to macrophages, numerous T lymphocytes, with an abundance of CD8$^+$ cells (suppressor/cytotoxic cells) are present in the human epididymis. It has been proposed that these cells serve an immunosuppressive role at this site and prevent immunologic reactions directed against sperm antigens [Ritchie et al., 1984]. Regions of the normal human epididymal epithelium express the human leukocyte antigen HLA-DR and may have an antigen-presenting role at this site [Ritchie et al., 1984]. We have also detected numerous macrophages and lymphocytes in the subepithelial space surrounding the vas deferens. The functions of these cells are totally unknown. The epididymis and vas deferens are storage sites of sperm; therefore, spermatozoa may be exposed to these white blood cells and their products for extended periods of time. It is possible that cytokine production in this location benefits sperm function. For example, a recent study has indicated that platelet-activating factor (PAF), a cytokine produced during inflammatory responses, promotes sperm motility [Rickler et al., 1989]. On the other hand, an imbalance in local cell types and cytokines present in the epididymis/ vas deferens caused by a local subclinical infection or other occurrence of epididymitis could result in adverse effects on spermatogenesis. We and others have reported that elevated numbers of white blood cells in semen are associated with infertility [Wolff and Anderson, 1988; Phadke and Phadke, 1961; Talbert et al., 1987; Caldamone et al., 1980]. We have also found that cytokine-positive white blood cells can be recovered from semen of infertility patients [Takahasi et al., 1989]. Recent evidence indicates that the lymphokine γ-interferon and the monokine tumor necrosis factor adversely affect human sperm motility [Hill et al., 1987] and the ability of human sperm to penetrate hamster eggs in vitro [Hill et al., 1989]. Furthermore, it is well established that products of polymorphonuclear leukocytes (i.e., H_2O_2, free oxygen radicals) are extremely toxic to sperm [reviewed in Anderson and Hill, 1988]. It is therefore likely that cytokines and other white blood cell products released during genital tract inflammation or cellular immune reactions to sperm or to viral or microbial antigens may be a cause of male infertility.

IMMUNE CELLS, CYTOKINES, AND
FEMALE REPRODUCTION

There is a growing appreciation that the female reproductive tract is an immunologically dynamic region. Abundant T lymphocytes, natural killer cells, and macrophages, mediators of cell-mediated immunologic responses, are present in the human endometrium during the secretory phase of the menstrual cycle (time of implantation) and throughout pregnancy [Kamat and Isaacson, 1987; Bulmer and Sunderland, 1984]. White blood cell numbers are dramatically increased in the reproductive tissues of women with endometriosis or reproductive tract infection [Wheeler, 1982; Blaustein, 1985]. Elevated numbers of lymphocytes and macrophages have also been detected in endometrial biopsy specimens of some infertile women [Lint, 1980; Monif, 1982; Xu et al., 1987].

Immunologic cytokines and other products of inflammatory cells in the female reproductive tract could adversely affect female fertility by inhibiting sperm function as described above. Furthermore, the preimplantation and implanting embryos appear to be particularly vulnerable targets of cytokine effects. Human mixed lymphocyte culture supernatants, which contain a variety of products from activated lymphocytes and macrophages, inhibited mouse embryo development and human trophoblast (choriocarcinoma) proliferation in vitro [Hill et al., 1987; Berkowitz et al., 1988]; cultured mouse lymphocyte and macrophage culture supernatants inhibited preimplantation embryo development [Hill et al., 1987] but, conversely, stimulated trophoblast outgrowth from mouse blastocysts that had attached to fibrinectin-coated petri dishes [Haimovici et al., 1990; Fenderson et al., 1983]. These data suggest that lymphocyte and/or macrophage products can have negative or positive effects on early pregnancy. A number of animal studies support this concept. On the "beneficial effects of cytokines" side are reports that 1) hybrid placentas and fetuses are larger than syngeneic placentas and fetuses [Billington et al., 1964]; 2) increased numbers of embryos develop in pregnant animals whose uterine horns have been presensitized against paternal histocompatibility antigens and have expressed a local "recall flare" reaction [James, 1967]; and 3) mice that have been treated with anti-T-cell antisera during pregnancy have smaller placentae than untreated mice [Athanassakis et al., 1987]. On the negative side, a number of studies in experimental animals have demonstrated an association between uterine leukocytosis and early abortion [Anderson and Alexander, 1979; Parr and Sirley, 1976]. We have recently determined that mice receiving syngeneic sperm-activated T lymphocytes by passive transfer demonstrate reduced litter sizes and an increased abortion rate [Haimovici et al., 1990]. It is possible that the timing and levels of specific cytokines in early gestation underlie adverse or beneficial effects of such factors in pregnancy.

Studies have been performed to examine the role of individual immunologic cytokines in pregnancy. It has been reported that trophoblast cells express receptors for cerebrospinal fluid (CSF)-1 [Muller et al., 1983] and γ-interferon [Gray et al., 1989] and therefore may be regulated by such factors in pregnancy. Athanassakis et al. [1987] reported growth-stimulating effects of granulocyte, macrophage-colony stimulating factor (GM-CSF) on cells isolated from the mouse placenta, and Gudas et al. [1983] reported growth-stimulating effects of platelet-derived growth factor on embryonal teratocarcinoma cells. We have found that some concentrations of Il-1, Il-2, and Il-4 significantly stimulated choriocarcinoma growth in vitro [Berkowitz et al., 1988]. On the other hand, γ-interferon, tumor necrosis factor-α and GM-CSF have been found to inhibit mouse embryo development and choriocarcinoma cell proliferation in vitro [Hill et al., 1987; Berkowitz et al., 1988], and γ-interferon also inhibited trophoblast outgrowth of mouse blastocysts in vitro [Haimovici et al., 1990].

SUMMARY AND CONCLUSIONS

The subspecialty of reproductive immunology that deals with immunologic cytokines and the role of cell-mediated immunologic reactions in fertility is a new and extremely exciting field. Evidence to date indicates that reproductive cells are sensitive to immunologic cytokines and other white blood cell products. These cell products may have beneficial or adverse effects on several reproductive functions, depending on concentration, timing of exposure, and synergy with other factors. This subspecialty promises to continue to provide valuable insights into immunologic control of events of reproduction.

ACKNOWLEDGMENTS

This work was supported by grants CA42738 and HD23775 from the National Institutes of Health and contract 010 from the Contraceptive Research and Development (CONRAD) Program, under a cooperative agreement with the United States Agency of International Development (U.S.A.I.D.). The views expressed by the authors do not necessarily reflect the views of the U.S.A.I.D. or CONRAD.

REFERENCES

Anderson DJ, Alexander NJ (1979): Induction of uterine leukocytosis and its effect on pregnancy in rats. Biol Reprod 21:1143–1152.

Anderson DJ, Hill JA (1988): Cell-mediated immunity in infertility. Am J Reprod Immunol Microbiol 17:22–30.

Athanassakis I, Bleackley RC, Paetkau V, Guilbert L, Barr PJ, Wegmann TG (1987): The immunostimulatory effect of T cells and T cell lymphokines on murine fetally derived placental cells. J Immunol 138:37–44.

Berkowitz RS, Hill JA, Kurtz CB, Anderson DJ (1988): Effects of products of activated leukocytes (lymphokines and monokines) on the growth of malignant trophoblast cells in vitro. Am J Obstet Gynecol 158:199–205.

Billington WD (1964): Influence of immunological dissimilarity of mother and fetus on size of placenta in mice. Nature 202:317–318.

Blaustein A (1985): Interpretation of Endometrial Biopsies, 2nd ed. New York: Raven Press, pp 88–107.

Bulmer JN, Sunderland CA (1984): Immunohistological characterization of lymphoid cell populations in the early human placental bed. Immunology 52:349–356.

Caldamone AA, Emilson LBV, Al-Juburi A, Cockett ATK (1980): Prostatitis: Prostatic secretory dysfunction affecting fertility. Fertil Steril 34:602–610.

Calkins JH, Sigel MM, Nankin HR, Lin T (1988): Interleukin-1 inhibits Leydig cell steroidogenesis in primary culture. Endocrinology 123:1605–1610.

Fenderson BA, Bartlett PF, Edidin M (1983): Maternal immunostimulation of a teratocarcinoma-derived cell line TerCs, J Reprod Immunol 5:287–293.

Gray PW, Leong S, Fennie EH, Farrar MA, Pingel JT, Fernandex-Luna J, Schreiber RD (1989): Cloning and expression of the cDNA for the murine interferon gamma receptor. Proc Natl Acad Sci USA 86:8497–501.

Gudas LJ, Singh JP, Stiles CD (1983): Secretion of growth regulatory molecules by teratocarcinoma stem cells. In Silver L, Martin G, Strickland S (eds): Teratocarcinoma Stem Cells. Cold Spring Harbor Conferences on Cell Proliferation, Vol 10. Cold Spring Harbor, NY: Cold Spring Harbor Laboratory, pp 229–236.

Gustafsson K, Soder O, Pollanen, Ritzen EM (1988): Isolation and partial characterization of an interleukin-1-like factor from rat testis interstitial fluid. J Reprod Immunol 14:139–150.

Haimovici F, Hill JA, Anderson DJ (1990): Effects of soluble products of activated lymphocytes and macrophages on mouse blastocyst implantation in vitro. Biol Reprod (in press).

Haimovici F, Takahashi K, Anderson DJ (1990): Infertility and abortion in mice receiving passive transfer of T-lymphocytes from sperm-immunized mice. Submitted.

Hill JA, Cohen J, Anderson DJ (1989): The effects of lymphokines and monokines on human sperm fertilizing ability in the zona-free hamster egg penetration test. Am J Obstet Gynecol 160:1154–1159.

Hill JA, Haimovici F, Anderson DJ (1987): Products of activated lymphocytes and macrophages inhibit mouse embryo development in vitro. J Immunol 139:2250–2259.

Hill JA, Haimovici F, Politch JA, Anderson DJ (1987): Effects of soluble products of activated lymphocytes and macrophages (lymphokines and monokines) on human sperm motion parameters. Fertil Steril 47:460–465.

James DA (1967): Some effects of immunological factors on gestation in mice. J Reprod Fertil 14:265–270.

Kamat BR, Isaacson PG (1987): The immunocytochemical distribution of leukocyte subpopulations in human endometrium. Am J Pathol 118:76–84.

Lint TF (1980): Complement. In Dhindsa DS, Schumacher GFB (eds): Immunological Aspects of Infertility and Fertility Regulation. New York: Elsevier-North Holland, pp 13–21.

Monif GRG (1982): Infectious Diseases in Obstetrics and Gynecology. Philadelphia: Harper and Row.

Muller R, Slamon DJ, Adamson Ed, Tremblay JM, Muller D, Cline MJ, Verma IM (1983): Transcription of c-onc genes c-rasKi and c-fms during mouse development. Mol Cell Biol. 3(6):1062–1069.

Parr EL, Sirley RL (1976): Embryotoxicity of leukocyte extracts and its relationship to intrauterine contraception in humans. Fertil Steril 27:1067–1077.

Phadke AM, Phadke GM (1961): Occurrence of macrophage cells in the semen and in the epididymis in cases of male infertility. J Reprod Fertil 2:400–404.

Rickler DD, Minhas BS, Kumar R, et al. (1989): The effects of platelet-activating factor on the motility of human spermatozoa. Fertil Steril 52(4):655–658.

Ritchie AWS, Hargreave TB, James K, Chisholm GD (1984): Intraepithelial lymphocytes in the normal epididymis: A mechanism for tolerance to sperm autoantigens? Br J Urol 56:79.

Syed V, Soder O, Arver S, Lindh M, Khan S, Ritzen EM (1988): Ontogeny and cellular origin of an interleukin-1-like factor in the reproductive tract of the male rat. Int J Androl 11:437–448.

Takahashi K, Wolff H, Anderson DJ (1989): Immunohistologic detection of cytokine production by white blood cells in leukocytospermic semen samples. Abstract 109. J Androl (Suppl).

Talbert IM, Hammond MG, et al. (1987): Semen parameters and fertilization of human oocytes in vitro: A multivariable analysis. Fertil Steril 48:270.

Warren DW, Pasupuleti V, Lu Y, Platler B, Horton R (1989): Stimulatory effects of tumor necrosis factor and interleukin-1 on adult rat Leydig cells in culture. Abstract 137. J Androl (Suppl).

Wheeler JE (1982): Pathology of the fallopian tube. In Blaustein A (ed): Pathology of the Female Genital Tract. New York: Springer-Verlag, pp 393–415.

Wolff H, Anderson DJ (1988): Immunohistologic characterization and quantitation of leukocyte subpopulations in human semen. Fertil Steril 49:497–504.

Xu C, Hill JA, Anderson DJ (1987): Identification of T-lymphocyte subpopulations in normal and abnormal human endometrial biopsies, abstracted. Soc Gynecol Invest.

DISCUSSION

DR. JONES: Do you think that the high incidence of seminal leukocytosis that you have observed in men is a reflection of subclinical infection, or is it an immune response to sperm?

DR. ANDERSON: Our preliminary data indicate that about half the men "clear up" with aggressive antibiotic therapy and half do not. It seems that a subpopulation of these men do have chronic cell-mediated immunity but it is not known whether this is against sperm or against colonized microbial infection.

DR. JONES: It would be important to resolve this issue, as the clinical implications are substantial.

DR GUPTA: Have you also found circulating antisperm antibodies in these men?

DR. ANDERSON: We recently completed a study of about 200 infertile patients and 50 fertile men. In the study, we looked for a correlation between leukocytospermia, the presence of specific white blood cell types, and the presence of antisperm antibodies. We did observe a trend toward increased antisperm antibodies in the infertile group, but it was not significant because of the small patient population. I think only 12 of the 200 patients had antisperm antibodies. We are continuing with this study because I think it addresses an important issue.

DR. GUPTA: Have you also looked for antibodies in the seminal plasma?

DR. ANDERSON: Yes. We compared the levels of antisperm antibodies in the seminal plasma and serum using immunobead tests.

DR. GUPTA: Does the same situation occur in females, and, if so, where do you find infiltration of these leukocytes?

DR. ANDERSON: That's an interesting question. In women, Dr. Joe Hill, one of our clinicians, has been studying cervical mucous samples obtained before and after postcoital testing. He has found that a significant number of infertile females have a large number of white blood cells in their cervical mucus. It is known that the cervix can contain T cells and that a large number of women appear to have inflammation and/or low-grade cell-mediated immunity at this location. It is certainly an issue that warrants further research.

DR. GUPTA: Did these female patients have antisperm antibodies?

DR. ANDERSON: We haven't investigated this factor in the study yet, but it is clearly an important issue.

DR. LUSTIG: Did you ever observe, by immunohistochemical techniques, expression of class II histocompatibility antigens (MHC II) on Sertoli cells from stem cells?

DR. ANDERSON: We investigated this while studying HLA expression on sperm and on germ cells. However, there is so much MHC II expressed by the macrophages that are residing right next to the Sertoli cells that it makes it difficult to ascertain to what extent the Sertoli cells are also expressing these antigens. We have never seen a noticeable expression of class II antigens on Sertoli cells.

DR. LUSTIG: The reason I asked this question is that in some pathologic conditions, such as orchitis, there is an apparent increase in MHC II expression on Sertoli cells.

DR. ANDERSON: That is a very interesting finding.

DR. SWERDLOFF: Do you think that the infiltrates that are near or around the rete testes have different types of cells than those in the interstitial testes?

DR. ANDERSON: The infiltrates that we have seen and those reported by Dr. Hargreave in infertile men had a T-cell component. It is particularly striking, because you rarely see these in the testes in the interstitial spaces. It suggests a focal T-cell response.

DR. SWERDLOFF: Most investigators have also seen increased amounts of leukocytes in men who were presumably infertile. Our experience in trying to alter the leukocyte numbers in semen with antibiotics has been very disappointing. Similarly, when we treated patients who had gonadotropin insufficiency with exogeneous gonadotropins, they exhibited a rather marked presence of leukocytes, predominantly granulocytes, in their semen. As to the reason for this response and whether it has any parallel during normal germ cell maturation, I am not certain.

DR. HANDELSMANN: How reproducible are your leukocyte findings in controls and in patients?

DR. ANDERSON: Regarding the healthy sperm donors who we have sampled over time, the technicians claim that they can identify a sperm donor by the white blood cell profile in the sample. So, in the usual semen sample, it is a fairly stable condition. However, some of our sperm donors have acute elevations of white cells that seem to be associated with certain subclinical infections. In our infertility patients, we haven't carried out many serial follow-up studies, but these are currently underway in our antibiotic treatment trial.

DR. HANDELSMANN: In the antibiotic trial, do you have a placebo or a nontreated group?

DR. ANDERSON: We have a nontreated group, and the trial has a double-blind crossover design.

MR. GRIFFIN: Could you speculate on the significance of the antifertility effect you observed in your mice, which seemed to be due to an increased number of postimplantation resorptions. Does this have implications for this type of immunity in terms of an antisperm vaccine?

DR. ANDERSON: I think you are going to have to do a great deal of soul searching if you want a T-cell component in an antisperm vaccine. It is quite possible that, in a species in which gestation lasts longer, resorption may occur even before pregnancy is noticed. So, it may be a very effective back-up mechanism to an antisperm vaccine.

MR. GRIFFIN: I was thinking more in terms of a sublethal effect on the sperm that would lead to teratogenicity as well as being curious as to whether a low-level cell-mediated immune response would be hazardous?

DR. ANDERSON: There is that possibility. A paper was published in the *Proceedings of the National Academy of Science* 3 or 4 years ago reporting that rats that had epididymitis produced offspring with teratologic defects.

DR. MITCHISON: In connection with your suggestion that those lymphocytes may be helping fertility, I wonder if you have any comment about either congenital or acquired deficiencies? I am particularly interested in things that affect macrophages, for example, granulomatous disease. Do you known anything about fertility in congenital/chronic granulomatous disease?

DR. ANDERSON: I went to a meeting in Banff, Alberta, last January in which the subject was immunotropism of pregnancy. One of the speakers presented data concerning pregnancies in immunodeficient mice and reported that they were essentially normal.

DR. GOLDBERG: I had the good fortune this past year to spend some time in Australia conducting a collaborative study with Dr. Barry Boettcher, Tim Roberts, and Chu Ching Chee. We screened the human testes cDNA library with a panel of antisera from infertile patients. These sera agglutinated, or immobilized, sperm. Although I was only there for about 4 months, we were able to isolate approximately 10 clones from this library. We isolated the DNA from one of these clones from which we have now sequenced a 600 nucleotide fragment. It doesn't show any sequence similarities to any other known piece of DNA. As it turns out, it has 60 nucleotides of open reading frame at the 3' end and may be useful for identifying other sperm antigens.

DR. MITCHISON: I would like to comment on the subject of identifying a C3b-like reactivity as C3b. As Dr. Anderson rightly said, it is too early to say that what she has observed is a C3b molecule. I would just like to draw attention to the wealth of available antobidies, not all of them monoclonal, that are directed against particular C3b sites. In particular, I would like to draw attention to nephrotoxic factor. This has been identified as a polyclonal antibody, but it has very precise reactivity against the well-defined peptide that we have revealed when C3 is cleaved to C3b. It is also an important part of the immunopathology of certain renal diseases that have been thoroughly studied from that point of view. These are exactly the types of reagents that are available for characterizing a reactivity prior to carrying out the molecular biology to determine antigenic structures.

14

Role of Acrosin and Antibodies to Acrosin in Gamete Interactions

A.E. De Ioannes, M.I. Becker, C. Pérez, C. Capote, and C. Barros

Acrosin is a serine protease localized in the mammalian sperm acrosome. It is present as proacrosin, from the early spermatid stage [Polakoski and Parrish, 1977; Kallajoki et al., 1986]. Because of its proteolytic activity, this enzyme is believed to play an important role in the binding and penetration of spermatozoa into the zona pellucida [Saling, 1981; Bleil and Wassarman, 1988; Jones et al., 1988]. Acrosin is also involved in the acrosome reaction and in the dispersion of the acrosomal matrix [Dunbar et al., 1985; Urch et al., 1985].

It has been difficult to relate the proteolytic activity of acrosin to sperm binding to the zona, because acrosin is exposed after the acrosomal reaction, which in turn occurs after primary gamete binding [Saling, 1989]. However, Bleil and Wassarman [1986, 1988] have demonstrated that gamete binding to the mouse zona can be considered in two steps. The first involves the interaction of a receptor located on the sperm plasma membrane with ZP3, a zona glycoprotein, that probably induces acrosomal reaction. A receptor located on the inner acrosomal membrane, ZP2, is exposed after the acrosomal reaction and is the second step. As a result of the acrosome reaction, the receptor to ZP3 is released together with the sperm plasma membrane and the sperm remain bound to the zona through the ZP2 receptor.

We propose that acrosin participates in the controlled digestion of ZP3 and ZP2; thus a tight interaction with sperm receptors present either on the sperm inner acrosomal membrane or on the remaining

Gamete Interaction: Prospects for Immunocontraception, pages 185–195

acrosomal matrix results on better exposure of the oligosaccharides present in ZP2. This model predicts that acrosin exerts selective degradation over the zona glycoproteins. We expect that ZP2 would be more sensitive to degradation than ZP3. This prediction fits with the evidence presented by Dunbar et al. [1985] and by Brown and Cheng [1985], who used porcine zona as a substrate for boar acrosin.

We studied the functional role of acrosin on gamete binding using the enzyme inhibitory effect of soybean trypsin inhibitor and a monoclonal antibody to acrosin. Gamete binding was assessed by phase-contrast microscopy employing Nomarski optics and scanning electron microscopy. Our results show that, during gamete coincubation, the soybean trypsin inhibitor precluded penetration, although it did allow sperm attachment as judged by the presence of numerous acrosomal ghosts and sperm tracks on the hamster zona pellucida. The binding of homologous sperm to hamster and human zona pellucidae was not maintained in the presence of soybean trypsin inhibitor. A similar effect was observed when the monoclonal antibody to acrosin, ACRO-C2E5, was added to the gamete coincubation medium in the in vitro fertilization system of hamster eggs. The evidence supports an important role of the enzyme in sperm binding to the zona pellucida. A model accounting for these observations is proposed.

MATERIALS AND METHODS

Monoclonal Antibodies to Acrosin

Purification of human acrosin from human semen samples was performed according to Leyton et al. [1986]. Monoclonal antibodies ACRO-C2E5 and ACRO-B4F6 were used. Data from enzyme-linked immunosorbent assays, immunoblots, immunoprecipitation, and indirect immunofluorescence on sperm cells indicate that ACRO-B4F6 binds only to bovine acrosin, whereas ACRO-C2E5 binds to bovine, hamster, mouse, and human acrosin [Elce et al., 1986].

Gametes

In vitro capacitation of hamster spermatozoa. Hamster spermatozoa were capacitated as described by Barros et al. [1984]. Briefly, caudal epididymal spermatozoa were incubated for 2 hr at 37°C in drops of 100 µl of tyrode albumin pyruvate lactate culture medium (TAPL-10K culture medium) [Yanagimachi, 1982]. Drops of medium containing spermatozoa were placed in a tissue culture petri dish and then covered with mineral oil. Drops of 20 μl containing 2–3 × 10^4 spermatozoa were used to inseminate oocytes.

Hamster oocyte preparation. Oocytes were obtained as described by Barros et al. [1984]. Briefly, superovulated mature golden hamster females were killed, and the oviducts were isolated and placed in a tissue culture petri dish with TAPL-10K culture medium. Oocytes in cumulus were recovered from the ampulla and treated with 0.1% hyaluronidase in Biggers medium (BWW medium) [Biggers et al., 1971], to eliminate the cumulus cells; they were then thoroughly washed by three changes of fresh BWW medium. Each group of oocytes was placed under mineral oil, in a drop of 100 μl of BWW medium, and was inseminated with 2–3 × 10^4 spermatozoa preincubated in TAPL-10K medium.

Human zona pellucida preparation. Human dead oocytes were collected from human ovaries from deceased women. The eggs were released into BWW medium [Biggers et al., 1971] containing 0.3% BSA, 0.1 mM soybean, 10 μg/ml lima bean trypsin inhibitor. The released human zonae were kept for 4 to 8 weeks in medium containing 2 M $(NH_4)_2SO_4$, 40 mM Hepes, and 0.5% dextran to a final pH of 7.0 [Yanagimachi et al., 1979]. Before use, they were thoroughly washed in culture medium as described elsewhere [Yoshimatsu et al., 1988].

Human sperm preparation. Human semen samples from fertile donors were washed twice in BWW culture medium; the pellet was then covered with 0.5 ml fresh culture medium and left in the incubator for 30 min to allow progressively moving spermatozoa to swim up into the culture medium. The selected spermatozoa were recovered and incubated for 3 hr in BWW to capacitate them [Barros and Jedlicki, 1985].

Preparation of the specimens for scanning electron microscopy. The eggs were fixed as described elsewhere [Barros et al., 1984] in 2% gluteraldehyde prepared in cacodylate buffer 0.25 M, pH 7.4, and postfixed in 1% osmium tetroxide in cacodylate buffer 0.25 M, pH 7.4. They were then dehydrated in a series of acetones at increasing concentrations, critical-point dried, mounted on specimen holders, sputtered with gold–palladium target, and observed with Jeol JSM 25 SII.

Bioassays

Effect of serine protease inhibitors and antiacrosin monoclonal antibodies on sperm–zona pellucida interaction in hamster. Hamster spermatozoa were incubated in capacitating medium for 2 hr and the samples divided into 3 drops. Soybean and ovomucoid trypsin inhibitors were added to the first and second drops, respectively, to final concentrations of 70 and 125 μM, respectively. The third drop was uses as a control and received only culture medium. After 15 min, zona-intact hamster oocytes were added to each of the sperm suspensions, and incubation proceeded for an additional period of 3 hr. At the end of the incubation, the eggs were prepared for their examination by phase contrast microscopy to evaluate the fertilization rate and for scanning electron microscopy to evaluate the characteristics of the outer surface of the zona pellucida.

The effects of ACRO-C2E5 and ACRO-B4F6 monoclonal antibodies on the sperm–zona association was studied by adding the monoclonal antibodies to capacitated spermatozoa at final concentrations ranging from 3 to 26 μM. The experiments were evaluated by phase-contrast microscopy to score the rate of fertilization and by scanning electron microscopy to study the surface characteristics of the zona pellucida.

Effect of serine protease inhibitors on human sperm association with human zona pellucida from nonviable oocytes. Human spermatozoa were preincubated at 37°C for 2.5 hr at a sperm concentration of 10^6/ml. Soybean or ovomucoid trypsin inhibitors were added in independent drops to a final concentration of 70 and 120 μM, respectively, and incubated for an additional 30 min. Salt-stored human zonae pellucidae were then added to the sperm suspension. The gamete mixture was incubated for 3 hr more, and at the end of the incubation period the eggs were examined by phase-contrast microscopy to evaluate the number of spermatozoa bound to the zona.

RESULTS AND DISCUSSION

To approach the functional significance of acrosin in the process leading to fertilization, we took advantage of the inhibitory effect of the ACRO-C2E5 monoclonal antibody on the enzymatic activity [Leyton et al., 1986]. This antibody inhibits the dissolution of the hamster zona pellucida by purified acrosin without the need of secondary antigen–antibody reactions [Elce et al., 1986], perhaps through steric hindrance.

The presence of the monoclonal antibody ACRO-C2E5 during gamete coincubation decreased the number of hamster sperm attached to the homologous zonae as compared with controls (Table 1). Scanning electron microscopy revealed that the number of tracks left by

TABLE 1. Effect of Antiacrosin Monoclonal Antibody ACRO-C2E5
on Hamster Sperm Penetration Through the Hamster Zona
Pellucida, Evaluated by Phase-Contrast Microscopy

Antibody	Concentration (μM)	Mean of bound spermatozoa	Percent zona penetration
ACRO-C2E5	26	5	0
ACRO-C2E5	13	17	31
ACRO-C2E5	3	>200[a]	100
ACRO-B4F6	26	>200	100
ACRO-B4F6	13	>200	100
ACRO-B4F6	3	>200	100
NONE		>200	100

[a]Over 200 bound spermatozoa. The specific monoclonal antibody ACRO-C2E5 reduced the number of bound spermatozoa to the zonae pellucidae and precluded zona penetration.

the sperm on the zona were clearly reduced, suggesting that the antibody affected the early stages of zona penetration (Fig. 1).

The idea that serine proteases are key factors involved in the early steps of gamete interactions is supported by the inhibitory effect of the soybean trypsin inhibitor (SBTI) when added to the gamete co-incubation medium [Saling, 1981; Jones et al., 1988]. Recently, Bleil and Wassarman [1988] demonstrated that the presence of the inhibitor in the gamete coincubation medium precludes the secondary binding of mouse sperm to the zona pellucida. To investigate further the mechanism of action of serine protease inhibitors in blocking gamete interactions, we tested the inhibitory effects of SBTI on the binding of human and hamster sperm to homologous zonae. After this treatment a significant inhibitory effect was observed in hamster (Table 2, Fig. 2) and human (Table 3, Fig. 3), indicating that a serine protease is involved at the level of the sperm binding to the zona pellucida in hamster and humans as well as previously described in mouse [Saling, 1981; Bleil and Wassarman, 1988] and pig [Jones et al., 1988]. After coincubating hamster zonae pellucidae with sperm in the presence of 125 μM SBTI no spermatozoa were found attached to the outer surface of the zona pellucida; however, acrosome ghosts and small sperm tracks were seen by scanning electron microscopy. They would correspond to the binding site of sperm that released the enzyme as the outcome of the acrosome reaction (Fig. 2). The massive release of the enzyme during the acrosome reaction may allow partial hydrolysis of the zonae; however, the presence of the inhibitor at a high concentration precludes further penetration and secondary binding to the zona.

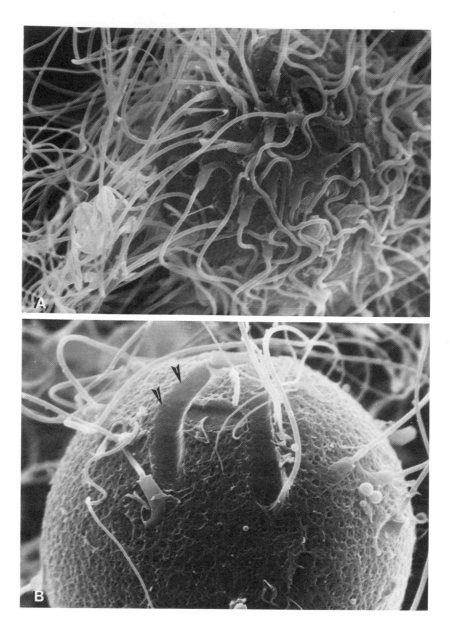

Fig. 1. Scanning electron microscopic micrographs of hamster eggs inseminated in vitro with capacitated hamster spermatozoa. **A:** Eggs coincubated with
spermatozoa in the presence of 13 μM of the nonspecific monoclonal antibody
ACRO-B4F6. Note that countless spermatozoa are bound to the outer surface of
the zona pellucida, and many are in the process of zona penetration. ×1,700. **B:**
Hamster eggs coincubated with spermatozoa in the presence of 13 μM of the
specific monoclonal antibody ACRO-C2E5. Note that only a few spermatozoa
are bound to the outer surface of the zona pellucida. A few spermatozoa made
a long, deep track but failed to penetrate it (arrowheads). ×2,300.

TABLE 2. Effect of SBTI and Ovomucoid Trypsin Inhibitors on Homologous Sperm Binding to Hamster Zonae Pellucida and on In Vitro Fertilization, Evaluated by Phase-Contrast Microscopy[a]

Inhibitor	Concentration (µM)	No. of eggs observed	Mean of bound spermatozoa	Percent fertilization
SBTI	125	73	2	1,4
Ovomucoid	125	83	16	57
None		55	41	92

[a]Results are means of five experiments. Soybean trypsin inhibitor inhibited sperm binding and sperm penetration through the zona pellucida.

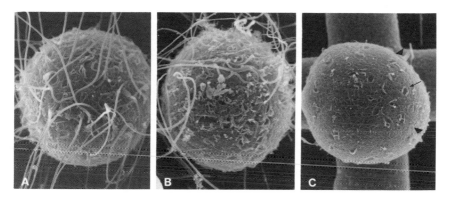

Fig. 2. Scanning electron microscopic micrographs of hamster eggs inseminated in vitro with capacitated spermatozoa. **A:** Eggs coincubated with spermatozoa in culture medium alone. ×900. **B:** Eggs coincubated with spermatozoa in the presence of ovomucoid trypsin inhibitor. ×910. **C:** Eggs coincubated with spermatozoa in the presence of soybean trypsin inhibitor. Note that there are no spermatozoa bound to the zona in spite of the fact that there are acrosomal ghosts and sperm (arrow) tracks (arrowheads). ×900.

Attempts to reduce fertility by passive transfer of the monoclonal antibody ACRO-C2E5 to fertile female mice have not resulted in inhibition of fertilization and preimplantation development (De Ioannes, unpublished results). The lack of antifertility effects of the monoclonal antibody ACRO-C2E5 in vivo is not in keeping with the in vitro inhibitory effects of the same antibody reported here. However, it is possible that the massive release of the enzyme during the acrosome reaction would allow high local concentrations that cannot be neutralized by the antibody in vivo, thus allowing sperm binding to the zona and the eventual fertilization of the eggs. Besides its role in penetration by the digestion of ZP1 [Dunbar et al., 1985], proacrosin has been recently shown to interact with carbohydrate moieties of zona glycoproteins, suggesting a receptor role for acrosin during

TABLE 3. Effect of SBTI on the Binding of Human Spermatozoa to Human Zonae Pellucidae, Evaluated by Phase-Contrast Microscopy[a]

Inhibitor	Concentration (μM)	No. of eggs observed	Mean of bound spermatozoa
SBTI	70	6	5.6
Ovomucoid	75	6	43.3
None		7	>200

[a]Results are means of three experiments. SBTI significatively inhibited human sperm binding to the homologous zonae pellucidae.

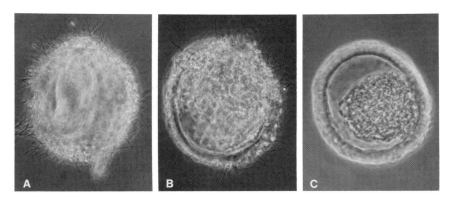

Fig. 3. Phase-contrast microscopic micrographs of human zonae pellucidae inseminated with capacitated human spermatozoa. **A:** Zona inseminated with capacitated spermatozoa and coincubated in culture medium without inhibitors. Note the large number of spermatozoa bound to the outer surface of the zona pellucida. ×525. **B:** Zona inseminated with capacitated spermatozoa and coincubated in the presence of ovomucoid trypsin inhibitor ×675. **C:** Zona inseminated with capacitated spermatozoa and coincubated in the presence of soybean trypsin inhibitor. Note the absence of spermatozoa bound to the zona. ×650.

the secondary binding of reacted sperm to the zona through a fucose-binding site [Jones et al., 1988]. However, the high concentration required for a full inhibitory effect of active site inhibitors such as SBTI, in contrast to the potent inhibitory effects, at low concentrations, of L-fucose and fucose containing glycan chains [Ahuja, 1982; Huang et al., 1982; Peterson et al., 1984; Shalgi et al., 1986], suggests that the fucose-binding site and the catalytic site are located at some distance. From this perspective, the enzymatic properties of acrosin would allow the sperm to open its way by breaking the network of the zona through a selective hydrolysis of ZP1 [Dunbar et al., 1985], which holds together the ZP filaments made of ZP2 and ZP3. In turn, the hydrolysis of ZP2 by acrosin may expose carbohydrate moieties for a further interaction with the proacrosin still bound to the remnants of the acrosome matrix, through the fucose-binding site [Jones et al., 1988]. This idea is supported by the work of Capote et al. [1989], showing that acrosin is present over the inner acrosomal membrane of acrosome-reacted spermatozoa using the immunogold technique with the monoclonal antiacrosin antibody ACRO-C2E5.

Thus acrosome-reacted sperm remain bound to the zona by a combination of the mechanic drive of the flagellar beating and the molecular interaction between proacrosin and zona carbohydrates. This is a dynamic process because, as the sperm progresses, the matrix dissolves and the zona is degraded through the conversion of proacrosin into acrosin [Töpfer-Peterson and Henschen, 1987]. Taking these facts together and considering that this enzyme is present in the sperm of all mammalian species studied to date, we underline the fundamental role of acrosin in gamete interactions leading to fertilization.

ACKNOWLEDGMENTS

We thank Dr. John Elce for providing the monoclonal antibody ACRO-C2E5, Dr. Horacio Croxatto for suggestions and comments, Horacio Vera for revision, Ignacia Aguirre for assistance in preparing the manuscript, and María Teresa Pino for typing the manuscript. This work was supported by Subproject Agreement CSA-89-040 from Contraceptive Research and Development Program (CONRAD); grants 495-89 and 577-89 from Fondo Nacional de Ciencias y Tecnología de Chile (FONDECYT); grant 3-P-86-1018-02 from International Development Research Center (IDRC); and grant GA-PS 87/10 from the Rockefeller Foundation.

REFERENCES

Ahuja KK (1982): Fertilization studies in the hamster: The role of cell surface carbohydrates. Exp Cell Res 140:353–362.

Barros C, Jedlicki A (1985): Human sperm fertilizing ability: Quality criteria. In Testact J, Frydamn R (eds): Human In Vitro Fertilization: Actual Problems and Prospects. Amsterdam: Elsevier Science Publishers, pp 79–91.

Barros C, Jedlicki A, Bize I, Aguirre E (1984): Relationship between the length of sperm pre-incubation and zona penetration in the golden hamster: Scanning electron microscopy study. Gamete Res 9:31–43.

Biggers JA, Whitten WK, Whittingham AG (1971): The culture of mouse embryos in vitro.

In Daniel JC (ed): Methods in Mammalian Embryology. San Francisco: W.H. Freeman, pp 86–116.

Bleil J, Wassarman PM (1986): Autoradiographic visualization of the mouse egg's sperm receptor bound to sperm. J Cell Biol 102:1363–1371.

Bleil JD, Wassarman PM (1988): Identification of a secondary sperm receptor in the mouse egg zona pellucida: Role in maintenance of binding of acrosome-reacted sperm to egg. Dev Biol 126:376–385.

Brown CR, Cheng TK (1985): Limited proteolysis of the porcine zona pellucida by homologous sperm acrosin. J Reprod Fertil 74:257–260.

Capote C, Pérez C, De Ioannes AE, Barros C (1989): Papel de la acrosina en la fecundación. Arch Biol Med Exp 22:R239.

Dunbar BS, Dudkiewicz AB, Bundman DS (1985): Proteolysis of specific porcine zona pellucida glycoproteins by boar acrosin. Biol Reprod 32:618–630.

Elce JS, Braham EJ, Zboril G, Leyton L, Pérez E, De Ioannes AE (1986): Monoclonal antibodies to bovine and human acrosin. Biochem Cell Biol 64:1242–1248.

Huang TTF, Ohzu E, Yanagimachi R (1982): Evidence suggesting that L-fucose is part of a recognition signal for sperm–zona pellucida attachment in mammals. Gamete Res 5: 355–361.

Jones R, Brown CR, Lancaster T (1988): Carbohydrate-binding properties of boar sperm proacrosin and assessment of its role in sperm–egg recognition and adhesion during fertilization. Development 102:781–792.

Kallajoki M, Parvinen M, Suominen J (1986): Expression of acrosin during mouse spermatogenesis: A biochemical and immunocytochemical analysis by a monoclonal antibody C11H. Biol Reprod 35:157–165.

Leyton L, De Ioannes AE, Croxatto HB, Graham EJ, Elce JS (1986): Two satisfactory methods for purification of human acrosin. Biochem Cell Biol 4:1020–1024.

Peterson RN, Russell LD, Hunt WP (1984): Evidence for specific binding of uncapacitated boar spermatozoa to porcine zonae pellucida in vitro. J Exp Zool 231:137–147.

Polakoski KL, Parrish RF (1977): Boar proacrosin: Purification and preliminary activation studies on proacrosin isolated from ejaculated boar sperm. J Biol Chem 252:1888–1894.

Saling PM (1981): Involvement of trypsin-like activity in binding of mouse spermatozoa to zonae pellucidae. Proc Natl Acad Sci USA 78:6231–6235.

Saling PM (1989): Mammalian sperm interaction with extracellular matrices of the egg. Oxford Rev Reprod Biol 11:339–388.

Shalgi R, Matityahu A, Nebel L (1986): The role of carbohydrates in sperm–egg interaction in rats. Biol Reprod 34:446–452.

Töpfer-Petersen E, Henschen A (1987): Acrosin shows zona and fucose binding, novel properties for a serine proteinase. FEBS Lett 226(1):38–42.

Urch U, Wardrip N, Hedrick J (1985): Limited and specific proteolysis of the zona pellucida by acrosin. J Exp Zool 233:479–483.

Yanagimachi R (1982): In vitro sperm capacitation and fertilization of golden-hamster eggs in a chemically defined medium. In Hafez ESE, Semm K (eds): In Vitro Fertilization and Embryo Transfer. Lancaster: MTP Press Limited, pp 65–76.

Yanagimachi R, Lopata A, Odom C, Bronson R, Nicolson MC (1979): Retention of biologic characteristics of zona pellucida in highly concentrated salt solution: The use of salt-stored eggs for assessing the fertilizing capacity of spermatozoa. Fertil Steril 31:562–574.

Yoshimatsu N, Yanagimachi R, Lopata A (1988): Zonae pellucidae of salt-stored hamster and human eggs: Their penetrability by homologous and heterologous spermatozoa. Gamete Res 21:115–126.

DISCUSSION

DR. ANDERSON: There has always been some question as to whether acrosin is truly sperm specific. Are there any recent data on this?

DR. DE IOANNES: Two years ago, we performed some experiments using polyclonal antisera to acrosin generated in our laboratory. We found some very odd activity in areas such as the pancreas and salivary glands. However, we could not find a protein that could be identified as kallikrein or another serum protease by Western blotting. It is possible that some epitope may be shared with other serine proteases.

DR. MOORE: With your monoclonal antibody, where did you get localization on acrosome-reacted sperm?

DR. DE IOANNES: We are performing experiments using immunogold. We found that, in the hamster, when the outer plasma membrane is removed, most of the acrosin is associated and is also removed. A little bit of acrosin may remain bound to the equatorial region. I think we need to repeat this work with more timed experiments to be more conclusive.

DR. MOORE: When the sperm is penetrating through the zona pellucida, it is the inner acrosomal membrane that is really in contact with zona matrix rather than other regions, such as the equatorial segment. How would that fit this in with your model of zona penetration?

DR. DE IOANNES: Well, the thing we hypothesize is that, as the plasma membrane and outer acrosomal membrane is fenestrated and as it is leaving the sperm surface, the matrix is progressively melting, so that there is still some acrosin, even after the end of the penetration.

15

Sperm Acrosin and Binding to the Zona Pellucida

E. Töpfer-Petersen, A.E. Friess, A. Henschen,
D. Cechova, and M. Steinberger

The fusion of the sperm and egg involves a series of highly complex molecular interactions at the level of the sperm–zona interface. Before penetration, the spermatozoa must bind to the surface of the zona pellucida and complete the acrosome reaction. Several lines of evidence suggest that complementary receptor molecules on both gametes are of decisive importance for these interactions [O'Rand, 1988].

In the female gamete, specific carbohydrate structures responsible for gamete binding and recognition are present in the zona pellucida [for review, see Wassarman et al., 1989], suggesting that the complementary carbohydrate-binding factor is part of the spermatozoon. Once bound to the zona, spermatozoa undergo the acrosome reaction, allowing the release of the lytic portion of the sperm acrosome, enabling the sperm to traverse the zona pellucida [for review, see Yanagimachi, 1988]. The acrosomal serine proteinase acrosin is one of the hydrolases released as a consequence of the acrosome reaction. Acrosin may be the most likely candidate for a "lysin," which contributes to penetration by specific and limited proteolysis of the zona glycoprotein matrix [Urch et al., 1985; Dunbar et al., 1985], thus facilitating the entry of the motile sperm into the zona pellucida. Acrosin has distinct structural features as compared with other serine proteinases and these may be related to its special function in fertilization [for review, see Hedrick et al., 1988].

Gamete Interaction: Prospects for Immunocontraception, pages 197–212
© 1990 Wiley-Liss, Inc.

FUCOSE-BINDING SITES ARE INVOLVED IN SPERM–EGG INTERACTION IN THE PIG

Fucoidan strongly inhibits sperm–zona binding not only in mammals but also in various lower organisms [Ahuja, 1985; Huang et al., 1982; Peterson et al., 1984; Rossignol et al., 1984]. Fucose in a similar conformation as in fucoidan has been suggested to be part of the recognition signal between gametes [Huang and Yanagimachi, 1984].

To detect fucose-binding activity in spermatozoa, fucosylated peroxidase (Fuc-HRP) was used as a standard carbohydrate ligand. The coupling of the carbohydrate ligand with colloidal gold as an electron-dense marker allows the precise ultrastructural localization of fucose-binding sites by transmission electron microscopy. In intact spermatozoa, fucose-binding sites are concentrated at the rostral region of the boar sperm head [Töpfer-Petersen et al., 1985]. After induction of the acrosome reaction by the ionophore A23187, a dramatic exposure and/or activation of fucose-binding sites occurs. The complete acrosomal region becomes heavily labeled (Fig. 1b) [Friess et al., 1987a]. Ultrathin sections of the acrosome-reacted spermatozoa show a preferential labeling of the fuzzy material adhering to the outer acrosomal membrane, whereas the inner acrosomal membrane shows only moderate but distinct labeling (Fig. 1c) [Friess et al., 1987a]. This labeling pattern indicates that fucose-binding activity may be associated with components of the acrosomal content. By a special fracture labeling technique [Aguas and Pinto da Silva, 1983] the intra-acrosomal occurrence of fucose-binding could be confirmed. Fracture faces through different regions of the acrosome show a clear labeling for fucose-binding in the acrosomal matrix (Fig. 1a) [Friess et al., 1987b]. Although fucose-binding sites are present at the sperm surface, the ultrastructural data demonstrate that the bulk of fucose-binding sites localized inside the acrosome are exposed during the course of the acrosome reaction. This unexpected distribution of fucose binding in spermatozoa raises the question as to the function of these fucose-binding sites during fertilization. If the fucose-binding sites do participate at one stage of sperm–zona binding, the binding of the zona proteins to the spermatozoa should be inhibited by fucose conjugates, and conversely the binding of Fuc-HRP should be blocked by the zona glycoproteins.

To examine the nature of the sperm–zona binding on a more molecular level, a novel approach has been developed on the basis of the biotin–avidin system. Utilizing biotinylated zona glycoproteins labeled with FITC–avidin for fluorescence microscopy, the topography of zona-binding sites on spermatozoa has been documented.

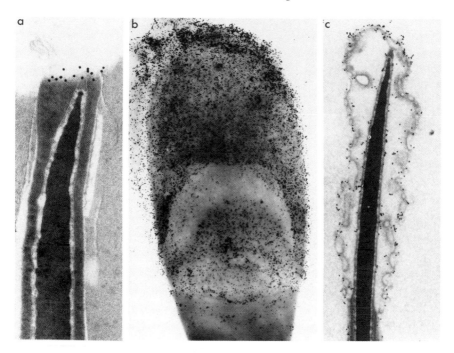

Fig. 1. Topography of fucose-binding sites in boar spermatozoa. Transmission electron microscopy of spermatozoa labeled with Fuc-HRP-colloidal gold. **a:** Fracture labeling of ejaculated spermatozoa. **b:** Total specimen preparation of acrosome-reacted spermatozoa. **c:** Ultrathin section of acrosome-reacted spermatozoa. (From Friess et al. [1987a,b], with permission of the publisher.)

The zona-binding pattern shows a striking similarity with the fucose-binding pattern (Figs. 1, 2). In live spermatozoa, zona-binding sites are concentrated at the apical part of the sperm head [Töpfer-Petersen and Schill, 1989]. However, zona binding appears to be mainly located within the acrosomal matrix. After fixation a significant increase in fluorescence over the entire acrosomal region was observed, indicating the intra-acrosomal occurrence of zona-binding activity (Fig. 2c). The binding is completely inhibited by different fucosyl conjugates such as fucoidan (Fig. 2d), Fuc-HRP, and fucosyllactose. Fucose and lactose alone show only small inhibitory effects, indicating that fucose in a more complex organization may be needed to compete with the zona glycoproteins. As was shown for fucoidan [Töpfer-Petersen, 1988], fucosyllactose also effectively inhibits the binding of capacitated spermatozoa to the zona pellucida in an in vitro sperm–egg binding assay (Fig. 3).

Furthermore, when assayed by a specific solid-phase binding as-

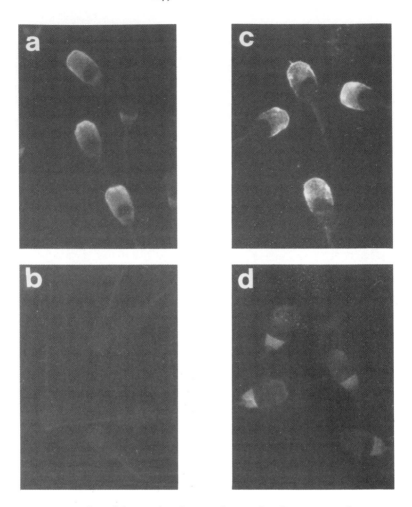

Fig. 2. Topography of fucose-binding and zona-binding sites in boar spermatozoa. Fluorescence microscopy of fixed spermatozoa. a: Labeled with FITC-Fuc-HRP. **b:** In the presence of fucoidan (1 mg/ml). **c:** Labeled with biotinylated zona pellucida and FITC-streptavidin. **d:** In the presence of fucoidan (1 mg/ml).

say [Töpfer-Petersen et al., 1985], the binding of Fuc-HRP to spermatozoa immobilized on ELISA plates was inhibited by heat-solubilized zona pellucida in a dose-dependent manner (Fig. 4), indicating that the zona glycoproteins compete with the standard fucose ligand for the same binding sites on the spermatozoon.

Taken together, these data indicate that fucose-receptor molecules on spermatozoa recognize specific fucose-containing carbohydrate structures on the zona pellucida and may therefore be involved in

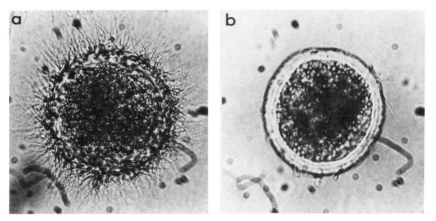

Fig. 3.   In vitro sperm binding assay [Saxena et al., 1986]. Light micrographs illustrating the binding of capacitated boar spermatozoa to the zona pellucida of porcine eggs in vitro **(a)** and in the presence of 150 mM fucosyllactose **(b)**.

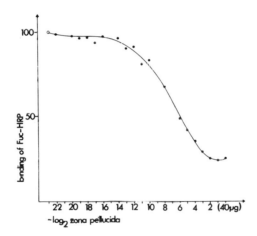

Fig. 4.   Inhibition of the binding of Fuc-HRP by decreasing amounts of heat-solubilized zona pellucida from (40 μg/ml). Determination of the remaining Fuc-HRP–binding capacity by the solid-phase binding assay (mod. ELLA) on ELISA plates with 10^5 sperms/well.

the complex sequence of sperm–zona interactions leading to fertilization.

THE MAJOR FUCOSE-BINDING PROTEIN IS IDENTICAL TO THE SPERM PROTEINASE ACROSIN

Predominantly a protein with an apparent molecular mass of 53 kd, and to some extent a 17 kd protein, has been shown to account

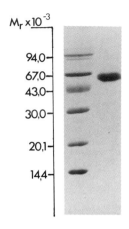

$M_r \times 10^{-3}$

94,0–

67,0–

43,0–

30,0–

20,1–

14,4–

Fig. 5.   SDS-PAGE of the major boar fucose-binding protein, i.e., α-acrosin.

for the fucose-binding activity of boar spermatozoa [Töpfer-Petersen et al., 1985]. The major fucose-binding protein (53 kd) has been isolated to apparent homogeneity by a two-step procedure, including high-resolution gel filtration and reverse-phase chromatography (Fig. 5) [Töpfer-Petersen and Henschen, 1987]. As expected, the isolated 53 kd protein shows strong affinity to the zona glycoproteins when Western blots were tested with the biotinylated zona proteins visualized with avidin–peroxidase (Fig. 6).

Amino acid sequence analysis by Edman degradation [Edman and Henschen, 1975] disclosed that the 53 kd protein contains two polypeptide chains with the N-termini starting with Arg-Asp-X-Ala-Thr and Val-Val-Gly-Gly-Met (Fig. 7). These sequences have been shown to be identical with those at an N-terminus of the sperm proteinase acrosin [Fock-Nüzel et al., 1980, 1984]. Furthermore, the isolated protein shows the same elution characteristic on reverse-phase chromatography as acrosin and exhibits a considerable amidolytic activity [Töpfer-Petersen and Henschen, 1988]. The structural data extended by the observation that the protein under investigation displays an excellent cross-reactivity with antibodies directed against acrosin (unpublished data) clearly demonstrate the identity of the fucose-binding protein with the acrosomal serine proteinase acrosin. Rather recently Jones and Brown [1987] identified the major zona-binding protein of 53 kd from boar spermatozoa as proacrosin/acrosin by means of its cross-reactivity with antibodies directed against acrosin.

ACROSIN IS A MULTIFUNCTIONAL PROTEIN

Acrosin is a serine proteinase with a light chain (A chain: Arg-Asp-Asn[carbohydrate]-Ala) and a heavy chain (B chain: Val-Val-

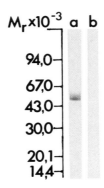

Fig. 6. Zona-binding of the major boar fucose-binding protein, i.e., α-acrosin. **a:** Western blots were probed with biotinylated zona pellucida and streptavidin-peroxidase and visualized by enzymatic amplification with 4-chloro-1-naphthol. **b:** Control, in the presence of nonlabeled zona pellucida.

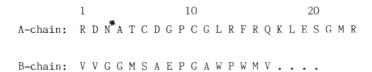

Fig. 7. N-terminal amino acid sequences in the major boar fucose-binding protein, identical with those in boar acrosin. Asterisk indicates N with carbohydrate side chain.

Gly-Gly) linked by two disulfide bridges. Its structure is clearly homologous to that of other proteinases. The heavy chain presenting the typical N-terminal sequence of an active serine proteinase comprises the catalytic triad of the enzyme, and the light chain of 23 amino acids corresponds to the propart. However, in comparison with other serine proteinases, acrosin exhibits a considerably higher molecular weight and contains a strikingly high proportion of hydrophobic amino acids [Fock-Nüzel et al., 1980; Zelezna et al., 1989].

In intact spermatozoa, acrosin occurs in an inactive zymogen form, proacrosin, with a molecular mass of 53–55 kd [Cechova et al., 1988; Baba et al., 1989a]. Proacrosin is a single-chain molecule that has the N-terminus of the 23 amino acids of the acrosin light chain and its sequence continues with the N-terminus of the heavy chain (Fig. 8). By a single proteolytic clip in the N-terminal region, proacrosin is autoactivated to the active enzyme now presenting the N-terminal sequence Val-Val-Gly-Gly of an activated serine proteinase

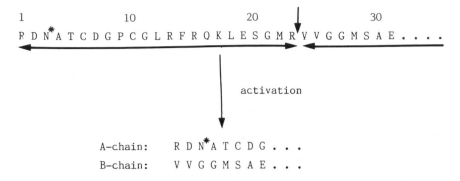

Fig. 8.   N-terminal amino acid sequence of boar proacrosin (53/55 kd), identical with the total A-chain and N-terminal B-chain sequences. Activation leads to the appearance of two N-termini because of the presence of the A-chain (light chain) and B-chain (heavy chain). Asterisk indicates N with carbohydrate side chain.

in addition to the N-terminus of the light chain (Fig. 8) [Cechova et al., 1988]. The proacrosin–acrosin conversion is believed to proceed by an intrazymogen mechanism rather than by the influence of an activating proteinase [Kennedy and Polakoski, 1981]. Nonproteolytic agents such as phospholipids and sulfated polysaccharides such as heparin, chondroitin sulfate, and fucoidan stimulate the activation [Parrish et al., 1980]. In this context it may be of biological significance that heat-solubilized zona pellucida exerts a similar effect on the proacrosin autoactivation [Töpfer-Petersen and Cechova, 1989]. Sulfated carbohydrate structures that are common to the sulfated polysaccharides and the zona glycoproteins may function as conversion activators. It could be speculated that upon binding to the sulfated carbohydrate structures proacrosin undergoes a conformational change that increases the susceptibility to cleavage of the Arg–Val bond.

The active enzyme formed by this major activation event consists of the light chain and a full-length heavy chain. Further proteolytic processing of the high-molecular-mass form (53–55 kd), designated α-acrosin results in the formation of the lower-molecular-mass β-form (38 kd), which seems to be the most stable form of the enzyme (Fig. 9). The two enzymatically active forms of acrosin possess the two identical N-termini because of the presence of the heavy and light chains. The processing of the higher molecular mass form to the "mature" form of acrosin (38 kd) results in the liberation of approximately 85 amino acids from the C-terminal part of the heavy chain. One-third of the residues has been shown to be proline [Zelezna et al., 1988]. Very recently the complete structures of boar and human

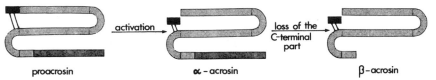

proacrosin   α – acrosin   β – acrosin

Fig. 9. Scheme of the proacrosin activation pathway. Proacrosin (53/55 kd) is activated by N-terminal cleavage of the Arg–Val bond, giving rise to the high-molecular-mass α-acrosin (53/55 kd). Further processing by C-terminal cleavage results in the formation of the lower molecular mass α-acrosin (38 kd).

proacrosin have been established by molecular cloning, confirming the unusual clustering of prolines, particularly in the C-terminal part of the molecule [Adham et al., 1989; Baba et al., 1989b]. The high proline content of acrosin and especially of the conversion peptide could account for the pronounced affinity of acrosin to membranes and other surfaces [Zelezna and Cechova, 1982; Zelezna et al., 1989].

The ability to bind carbohydrates seems to be another unique property of acrosin. Other serine proteinases such as thrombin, trypsin, urokinase, and elastase lack a comparable fucose- and zona-binding property. Neither Fuc-HRP as the standard fucose ligand nor the biotinylated zona pellucida bind to ordinary serine proteinases when tested by the solid-phase binding assay [Töpfer-Petersen, 1989].

STRUCTURAL ASPECTS OF THE ACROSIN–ZONA BINDING

Acrosin combines several functional properties within a single molecule—the catalytic triad of the proteinase, hydrophobic domains responsible for the special membrane-associating character of the enzyme, and the carbohydrate-binding sites by which the molecule can bind to the zona pellucida. An interesting approach to the study of structure–function relationships in acrosin is the isolation of the special structures responsible for the distinct function of acrosin.

The proteolytic property of a serine proteinase can be selectively destroyed by diiosopropyl fluorophosphate (DFP) blocking of the serine residue in the active center. Treatment of acrosin with DFP abolishes the enzymatic activity but not the zona- and fucose-binding properties [Töpfer-Petersen and Henschen, 1988]. It may be suggested that the functional properties are distributed between the two chains. Thus the binding ability might be associated with the acrosin light chain, which remains linked to the active enzyme after activation. The two chains can be separated by mercaptolysis and S-pyridylethylation of the active two-chain molecule followed by re-

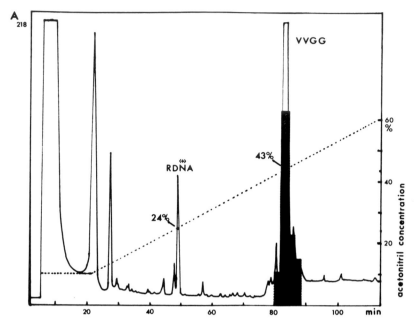

Fig. 10. Reverse-phase chromatography of α-acrosin (53/55 kd) after mercapatolysis and S-pyridylethylation. Zona binding was tested by the solid-phase binding assay with biotinylated zona pellucida using the avidin–biotin system.

verse-phase chromatography and then tested separately. However, the heavy chain but not the light chain shows strong binding to both fucose and zona pellucida (Fig. 10). Thus the carbohydrate-binding sites are located on the acrosin heavy chain. The carbohydrate affinity is independent of the inherent proteolytic activity of the enzyme [Töpfer-Petersen and Henschen, 1988].

Autoproteolysis of acrosin gradually destroys not only its enzymatic activity [Parrish and Polakoski, 1978] but also its zona-binding property. However, by limited autoproteolysis of the active 53 kd acrosin, a peptide is released that binds to the zona pellucida. Western blots of the autolyzed acrosin probed with biotinylated zona proteins show a strong affinity for the 53 kd protein corresponding to the active α-form, for the 38 kd protein corresponding to the active β-form, and for a 15 kd peptide corresponding to one of the low-molecular-weight fragments [Töpfer-Petersen et al., 1989]. The peptide has been isolated in low amounts by reverse-phase chromatography (Fig. 11). It may be suspected that the C-terminal part, i.e., the region of the acrosin molecule that displays the most unusual struc-

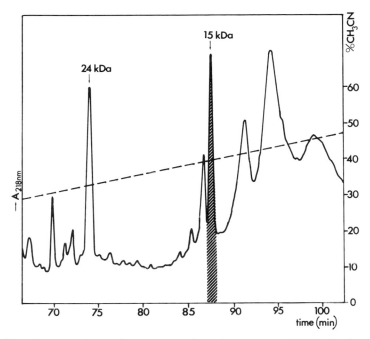

Fig. 11.   Reverse-phase chromatography of α-acrosin (53/55 kd) after limited autoproteolysis. Zona binding was tested by the solid-phase binding assay with biotinylated zona pellucida using the biotin-avidin system.

tural features, also carries the carbohydrate-binding sites. The zona-binding fragment, however, is not identical with the C-terminal peptide formed during the early stage of α-acrosin to β-acrosin conversion. Edman degradation of the isolated peptide revealed a contiguous sequence of 30 amino acids of the N-terminal part of the heavy chain [Töpfer-Petersen et al., 1989], starting with the N-terminal tetrapeptide Val-Val-Gly-Gly. The 15 kd peptide represents the first 100–110 amino acid residues of the heavy chain. This region is highly homologous with other serine proteinases containing two of the amino acids that are part of the catalytic triad of the proteinase [Fock-Nüzel, 1983; Adham et al., 1989]. Therefore, it seems likely that short segments of the sequence may account for the fucose- and zona-binding properties of the sperm proteinase acrosin.

CONCLUSIONS

The penetration of the zona pellucida is a crucial step during fertilization. The mechanism by which the spermatozoa overcome this barrier is not completely understood. However, a combination of forces produced by the hyperactivated spermatozoon and enzymatic digestion is proposed to be necessary for sperm penetration to occur [Green, 1987]. Acrosin may be the most likely candidate for an enzyme that contributes to sperm penetration by specific and limited proteolysis of the zona glycoproteins [Urch et al., 1985; Dunbar et al., 1985]. The unique structural and functional properties of acrosin may be related to its function to assist the motile sperm to traverse the zona pellucida. We have demonstrated that acrosin combines three different functional units in its heavy chain: the catalytic triad of an activated serine proteinase, the membrane-associating domain(s) in the C-terminal part, and the carbohydrate binding sites in the N-terminal part. Via autolysis different active acrosin forms or inactive fragments are generated that combine the acrosin functions in different manners. The carbohydrate affinity can be separated from the hydrophobic activity by C-terminal processing without concomitant loss of enzymatic activity or alternatively by N-terminal processing creating fragments that have lost their enzymatic activity.

Rather recently O'Rand and coworkers [1986] described a model in which alternating cycles of binding to, digestion of the zona proteins, and release from the zona pellucida together with the forward motility of the spermatozoon would be required to achieve penetration. Acrosin may be instrumental in all three stages: the binding, digestion, and release reactions. Thus, once bound to the zona pellucida, spermatozoa undergo the acrosome reaction and proacrosin is activated to acrosin containing a full-length heavy chain. Via its membrane-associating domains and the carbohydrate-binding sites, acrosin may function as the binding link between the acrosome-reacted spermatozoon and the zona pellucida. Acrosin may then locally digest the zona glycoproteins. Processing of acrosin in the way that the enzyme is released from the C-terminal membrane-associating attachment sites, allows the released spermatozoon to move deeper into the zona pellucida; subsequently these steps are repeated until the spermatozoon has completed penetration.

We do not know how acrosin undergoes autoproteolysis in vivo. However, it is reasonable to suggest that specific processing of acrosin will be of functional importance for sperm penetration to occur and that these events are regulated by the zona pellucida.

ACKNOWLEDGMENTS

The authors are indepted to Ms. A. Scharf, C. Ebner von Eschenbach, and U. Cerwony for excellent technical assistence and to Prof.

W.-B. Schill for support. The provision of a research fellowship (D.C.) by the Alexander-von-Humboldt-Stiftung is gratefully acknowledged. The work was supported by the Deutsche Forschungsgemeinschaft (To 114/1-1, He 1072/6-2, and Schi 86/6-2).

REFERENCES

Adham IM, Klemm U, MaierW-M, Hoyer-Fender S, Tsaousidou S, Engel W (1989): Cloning of preproacrosin and analysis of its expression pattern in spermiogenesis. Eur J Biochem 182:563–568.

Aguas AP, Pinto da Silva P (1983): Regionalization of transmembrane glycoproteins in the plasma membrane of boar sperm head by fracture labelling. J Cell Biol 97:1356–1364.

Ahuja KK (1985): Carbohydrate determinants involved in mammalian fertilization. Am J Anat 174:207–223.

Baba T, Michikawa Y, Kawakura K, Arai Y (1989a): Activation of boar proacrosin is effected by processing at both N-terminal and C-terminal portions of the zymogen molecule. FEBS Lett 244:132–136

Baba T, Watanabe K, Kashiwabara S, Arai Y (1989b): Primary structure of human proacrosin deduced from cDNA sequence. FEBS Lett 244:296–300.

Cechova D, Töpfer-Petersen E, Henschen A (1988): Boar acrosin is a single-chain molecule which has the N-terminus of the acrosin A-chain (light chain). FEBS Lett 241:136–140.

Dunbar DS, Dudkiewicz AB, Bundman DS (1985): Proteolysis of specific porcine zona pellucida glycoproteins by boar acrosin. Biol Reprod 32:619–630.

Edman P, Henschen A (1975): Sequence determination. In Needleman SB (ed): "Sequence Determination." Berlin: Springer Verlag, pp 232–279.

Fock-Nüzel R (1983): Studien zur Primarstruktur des Eberakrosins. Ph.D. thesis, Max-Planck-Institute for Biochemistry, Martinsried, FRG.

Fock-Nüzel R, Lottspeich F, Henschen A, Müller-Esterl W (1980): N-terminal amino acid sequence of boar sperm acrosin. Hoppe Seyler Z Physiol Chem 3261:1381–1388.

Fock-Nüzel R, Lottspeich F, Henschen A, Müller-Esterl W (1984): Boar acrosin is a two-chain molecule. Isolation and primary structure of the light chain: Homology with the propart of other serine proteinases. Eur J Biochem 141:441–446.

Friess AE, Töpfer-Petersen E, Schill W-B (1987a): Electron microscopic localization of a fucose-binding protein in acrosome-reacted spermatozoa by the fucosyl-peroxidase-gold-method. Histochemistry 86:297–303.

Friess AE, Töpfer-Petersen E, Schill W-B (1987b): Fracture labelling of boar spermatozoa for the fucose-binding protein (FBP). Histochemistry 87:181–183.

Green DPL (1987): Mammalian sperm cannot penetrate the zona pellucida solcy by force. Exp Cell Res 169:31–38.

Hedrick JL, Urch UA, Hardy DM (1988): The structure–function properties of the sperm enzyme acrosin. In Shoemaker S, Sonnet P, Whitaker J (eds): Enzymes in Agricultural Biotechnology. Washington, DC: ACS Books, pp 1–11.

Huang TTF, Ohzu E, Yanagimachi R (1982): Evidence suggesting that L-fucose is part of the recognition signal for sperm–zona pellucida attachment in mammals. Gamete Res 5:355–361.

Huang TTF, Yanagimachi R (1984): Fucoidan inhibits attachment of guinea pig spermatozoa to the zona pellucida through binding to the inner acrosomal membrane and equatorial segment. Exp Cell Res 153:363–373.

Jones R, Brown CR (1987): Identification of a zona binding protein from boar spermatozoa as proacrosin. Exp Cell Res 71:503–508.

Kennedy WP, Polakoski KL (1981): Evidence for an intrazymogen mechanism in the conversion of proacrosin into acrosin. Biochemistry 20:2240–2245.

O'Rand MG (1988): Sperm–egg recognition and barriers to interspecies fertilization. Gamete Res 19:315–328.

O'Rand MG, Welch JE, Fisher SJ (1986): In Dhindsda DS, Bahl O (eds): Molecular and Cellular Aspects of Reproduction. New York: Plenum Press, pp 131–144.

Parrish RF, Polakoski KL (1978) Boar-acrosin: Purification and characterization of the initial active enzyme resulting from the conversion of boar acrosin to acrosin. J Biol Chem 253:8428–8432.

Parrish RF, Wincek TJ, Polakoski KL (1980): Glycosaminoglycan stimulation of in vitro conversion of boar proacrosin into acrosin. J Androl 1:89–95.

Peterson RN, Russell LD, Hunt WP (1984): Evidence for specific binding of uncapacitated boar spermatozoa to porcine zona pellucida in vitro. J Exp Zool 231:137–147.

Rossignol DP, Decker GL, Lennarz WJ (1984): Cell–cell interactions and membrane fusion during fertilization in sea urchin. In Beers RF, Bassett EG (eds): Cell Fusion: Gene Transfer and Transformation. New York: Raven Press, pp 5–26.

Saxena N, Peterson RN, Sharif S, Saxena NK, Russell LD (1986): Changes in the organization of surface antigens during capacitation of boar spermatozoa as detected by monoclonal antibodies. J Reprod Fertil 78:601–614.

Töpfer-Petersen E (1988): Sperm–egg interaction in the pig—A model for mammalian fertilization. In Holstein AF, Bettendorf G, Hölzer KH, Leidenberger F (eds): "Carl Schirren Symposium—Advances in Andrology. Berlin: Diesbach Verlag, pp 251–260.

Töpfer-Petersen E (1989): Molecular events during fertilization. In Kotyk A, Skoda J, Paces V, Kostka V (eds): Highlights in Modern Biochemistry. Zeist: VSP, pp 1131–1141.

Töpfer-Petersen E, Cechova D (1990): Zona pellucida induces proacrosin-to-acrosin conversion. Int J Androl 13:190–196.

Töpfer-Petersen E, Friess AE, Nguyen H, Schill W-B (1985): Evidence for a fucose-binding protein in boar spermatozoa. Histochemistry 83:139–145.

Töpfer-Petersen E, Henschen A (1987): Acrosin shows zona and fucose binding, novel properties for a serine proteinase. FEBS Lett 226:38–42.

Töpfer-Petersen E, Henschen A (1988): Zona pellucida–binding and fucose-binding of boar sperm acrosin is not correlated with proteolytic activity. Biol Chem Hoppe Seyler 369:69–76.

Töpfer-Petersen E, Schill W-B (1989): The sperm surface and sperm–egg interaction in the pig. In Holstein AF, Voigt KD, Grässlin D (eds): Reproductive Biology and Medicine. Berlin: Diesbach, pp 78–90.

Töpfer-Petersen E, Steinberger M, Ebner von Eschenbach C, Zucker A (1989): Zona pellucida binding of boar sperm acrosin is associated with N-terminal part of the acrosin B-chain (heavy chain). FEBS Lett 265:51–54.

Urch UA, Wardrip NJ, Hedrick JL (1985): Limited and specific proteolysis of the zona pellucida by acrosin. J Exp Zool 233:479–483.

Wassarman P, Bleil J, Fimiani C, Florman H, Greve J, Kinloch R, Moller C, Mortillo S, Roller R, Salzmann G, Vazquez M (1989): The mouse egg receptor for sperm: A multifunctional zona glycoprotein. In Dietl J (ed): The Mammalian Egg Coat. Berlin: Springer-Verlag, pp 18–37.

Yanagimachi R (1988): Mammalian fertilization. In Knobil E, Neill JD, Ewing LL, Greenwald GS, Market CL, Pfaff DW (eds): The Physiology of Reproduction, Vol 1. New York: Raven Press, pp 135–185.

Zelezna B, Cechova D (1982): Boar acrosin: Isolation of two active forms of boar ejaculated sperm. Hoppe Seyler Z Physiol Chem 363:757–766.

Zelezna B, Cechova D, Henschen A (1989): Isolation of the boar sperm acrosin peptide released during the conversion of α-form into β-form. Biol Chem Hoppe Seyler 370: 323–327.

DISCUSSION

DR. DEAN: Do you have any idea what macromolecule in the zona pellucida might be responsible for autocatolytic functions or to which acrosin binding may occur?

DR. TÖPFER-PETERSEN: It is not easy to separate the pig zona pellucida, so I don't know which it is. But it is not exclusively to a 55 kd protein; we also found binding with a 90 kd peptide.

DR. DEAN: Are all of the zona proteins in the pig glycosylated, as they are in women?

DR. TÖPFER-PETERSEN: I don't know. We tried to separate the different zona proteins, but, unfortunately, we were not successful. When we digest the complete zona, we find specific peptides that inhibit acrosin–zona binding. I hope very soon to see a peptide sequence of all the zona proteins so that we can fit the sequence of such a peptide into a pattern.

DR. O'RAND: Have you detected acrosin on the surface of living sperm before the acrosome reaction with any of your antibodies. I think that Jerry Hedrick reported that he had done that, and I wondered if you had seen anything similar.

DR. TÖPFER-PETERSEN: We have detected fucose-binding sites on the sperm plasma membrane. Initially, we though that it might be one of the peptides associated with acrosin. But the sequence is completely different. It has nothing to do with acrosin. It comes from and is coated by or absorbed from the seminal plasma. So we do not have much evidence that acrosin is on the surface.

DR. PRIMAKOFF: You proposed that acrosin may have a role in zona binding and zona penetration. I wonder if there is any new information about acrosin inhibitors. I know that some years ago Dr. Saling published that, in the mouse, inhibitors of the protease site do not inhibit penetration. This indicated that acrosin is not required. I am wondering if there is any evidence in a sperm–zona-binding assay that acrosin has a binding activity.

DR. TÖPFER-PETERSEN: What we have found is that heavy chain acrosin—not activated acrosin—inhibits sperm binding and sperm penetration. The question of the inhibitors is critical. I think we must try natural inhibitors. We have some evidence that there is a intra-acrosomal inhibitor inside the acrosome. And, in a special group of infertile men, we found that acrosin activity is suppressed. That means there is enough acrosin available, but the conversion to acrosin is incomplete. I think that there is a very special regulation of the inhibitors and acrosin.

DR. VASQUEZ: Based on the results in the mouse concerning changes in the structure of the zona pellucida after fertilization, have you tried to see the effect acrosin on activated eggs?

DR. TÖPFER-PETERSEN: No, I haven't.

16

Receptors for Zona Pellucida on Human Spermatozoa

M.G. O'Rand, E.E. Widgren, B.S. Nikolajczyk,
R.T. Richardson, and R.B. Shabanowitz

The basis for the specificity of gamete recognition and fusion lies in the molecular structures of the interacting molecules. To understand these interacting molecules, they must first be carefully identified and their functions characterized. Currently there appear to be several different candidates for a sperm zona-binding protein (ZBP) that interacts with the zona. These would include both enzymatic and lectin-like molecules. The enzyme galactosyltransferase [Lopez et al., 1985; Macek and Shur, 1988] has been examined in detail for its role as a sperm ZBP. The acrosomal enzyme acrosin has also been examined as a ZBP both in its traditional role as a serine protease that acts on the zona as a substrate and as a lectin [Töpfer-Petersen and Henschen, 1988]. Trypsin-like protease activity has been reported to be involved in zona binding in the mouse [Saling, 1981; Benau and Storey, 1988], although a specific enzyme molecule has yet to be identified. However, a mouse ZBP that binds a seminal plasma proteinase inhibitor has been described [Poirier et al., 1986; Richardson et al., 1987] and α-D-mannosidase has been reported to play a role in sperm–zona binding in rat sperm [Tulsiani et al., 1989]. In addition to enzymes, lectins also function as ZBPs. As noted above, acrosin has lectin activity, as does the rabbit sperm autoantigen RSA. RSA is a lectin-like molecule that binds to zonae with high affinity; its properties are similar to those of sea urchin bindin [O'Rand et al., 1988; O'Rand and Widgren, 1989]. Finally, a 95 kd mouse ZBP that also binds antiphosphotyrosine antibodies and may therefore be a tyrosine kinase substrate has recently been reported by Leyton and Saling [1989].

Gamete Interaction: Prospects for Immunocontraception, pages 213–224
© 1990 Wiley-Liss, Inc.

The oocyte's receptor, on the other hand, appears to be one or more carbohydrate moieties of the zona pellucida's ZP3 and ZP2 components [see O'Rand, 1988, for review]. Because the exquisite specificity of fertilization requires interactions that will result in penetration and successful fertilization, it seems likely that several different interacting molecules will be required. Consequently the phrase "avidity of fertilization" has been introduced [O'Rand, 1988] to describe the concept that it is the sum of the affinities of all the sperm's binding proteins for the oocyte's extracellular coats and plasma membrane that will determine the specificity of fertilization.

In the case of human spermatozoa and human zonae pellucidae, the zona components have been studied in more detail than those of the sperm. Over the past decade the structure of the human zona pellucida has been defined [Sacco and Palm, 1977; Sacco et al., 1984, 1986; Shabanowitz and O'Rand, 1988a,b] and shown to contain the three basic glycoprotein components found in other mammals, namely, ZP1, ZP2, and ZP3. After SDS-PAGE under nonreducing conditions, human ZP1 and ZP2 comigrate as a single band of $M_r = 92$–120 kd, while ZP3 migrates to $M_r = 57$–73 kd [Shabanowitz and O'Rand, 1988b]. If the zona glycoproteins are first reduced, then ZP1 and ZP2 are separated into ZP1 at $M_r = 97$ kd and ZP2 at $M_r = 82$ kd. ZP3 migrates to approximately $M_r = 70$ kd after reduction. Two-dimensional IEF/SDS-PAGE has shown that all three zona glycoprotein components have acidic pI values and contain multiple charged species [Shabanowitz and O'Rand, 1988b].

The binding of spermatozoa to the zona pellucida also induces the acrosome reaction. Studies by Cross et al. [1988] have shown that human sperm are induced to undergo acrosome reactions by intact and solubilized zonae. The peptide portion of ZP3 in the mouse was shown to be necessary for inducing the acrosome reaction [Wassarman et al., 1986]. Similarly, rabbit [O'Rand and Fisher, 1987], hamster [Cherr et al., 1986], and bovine [Florman and First, 1988] zonae induce the sperm acrosome reaction.

Western blotting of sperm proteins probed with ^{125}I-heat solubilized zonae resulted in the initial identification of the ZBP of spermatozoa [O'Rand et al., 1985]. More recent studies on boar [Brown and Jones, 1987], human [Shabanowitz and O'Rand, 1988b], and mouse [Leyton and Saling, 1989] have confirmed the technique to be a useful one for visualization of ZBP. However, as pointed out by O'Rand et al. [1985], limitations of the method include the obvious fact that proteins must survive SDS treatment and, in some cases, boiling before electrophoresis and transfer to a membrane. It is unlikely that ZPBs that depend on subunits or conformations for binding would survive such treatments. Additionally, proteins present in the sample in small amounts (<1 μg) may be difficult to detect above background because of the signal-to-noise ratio on the membrane. It should also be considered that the specificity and method of preparation of the probe will effect the outcome of its interaction with the ZBP on the membrane [Shabanowitz and O'Rand, 1988b; Leyton and Saling, 1989]. Nevertheless, human ZBPs of 16, 18, 19, 35, and 60 kd have been identified. Both human ZP1–2 and ZP3 bind to all of these sperm proteins [O'Rand et al., 1985; Shabanowitz and O'Rand, 1988b].

Studies on the binding of human spermatozoa to human zona pellucida have revealed that spermatozoa can be saturated with ^{125}I-labeled, heat-solubilized human zona pellucida (HSHZP) [Shabanowitz and O'Rand, 1988b]. These results indicate that the sperm surface contains receptor(s) for zona pellucida. Similar results have been found in other species. For example, in the mouse zona pellucida, of the three glycoproteins that have been identified (ZP1, ZP2, and ZP3), ZP3 (M_r = 83 kd) has been identified as being responsible for sperm binding and for the induction of the acrosome reaction [Bleil and Wassarman, 1980, 1983]. ZP2 (M_r = 120 kd) also binds spermatozoa, but only after the acrosome reaction [Bleil and Wassarman, 1986]. In the pig, ZP3 of M_r = 55 kD (55–60 kd range) has been identified as the boar sperm receptor [Sacco et al., 1984, 1986; Peterson et al., 1985]. Further work on the boar has shown that both the 90 and 55 kd (α) zona components bind sperm [Berger et al., 1989]. In the rabbit M_r = 87 kd component of the zona, which contains both ZP2 and ZP3 as assessed by two-dimensional SDS-PAGE [O'Rand et al., 1988] has been identified as the receptor for the sperm protein RSA.

Investigations into the carbohydrate moieties of the zona have indicated a number of possibilities. In the mouse zona, Florman and Wassarman [1985] identified a glycopeptide from the ZP3 molecule with an O-linked carbohydrate moiety that was responsible for the binding of the sperm to the zona. Galactose was subsequently identified as the key sugar in this interaction [Bleil and Wassarman, 1988]. In the pig, N-acetylglucosamine has been implicated as the key sugar [Berger et al., 1989]. In the rabbit, the lectin-like sperm protein RSA has been found to bind zona with a dissociation constant of 5.6 × 10^{-13} M. Such strong binding is inhibited by the sulfated carbohydrates fucoidin, chondroitin sulfate B, and heparin, but not by chondroitin sulfates A and C [O'Rand et al., 1988]. Only very high concentrations (>10 mM) of monosaccharides will inhibit RSA–zona interaction. The spatial orientation (α 1–3 linkage) of the monosaccharides (fucose, galactose, or glucose) and the position of the sulfate on the C4 carbon along the backbone of the polymer molecule are probably more important than the specific monosaccharide. Based on the evidence to date, it is likely that the sperm's most adhesive ZBP is a lectin or a lectin-like molecule that is similar to sea urchin bindin [Vacquier and Moy, 1977; Glabe et al., 1982] in its physical and chemical properties [O'Rand and Widgren, 1989; see O'Rand, 1988, for review].

Recent structural work on RSA peptides has shown that a 10 amino acid peptide sequence (P10G; PGGGTLPPSG), obtained from the 14,000 dalton RSA family member, is an autoantigenic epitope specifically binding rabbit antirabbit sperm autoantisera [O'Rand and Widgren, 1989]. Moreover, P10G is a sequence with similarities to five different bindin segments [O'Rand and Widgren, 1989]. Consequently, the presence of P10G in human spermatozoa is of interest, particularly in light of our earlier work with monoclonal antibodies to RSA that revealed cross-reactivity to human sperm proteins of 17, 18, and 87 kd [O'Rand and Irons, 1984]. The three human ZBPs of 16, 18, and 19 kd may, therefore, prove to have interesting similarities to P10G and RSA.

Figure 1A shows the presence of immunologically cross-reactive RSA-like molecules of 65–70 kd in human (lane 7) and pig (lane 8) spermatozoa. Rabbit spermatozoa are shown in lane 9. The arrowheads indicate the major bands at 70 and 65 kd. These bands represent aggregated forms of RSA [O'Rand et al., 1988]. Control blots with only second antibody (goat antimouse, lanes 4, 5, 6) are negative. For comparison, purified RSA is shown in Figure 1B, lanes 1, 3, and 5, using the same antisera as in Figure 1A. In this case the antiserum detects one of the lower molecular forms (16 kd) and the aggregated forms (65–70 kd) on the blot (lane 3). In rabbit spermatozoa (lanes 2, 4, 6), the antiserum detects the aggregate forms (lane 4).

The reactivity of anti-RSA antisera with human spermatozoa can also be demonstrated by ELISA (Fig. 2). Figure 2 shows that anti-RSA antiserum has a significant titer ($\leq 1/640$) against human sperm lysate. Because P10G is an epitope within RSA, it would be expected that antibodies to P10G would also react against human spermatozoa. Figure 2 also shows the reactivity of affinity-purified anti-P10G antibodies on human sperm lysate.

Figure 3 shows the immunofluorescent localization of anti-RSA antisera on human spermatozoa. Fluorescence can be seen localized around the entire head plasma membrane (Fig. 3A) and may on some sperm be concentrated in the postacrosomal and neck regions

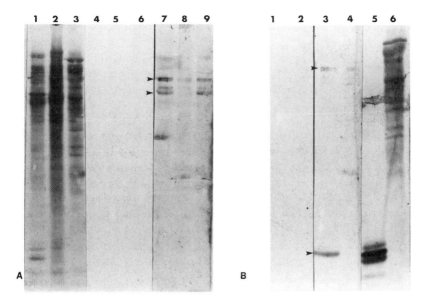

Fig. 1. **A:** Western blots of SDS-PAGE of human **(lanes 1, 4, 7)**, pig **(lanes 2, 5, 8)**, and rabbit **(lanes 3, 6, 9)** sperm lysates. Two hundred micrograms of protein was loaded in each lane. Lanes 1, 2, 3 stained with amido black; lanes 4, 5, 6 (control) stained with biotin-labeled goat antimouse immunoglobulins A, G, and M, heavy-chain-specific (GAM-b), followed by avidin-alkaline phosphatase (AAP) and NBT/BCIP substrates; and lanes 7, 8, 9 stained with mouse anti-RSA, GAM-b, AAP, and NBT/BCIP. Arrowheads indicate bands at 70 and 65 kd in lane 7. **B:** Western blots of SDS-PAGE of purified RSA **(lanes 1, 3, 5)**, 43 μg protein loaded in each lane and rabbit sperm lysate **(lanes 2, 4, 6)**, 200 μg protein loaded in each lane. Lanes 1, 2, control; lanes 3, 4, mouse anti-RSA; and lanes 5, 6, amido black. Blots were stained as in A. Arrowheads show the 16 kd and aggregate forms of RSA.

(Fig. 3B). Spermatozoa treated with adjuvant control sera stain only very weakly (Fig. 3C). The phase contrast images are shown in Figure 3D–F. Similar localizations are seen on rabbit spermatozoa [O'Rand and Romrell, 1981; Esaguy et al., 1988].

Because P10G is an autoantigenic epitope, antisera from vasectomized men as well as sera from men attending an infertility clinic were tested for reactivity to P10G. Figure 4 shows the results of an ELISA on two samples from vasectomized men (V1 and V2) and 10 different sera from male patients attending an infertility clinic. Reactivity to human sperm lysate is also shown for comparison. In both vasectomized sera, antibodies to P10G were detected, and, in every case in which antisperm antibodies were seen, the serum was also positive for P10G. Infertile sera without strong antisperm antibody activity were also positive. The mean ELISA value for reactivity to

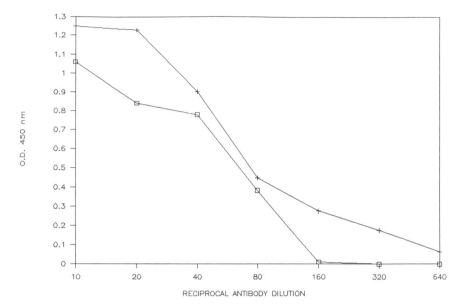

Fig. 2.   ELISA of mouse anti-RSA (+) and affinity-purified rabbit anti-P10G (□) on human sperm lysate. Control values for preimmune sera were subtracted from the ELISA values at each dilution. Each point is the mean of a triplicate determination.

P10G (0.01625 ± 0.0234 S.D.) is based on four serum samples from normal fertile females who were negative for the antisperm antibody bead test [Bronson et al., 1985]. Of the 10 male samples, 7 were >2 S.D. (+0.0468) above the mean ELISA value (0.01625) of reactivity to P10G. The antisperm antibody ELISA values have had the mean ELISA value of the four normal sera (negative bead test) subtracted from them.

Figure 5 shows the results of an ELISA on 14 different sera samples from female infertility patients. Two of the fourteen (Nos. 6 and 12) had antisperm antibodies but did not react with P10G. Of the 14 sera, 6 were >2 S.D. (+0.0468) above the mean ELISA value (0.01625) of reactivity to P10G. The mean P10G ELISA value is the same as used in Figure 4. The antisperm antibody ELISA values have been corrected as in Figure 4.

Obviously many more sera will need to be tested before general conclusions about P10G immunogenicity can be made. However, initially at least, we conclude that a P10G epitope is contained in human sperm and that males with antisperm antibodies react immunologically to it. Females also react to P10G, but all female pa-

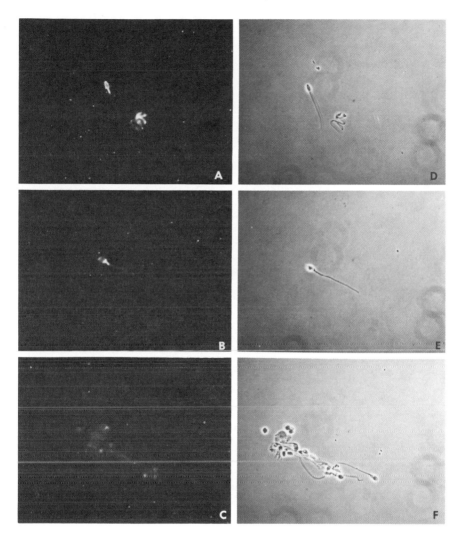

Fig. 3. Indirect immunofluorescence of mouse anti-RSA antisera on human spermatozoa **(A,B)** and matched phase-contrast images **(D, E)**. Adjuvant control sera immunofluorescence **(C)** and phase contrast **(F)**.

tients with antisperm antibodies have not necessarily reacted with P10G.

The reactivities of the anti-RSA and anti-P10G sera to human spermatozoa are indicative of a human protein analogous to RSA. Because RSA is a ZBP and because the presence of 16, 18, and 19 kd ZBPs in human sperm has been described, it is likely that the human sperm 16, 18, and 19 kd lower molecular weight proteins are analo-

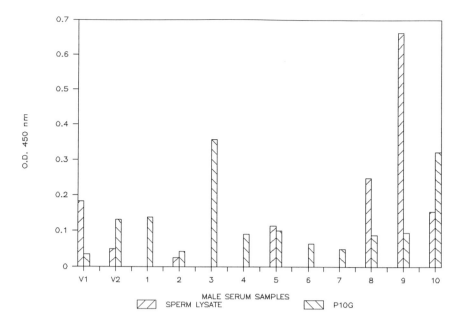

Fig. 4. ELISA of sera from vasectomized (V1, V2) and infertile males (Nos. 1–10) on P10G and human sperm lysate.

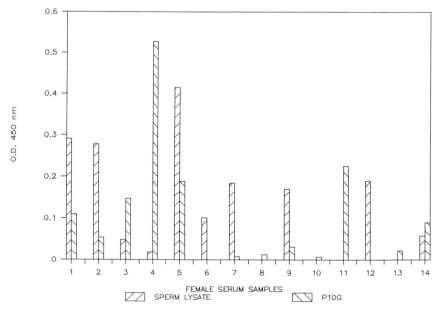

Fig. 5. ELISA of sera from infertile females (Nos. 1–14) on P10G and human sperm lysate.

gous to the lower molecular weight forms of RSA. Direct isolation of ZBP 16 kd from human sperm and its peptide sequence should confirm its structural similarity to both RSA and P10G. Functional tests of its zona-binding activity in solution will determine its similarity to RSA and bindin.

ACKNOWLEDGMENTS

This study was supported by NIH grant HD-14232 to M.G.O. R.T.R. was supported by reproductive biology NIH postdoctoral training grant HD07315.

REFERENCES

Benau DA, Storey BT (1988): Relationship between two types of mouse sperm surface sites that mediate binding of sperm to the zona pellucida. Biol Reprod 39:235–244.

Berger T, Davis A, Wardrip NJ, Hedrick JL (1989): Sperm binding to the pig zona pellucida and inhibition of binding by solubilized components of the zona pellucida. J Reprod Fertil 86:559–565.

Bleil JD, Wassarman PM (1980): Structure and function of the zona pellucida: Identification and characterization of the proteins of the mouse oocyte's zona pellucida. Dev Biol 76:185–203.

Bleil JD, Wassarman PM (1983): Sperm–egg interactions in the mouse: Sequence of events and induction of the acrosome reaction by a zona pellucida glycoprotein. Dev Biol 95: 317–324.

Bleil JD, Wassarmann PM (1986): Autoradiographic visualization of the mouse egg's sperm receptor bound to sperm. J Cell Biol 102:1363–1371.

Bleil JD, Wassarman PM (1988): Galactose at the nonreducing terminus of O-linked oligosaccharides of mouse egg zona pellucida glycoprotein ZP3 is essential for the glycoprotein's sperm receptor activity. Proc Natl Acad Sci USA 85:6778–6782.

Bronson RA, Cooper G, Hjort T, Ing R, Jones WR, Wang SX, Mathur HO, Williamson Ho, Rust PF, Fudenberg HH, Mettler L, Czuppon AB, Sudo N (1985): Anti-sperm antibodies detected by agglutination, immobilization, autocytotoxicity and immunobead-binding assays. J Reprod Immunol 8:279.

Brown CR, Jones R (1987): Binding of zona pellucida proteins to a boar sperm polypeptide of Mr 53,000 and identification of zona moieties involved. Development 99:333–339.

Cherr GN, Lambert H, Meizel S, Katz DF (1986): In vitro studies of the golden hamster sperm acrosome reaction: Completion on the zona pellucida and induction by homologous soluble zonae pellucidae. Dev Biol 114:119–131.

Cross NL, Morales P, Overstreet JW, Hanson FW (1988): Induction of acrosome reactions by the human zona pellucida. Biol Reprod 38:235–244.

Esaguy N, Welch JE, O'Rand MG (1988): Ultrastructural mapping of a sperm plasma membrane autoantigen before and after the acrosome reaction. Gamete Res 19:387–399.

Florman HM, First NL (1988): The regulation of acrosomal exocytosis. I. Sperm capacitation is required for the induction of acrosome reactions by the bovine zona pellucida in vitro. Dev Biol 128:464–473.

Florman HM, Wassarman PM (1985): O-linked oligosaccharides of mouse egg ZP3 account for its sperm receptor activity. Cell 41:313–324.

Glabe CG, Grabel LB, Vacquier VD, Rosen SD (1982): Carbohydrate specificity of sea urchin sperm bindin: A cell surface lectin mediating sperm–egg adhesion. J Cell Biol 94:123–128.

Leyton L, Saling P (1989): 95kd sperm proteins bind zp3 and serve as tyrosine kinase substrates in response to zona binding. Cell 57:1123–1130.

Lopez LC, Bayna EM, Litoff D, Shaper NL, Shaper JH, Shur BD (1985): Receptor function of mouse sperm surface galactosyltransferase during fertilization. J Cell Biol 101:1501–1510.

Macek MB, Shur BD (1988): Protein carbohydrate complementarity in mammalian gamete recognition. Gamete Res 20:93–109.

O'Rand MG (1988): Sperm–egg recognition and barriers to interspecies fertilization. Gamete Res 19:315–328.

O'Rand MG, Fisher SJ (1987): Localization of the zona pellucida binding sites on rabbit spermatozoa and induction of the acrosome reaction by solubilized zonae. Dev Biol 119:551–559.

O'Rand MG, Irons GP (1984): Monoclonal antibodies to rabbit sperm autoantigens. II. Inhibition of human sperm penetration of zona-free hamster eggs. Biol Reprod 30:731–736.

O'Rand MG, Matthews JE, Welch JE, Fisher SJ (1985): Identification of zona binding proteins of rabbit, pig, human and mouse spermatozoa on nitrocellulose blots. J Exp Zool 235:423–428.

O'Rand MG, Romrell LJ (1981): Localization of a single sperm membrane autoantigen (RSA-1) on spermatogenic cells and spermatozoa. Dev Biol 84:322–331.

O'Rand MG, Widgren EE (1989): Molecular biology of a sperm antigen: Identification of the sequence of an autoantigenic epitope. In Mettler L, Billington WD (eds): Reproductive Immunology. Amsterdam: Elsevier, pp 61–67.

O'Rand MG, Widgren EE, Fisher SJ (1988): Characterization of the rabbit sperm membrane autoantigen, RSA, as a lectin-like zona binding protein. Dev Biol 129:231–240.

Peterson RN, Henry L, Hunt W, Saxena N, Russell LD (1985): Further characterization of boar sperm plasma membrane proteins with affinity for the porcine zona pellucida. Gamete Res 12:91–100.

Poirier GR, Robinson R, Richardson R, Hinds K, Clayton D (1986): Evidence for a binding site on the sperm plasma membrane which recognizes the murine zona pellucida: A binding site on the sperm plasma membrane. Gamete Res 14:235–243.

Richardson R, Buckingham T, Boettger H, Poirier GR (1987): A monoclonal antibody to a zona pellucida–proteinase inhibitor binding component on murine zona pellucida. J Reprod Immunol 11:101–116.

Sacco AG, Palm VS (1977): Heteroimmunization with isolated pig zonae pellucidae. J Reprod Fertil 51:165–168.

Sacco AG, Subramanian MG, Yurewicz EC (1984): Association of sperm receptor activity with a purified pig zona antigen (PPZA). J Reprod Immunol 6:89–103.

Sacco AG, Yurewicz EC, Subramanian MG (1986): Carbohydrate influences the immunogenic and antigenic characteristics of ZP3 macromolecule (Mr 55,000) of the pig zona pellucida. J Reprod Fertil 76:575–586.

Saling P (1981): Involvement of trypsin-like activity in binding of mouse spermatozoa to zona pellucida. Proc Natl Acad Sci USA 78:6231–6235.

Shabanowitz RB, O'Rand MG (1988a): Characterization of the human zona pellucida from fertilized and unfertilized eggs. J Reprod Fertil 82:151–161.

Shabanowitz RB, O'Rand MG (1988b): Molecular changes in the human zona pellucida associated with fertilization and human sperm/zona interactions. Ann NY Acad Sci 541: 621–632.

Töpfer-Petersen E, Henschen A (1988): Zona pellucida-binding and fucose-binding of boar sperm acrosin is not correlated with proteolytic activity. Biol Chem Hoppe Seyler 369: 69–76.

Tulsiani DRP, Skudlarek MD, Orgebin-Crist MC (1989): Novel alpha-D-mannosidase of rat sperm plasma membranes: characterization and potential role in sperm–egg interactions. J Cell Biol 109:1257–1267.

Vacquier VD, Moy GW (1977): Isolation of bindin: The protein responsible for adhesion of sperm to sea urchin eggs. Proc Natl Acad Sci USA 74:2456–2460.

Wassarman PM, Bleil JD, Florman HM, Greve JM, Roller RJ, Salzmann GS (1986): Nature of the mouse egg's receptor for sperm. In JL Hedrick (ed): "The Molecular and Cellular Biology of Fertilization." New York: Plenum Pres, pp 55–77.

DISCUSSION

DR. ALEXANDER: In rabbits, is the P10G antigen from the epididymis or from the testes?

DR. O'RAND: In rabbits, we found that the antigen is present in the testes, and the message for the protein is made in pachytene spermatocytes. Now, whether that is also true in other species, we do not know. It might be that there is cross-reactivity with proteins that are made in the epididymis as is the case in human sperm.

DR. ISOJIMA: You say that some infertile women have antibody against the P10G. Have you ever tried the other biological tests, such as immobilization or agglutination tests?

DR. O'RAND: In some of the patients who were observed clinically, there was agglutination and sperm immobilization. But not all of the patients had all of these characteristics. Some who were immobilization negative also reacted with this antigen, and some who did not appear to have any agglutination also reacted.

DR. ISOJIMA: Was this observed in the male also?

DR. O'RAND: I am not sure about the males.

DR. ANDERSON: I have worked a lot with sperm ELISA and it is important to run a negative control plate to rule out the possibility that you are pulling IgG nonspecifically from sera of men with high levels of IgG that may not be specific for sperm antigen.

DR. O'RAND: Each plate that we ran has within it a positive and a negative control. We subtract the control values, because we found that, for example, to run a series of unknowns on one plate and have your knowns on the next plate allows variation from plate to plate. Thus every plate has its own positive and negative control.

DR. ANDERSON: Serum controls or antigen controls?

DR. O'RAND: When we are doing P10G, we conjugated it to thyroglobulin and ran thyroglobulin without the P10G as the antigen control. Then we subtracted those values from what we measured when the peptide was present. When we are doing sperm lysates on the plate, it is more difficult and thus necessary to have some good control sera for subtracting.

17

Regulation of Acrosomal Exocytosis by Sperm Binding to the Zona Pellucida

L. Leyton, D. Bunch, P. Le Guen, M. Selub, and P. Saling

During the interactions between gametes leading to fertilization, the occurrence of the sperm's acrosome reaction (AR) appears to be regulated carefully. In the usual sequence of cellular events, studied in greatest detail using mouse gametes, it has been found that fully acrosome-intact sperm penetrate the cumulus matrix and bind to the egg's extracellular coat, the zona pellucida (ZP). After binding, exocytosis of the acrosome (the AR) occurs; thereafter, the sperm penetrates through the ZP matrix and gains direct access to the egg's plasma membrane, to which it first binds and then fuses [reviewed in Saling, 1989]. Numerous studies over many years have revealed the necessity of the AR for fertilization in all species examined: Even when presented with a naked egg plasma membrane, sperm that have not undergone an AR are unable to fuse [reviewed in Yanagimachi, 1988]. Furthermore, sperm that undergo an AR prematurely, prior to reaching the ZP surface, appear to be excluded from further participation in fertilization. Those sperm that undergo an AR before reaching the outer margin of the cumulus layer are unable to enter that matrix [Cherr et al., 1986; Cummins and Yanagimachi, 1986], whereas those sperm that lose their acrosomes while traversing the cumulus layer appear to adhere firmly to adjacent cumulus cells [Cherr et al., 1986]. Thus it appears important that acrosomal exocytosis occurs in a restricted location, and it would not be unlikely

Gamete Interaction: Prospects for Immunocontraception, pages 225–238
© 1990 Wiley-Liss, Inc.

that specific mechanisms exist to facilitate and regulate this event. An understanding of the molecular mechanisms that bring about the AR should allow us to control the fertilization process itself.

In considering mechanisms that might govern acrosomal exocytosis, it may be useful to remove sperm–ZP interaction, intellectually, from the specific case of fertilization and, instead, examine this event in a more generalized context. Does this particular interaction resemble other intercellular interactions about which more is understood? Could such alternative systems serve as models for examining hypotheses concerning the molecular mechanism of regulated acrosomal exocytosis? It may be appropriate to consider briefly what is known about sperm–ZP interaction in these terms.

SPERM INTERACTION WITH AN EGG EXTRACELLULAR MATRIX, THE ZONA PELLUCIDA

The murine ZP has been well characterized; it is an extracellular matrix secreted by the egg and consists principally of three glycoproteins, ZP1, ZP2, and ZP3 [Bleil and Wassarman, 1980a,b; Greve and Wassarman, 1985]. Considerable evidence suggests that ZP-3 serves not only as ligand for initial sperm binding, but also as the ZP component responsible for AR triggering [Bleil and Wassarman, 1983, 1986]. Although the affinity of ZP3 for its receptor in the sperm plasma membrane has not yet been reported, binding appears to be both specific and saturable, characteristics of typical ligand–receptor interactions [Bleil and Wassarman, 1983, 1986]. Dissection of the bifunctional role of murine ZP3 has revealed that ligand activity depends little on the polypeptide backbone of the molecule, but resides in its O-linked oligosaccharides [Florman et al., 1984; Florman and Wassarman, 1985]. Pronase digestion of ZP3 results in small glycopeptides (1.5–6 kd) that bind to sperm and are as effective as undigested ZP3 in competitively inhibiting sperm binding to intact ZP [Florman et al., 1984; Florman and Wassarman, 1985]. However, these small ZP glycopeptides do not trigger the AR, suggesting that the polypeptide chain or intact molecule plays a role in the latter activity.

The acrosome, a Golgi-derived organelle that develops during spermiogenesis, can be considered a secretory granule situated at the apex of the sperm head [Harrison, 1983]. During the AR, the sperm's plasma and outer acrosomal membranes fuse at multiple sites, resulting in the release of the acrosomal contents. Such polarized fusion at multiple sites in a single cell is not unique to sperm and may be observed in other secretory systems, such as the exocytosis of histamine by mast cells [Lawson et al., 1978]. In the latter case, the cross-linking or aggregation of receptors in the mast cell plasma membrane by IgE is an initiating signal in the cascade, resulting in exocytosis [Ishizaki et al., 1978].

Phosphorylation by a variety of endogenous protein kinases represents an important mode of receptor regulation for many types of secretory cells [Roberts and Butcher, 1983; Spearman et al., 1983; Browning et al., 1985; Sibley and Lefkowitz, 1985; Huganir et al., 1986]. Some of the kinase substrates are represented by receptors [Hempstead et al., 1983], ion channels in the cell membrane [Ewald et al., 1985], or other signalling mediators, such as phospholipase C-II [Margolis et al., 1989; Meisenhelder et al., 1989]. The response of sea urchin sperm to egg jelly peptides, which results in the AR, is a pertinent example of exocytotic regulation via phosphorylation [Ward et al., 1985, 1986; Bentley et al., 1986; Singh et al., 1988].

The receptors for several hormones and growth factors (e.g., insulin, EGF, and PDGF) are protein-tyrosine kinases (PTK) [Hunter, 1987]. PTK genes and their products are highly conserved across eukaryotic cells, and PTKs are thought to be critical regulators of many cellular responses [Hunter and Cooper, 1985]. These kinases are activated by ligand binding. An unusual aspect of this signal transduction system is receptor autophosphorylation, which often depends on receptor aggregation [Yarden and Ullrich, 1988]. The significance of autophosphorylation is not yet fully clarified, but has been shown to regulate ion channels directly [Hopfield et al., 1988] and to couple insulin receptors to G proteins [Czech et al., 1988]. Another interesting aspect of several of the PTK receptors, such as EGF receptor, is the finding that receptor oligomerization is an early event in the signalling cascade [Yarden and Schlessinger, 1987].

TRIGGERING OF THE ACROSOME REACTION INVOLVES AGGREGATION OF SPERM RECEPTORS FOR ZP3

Findings from a diverse array of systems that involve ligand-dependent cellular responses suggest that a common element in the signalling pathway may be ligand-dependent receptor aggregation. Among those systems that may use such a mechanism are mast cells in response to IgE [Ishizaka et al., 1978]; many different cell types in response to EGF [Yarden and Schlessinger, 1987] and insulin [Heffetz and Zick, 1986]; acetylcholine receptors in rat myotubes [Pumplin et al., 1987]; and T lymphocytes during the initiation of the immune response [Ledbetter et al., 1987]. Because of the observed difference in cellular response of capacitated sperm following exposure to ZP3 glycopeptide as opposed to exposure to whole ZP3 molecule, it seemed possible that acrosomal exocytosis could also be triggered by receptor aggregation. In this specific case, it could be postulated that it is the aggregation of ZP3 receptors in the plasma membrane overlying the acrosome that provides the exocytotic stimulus.

To test this hypothesis, we generated monospecific polyclonal antibodies against ZP2 and ZP3, and examined the effects of these probes on capacitated sperm incubated in the absence or presence of various ZP protein preparations [Leyton and Saling, 1989a]. For some experiments, we used ZP glycopeptides, a preparation known to retain specific binding, but not AR-triggering, activity [Florman et al., 1984; Florman and Wassarman, 1985]. In other experiments, a preparation of ZP proteins modified by previous exposure of ZP-enclosed oocytes to the phorbol diester 12-O-tetradecanoyl-phorbol-13-acetate, was used; ZP3 recovered from such preparations, termed $ZP3_{pm}$, display ZP ligand activity, but not full AR-triggering activity [Endo et al., 1987].

Monospecific polyclonal antibodies (pAbs) were raised in rabbits using purified ZP proteins as immunogen. ZP were isolated from mouse ovaries [Bleil and Wassarman, 1986; Lakoski et al., 1988; Leyton et al., 1989] and the proteins separated by SDS-PAGE under nonreducing conditions [Bleil and Wassarman, 1980b]. Separated ZP proteins were transferred electrophoretically to nitrocellulose [Towbin et al., 1979], identified according to their M_r, and the individual proteins immobilized to nitrocellulose were used for immunization according to Knudsen [1985]. In total, each rabbit received approximately 5 μg of purified ZP protein as immunogen [Leyton and Saling, 1989a]. Each pAb preparation, and its corresponding preimmune serum, was characterized for specific binding to the appropriate ZP protein by ELISA, dot blot, and Western blot analysis. pAb interaction with native solubilized ZP proteins, with SDS-denatured and electrophoresed ZP proteins, and with pronase-digested ZP glycopeptides was assessed; it was found that both anti-ZP2 Ab and anti-ZP3 Ab, and their respective univalent fragments, recognize the appropriate ZP protein specifically and to the same extent [Leyton and Saling, 1989a].

Capacitated mouse sperm were exposed to ZP glycopeptides followed by pAbs against either ZP2 or ZP3. The sperm's acrosomal status was monitored by the chlortetracycline (CTC) fluorescence assay [Saling and Storey, 1979; Ward and Storey, 1984]. At the start of the experiment, nearly 80% of the sperm display intact acrosomes. Treatment of such a sperm population with solubilized whole ZP triggers the AR in the majority of sperm. In contrast, treatment with ZP glycopeptides fails to trigger the appearance of the AR pattern even though the glycopeptides bind to sperm. However, exposure of sperm to ZP glycopeptides followed by anti-ZP3 IgG results in ARs to the same extent as exposure to whole ZP. This induction of the AR is specific for anti-ZP3 IgG, and no ARs are observed if the ZP glycopeptides are omitted or if glycopeptide-treated sperm are incubated subsequently with anti-ZP2 pAb. Importantly, ZP glycopeptide-treated sperm do not undergo ARs in the presence of univalent anti-ZP3 Fab fragments. But, if cells from this preparation are incubated subsequently with goat anti-rabbit IgG, ARs are observed in the majority of the population. The use of ZP_{pm} in place of ZP glycopeptides generates similar results [Leyton and Saling, 1989a].

These findings are consistent with the hypothesis that aggregation of sperm molecules recognized by ZP3 glycopeptides triggers the events leading to acrosomal exocytosis. The results also provide indirect evidence for the importance of the ZP3 polypeptide in triggering ARs by cross-linking the plasma membrane components recognized by ZP3.

IDENTIFICATION OF SUBSTRATES FOR PROTEIN-TYROSINE KINASE(S) AND THEIR RELATIONSHIP TO ZP BINDING

Considering ZP3's ligand activity [Bleil and Wassarman, 1980a; Florman et al., 1984; Florman and Wassarman, 1985], its consequent AR triggering by the aggregation of ZP3 receptor in the mouse sperm plasma membrane [Leyton and Saling, 1989a], and the finding that a class of conserved cell surface receptors for various extracellular ligands are PTKs [Hunter and Cooper, 1985; Yarden and Ullrich, 1988], we wondered whether triggering of the AR might elevate PTK activity. Although a variety of methods could be considered to measure PTK activity, one of the simplest makes use of antiphosphotyrosine antibodies to detect the presence and relative amount of phosphotyrosine (PY) residues on cellular proteins. Monospecific anti-PY Abs reacted on immunoblots with three mouse sperm proteins, with M_r = 52, 75, and 95 kd (p52, p75, and p95, respectively) [Leyton and Saling, 1989b]. The PTK activity detected here does not appear to be related to sperm motility, because sperm immobilized by incubation in $LaCl_3$ at 4°C display anti-PY Ab reactivity equivalent to parallel samples of progressively motile sperm incubated in $CaCl_2$

at 37°C [Leyton and Saling, 1989b]. The phosphoproteins p52 and p75 are detected only in capacitated sperm, whereas p95 is detected in Ca^{2+}- or La^{3+}-exposed sperm and in capacitated sperm. Sperm extracts prepared in RIPA buffer [Kamps and Sefton, 1988] demonstrate high levels of anti-PY Ab reactivity; such reactivity depends on the presence of Na_3VO_4 during extraction to inhibit endogenous phosphatase. For p95, the level of immunoreactivity is enhanced twofold by capacitation and fourfold by sperm interaction with solubilized ZP proteins. These findings suggest that tyrosine residues of a 95 kd protein located in the acrosomal region of the sperm head are phosphorylated in response to ZP binding.

IDENTIFICATION OF A ZP3 RECEPTOR

Because specific ZP3–binding proteins of sperm (i.e., a ZP3 receptor) had not been reported previously, we carried out further investigations using a Western blot assay. Sperm samples used in these studies were prepared to preserve the plasma membrane overlying the acrosome optimally. Mouse sperm exposed briefly to Ca^{2+} using noncapacitating conditions demonstrate minimal levels of spontaneous ARs. Such preparations also display maximal ZP-binding activity regardless of capacitation status [Saling et al., 1978]. Sperm prepared using these conditions were dissolved in SDS and the proteins separated by SDS-PAGE. Western blots of these gels were probed directly with iodinated ZP proteins. When blots containing separated sperm proteins were probed directly with ^{125}I-whole ZP or ^{125}I-ZP3, two sperm proteins, with $M_r = 95$ and 42 kd, were detected; faint reactivity was observed with low-M_r components running near the dye front of the gel. ^{125}I-ZP2 did not bind to either the 95 or 42 kd proteins or to any other sperm protein, when sperm were prepared in this manner.

ARE THE 95 KD COMPONENT RECOGNIZED BY ZP3 AND THE 95 KD PY-CONTAINING COMPONENT THE SAME PROTEIN?

Having identified 95 kd mouse sperm proteins that display two types of activity related to ZP binding, we were eager to determine whether both activities reside in the same protein. Data obtained in two lines of investigation suggest that this is so. Indirect immunofluorescence studies using fixed sperm cells indicated that an anti-PY

Ab localized to the acrosomal region of the sperm head [Leyton and Saling, 1989b] in a distribution similar to that observed for ZP3 binding to mouse sperm heads [Bleil and Wassarman, 1986]. In addition, a dot blot assay tested whether 95 kd sperm proteins that bind to ZP are also recognized by anti-PY Abs.

For this assay, solubilized ZP proteins (0, 50, and 100 ZP) were blotted onto a nitrocellulose sheet. After a constant amount of sperm protein was applied to the wells of the dot blot and washed, the nitrocellulose sheet was probed for the presence of PY residues using, sequentially, a mouse monoclonal anti-PY Ab [Glenney et al., 1988], rabbit anti-mouse Ig, and ^{125}I-goat anti-rabbit IgG. For this experiment, capacitated sperm proteins were separated by SDS-PAGE; protein in the 95 kd region was electroeluted from the gel, the SDS was removed, and samples were applied to nitrocellulose, as described above. ^{125}I bound to individual spots was counted and used to estimate the extent of anti-PY Ab reactivity and thus the relative amount of PY residues present.

Compared with the absence of ZP, anti-PY Ab reactivity increased eightfold in the presence of 50 ZP and 20-fold in the presence of 100 ZP. No specific counts were associated with a variety of controls, including 1) the absence of anti-PY Ab, 2) the absence of sperm protein, or 3) the use of anti-PY Ab that had been incubated previously with the hapten PY. In this experiment, we interpret the increase in anti-PY Ab reactivity with increased amount of ZP protein as a consequence of the ability of more p95 to bind as the amount of available ZP is increased rather than any direct effect of ZP on PTK activity. The implication of this finding is that the 95 kd protein recognized by ZP3 and the 95 kd sperm protein that serves as a PTK substrate are likely to be the same protein. Although possible, it seems less likely that two or more proteins from the 95 kd region associate following electroelution and that these are responsible, separately, for the observed activities. Two-dimensional gel analysis is planned to address this question more directly.

PRELIMINARY CHARACTERIZATION OF P95

In other systems, such as with insulin and EGF, the cell surface receptor is itself a protein tyrosine kinase that is stimulated by ligand binding and that autophosphorylates. With regard to triggering of acrosomal exocytosis, we hypothesize that p95, a putative ZP3 receptor, is similar to insulin receptor and EGF receptor, with PTK activity that is stimulated upon receptor aggregation and that also autophosphorylates. We are currently pursuing two lines of investigation relevant to this hypothesis, namely, the determination of intrinsic kinase activity of p95 and the isolation of a bioactive membrane fraction containing p95.

If p95 is similar to other PTK receptors, it should itself be a tyrosine kinase capable of autophosphorylation. Our initial experiments to identify this activity suggest that, following transfer to nitrocellulose, a 95 kd sperm protein is capable of autophosphorylation when incubated in a solution containing ^{32}P-γ-ATP, Ca^{2+}, Mg^{2+}, and Mn^{2+}. Studies are underway presently to confirm this important result.

If p95 serves as a ZP3 receptor, previous results (see above) predict that it will be located in the sperm head plasma membrane. Using a simple vortexing technique to demembranate the cells, followed by fractionation of the resulting low-speed supernatant (1,000g sup) on a discontinuous sucrose gradient, we obtain two major fractions, band 2 and band 3, that are highly membrane enriched. Vectorial labeling of mouse sperm with ^{125}I prior to demembranation indicates that 90% of the label is found in band 2. When the ability of these preparations to compete with capacitated sperm for binding to intact ZP is tested, material in the 1,000g sup and in band 2 display significant, concentration-dependent inhibition of sperm binding to ZP. Band 3 contains inhibitory activity that amounts to 0–20% of that found in band 2 (Bunch and Saling, in preparation). To determine the presence of p95, we have probed sperm at various stages of demembranation with anti-PY Ab. Because demembranation is conducted using sperm that would not be expected to contain PY (no exposure to Ca^{2+}, capacitating conditions, or ZP), PTK must be activated in a cell-free system to enable detection of kinase substrates using the anti-PY Ab. For this purpose, the preparations of interest are incubated in an activation buffer that includes ATP and divalent cations. Western blots of these preparations, probed with anti-PY Ab, reveal that p95 cannot be detected in demembranated cells, but is present in the 1,000g sup at levels comparable to that found in an equivalent number of normally activated sperm. In addition, it should be noted that p95 is present solely in the particulate fraction of the 1,000g sup and cannot be detected in the soluble fraction. The results from this work-in-progress suggest that p95 fractionates in a plasma membrane-enriched preparation of mouse sperm that contains ZP-binding activity (Bunch, Le Guen, Leyton, and Saling, in preparation). We are hopeful that this type of analysis will facilitate future studies directed toward the isolation and characterization of p95, the first reported ZP3 receptor.

SUMMARY

Using bivalent and monovalent anti-ZP protein Abs [Leyton and Saling, 1989a], we find that treatment of the sperm surface with agents likely to cross-link ZP3 receptors leads to acrosomal exocytosis. We have also identified a 95 kd protein as a putative ZP3 receptor [Leyton and Saling, 1989b]. Additionally, we have found that, in response to ZP binding, the PY level of a 95 kd sperm protein is increased [Leyton and Saling, 1989b]. Using immunofluorescent localization or a dot blot assay, we have provided two lines of evidence, albeit indirect, to suggest that ZP3 receptor activity and PY residues are found in the same protein [Leyton and Saling, 1989b]. Finally, preliminary investigations suggest that a 95 kd mouse sperm protein is an autophosphorylating kinase and cofractionates with plasma membranes that are enriched in ZP-binding activity.

Based on the data presented here, and borrowing heavily from findings for various PTK receptors, we have formulated a novel view of the relationship between sperm binding to the ZP and triggering of the AR. We propose that acrosomal exocytosis is triggered by the aggregation of ZP3 receptor(s) in the sperm's plasma membrane. Aggregation increases the intrinsic PTK activity of the clustered ZP3 receptor, p95, and provides the initial signal for the cascade that eventually results in the AR. In noncapacitated sperm, ZP3 receptor may bind its ligand, ZP3, but will not be aggregated readily because of a relatively rigid membrane. A significant event of capacitation is increased fluidity of at least some domains of the sperm plasma membrane, which could facilitate the clustering of ZP3 receptor(s) by multivalent ZP3 molecules.

This model accounts for the observations that ZP3 glycopeptides bind readily to sperm but are unable to trigger ARs and that a substantial portion of the ZP3 peptide is required for AR activity. According to this view, ZP3 could be considered a kinetic regulator of the AR. Spontaneous ARs will occur in capacitated sperm because of the random collision of ZP3 receptor in fluid domains of the membrane. ZP3 may accelerate this process, greatly increasing the probability of AR occurrence at the ZP surface. If this interpretation is correct, PTK activity would be expected to increase with capacitation (responsible for increased spontaneous ARs) and to increase further following exposure to ZP3 (responsible for ZP3–promoted ARs). Experimental results are consistent with these predictions.

If this model is correct, it seems unlikely that mouse sperm will be unique in utilizing this type of highly conserved signal transduction system during interaction with the ZP. Indeed, as a consequence of capacitation, our preliminary studies indicate that proteins in human and bovine sperm also serve as substrates for PTK, suggesting that mammalian sperm from several different species may employ a similar molecular system to trigger the AR. We plan to determine whether alterations in PY levels occur in species other than the mouse following exposure to homologous ZP. Investigation of these and other related questions may facilitate our understanding of the molecular basis of regulated exocytosis at fertilization.

ACKNOWLEDGMENTS

The authors are grateful to Drs. S. Earp, P. Maness, and B. McCune of the University of North Carolina at Chapel Hill and to Dr. J. Glenney of the University of Kentucky for providing the antiphosphotyrosine antibodies used in these experimetns. Dr. K. Burridge of University of North Carolina at Chapel Hill graciously donated ^{125}I-labeled goat anti-rabbit Ig in addition to providing constructive comments on the experimental design. Ms. Athy Robinson participated skillfully in many aspects of this work, particularly in the isolation of mouse zonae pellucidae. The work was supported by grants from the NIH and the Andrew W. Mellon Foundation. Generous support was provided to L.L. from The Rotary Foundation of Rotary International and to P.L.G. from The Lalor Foundation.

REFERENCES

Bentley JK, Tubb DJ, Garbers DL (1986): Receptor-mediated activation of spermatozoan guanylate cyclase. J Biol Chem 261:14859–14862.

Bleil JD, Wassarman PM (1980a): Mammalian sperm–egg interaction: Identification of a glycoprotein in mouse egg zonae pellucidae possessing receptor activity for sperm. Cell 20:873–882.

Bleil JD, Wassarman PM (1980b): Structure and function of the zona pellucida: Identification and characterization of the proteins of the mouse oocyte's zona pellucida. Dev Biol 76:185–202.

Bleil JD, Wassarman PM (1983): Sperm–egg interactions in the mouse: Sequence of events and induction of the acrosome reaction by a zona pellucida glycoprotein. Dev Biol 95: 317–324.

Bleil JD, Wassarman PM (1986): Autoradiographic visualization of the mouse egg's sperm receptor bound to sperm. J Cell Biol 102:1363–1371.

Browning MD, Huganir R, Greengard P (1985): Protein phosphorylation and neuronal function. J Neurochem 45:11–23.

Cherr G, Lambert H, Meizel S, Katz D (1986): In vitro studies of the golden hamster sperm acrosome reaction: Completion on the zona pellucida and induction by homologous soluble zonae pellucidae. Dev Biol 114:119–131.

Cummins J, Yanagimachi R (1986): Development of ability to penetrate the cumulus oophorus by hamster spermatozoa capacitated in vitro. Gamete Res 15:187–212.

Czech MP, Klarland J, Yagaloff K, Bradford A, Lewis R (1988): Insulin receptor signaling. J Biol Chem 263:11017–11020.

Endo Y, Mattei A, Kopf GS, Schultz RA (1987): Effects of a phorbol ester on mouse eggs: Dissociation of sperm receptor activity from acrosome reaction-inducing activity of the mouse zona pellucida protein, ZP3. Dev Biol 123:574–577.

Ewald DA, Williams A, Levitan IB (1985): Modulation of single Ca^{2+}-dependent K^+-channel activity by protein phosphorylation. Nature 315:503–506.

Florman HM, Bechtol KB, Wassarman PM (1984): Enzymatic dissection of the functions of the mouse egg's receptor for sperm. Dev Biol 106:243–255.

Florman HM, Wassarman PM (1985): O-linked oligosaccharides of mouse egg ZP3 account for its sperm receptor activity. Cell 42:313–324.

Glenney JR, Zokas L, Kamps MP (1988): Monoclonal antibodies to phosphotyrosine. J Immunol Methods 109:277–285.

Greve JM, Wassarman PM (1985): Mouse egg extracellular coat is a matrix of interconnected filaments possessing a structural repeat. J Mol Biol 181:253–264.

Harrison RAP (1983): The acrosome, its hydrolases, and egg penetration. In Andre J (ed): The Sperm Cell. The Hague: Martinus Nijhoff, pp 259–273.

Heffetz D, Zick Y (1986): Receptor aggregation is necessary for activation of the soluble insulin receptor kinase. J Biol Chem 261:889–894.

Hempstead BL, Parker CW, Kulczycki A (1983): Selective phosphorylation of the IgE receptor in antigen-stimulated rat mast cells. Proc Natl Acad Sci USA 80:3050–3053.

Hopfield JF, Tank D, Greengard P, Huganir R (1988): Functional modulation of the nicotinic acetylcholine receptor by tyrosine phosphorylation. Nature 336:677–680.

Huganir RL, Delacour AH, Greengard P, Hess GP (1986): Phosphorylation of the nicotinic acetylcholine receptor regulates its rate of desensitization. Nature 321:774–776.

Hunter T (1987): A thousand and one protein kinases. Cell 50:823–829.

Hunter T, Cooper JA (1985): Protein-tyrosine kinases. Annu Rev Biochem 54:897–930.

Ishizaki T, Ishizaki K, Conrad DH, Froese A (1978): A new concept of triggering mechanisms of IgE-mediated histamine release. J Allergy Clin Immunol 61:320–330.

Kamps MP, Sefton B (1988): Identification of multiple novel polypeptide substrates of the v-src, v-yes, v-fps, v-fos, and v-erb-B oncogenic tyrosine protein kinases utilizing antisera against phosphotyrosine. Oncogene 2:305–315.

236   *Leyton et al.*

Knudsen K (1985): Proteins transferred to nitrocellulose for use as immunogen. Anal Biochem 147:285–288.

Lakoski KA, Carron CP, Cabot CL, Saling PM (1988): Epididymal maturation and the acrosome reaction in mouse sperm: Response to zona pellucida develops coincident with modification of M42 antigen. Biol Reprod 38:221–233.

Lawson D, Fewtrell C, Raff M (1978): Localized mast cell degranulation induced by concanavalin A–Sepharose beads. J Cell Biol 79:394–400.

Ledbetter JA, June CH, Grosmaire LS, Rabinovitch PS (1987): Crosslinking of surface antigens causes mobilization of intracellular ionized calcium in T lymphocytes. Proc Natl Acad Sci USA 84:1384–1388.

Leyton L, Robinson A, Saling P (1989): Relationship between the M42 antigen of mouse sperm and the acrosome reaction induced by ZP3. Dev Biol 132:174–178.

Leyton L, Saling PM (1989a): Evidence that aggregation of mouse sperm receptors by ZP3 triggers the acrosome reaction. J Cell Biol 108:2163–2168.

Leyton L, Saling PM (1989b): 95 kD sperm proteins bind ZP3 and serve as substrates for tyrosine kinase in response to zona binding. Cell 57:1123–1130.

Margolis B, Rhee SG, Felder S, Mervic M, Lyall R, Levitzki A, Ullrich A, Zilberstein A, Schlessinger J (1989): EGF induces tyrosine phosphorylation of phospholipase C-II: A potential mechanism for EGF receptor signaling. Cell 57:1101–1107.

Meisenhelder J, Suh P-G, Rhee SG, and Hunter T (1989): Phospholipase C-γ is a substrate for the PDGF and EGF receptor protein-tyrosine kinases in vivo and in vitro. Cell 57:1109–1122.

Pumplin DW, Bloch BJ, Strong J (1987): Disruption and reformation of the acetylcholine receptor clusters of cultured rat myotubes occur in two distinct stages. J Cell Biol 104:97–108.

Roberts ML, Butcher FR (1983): The involvement of protein phosphorylation in stimulus-secretion coupling in the mouse exocrine pancreas. Biochem J 210:353–359.

Saling PM (1989): Mammalian sperm interaction with extracellular matrices of the egg. Oxford Rev Reprod Biol 11:339–388.

Saling PM, Storey BT (1979): Mouse gamete interactions during fertilization in vitro: Chlortetracycline as a fluorescent probe for the mouse sperm acrosome reaction. J Cell Biol 83:544–555.

Saling PM, Storey BT, Wolf DP (1978): Calcium-dependent binding of mouse epididymal spermatozoa to the zona pellucida. Dev Biol 65:515–525.

Sibley DR, Lefkowitz RG (1985): Molecular mechanisms of receptor desensitization using the beta-adrenergic receptor-coupled adenylate cyclase system as a model. Nature 317:124–129.

Singh S, Lowe DG, Thorpe DS, Rodriguez H, Kuang W, Dangott L, Chinkers M, Goedd D, Garbers DL (1988): Membrane guanylate cyclase is a cell-surface receptor with homology to protein kinases. Nature 332:708–712.

Spearman TN, Hurley KP, Olivas R, Ulrich RG, Butcher FR (1983): Subcellular location of stimulus-affected endogenous phosphoproteins in the rat parotid gland. J Cell Biol 99:1354–1363.

Towbin H, Staehlin TH, Gordon J (1979): Electrophoretic transfer of proteins from poly-acrylamide gels to nitrocellulose sheets: procedure and some applications. Proc Natl Acad Sci USA 16:4359–4364.

Ward CR, Storey BT (1984): Determination of the time course of capacitation in mouse spermatozoa using a chlortetracycline fluorescence assay. Dev Biol 104:287–296.

Ward GE, Garbers DL, Vacquier VD (1985): Effects of extracellular egg factors on sperm guanylate cyclase. Science 227:768–770.

Ward GE, Moy GM, Vacquier VD (1986): Phosphorylation of membrane-bound guanylate cyclase of sea urchin spermatozoa. J Cell Biol 103:95–101.

Yanagimachi R (1988): Mammalian fertilization. In Knobil E, Neill J (eds): Physiology of Reproduction, Vol 1. New York: Raven Press, pp 135–185.

Yarden Y, Schlessinger J (1987): Epidermal growth factor induces rapid, reversible aggre-gation of the purified epidermal growth factor receptor. Biochemistry 26:1443–1451.

Yarden Y, Ullrich A (1988): Growth factor receptor tyrosine kinases. Annu Rev Biochem 57:443–478.

DISCUSSION

DR. CUASNICÚ: There is no doubt that zona pellucida induces the acrosome reaction in different species. However, many other mole-cules are present in the cumulus or in follicular fluid. According to a report by Dr. Bedford and myself, you can induce a functional ac-rosome reaction and oocyte penetration in the oviduct in the absence of the zona pellucida. This indicates that the zona pellucida is not completely necessary. What is your feeling about this?

DR. SALING: I think that there are several answers to that ques-tion. First, I think it is not unlikely that there is one mechanism for causing the acrosome reaction. If I go back to the model that we are using, we are thinking about receptor clustering. Now it may be that there are a variety of agents that can cause receptor clustering, but events that are subsequent to that clustering are likely to be highly conserved. It is clear that spontaneous acrosome reactions occur. This may be due to a spontaneous collision of the appropriate num-ber and variety of receptors in the sperm membrane that then trig-gers an acrosome reaction in that cell. In addition, I view ZP-3 not as the one and only inducer but rather as an accelerator of the reaction. Thus it is actually a kinetic property that is altered in the cells that allows the acrosome reaction to occur at the place where it is most useful.

DR. AITKEN: The insulin receptor is a tyrosine kinase. You can activate it by receptor clustering. You can also directly activate the tyrosine kinase entity with hydrogen peroxide. You take an insulin-dependent cell, expose it to hydrogen peroxide, and the response is similar. Now we know in the human that a variety of reagents will induce the acrosome reaction. Ionophores, antibodies, and diesterol analogs are all promoters first because of hydrogen peroxide production. As I recall, Bayard Storey once reported that mouse sperm are capable of generating hydrogen peroxide. I wonder if you know of any studies that might tie these observations together in the mouse, that might suggest that there is also a reactive oxygen species activation of the tyrosine kinase.

DR. SALING: No, I don't know of any information that directly relates all those elements that have been observed in a variety of different systems, including sperm. But, I think that we are viewing the role of tyrosine kinase here in a very proximal stage of acrosome reaction induction, whereas it may be that some of the events that you are speaking about would involve the activation of a kinase at a much more distal time frame. Thus, if this is the case, we may be talking about apples and oranges. I don't really have the answer to that question.

DR. HECHT: Have you experimented with the antibodies to any of the proto-oncogene products known to be tyrosine kinases?

DR. SALING: No, but we are about to begin those experiments.

DR. AHUJA: The 95 kd proteins are localized in the acrosome region. I am also aware that the galactosyl transferase is present in the same region, and possibly the same binding site, as something like 13 different lectins that are thought to be present exclusively in the acrosome region. I just wonder whether the 95 kd proteins have any galactosyl transferase activity? Would you care to speculate?

DR. SALING: Since we haven't looked at that thus far, it would be premature to speculate. The galactosyl transferase activity that Barry Shur reports is of a very different molecular weight, so on that basis alone one would suspect that we are talking about different proteins.

18

Fertilization: Changes in Sperm and Zona Carbohydrates

Kamal K. Ahuja

Fertilization involves a sequence of highly complex interactions between the haploid male and female germ cells that leads to the formation of a zygote, marking the beginning of a new individual. Both spermatozoa and oocytes are released as highly differentiated cells from gonads and then mature in the secretions of the reproductive tracts and accessory sexual glands. Ejaculated or epididymal spermatozoa go through a sequence of physiological changes, called *capacitation*, and then produce a prominent change in motility, called *hyperactivation*, that is associated with the sperm's ability to fertilize the oocyte.

The fully capacitated spermatozoa pass through several layers of somatic cells before reaching the zona pellucida, an acellular translucent layer surrounding the oocyte. The zona pellucida presents a formidable barrier to spermatozoa before they fuse with the egg membrane. This fusion is generally achieved initially by the establishment of a strong adhesive bond between the two surfaces (sperm–zona binding), followed by sperm passage through the zona pellucida. This is aided by the exocytotic release of enzymes from a secretory granule, the acrosome, located in the sperm head. Immediately after the spermatozoon makes contact with the egg membrane and fuses, exocytosis of another set of secretory granules, the cortical granules, is triggered. The contents of these granules modify the egg membrane and the zona pellucida so that any further penetration by spermatozoa is prevented, the so-called block to

Gamete Interaction: Prospects for Immunocontraception, pages 239–258
© 1990 Wiley-Liss, Inc.

polyspermia. The net effect of these exocytotic reactions is that a single haploid genome is transferred into the oocyte, eventually resulting in the formation of a zygote.

SURFACE CARBOHYDRATES MEDIATING
SPERM–ZONA INTERACTIONS

Sufficient experimental evidence is now available to suggest that, similar to cellular interactions in many other biological systems, sperm–egg interactions are also mediated by surface glycoconjugates and related enzymes. Unlike many other systems, however, the molecular events underlying fertilization are still poorly understood primarily for three reasons. First, the poor availability of cells under question, particularly the oocytes, has not allowed large-scale biochemical studies. Second, spermatozoa, whether epididymal or ejaculated, are an extremely heterogeneous population of cells that matures asynchronously. Many key changes on the sperm surface occur either in the vicinity of the zona pellucida or are triggered by zona components. It is therefore quite difficult to synchronize these changes in a sufficiently large number of cells to perform effective biochemical analyses. Furthermore, some of these changes are too subtle to be carried out on stripped-out surface molecules. Third, many animal species have been used for a variety of experiments, thus making it difficult to construct a unifying model on which one can base the reasoning behind a certain line of experiments.

Despite these problems, our understanding of the nature and role of glycoconjugates and related substances localized on gamete surfaces that may play a key role in fertilization has advanced significantly (Table 1). These components can be categorized as glycoconjugates, glycosyltransferases, and hydrolases. The relative merits of these components in a given species have been discussed previously [Ahuja, 1985a,b; Fraser and Ahuja, 1988]. The purpose of this paper is to utilize the existing information on the role of these substances in sperm–egg and other cellular interactions to propose a working model that will provide a unifying focus for many experimentally testable hypotheses in different species. Some recent examples of the modifications of the zona components caused by exocytoses in the male or female gamete, as well as the oviductal secretions, will be discussed in the context of the proposed models.

TABLE 1. Indications of Surface Components Involved in Sperm–Egg Adhesion in Mammals

Species	Sperm	Zona pellucida	References
Guinea pig	Fucose-binding component	—	Huang and Yanagimachi [1985]
Hamster	Fucosylated moieties	—	Ahuja [1982]
	Glycosyltransferases	—	Ahuja [1985b]
	Glycosulfatases	—	Ahuja and Gilburt [1985]
Mouse	Galactosyltransferase	N-acetylglucosamine residues (ZP3)	Lopez and Shurr [1987]
	Trypsin-like enzyme	—	Saling [1981], Saling et al. [1989]
	50 kd protein	—	Muller [1989]
	—	83 kd glycoprotein (ZP3)	Florman and Wassarman [1985]
Pig	—	58 kd protein	Sacco et al. [1984]
	53 kd glycoprotein	All major zona proteins	Brown and Jones [1987]

Localization

SPERM–ZONA INTERACTIONS: EXPERIMENTALLY TESTABLE MODELS

A working model depicting the three categories of components is given in Figure 1. The maturational changes, including capacitation and hyperactivation, the sperm passage through the cumulus oophorous, and the early stages of acrosomal reaction, lead to the close proximation of the spermatozoon with the zona pellucida. The early contact between the two interacting surfaces coincides with the removal of coating factors from the sperm surface [Shur and Hall, 1982] and the zona pellucida [Hartmann and Hutchinson, 1980]. This causes the exposure of sperm glycosyltransferases as well as the saccharide chains on the two surfaces, complete with terminal sugars that are now able to bind with their corresponding counterparts (i.e., glycosyltransferase), thus bringing about an even closer union between the two cells. In the mouse, the binding between a sperm surface galactosyltransferase and the N-acetylglucosamine residues of ZP3 has been suggested to result in an enzyme–substrate complex that initiates sperm–zona binding [Lopez and Shur, 1987].

The timing of coating substance removal is critical, as is the met-

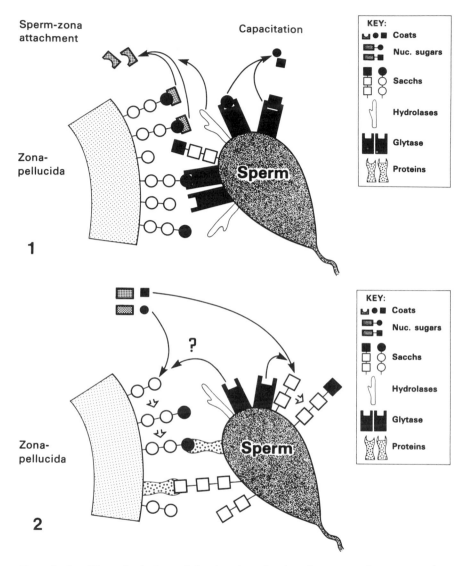

Figs. 1, 2. Hypothetical models showing the involvement of sperm surface components in mediating interactions with the zona pellucida. See text for details.

abolic activation of sperm surface enzymes. A combined interplay between the synthetic and hydrolyzing enzymes ensures the sequential exposure of the saccharide chains of the inner layers of the zona pellucida (ZP2?; see below), which, in turn, can bind to other sperm glycosyltransferases. Aided by the mechanical thrust produced by flagellar movement, these enzyme–substrate interactions eventually achieve sperm passage through the matrix of the zona pellucida. The key feature of this proposal is the lectin-like binding of the sperm surface glycosyltransferases to zona saccharides (Fig. 1).

Alternatively, during sperm–zona binding, the sperm surface glycosyltransferases could act purely as synthetic enzymes, leaving the function of binding to saccharide chains to an entirely separate class of proteins (lectins?) present on the two interacting surfaces (Fig. 2). According to this model, the sperm glycosyltransferases are activated on the zona surface to effect the further N-glycosylation of incomplete saccharide chains on the sperm and zona surfaces (cis- and trans-glycosylation, respectively) via nucleotide sugar donors. The association of the terminal sugars of the fully glycosylated chains with the corresponding proteins results in a higher affinity binding and closer approximation between the two surfaces. Activation of specific hydrolases would be required to dissolve these bonds so that the whole procedure could be repeated again, probably involving another set of transferases and saccharides, as described above. The repeated "glycosylation–binding to proteins–hydrolysis" reactions are aided by the mechanical forces generated by the flagellar beating to achieve a sequence of binding–unbinding reactions. Under the influence of metabolic changes occurring within spermatozoa, a variety of surface-linked ectoglycosyltransferases might be involved to achieve the correct timing and species specificity of fertilization.

In this model, the major function of the coating substances would be to protect the nascent oligosaccharides on the interacting surfaces from premature hydrolysis or glycosylation. Both the glycosyltransferases and the nucleotide sugars would be expected to be present on the inner acrosomal membrane, which is derived from the endoplasmic reticulum–Golgi complex, the conventional site for the synthesis and processing of glycopeptides in many cell studies to date [reviewed by Ahuja, 1985]. In many lower organisms it has been shown that the newly glycosylated moieties rather than the glycosyltransferases achieve an effective binding with the corresponding proteins [reviewed in Ahuja, 1985a]. In mammals any future studies undertaken to test the validity of this model will obviously incorporate, among others, the localization of nucleotide sugars and glycosyltransferases on the interacting surfaces, the nature of glycosylation reactions (cis or trans), the strength of binding between the enzymes and substrates, and the nature and extent of hydrolyzing reactions. Advances in molecular biology will allow the dissection of a highly complicated dynamic process in a given experimental model, but of equal importance will be the universality of a particular observation that will facilitate the emergence of a unifying hypothesis of fertilization in mammals.

The studies designed to ascertain the topographical localization of active surface carbohydrates involved in fertilization will also be very important. In view of the complex shapes and forms of the mammalian gametes, a correct geometrical compatibility between the interacting cells is as important as their chemical compatibility. It should not be surprising if the active components are found to undergo topographical changes during fertilization because of changing positions of cells with regard to each other. Changes during capacitation in the distribution of UEA (*Ulex europeaus agglutinin*) I–binding sites on mouse spermatozoa [Lee and Ahuja, 1988] and PH-20 antigen on guinea pig spermatozoa [Primakoff et al., 1985] are clear examples of this phenomenon. A specific example of various zona components playing different roles is available in the mouse, where the low-molecular-weight (MW) ZP3 is involved in the "attachment" phase, whereas the higher MW ZP2 seems to be responsible for the "binding" phase [Bleil et al., 1988; Florman and Wasserman, 1985].

POSSIBLE MODIFICATIONS OF ZONA INTRINSIC PROTEINS

While considering the advantages of unifying models of sperm–egg interactions as outlined above, it is also important to highlight their limitations. Figures 1 and 2 essentially contain a summary of present knowledge of surface carbohydrates and related enzymes in gametes based on a variety of biochemical and microscopic studies. Very few of these studies have addressed the possibility that the cells have the capacity to change each other's or their own saccharide environment or be influenced by saccharides associated with the secretions of the genital tract *while* undergoing fertilization. This is very important, because, in a complicated and dynamic process such as mammalian fertilization, a multiple set of carbohydrate receptors might have been evolved to meet the unique requirement of gamete selection, maturation and species-specific fertilization. Before fusing with the egg, the highly differentiated spermatozoon is required to pass through the zona's nonliving glycoproteinaceous coat, a process that can take between 4 and 25 min and can involve a variety of subtle but important changes that confer on the gametes their ability to form the beginning of a new individual. It is noteworthy that sperm microinjection experiments performed to date have produced ambiguous results in the mouse and human probably because sperm–egg fusion is attempted without allowing for the surface and

TABLE 2. Modifications of Eggs by Oviductal Components

Species	Site	Nature	References
Hamster	Zona pellucida	Antigen deposits on outer surface	Fox and Shivers [1975]
Mouse	Zona pellucida	Glycosaminoglycan deposits	Fowler and Grainge [1985]
	Oolemma	Binding with a soluble antigen	Gaunt [1985]
	Perivitelline space	Accumulation of a 215 kd protein	Kapur and Johnson [1985]
Pig	Zona pellucida	Addition of a 250 kd protein	Brown and Cheng [1986]

associated metabolic changes on gametes to occur. In many of the biochemical studies indicated in Table 1 these changes would have remained undetected, because they were carried out either on fixed spermatozoan or oocytes or with substances previously isolated from a heterogenous population of cells changing asynchronously.

Any examination of the involvement of carbohydrates in sperm–zona interactions must taken into consideration the extrinsic carbohydrates or other factors that might affect the functioning of the intrinsic zona saccharides. Three such sources of saccharides with the possibility of a key role in mediating fertilization are considered here: 1) oviductal glycoproteins, 2) sperm membrane associated glycoproteins, and 3) cortical glycoproteins.

In the remainder of this paper, a brief summary will be given of the representative experiments in these three areas that are currently being performed in the author's laboratory. Much of the work described below has been carried out with more than one mammalian model (mouse, hamster, and human), but only the representative data from one species will be presented.

Oviductal Glycoproteins

It has been shown in at least four mammalian species that, similar to the case in many lower animals, the egg surface is modified by the oviductal secretions immediately before fertilization (Table 2). The bulk of the modifications of the zona pellucida are caused by the acquisition of mucinous antigens from oviductal secretions. In the hamster, these deposits not only confer a degree of heterogeneity on the zona pellucida but also enhance the ability of this layer to induce the acrosome reaction and allow faster sperm penetration [Fraser

TABLE 3. Zone Modifications by Oviductal Secretions in the Pig[a]

Hours post ovulation	Location	Stages of development	Zona removed in 0.05% pronase (min)
0	Ovary	Oocytes	<5
24	Oviduct	1 Cell	>300
48	Oviduct	2–4 Cells	>300
72	Oviduct	4–8 Cells	<5

[a]Oocytes and embryos were obtained from the reproductive tracts of inseminated pigs. After extensive washing in saline they were exposed to 0.05% pronase for dissolution of the zona pellucida (Trounson and Polge, personal communication).

and Ahuja, 1988; Kan et al., 1988]. The physical properties of the pig zona, as determined by its dissolution in pronase, are also changed following its modification with the oviductal components (Table 3). In the mouse, the fertilization rates in vitro are significantly higher in oviductal eggs than in ovarian eggs, and, upon transfer to pseudopregnant recipients, the former result in significantly higher implantation rates (Wood, personal communication).

Monoclonal antibodies of defined carbohydrate specificity were used to determine whether specific carbohydrates are deposited onto the zona pellucida by oviductal secretions. Four monoclonal antibodies (IgM) specific for fucosylated saccharide terminals (Table 4) were chosen for these experiments because of the previously demonstrated importance in the hamster fertilization of saccharides rich in fucose, galactose, and acetylated amino sugars [Ahuja, 1982]. Eggs obtained from either the ovary or the oviduct were treated for 30 min with specific antibodies washed extensively in phosphate-buffered saline containing BSA and then stained with FITC-conjugated second antibody (1:50 dilution of goat antimouse IgG) before observation against UV light. In parallel experiments the frozen sections of the hamster oviduct were similarly treated with these antibodies.

The outer surface of the zonae pellucidae of oviductal eggs treated with anticarbohydrate antibodies showed bright, uniform fluorescence, whereas the ovarian eggs did not show any fluorescence (Table 4). The epithelial cells lining the oviductal cavity also fluoresced strongly with all four antibodies. The ovarian eggs exposed to the aqueous flushings of the hamster oviducts also showed strong fluorescence on the outer surface of the zona pellucida, indicating strongly that the fucosylated glycoconjugates detected on the zona surface possibly originate from the secretions of the oviduct.

The studies involving the binding of these fucosylated saccharides to sperm and egg membranes are still in progress, but a further

TABLE 4. Monoclonal Antibodies Used to Label Hamster Eggs and Oviduct

Antibody	Known specificity		Antibody binding to zona		Epithelial cells of oviduct
			Ovarian	Oviductal	
H001	$\overset{\displaystyle Fuc^a}{\overset{\displaystyle \vert}{Gal}}$ ⎯⎯⎯ $\overset{\displaystyle Fuc}{\overset{\displaystyle \vert}{GlcNac}}$		−	+ + +	+ + +
A003	$GalNAc$ ⎯⎯⎯ $\overset{\displaystyle Fuc}{\overset{\displaystyle \vert}{Gal}}$		−	+ + +	+ + +
B006	Gal ⎯⎯⎯ $\overset{\displaystyle Fuc}{\overset{\displaystyle \vert}{Gal}}$		−	+ + +	+ + +
9E9	$\overset{\displaystyle Fuc}{\overset{\displaystyle \vert}{Gal}}$ ⎯⎯⎯ $GlcNAc$		−	+ + +	+ + +

[a]Fuc, fucose; Gal, galactose; GalNAc, N-acetylgalactosamine; GlcNAc, N-acetylglucosamine. See text for further details.

degree of specificity in binding, as shown in Table 4, is indicated by the observations that the other monoclonals specific for nonfucosylated saccharides exhibited no binding toward the zona pellucida or the oviductal epithelial layer (Ahuja and Gilburt, unpublished observations). Whether the newly deposited fucosylated saccharides on the zona pellucida have a role in zona-mediated influences on the penetrating spermatozoa or on the subsequent block to polyspermy is not known.

Sperm Glycoproteins

Many previous studies with lectins and other carbohydrate-specific probes have confirmed that the sperm head, particularly the acrosomal region, is strikingly rich in a variety of saccharides [reviewed in Ahuja, 1984; Lee and Ahuja, 1988]. While the distribution of these saccharides on the surface of capacitating and acrosome-reacting spermatozoa has been a favorite topic of research to date, their behavior *during* interactions with the zona pellucida and how they might affect the latter locally have been surprisingly neglected.

A morphological examination of the local changes in saccharides during sperm–zona binding would necessitate the use of probes that are sperm specific, i.e., show no binding toward zona pellucida and are predominantly confined to the head region of the capacitated spermatozoa. Using a number of lectins [Lee and Ahuja, 1988] and anticarbohydrate monoclonal antibodies (Ahuja, unpublished data),

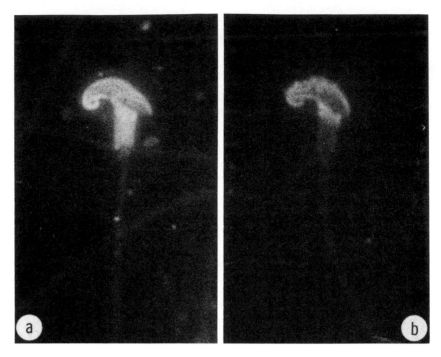

Fig. 3. Binding of a monoclonal antibody (mAb) against a sperm membrane 27 kd glycoprotein to hamster spermatozoa before **(a)** and after **(b)** capacitation. Note the aggregation of antibody-binding sites to the acrosomal region of the capacitated spermatozoa.

we have shown that in mouse, hamster, and human eggs the outer surface of the zona pellucida is significantly modified by saccharides originating from the membranes of penetrating spermatozoa in homologous or heterologous species combinations.

For example, a monoclonal antibody raised against a 27 kd glycoprotein associated with sperm membrane bound exclusively to the acrosomal membranes of capacitated hamster spermatozoa (Fig. 3). The antibody showed no reaction toward the zona pellucida. Following a brief incubation of hamster oocytes or zona fragments with capacitated spermatozoa, when the sperm–egg complexes were gently washed and then exposed to the monoclonal antibody and the FITC-goat antimouse IgG, a very specific pattern of zona staining was observed (Fig. 4). During the first 5 min or so only small patches of fluorescence were seen on the zona surface, with the bulk of it still associated with the acrosomal swellings or recently deposited acrosomal shrouds on the zona surface. At 60 min, however, the outer surface of the zona was uniformly labeled with this antibody, and the pattern was remarkably similar to that observed with the anti-zona antibodies [Ahuja and Tzartos, 1981].

A closer examination of the penetrated eggs indicated that a part of the label had not only transferred firmly to the outer zona surface but also migrated to the perivitelline space via the sperm penetration slit. The binding of the label to the outer zona surface was not random, because 1) it did not come off the zona for many hours after fertilization, 2) it exhibited a distinct mosaic pattern, 3) it did not bind to a mass of cumulus cells, 4) the binding was inhibited in the presence of fucoiden, 5) other anticarbohydrate that specifically binds to the head or the flagellar regions of spermatozoa did not show this pattern of antigen transfer to the zona, and 6) the ultrastructural studies using indirect labeling of sperm–egg complexes by biotinylated UEA/streptavidin gold confirm this observation (Lee and Ahuja, unpublished data). Similar observations were made with the mouse gametes and the heterologous combinations of hamster, mouse, and human gametes, although the intensity of labeling of the zona was reduced and comparatively irregular in these studies.

This highly specific transfer of sperm-related saccharides to the zona pellucida was unlikely to be a nonspecific artifact of the in vitro culture conditions, because hamster eggs fertilized in vivo exhibited a similar pattern of sperm antigen transfer to the zona pellucida (data not shown). While it is unclear at the present time whether the newly deposited sperm glycoconjugates mediate more than a firm association with the zona pellucida, it is clear that they are capable of significantly influencing the local saccharide environment of the fertilization site on the zona pellucida.

Cortical Glycoproteins

Following the entry of a fertilizing spermatozoon, the secretory granules lying in the egg cortex exocytose their contents into the perivitelline space, thus modifying the properties of the oocyte plasma membrane and the zona pellucida. This prevents the entry of further spermatozoa into the oocyte and establishes the so-called block to polyspermia, although the nature of cortical substances and the biochemical mechanism underlying these changes are poorly understood [Yanagimachi, 1988].

A study of the nature and kinetics of the cortical exocytosis is important because of not only the postfertilization changes induced by the cortical contents but also the prefertilization. A considerable number of cortical granules are discharged into the perivitelline space long before fertilization occurs, probably to influence and prepare the perivitelline environment as well as the zona pellucida for the encounter with spermatozoa [Okada et al., 1986]. Encouraged by the knowledge that in many lower animals cortical granules are rich in lectins and lectin-binding substances [Schuel, 1978], we examined the cortex of mammalian eggs for the presence of glycoconjugates. The results obtained to date confirm that, in the hamster, mouse, and human oocytes, fucosyl- and sialyl-rich glycoconjugates are released into the perivitelline space following sperm–egg fusion or parthenogenetic activation of the egg [Lee et al., 1989].

Unfertilized mouse oocytes treated with FITC-conjugated lectins LPA, FBP, and UEA I did not show any binding, but after fertilization or calcium ionophore 23187 activation of the oocyte the egg membrane was found to be stained in a punctate manner (Fig. 5) [Lee et al., 1989]. The binding was due to cortical granule release of sialyl- or fucosyl-rich glycoconjugates on the egg surface, because it did not occur in the presence of appropriate sugars. Further ultrastructural studies also confirmed these findings (Lee and Ahuja, unpublished data). The appearance of the glycoconjugates on the egg membrane was associated with the release of cortical granules and was uniform except for the area overlying the second meiotic spindle. As judged by the size of the granules, the lectin binding was at its maximum within 25 min after sperm–egg fusion. By the time the embryo had reached the pronucleate stage the granules had become larger and fewer because of the aggregation of the cortical substances. By the time the first cleavage division began, there was only one large clump of lectin-labeled material left that surrounded the cleavage furrow of the early two-cell embryo. By the late two-cell stage or early four-cell stage much of the staining had completely disappeared [Lee et al., 1988]. Similar observations were made in the hamster (Ahuja and Gilburt, unpublished data) and the human oocytes (Ahuja and Lee, unpublished data).

Although it is premature to speculate on the functional significance of these observations in early mammalian development, it is tempting to conduct further experiments designed to investigate the role of the newly released perivitelline saccharides in establishing the block to polyspermia and their contribution to a proper launch of the embryo toward early cleavage divisions [see Lee and Ahuja, 1988, for details]. The finding that a variety of glycoconjugates of cortical origin might be available in the perivitelline space of the oocyte before, during, and after fertilization raises an exciting possibility. The glycoconjugates associated with the sperm membranes and the oviductal secretions and the glycoconjugates released by the cortical granules of the oocytes are all capable of significantly influencing the

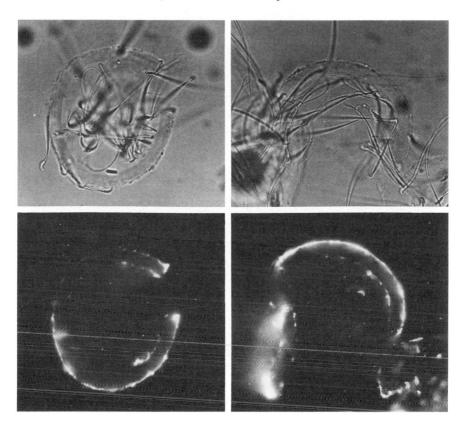

Fig. 4. The specific transfer of a sperm membrane antigen to the outer surface of the zona pellucida. The zona fragments collected from ovulated oocytes were exposed to capacitated spermatozoa for 60 min, washed, and then labeled with the mAb and the FITC-conjugated second antibody. The outer surface of the zona was labeled uniformly, but neither the inner zona surface nor zona-adherent spermatozoa showed any binding.

zona pellucida, the most formidable barrier that the spermatozoon has to negotiate before fusing with the oocyte. The labeling studies carried out to date have not suggested the absorption or incorporation of cortical glycoconjugates into the egg membrane or the zona pellucida, but this may be a reflection of the limitation of the techniques or the probes used to date. Analogous to the situation in some amphibians [Hendricks and Katagiri, 1988], the mammalian cortical granules may also contain a glycoprotein that is rich in fucose and galactose, has a low species specificity, and reacts with the components of the zona pellucida. Depending on the time of its release, it may influence the pre- as well as the postfertilization changes.

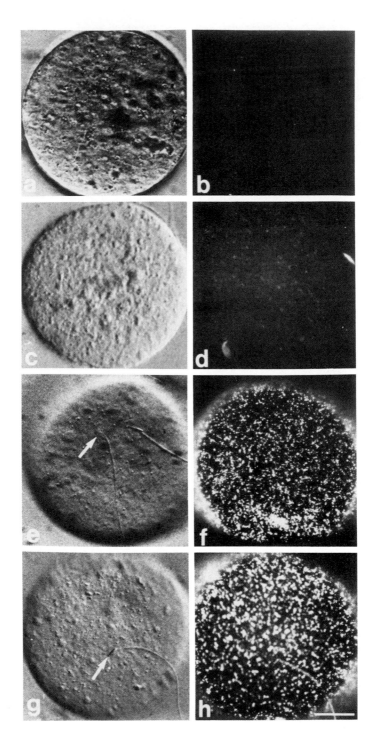

CONCLUSIONS

The purpose of this paper was to summarize the present state of knowledge of the changes in surface carbohydrates during fertilization. The information obtained from biochemical and morphological studies conducted in many laboratory species has been used to propose a unifying model on which many experimentally testable hypotheses can be based. While one can argue that the species diversity favors the multiplicity of mechanism over and above a unifying working theme, it is noteworthy that at the molecular level there are many similarities between mammals (calcium-induced activation of oocytes and spermatozoa, for example). Some of the differences reported to occur between the species may at least in part be due to the different types of approaches used by different investigators.

The idea of a multiple set of saccharide receptors on the gamete surfaces [Ahuja, 1985a; O'Rand, 1988] might be a serious reflection of the different saccharides whose timely appearance on the theater stage, the zona pellucida, creates a carbohydrate-rich microenvironment that is constantly changing to achieve species-specific fertilization (Fig. 6). The intrinsic glycoproteins of the zona pellucida are likely to be under the influence of saccharide-rich substances contributed by the spermatozoon, the cortical granules, and the oviductal secretions. Some of the saccharides originating from the egg cortex and the oviductal secretions are likely to be present in the perivitelline space of the oocyte before, during, and after fertilization. In a dynamic situation the failure in the timely release/addition of any of these components may result in suboptimal or failed fertilization. Clearly the biochemical and morphological studies undertaken to assess the roles of carbohydrates intrinsically associated with the surfaces must also taken into consideration the influence of additional saccharides that appear at specific time intervals during fertilization. The experiments that fail to acknowledge the role of

---

Fig. 5.   The distribution of labeled glycoconjugates on the surface of zona-free oocytes sampled at various times after exposure to capacitated spermatozoa. Samples of oocytes were labeled with FITC-UEA I at 0 (**a,b**), 10 (**c,d**), 15 (**e,f**), and 30 min (**g,h**) after the addition of spermatozoa. Note the absence of labeling in the oocytes incubated without spermatozoa (a,b) or during the early stages of incubation (c,d). Consecutive stages of fusion with spermatozoa (arrows) are shown in e to h. The aggregates of glycoconjugates discharged during the later stages (g, h) appeared to be of greater size than those spots of earlier stages (c,f). Similar results were obtained with FITC conjugated FBP (*Lotus tetragonolobous*) and LPA (*Limulus polyphemus*) lectins (pictures not shown). Scale bar = 20 μm. (Reproduced from Lee et al., 1988, with permission of the publisher.)

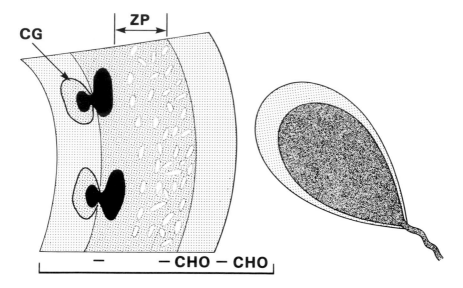

Fig. 6.   A schematic representation of the carbohydrate-rich microenvironment of sperm–zona interactions. Note the cortical, oviductal, and sperm carbohydrates being added onto the zona components. ZP, zona pellucida; CG, cortical granules; CHO, carbohydrate groups.

these substances are therefore unlikely to represent a complete picture.

ACKNOWLEDGMENTS

I gratefully acknowledge the expert technical assistance provided by Mr. David Gilburt during the course of these studies.

REFERENCES

Ahuja KK (1982): Fertilization studies in the hamster: The role of cell surface carbohydrates. Exp Cell Res 140:353–362.

Ahuja KK (1984): Lectin-coated beads in the investigation of sperm capacitation in the hamster. Dev Biol 104:131–142.

Ahuja KK (1985a): Carbohydrate determinants involved in mammalian fertilization. Am J Anat 174:207–224.

Ahuja KK (1985b): Inhibitors of glycoprotein biosynthesis block fertilization in the hamster. Gamete Res 11:179–189.

Ahuja KK, Gilburt DJ (1985): Involvement of sperm sulphatases in early sperm–zona interactions in the hamster. J Cell Sci 78:247–261.

Ahuja KK, Tzartos SJ (1981): Investigation of sperm receptors in the zona pellucida using univalent (Fab) antibodies to hamster ovary. J Reprod Fertil 61:257–264.

Bleil JD, Grieve JM, Wassarman PM (1988): Identification of a secondary sperm receptor in the mouse egg zona pellucida: Role in maintenance of binding of acrosome-reacted sperm to eggs. Dev Biol 128:376–385.

Brown CR, Cheng WKT (1986): Changes in composition of procine zona pellucida during development of the oocyte to the 2 to 4 cell embryo. J Embryol Exp Morphol 92:183–191.

Brown CR, Jones R (1987): Binding of zona pellucida proteins to a boar sperm polypeptide of 53k and identification of zona moieties involved. Development 99:333–339.

Florman HM, Wassarman PM (1985): O-linked saccharides of mouse egg ZP3 account for its sperm receptor activity. Cell 41:313–324.

Fowler RE, Grainge C (1985): A histochemical study of the changes occurring in the protein–carbohydrate composition of the cumulus–oocyte complex and zona pellucida in immature mice in response to gonadotrophin stimulation. Histochem J 17:1235–1249.

Fox LL, Shivers CA (1975): Detection and localization of specific antigens in the reproductive tracts of cycling pregnant and ovariectomized hamsters. Fertil Steril 26:579–598.

Fraser LR, Ahuja KK (1988): Metabolic and surface events in fertilization. Gamete Res 20:491–519.

Gaunt SJ (1985): In vivo and in vitro cultured mouse preimplantation embryos differ in their display of a teratocarcinoma cell surface antigen. J Embryol Exp Morphol 88:55–69

Hartmann JF (1984): Mammalian fertilization: Gamete surface interactions in vitro. In Hartman JF (ed): Mechanism and Control of Animal Fertilization. New York: Academic Press, pp 325–364.

Hendricks JL, Katagiri C (1988): *Bufo japonicus* and *Xenopus laevis* egg jellies contain structurally related antigens and cortical granule lectin ligands. J Exp Zool 245:78–85.

Huang TTF, Yanagimachi R (1985): Inner acrosomal membrane of mammalian spermatozoa: Its properties and possible functions in fertilization. Am J Anat 174:249–268.

Kan FWK, Sylvie SJ, Blean G (1988): Immuno-electron microscopic localization of an oviductal antigen in hamster zona pellucida by use of a monoclonal antibody. J Histochem Cytochem 36(11):1441–1447.

Kapur RP, Johnson LV (1985): An oviductal fluid glycoprotein associated with ovulated mouse ova and early embryos. Dev Biol 112:89–93.

Lee SH, Ahuja KK (1987): An investigation using lectins of glycocomponents of mouse spermatozoa during capacitation and sperm–zona binding. J Reprod Fertil 80:65–74.

Lee SH, Ahuja KK (1989): Fucosylated glycoconjugates are released on the oocyte surface during human fertilization. Abstract III–2: Symposium on Fertilization in Mammals, Boston, August 1–5, 1989. Serono Symposium Publications.

Lee SH, Ahuja KK, Gilburt DJ, Whittingham DG (1988): The appearance of glycoconjugates associated with cortical granules released during mouse fertilization. Development 102:595–604.

Lee SH, Ahuja KK, Whittingham DG (1989): An analysis of the oocyte surface after cortical granules release gamete interaction: Prospects for immunocontraception. WHO-CONRAD symposium bariloche, Argentina (Abstract).

Lopez LC, Shur BD (1987): Redistribution of mouse sperm surface galactosyltransferase after the acrosome reaction. J Cell Biol 105:1663–1670.

Muller CH (1989): Regulation of sperm fertilizing ability by modification of an epididymal glycoprotein. Symposium on Fertilization in Mammals, Boston, August 1–5, 1989. Serono Symposium Publications.

Okada A, Yanagimachi R, Yanagimachi H (1986): Development of a cortical granule free area of cortex and the perivitelline space in the hamster oocyte during maturation and following fertilization. J Submicrosc Cytol 18:223–247.

O'Rand MG (1988): Sperm–egg recognition and barriers to interspecific fertilization. Gamete Res 19:315–328.

Primakoff P, Hyatt H, Myles DG (1985): A role for the migrating sperm surface antigen pH-20 in guinea pig sperm binding to the egg zona pellucida. J Cell Biol 101:2239–2244.

Sacco AG, Subramanian MG, Yuvewicz EC (1984): Association of sperm receptor activity with a purified pig zona antigen (PPZA). J Reprod Immunol 6:89–103.

Saling PM (1981): Involvement of trypsin-like activity in binding of mouse spermatozoa to zona pellucida. Proc Natl Acad Sci USA 78:6231–6235.

Saling PM, Bunch D, LeGuer P, Leyton L (1989): ZP3-induced acrosomal exocytosis in mouse sperm. Symposium on Fertilization in Mammals, Boston, August 1–5, 1989. Serono Symposium Publications.

Schuel H (1978): Secretory functions of egg cortical granules in fertilization and development: A critical review. Gamete Res 1:299–382.

Shur BD, Hall NG (1982): A role for mouse sperm surface galactosyltransferase in sperm binding to the zona pellucida. J Cell Biol 95:574–579.

Yanagimachi R (1988): Mammalian fertilization. In Knobil E, Neill J (eds): Physiology of Reproduction. New York: Raven Press, pp 135–185.

DISCUSSION

DR. HECHT: My question concerns the sperm-specific epitope. Is that something that is made in the testis, in the epididymis, or is it from secretions?

DR. AHUJA: We can certainly stain spermatozoa from various regions of the epididymis. As to whether the epitope is present in the testis, we do not know.

DR. HECHT: Do you envision that the sperm epitope is a component of the membrane that is being lost as the sperm mature? What I find difficult to envision is the mechanism that allows it to be selectively released.

DR. AHUJA: During its binding with the zona?

DR. HECHT: Yes, during binding as well as during fertilization.

DR. AHUJA: That is not particularly hard to explain—although many of these studies are ongoing. If you look at the sperm and zona interaction as a three-phase phenomenon, you have the attachment phase (some of these substances are released, for example, membrane-bound sperm components at the outer surface of the zona) followed by a more intimate interactive phase with the matrix; perhaps sperm enzymes are released onto the zona at this stage. Third, you have zona penetration. During the first two phases, epitopes may afford sperm orientation to allow sperm to enter areas where enzyme release has occurred.

DR. MOORE: Have you looked at cumulus intact oocytes as well as at sperm attachment?

DR. AHUJA: All the sperm–egg attachment and binding experiments were done with cumulus enclosed eggs. When photographs were taken, the cumulus cells were removed.

DR. MOORE: In vivo, you probably would not have so many sperm around the egg. Don't you think that it is significant in terms of in vivo fertilization, as opposed to in vitro.

DR. AHUJA: We repeated our in vitro labeling experiments using in vivo fertilized eggs. Embryos from three different species revealed no differences. Of course, you will not see that precipitate ring around the zona when you use certain markers. What you will see is a large deposit just on the outside of the slit.

DR. SALING: Do you know what type of epitope the Basic 28K antibody binds to? Is it carbohydrate or protein?

DR. AHUJA: In all these studies, we used IgM preps, and the antibodies raised were against carbohydrate determinates, namely, blood antigens.

DR. SALING: So, the fluorescence you are picking up on the zona may be a modification of existing zona proteins, caused by sperm proteases? Or could it be from egg proteases released as a function of exposure to sperm?

DR. AHUJA: In that particular series of experiments, we did not expose the eggs to sperm. These eggs were flushed out of the oviduct, washed, and exposed to the antibodies. We didn't see that precipitation in follicular eggs. Another important point that I did not have time to explain is that the punctate distributions of carbohydrates defined initially with UEA and salic acid–specific lectins can also be defined by fucose-selected carbohydrate panels of antibodies.

DR. SALING: I'm a bit confused. I was speaking about the monoclonal against the 28 kd protein of the sperm.

DR. AHUJA: The only thing that I can tell you at the moment is that if you take zona fragments, where the inside as well as the outside are equally exposed to capacitating sperm, you only pick up the precipitation from the outside, not the inside.

DR. DACHEUX: Is the protein you observed on the zona pellucida from membrane components released by the sperm during the acrosome reaction?

DR. AHUJA: Yes. I think there was a slide that depicted proteins associated with the swelling in the head region where the sperm are attached to the zona. It's very easy to observe. I think that on that basis alone I would hypothesize that it is probably associated with acrosomal membranes. However, having said that, you can also detect the same protein in the penetration slit, as well as in the perivitelline space.

DR. KURPISZ: You pointed out the certain universalities of the carbohydrate moieties across species on zona pellucida. There are similar universalities, I think, on the sperm side. We have in evidence that in human sperm, for example, of terminal acetylgalactosamines and glucosamines. Competition experiments with monoclonal antibodies are tricky to perform consistently, because the sugar moieties have to be terminally located. Perhaps it would be more straightforward to see the effect of specific enzymatic digestions in respect to those sugars that you discussed and determine whether this digestion can prevent binding of the sperm to zona.

DR. AHUJA: We do plan to conduct that experiment. Thank you for your comments.

19

Development and Maturation of the Zona Pellucida

Anthony G. Sacco

The zona pellucida is an antigenically and biochemically complex, translucent extracellular glycoprotein matrix that surrounds the mammalian oocyte and preimplantation embryo [Austin, 1961; Piko, 1969; Dunbar and Wolgemuth, 1984; Wassarman, 1987, 1988; Dietl, 1989a]. It persists from the earliest stages of folliculogenesis until just prior to the time of implantation. Recently, it has gained considerable attention for reasons including increased interest in the molecular basis of mammalian sperm–egg interaction [O'Rand et al., 1986; Yanagimachi, 1988a,b; Katz et al., 1989], the zona's potential use as an immunocontraceptive target antigen [Sacco, 1987; Henderson et al., 1988; Sacco and Yurewicz, 1989], and the development of human in vitro fertilization technology [Jones et al., 1986]. The application of recent advances in the areas of molecular biology and genetic engineering and the introduction of new electrophoretic and purification techniques to investigations involving the zona pellucida have resulted in the generation of considerable new data that have elucidated the compositional structure of the zonae of several species [Sacco et al., 1981; Dunbar et al., 1981; Ahuja and Bolwell, 1983], particularly the mouse [Bleil and Wassarman, 1980a; Shimizu et al., 1983] and pig [Sacco et al., 1981; Dunbar et al., 1981; Hedrick and Wardrip, 1986, 1987; Yurewicz et al., 1987]. Although varying somewhat in composition among the different species, most zonae are comprised primarily of three to four major developmentally regulated glycoconjugates. Functionally, the zona has several roles, but the major of these concern its involvement in critical steps in the

Gamete Interaction: Prospects for Immunocontraception, pages 259–276
© 1990 Wiley-Liss, Inc.

fertilization process [Sacco, 1981; Dunbar and Wolgemuth, 1984; Wassarman, 1987]. Biological studies utilizing the isolated zona components that have recently become available are now revealing the functional roles of these various individual zona macromolecules [Bleil and Wassarman, 1980a,b; Sacco et al., 1984; Florman et al., 1984; Urch et al., 1985; Dunbar and Bundman, 1987].

One major area of zona pellucida research that has not made comparable progress to date and that still remains controversial is that regarding the origin and development of this structure. Very few studies concentrating specifically on the synthesis of zona pellucida macromolecules and their extracellular assembly have been performed. While early morphological and histochemical studies have indicated a major involvement of the oocyte in the formation of the zona pellucida, the precise role of follicle (granulosa) cells in the generation of this structure remains less clear [Dunbar et al., 1989; Dietl, 1989a,b]. Recent biochemical data have not adequately clarified this issue [Bleil and Wassarman, 1980c; Shimizu et al., 1983; Chamberlin et al., 1989; Nakano, 1989]. Thus the question of whether the zona is solely a product of the developing oocyte or a product of both the oocyte and follicle cells still remains to be answered with certainty. It is the purpose of this chapter to present a concise overview of those studies describing the origin and formation of the mammalian zona pellucida.

OVARIAN FOLLICULAR DEVELOPMENT

The basic morphological and functional compartment of the ovary is the follicle [Peters, 1978; Tsafriri, 1978; Centola, 1983; Geneser, 1986]. Distinct developmental stages of the follicle exist and are categorized as the 1) primordial (small) follicle; 2) primary follicle; 3) secondary follicle; and 4) tertiary, graafian, or preovulatory follicle [Pederson and Peters, 1968] (Fig. 1). The latter stage is further categorized according to size as small, medium, or large. The term *folliculogenesis* is restricted to the period of time encompassing the transformation of oocytes, which initially lie in clusters called cell *nests*, to the primordial follicle, which consists of an oocyte encircled by a single layer of squamous follicle (granulosa) cells resting on a basement membrane (Fig. 1A). No perivitelline space is present at the primordial follicle stage, and the follicle is surrounded by dense connective tissue. Primordial follicles are located in the ovarian cortex, just beneath the surface of the epithelium, usually in small groups. The transition of the primordial follicle into later stages is referred to as either follicular *growth, development, or maturation*.

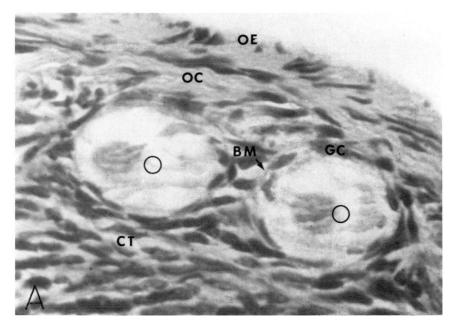

Fig. 1. Representative follicular stages in the squirrel monkey. **A:** Primordial follicles; **B:** primary follicle; **C:** multilayered primary follicles; **D:** secondary follicle; **E:** tertiary follicle. A, antrum; BM, basement membrane; CT, connective tissue; GC, granulosa cells; O, oocyte; OC, ovarian cortex; OE, ovarian epithelium; TE, theca externa; TF, theca folliculi; TI, theca interna; ZP, zona pellucida. A, ×2000. B, ×1533. C, ×480. D, ×228. E, ×242.

In the primary follicle (Fig. 1B,C), the oocyte has enlarged and the flattened follicular cells have grown in height to become first cuboidal in shape and then columnar. During this period the cytoplasm of these cells has assumed a granular appearance, and the cells are now referred to as *granulosa* cells. They proliferate by mitotic division and give rise to a stratified epithelium that is delimited from the surrounding connective tissue by a distinct basement membrane. It is during this period of granulosa cell proliferation that the zona pellucida is deposited. Also, during this period, the follicle moves deeper into the ovarian cortex, and the surrounding stroma cells are organized into a concentric sheath, termed the *theca folliculi*.

As the granulosa cells continue to proliferate and the follicle grows in size, small, irregular, fluid-filled spaces appear between the granulosa cells. These spaces enlarge and eventually coalesce to form a fluid-filled, crescent-shaped cavity, called the *antrum*. A follicle with a fully formed antrum is designated a *secondary* follicle (Fig. 1D). As the antrum enlarges, the oocyte, now surrounded by the fully

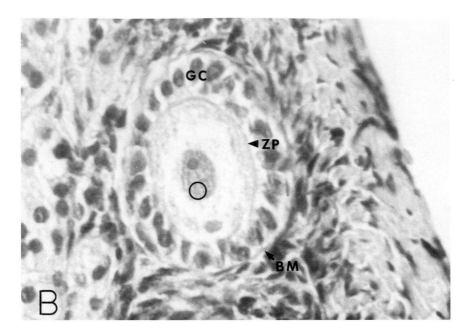

Fig. 1B.

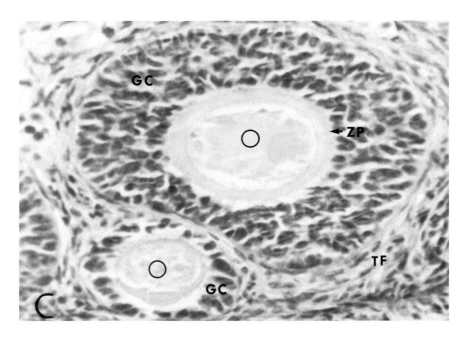

Fig. 1C.

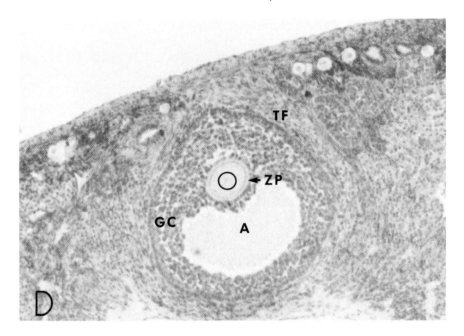

Fig. 1D.

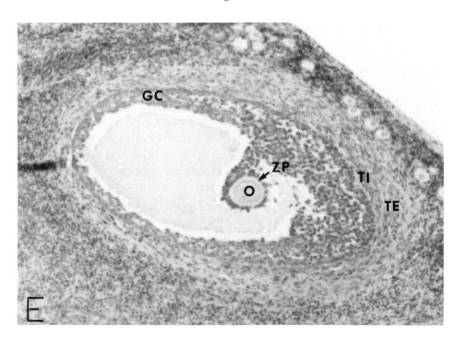

Fig. 1E.

formed and essentially mature zona pellucida, is gradually displaced
into an eccentric position and is surrounded by granulosa cells, forming a projection that extends into the antral cavity. The follicle is now
referred to as a *tertiary* follicle (Fig. 1E). It is also during this period
of antral growth that the theca folliculi differentiates into the highly
vascularized theca interna and the connective tissue–natured theca
externa.

MORPHOLOGICAL DEVELOPMENT OF THE
ZONA PELLUCIDA

Even a cursory review of the literature quickly reveals that significant variability exists among species regarding oocyte and, hence,
likely zona pellucida development and maturation [Tsafriri, 1978].
Nonetheless, a generalized description of the major morphological
events associated with zona pellucida development are as follows.

In the oocyte of the early primary follicle, most of the major cytoplasmic organelles such as the Golgi complex, mitochondria, endoplasmic reticulum, and lysosomes are concentrated in a crescent-
shaped juxtanuclear position, referred to as the *Balbiani vitelline body*
[Hertig, 1968]. As the primary follicle continues to develop, the
perivitelline space appears, but at some locations tight junctions re-
sembling desmosomes can still be observed between the vitelline
membrane and the granulosa cells. Extending into the perioocytic
space are numerous oocyte microvilli and some protrusions of the
granulosa cells. The location and appearance of the Golgi apparatus
has also changed during this later period of primary follicle development. The Golgi has moved from its juxtanuclear location to the
subcortical region, the majority of cisternae are now dilated, and the
number of Golgi vesicles has markedly increased and are now concentrated at the periphery of the oocyte. A filamentous material can
be observed in some of these larger vesicles, and in some locations
the ooplasma membrane and vesicles have fused in a manner resem-
bling exocytosis. Concurrently, a similar appearance and pattern of
events occurs in the Golgi apparatus of the follicle cells. Such
changes in these structures are suggestive that both the follicle cells
and the oocyte are involved in active synthesis.

Initially, the zona pellucida appears as small patches of opaque
material in the vicinity of microvilli of both the oocyte membrane and
adjacent granulosa cell membranes. Thus the zona pellucida is not
deposited as a continuous entity, but in discontinuous patches that
coalesce secondarily to form a complete and continuous layer encas-
ing the growing oocyte. Concomitant with the initial appearance of

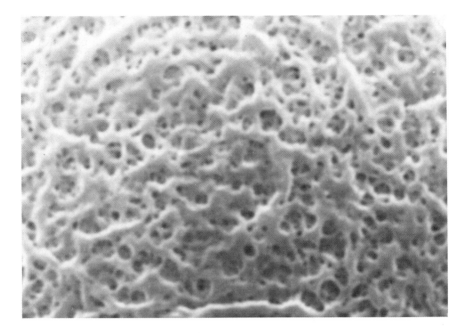

Fig. 2. Surface ultrastructure of the mouse zona pellucida as viewed by scanning electron microscopy. × 25,000.

zona pellucida material is an increase in the number of oocyte microvilli and granulosa cell protrusions. These structures extend into the substance of the developing zona. The oocyte microvilli tend to be more numerous and more evenly distributed over the surface of the oocyte than those associated with the follicular cells.

Once the zona pellucida has completely encircled the oocyte, the Golgi apparatus takes on a different appearance. At this point it now consists primarily of flattened cisternae, located in the periphery of the cytoplasm.

Morphological findings suggest that extracellular maturation of the zona pellucida begins with granular material that appears in close proximity to the developing zona matrix. Fine filamentous connections, perhaps serving as branch points, are also associated with the matrix. Collectively, their fibrillogranular material is responsible for the amorphous appearance of the zona, as observed in scanning and transmission electron micrographs. As the zona pellucida grows in thickness, a higher density of these fibrils becomes apparent, and the mature zona appears as an extensive fibrous network interspersed with numerous pores of varying size (Fig. 2). Differences in density within the mature zona pellucida do exist [Dietl and Czuppon, 1984], however, with the inside (oocyte side) typically appearing more electron dense than the outside (granulosa cell side).

As the follicle continues to progress toward the tertiary stage, the zona matrix becomes wider and denser, and numerous granulosa cell protrusions and microfilaments can be observed traversing its width. As the follicle advances into the preovulatory stage, a gradual granulosa cell–zona dissociation occurs, and these cell protrusions with their associated microvilli retract as the zona reaches maturity.

BIOSYNTHETIC DEVELOPMENT OF THE ZONA PELLUCIDA

To date, detailed biosynthetic investigation of zona proteins has been limited to the mouse [Wassarman, 1988; Chamberlin et al., 1989]. Such studies strongly suggest that, at least for this species, zona proteins are expressed solely in an oocyte-specific manner. Several investigations [Bleil and Wassarman, 1980a,b; Greve et al., 1982; Shimizu et al., 1983] have indicated that the mouse zona pellucida is comprised of three major sulfated glycoproteins, termed ZP1, ZP2, and ZP3. In vitro metabolic labeling experiments involving the incorporation of radiolabeled methionine and fucose into follicle cell–denuded oocytes demonstrate that the growing oocyte is capable of synthesizing all three of these glycoproteins. More recent studies [Philpott et al., 1987], involving the use of antisense RNA probes, also detected ZP3 transcripts only in growing oocytes and not in granulosa cells and thus supports the conclusion of the earlier studies that the mouse zona is solely a product of the oocyte.

Such biosynthetic studies have revealed that ZP1 is the largest of the mouse zona proteins, with an apparent molecular weight of 200 kd [Bleil and Wassarman, 1980a; Shimizu et al., 1983]. It is synthesized as a 135 kd molecular weight dimer to which high mannose-type oligosaccharides are added to give rise to a 150 kd molecular weight intermediate. Additional processing in the Golgi apparatus give rise to the mature 200 kd form. ZP2 (120 kd) is synthesized as an 81 kd core polypeptide chain with six N-linked oligosaccharide side chains [Greve et al., 1982] to yield a 91 kd ZP2 precursor molecule. Mature ZP2 is derived from this precursor by the processing and addition of as-yet-to-be-characterized O-linked sugars. Mouse ZP3 (83 kd) is at first synthesized as a 44 kd polypeptide to which three to four N-linked oligosaccharides are attached, yielding 53 and 56 kd glycoprotein intermediates. These precursors are then processed, and O-linked oligosaccharides are bound to produce the mature 83 kd form.

The rate of mouse zona biosynthesis has been measured with a follicle culture system and radiolabeled precursors [Shimizu et al., 1983]. During the first day of culture, 7–8% of the total proteins synthesized were incorporated into the zona, but by the sixth day of culture this percentage had dropped to 2–3%. These values correspond quantitatively to the decrease in ZP3 transcripts observed in the later stages of oocyte growth as reported by Philpott et al. [1987]. Fully grown oocytes [Bleil and Wassarman, 1980b; Flechon et al., 1984] and superovulated oocytes [Shimizu et al., 1983], although synthesizing protein, do not synthesize zona proteins. Thus the pattern of zona protein synthesis is closely correlated to the abundance of zona gene transcripts and appears restricted to the early stages of follicle/oocyte growth, and the recent biosynthesis data are apparently in agreement with morphological evidence.

The preovulatory mouse oocyte is surrounded by a zona pellucida approximately 7 μm in thickness, containing 4–5 ng of protein, with its constituent ZP1, ZP2, and ZP3 glycoproteins seemingly organized into a matrix of branched filaments [Greve and Wassarman, 1985]. Treatment of the zona with chymotrypsin and dithiothreitol reduces the branched conformation to individual ZP2 and ZP3 fibrils, suggesting that ZP1 is responsible for the branching appearance of the matrix. Thus, in the mouse, the mature zona pellucida of the preovulatory oocyte appears to be an ordered structure of ZP2 and ZP3 filaments held together by ZP1 [Greve and Wassarman, 1985].

CELLULAR ORIGIN OF THE ZONA PELLUCIDA

Years of morphological, cytochemical, immunohistochemical, autoradiographic, and, more recently, biochemical and molecular biology directed investigations have not as yet specifically clarified the issue of the precise cellular origin of the zona pellucida. Over this period, three theories have been formulated regarding the site of synthesis of this structure: Zona components are synthesized by 1) only the follicle cells, 2) only the oocyte, or 3) by both the oocyte and follicle cells (Table 1). The view that the zona pellucida is solely a product of the follicle cells was generated primarily from early morphological data and, in view of the recent biochemical data, can likely be eliminated from consideration. However, at present, strong evidence does exist for the involvement of oocytes and follicle (granulosa) cells in the synthesis of zona pellucida material. Thus the controversy regarding origin of the zona centers on whether, in vivo, it is produced solely by the oocyte or primarily by the oocyte in combination with contributions by the follicle cells.

TABLE 1. Studies Supporting Major Views of Cellular Origin of Zona Pellucida

Follicle cell	Oocyte	Oocyte and follicle cell
Chiquione [1959]	Franchi [1960]	Yamada et al. [1957]
Sotelo and Porter [1959]	Odor [1960]	Wartenberg and Stegner [1960]
Trujillo-Cenoz and Sotelo [1959]	Stegner and Wartenberg [1961]	Hadek [1965]
Chiquoine [1960]	Kang [1974]	Hope [1965]
Merker [1961]	Oakberg and Tyrell, [1975]	Hertig and Adams [1967]
Adams and Hertig [1964]	Haddad and Nagai [1977]	Hedrick and Fry [1980]
Blandau and Odor [1972]	Bleil and Wassarman [1980a]	Tesoriero [1984]
Guraya [1974]	Bleil and Wassarman [1980b]	Wolgemuth et al. [1984]
Verma and Verma [1980]	Bousquet et al. [1981]	Takeuchi and Takeuchi [1985]
	Greve et al. [1982]	Maresh and Dunbar [1987]
	Wassarman and Bleil [1982]	
	Shimizu et al. [1983]	
	Zamboni and Upadhyay [1983]	
	Flechon et al. [1984]	
	Wassarman et al. [1984]	
	Leveille et al. [1987]	
	Philpott et al. [1987]	
	Takagi et al. [1989]	

Recent biochemical evidence [Bleil and Wassarman, 1980a,b; Greve et al., 1982; Shimizu et al., 1983] does clearly indicate that the developing mouse oocyte is capable of synthesizing all components of its zona pellucida. Such biochemical data are also supported by morphological data from mouse studies [Zamboni and Upadhyay, 1983]. However, other biochemical evidence exists that suggests that the rates of synthesis of proteins by the oocyte are insufficient to account for its mature weight plus that of its zona [Loewenstein and Cohen, 1964; Schultz et al., 1979a,b]. In addition, some ultrastructural evidence is not supportive of the theory that the zona is syn-

TABLE 2. Major Evidence For and Against the Oocyte as the
Sole Site of Synthesis of Zona Pellucida

For	Against
Biochemical data indicating mouse oocyte can synthesize all zona components in vitro	Insufficient rates of protein synthesis
Development of zonae-encased oocytes at ectopic site	Inadequate intracellular organelles in oocyte
	In vitro studies lack extracellular regulatory mechanisms
Morphological, cytochemical, and immunohistochemical data associating zona material with developing oocyte	Association of zona material with follicle cells and follicle cell cultures

thesized in its entirety by the oocyte. The oocyte does not appear to possess the necessary intracellular organelles either in location, amount, or orientation and at the appropriate time to synthesize a structure comprising approximately 20% of its weight [Tesoriero, 1984]. Also, it may be justly argued that in such in vitro studies possible extracellular regulatory mechanisms are lost, thereby obscuring the natural sequence of events in zona pellucida synthesis.

Likewise, studies involving the long-term in vitro culture of granulosa cells isolated from primary and early secondary follicles have shown, with immunochemical techniques, that such cultures secrete zona pellucida material [Maresh and Dunbar, 1987]. There is also in vivo data that suggest that some zona pellucida proteins can be produced in the absence of oocytes [Skinner et al., 1984]. Thus studies such as these strongly implicate the involvement of follicle cells in zona synthesis. Furthermore, the evidence from the numerous morphological, cytochemical, and immunohistological studies performed throughout the years that demonstrate the association and localization of zona pellucida material with follicle cells cannot be ignored, although it can be argued that site of localization does not automatically designate or prove site of synthesis (Table 2).

Collectively, drawing from all these reports, it becomes obvious that the synthesis of the zona pellucida is a complex process likely involving numerous synthetic pathways that occur simultaneously and concurrently with numerous other synthetic processes in the developing and growing follicle. Moreover, it is apparent that the question of zona pellucida origin must not be oversimplified by assuming that a common synthetic pathway of zona synthesis applies to all species. Perhaps, as additional data become available, species-unique pathways of zona synthesis and maturation will emerge. Thus, for some species, the oocyte could be the sole contributor to the formation of this structure, whereas, for others, both the oocyte and follicle cells could be responsible, perhaps in some sequential fashion.

REFERENCES

Adams EC, Hertig AT (1964): Studies on guinea pig oocytes. I. Electron microscopic observations on the development of cytoplasmic organelles in oocytes of primordial and primary follicles. J Cell Biol 21:397–427.

Ahuja KK, Bolwell GP (1983): Probable asymmetry in the organization of components of the hamster zona pellucida. J Reprod Fertil 69:49–55.

Austin CR (1961): The Mammalian Egg. Springfield, IL: C.C. Thomas.

Blandau RJ, Odor DL (1972): Observations of the behaviour of oogonia and oocytes in tissue and organ culture. In Biggers JD, Schuetz AW (eds): Oogenesis. Baltimore: University Park Press, pp 301–330.

Bleil JD, Wassarman PM (1980a): Structure and function of the zona pellucida: Identification and characterization of the proteins of the mouse oocyte's zona pellucida. Dev Biol 76:185–202.

Bleil JD, Wassarman PM (1980b): Mammalian sperm–egg interaction: Identification of a glycoprotein in mouse egg zonae pellucidae possessing receptor activity for sperm. Cell 20:873–882.

Bleil JD, Wassarman PM (1980c): Synthesis of zona pellucida proteins by denuded and follicle-enclosed mouse oocytes during culture in vitro. Proc Natl Acad Sci USA 77:1029–1033.

Bousquet D, Leveille MC, Roberts KD, Chapdelaine A, Bleau G (1981): The cellular origin of the zona pellucida antigen in the human and hamster. J Exp Zool 215:215–218.

Centola GM (1983): Structural changes: Follicular development and hormonal requirements. In Serra GB (ed): The Ovary. New York: Raven Press, pp 95–111.

Chamberlin ME, Ringuette MJ, Philpott CC, Chamow SM, Dean J (1989): Molecular genetics of the mouse zona pellucida. In Dietl J (ed): The Mammalian Egg Coat: Structure and Function. Berlin: Springer-Verlag, pp 1–17.

Chiquoine AD (1959): Electron microscopic observations on the developmental cytology of the mammalian ovum. Anat Rec 133:258–259.

Chiquoine AD (1960): The development of the zona pellucida of the mammalian ovum. Am J Anat 106:149–196.

Dietl J (1989a): The Mammalian Egg Coat: Structure and Function. Berlin: Springer-Verlag.

Dietl J (1989b): Ultrastructural aspects of the developing mammalian zona pellucida. In Dietl J (ed): The Mammalian Egg Coat: Structure and Function. Berlin: Springer-Verlag, pp 49–60.

Dietl J, Czuppon AB (1984): Ultrastructural studies of the porcine zona pellucida during the solubilization process by Li-3,5-diiodosalicylate. Gamete Res 9:45–54.

Dunbar BS, Bundman DS (1987): Evidence for a role of the major glycoprotein in the structural maintenance of the pig zona pellucida. J Reprod Fertil 81:363–376.

Dunbar BS, Liu C, Sammons DW (1981): Identification of the three major proteins of porcine and rabbit zonae pellucidae by high resolution two-dimensional gel electrophoresis: Comparison with serum, follicular fluid and ovarian cell proteins. Biol Reprod 24: 1111–1124.

Dunbar BS, Maresh GA, Washenik K (1989): Ovarian development and formation of the mammalian zona pellucida. In Dietl J (ed): The Mammalian Egg Coat: Structure and Function. Berlin: Springer-Verlag, pp 38–48.

Dunbar BS, Wolgemuth DJ (1984): Structure and function of the mammalian zona pellucida, a unique extracellular matrix. Modern Cell Biol 3:77–111.

Flechon JE, Pavlok A, Kopecny V (1984): Dynamics of zona pellucida formation by mouse oocyte: An autoradiographic study. Biol Cell 51:403–406.

Florman HM, Bechtol KB, Wassarman PM (1984): Enzymatic dissection of the functions of the mouse egg's receptor for sperm. Dev Biol 106:243–255.

Franchi LL (1960): Electron microscopy of oocyte–follicle cell relationship in the rat ovary. J Biophys Biochem Cytol 7:397–398.

Geneser F (1986): Textbook of Histology. Philadelphia: Lea and Febiger, pp 589–670.

Greve JM, Salzmann GS, Roller RJ, Wassarman PM (1982): Biosynthesis of the major zona pellucida glycoprotein secreted by oocytes during mammalian oogenesis. Cell 31: 749–759.

Greve JM, Wassarman PM (1985): Mouse egg extracellular coat is a matrix of interconnected filaments possessing a structural repeat. J Mol Biol 181:253–264.

Guraya SS (1974): Morphology, histochemistry and biochemistry of human oogenesis and ovulation. Int Rev Cytol 37:121–152.

Haddad A, Nagai MET (1977): Radioautographic study of glycoprotein synthesis and renewal in the ovarian follicle of mice and the origin of the zona pellucida. Cell Tissue Res 117:347–369.

Hadek R (1965): The structure of the mammalian egg. Int Rev Cytol 19:29–68.

Hedrick JL, Fry GN (1980): Immunocytochemical studies on the porcine zona pellucida. J Cell Biol 87:163a.

Hedrick JL, Wardrip NJ (1986): Isolation of the zona pellucida and purification of its glycoprotein families from pig oocytes. Anal Biochem 157:63–70.

Hedrick JL, Wardrip NJ (1987): On the macromolecular composition of the zona pellucida from porcine oocytes. Dev Biol 121:478–488.

Henderson CJ, Hulme MJ, Aitken RJ (1988): Contraceptive potential of antibodies to the zona pellucida. J Reprod Fertil 83:325–343.

Hertig AT (1968): The primary human oocyte. Some observations of the fine structure of Balbianis vitelline body and the origin of the annulate lamellae. Am J Anat 122:107–138.

Hertig AT, Adams EC (1967): Studies on the human oocyte and its follicle. I. Ultrastructural and histochemical observations on the primordial follicle stage. J Cell Biol 34:647–675.

Hope J (1965): Fine structure of the developing follicles of the rhesus ovary. J Ultrastruct Res 12:592–610.

Jones HW, Jones GS, Hodgen GD, Rosenwaks Z (1986): In Vitro Fertilization. Baltimore: Williams & Wilkins.

Kang YH (1974): Development of the zona pellucida in the rat oocyte. Am J Anat 139: 535–566.

Katz DF, Drobnis EZ, Overstreet JW (1989): Factors regulating mammalian sperm migration through the female reproductive tract and oocyte vestments. Gamete Res 22:443–469.

Leveille MC, Roberts KD, Chevalier S, Chapdelaine A, Bleau G (1987): Formation of the hamster zona pellucida in relation to ovarian differentiation and follicular growth. J Reprod Fertil 79:173–183.

Loewenstein JE, Cohen AI (1964): Dry mass, lipid content and protein content of the intact and zona-free mouse ovum. J Embryol Exp Morphol 12:113–121.

Maresh GA, Dunbar BS (1987): Expression of specific proteins by ovarian primary follicles cultured in vitro. Biol Reprod (Suppl 1) 36:88a.

Merker HJ (1961): Electronen mikroskopische untersuchungen über die bildung der zona pellucida in den follikeln des kaninchenovars. Z Zellforsch Mikrosk Anat 83:375.

Nakano M (1989): Fractionation and characterization of the glycoproteins of zona pellucida. In Dietl J (ed): The Mammalian Egg Coat: Structure and Function. Berlin: Springer-Verlag, pp 75–98.

Oakberg EF, Tyrell PD (1975): Labeling the zona pellucida of the mouse oocyte. Biol Reprod 12:477–482.

Odor DL (1960): Electron microscopic studies on ovarian oocytes and unfertilized tubal ova in the rat. J Biophys Biochem Cytol 7:567–574.

O'Rand MG, Welch JE, Fisher SJ (1986): Sperm membrane and zona pellucida interactions during fertilization. In Dhindsa DS, Bahl OP (eds): Molecular and Cellular Aspects of Reproduction. New York: Plenum Press, pp 131–144.

Pedersen T, Peters H (1968): Proposal for the classification of oocyte and follicles in the mouse ovary. J Reprod Fertil 17:555–557.

Peters H (1978): Folliculogenesis in mammals. In Jones RE (ed): The Vertebrate Ovary. New York: Plenum Press, pp 121–144.

Philpott CC, Ringuette MJ, Dean J (1987): Oocyte specific expression and developmental regulation of ZP3, the sperm receptor of the mouse zona pellucida. Dev Biol 121:568–575.

Piko L (1969): Gamete structure and sperm entry in mammals. In Metz CB (ed): Fertilization. New York: Academic Press, Vol 2, pp 325–403.

Sacco AG (1981): Immunocontraception: Consideration of the zona pellucida as a target antigen. In Wynn RM (ed): Obstetrics and Gynecology Annual, Vol 10. New York: Appleton-Century-Crofts, pp 1–26.

Sacco AG (1987): The zona pellucida: Current status as a candidate antigen for contraceptive vaccine development. Am J Reprod Immunol Microbiol 15:122–130.

Sacco AG, Subramanian MG, Yurewicz EC (1984): Association of sperm receptor activity with a purified pig zona antigen (PPZA). J Reprod Immunol 6:89–103.

Sacco AG, Yurewicz EC (1989): Use of the zona pellucida as an immunocontraceptive target antigen. In Dietl J (ed): Berlin: Springer-Verlag, pp 128–153.

Sacco AG, Yurewicz EC, Subramanian MG, DeMayo FJ (1981): Zona pellucida composition: Species cross-reactivity and contraceptive potential of antiserum to a purified pig zona antigen (PPZA). Biol Reprod 25:977–1008.

Schultz RM, Letourneau GE, Wassarman PM (1979a): Program of early development in the mammal: Changes in patterns and absolute rates of tubulin and total protein synthesis during oogenesis and early embryogenesis in the mouse. Dev Biol 68:341–359.

Schultz RM, Letourneau GE, Wassarman PM (1979b): Program of early development in the mammal: Changes in the patterns and absolute rates of tubulin and total protein synthesis during oocyte growth in the mouse. Dev Biol 73:120–133.

Shimizu S, Tsuji M, Dean J (1983): In vitro biosynthesis of three sulfated glycoproteins of murine zonae pellucidae by oocytes grown in follicle culture. J Biol Chem 258:5858–5863.

Skinner SM, Mills T, Kirchick HJ, Dunbar BS (1984): Immunization with zona pellucida proteins results in abnormal ovarian follicular differentiation and inhibition of gonadotropin-induced steroid secretion. Endocrinology 115:2418–2432.

Sotelo JR, Porter KR (1959): An electron microscopic study of the rat ovum. J Biophys Biochem Cytol 5:327–342.

Stegner HE, Wartenberg (1961): Elektronmikroskopische und histotopochemische untersuchungen uber struktur und bildung der zona pellucida menschlichen eizellen. Z Zellforsch 53:702–713.

Takagi J, Dobashi M, Araki Y, Imal Y, Hiroi M, Tonosaki A, Sendo F (1989): The development of porcine zona pellucida using monoclonal antibodies: II. Electron microscopy. Biol Reprod 40:1103–1108.

Takeuchi IK, Takeuchi YK (1985): Use of tannic acid for ultrastructural visualization of zonae pellucidae in growing oocytes of rat ovarian follicle. Zool Sci 2:135–139.

Tesoriero JV (1984): Comparative cytochemistry of the developing ovarian follicles of the dog, rabbit and mouse: Origin of the zona pellucida. Gemete Res 10:301–318.

Trujillo-Cenoz O, Sotelo JR (1959): Relationships of the ovular surface with follicle cells and origin of zona pellucida in the rabbit oocytes. J Biophys Biochem Cytol 5:347.

Tsafriri A (1978): Ooocyte maturation in mammals. In Jones RE (ed): The Vertebrate Ovary. New York: Plenum Press, pp 409–442.

Urch UA, Wardrip NJ, Hedrick JL (1985): Limited and specific proteolysis of the zona pellucida by acrosin. J Exp Zool 233:479–483.

Verma GP, Verma KP (1980): Carbohydrate histochemistry of ovarian follicle with reference to the formation of zona pellucida in rabbit. Acta Histochem Cytochem 13:377–385.

Wartenberg H, Stegner HE (1960): Uber die elektronenmikroshopiche feinstruktur des menschlichen ovarialeises. Z Zellforsch 52:450–474.

Wassarman PM (1987): The zona pellucida: A coat of many colors. BioEssays 6:161–166.

Wassarman PM (1988): Zona pellucida glycoproteins. Annu Rev Biochem 57:415–442.

Wassarman PM, Bleil JD (1982): The role of zona pellucida glycoproteins as regulators of sperm-egg interactions in the mouse. In Frazier WA, Glaser L, Gottlieb DI (eds): Cellular Recognition. New York: Alan R. Liss, pp 845–863.

Wassarman PM, Greve JM, Perona RM, Roller RJ, Salzmann GS (1984): How mouse eggs put on and take off their extracellular coat. In Davidson EH, Firtel RA (eds): Molecular Biology of Development. New York: Alan R. Liss, pp 213–225.

Wolgemuth DJ, Celenza J, Bundman DS, Dunbar BS (1984): Formation of the rabbit zona pellucida and its relationship to ovarian follicular development. Dev Biol 106:1–14.

Yamada E, Muta T, Motomura A, Koga H (1957): The fine structure of the oocyte in the mouse ovary studied with electron microscope. Kurrume Med J 4:148–171.

Yanagimachi R (1988a): Sperm-egg fusion. In Duzgunes N, Bronner F (eds): Current Topics in Membranes and Transport, Vol 32: Membrane Fusion in Fertilization, Cellular Transport and Viral Infection. New York: Academic Press, pp 3–43.

Yanagimachi R (1988b): Mammalian fertilization. In Knobil E, Neill J (eds): The Physiology of Reproduction. New York: Raven Press, pp 135–185.

Yurewicz EC, Sacco AG, Subramanian MG (1987): Structural characterization of the M_r = 55,000 antigen (ZP3) of porcine oocyte zona pellucida. J Biol Chem 262:564–571.

Zamboni L, Upadhyay S (1983): Germ cell differentiation in mouse adrenal glands. J Exp Zool 228:173–193.

DISCUSSION

DR. AITKEN: With the various panels of monoclonal antibodies against the zona pellucida now available, do you know of any studies that show differentiation of the zona pellucida during folliculogenesis? Is it laid down in its final form in the very early follicle, and then does it just grow in the oocyte, or does it differentiate?

DR. SACCO: There are studies with monoclonal antibodies that show that the zona pellucida seems to be formed in a layered type of pattern, and some researchers suggest that this demonstrates that the oocyte is producing it.

DR. CUASNICU: Different studies in vivo and in vitro indicate that ovarian oocytes can be penetrated as well as tubal eggs are, indicating that zona pellucida maturation is not needed, at least for that event. Do you have any evidence that zona pellucida maturation is needed for any other specific event?

DR. SACCO: That's a good question. I don't really think that I can answer that. Most of the studies I have done have involved ovarian oocytes, and I am more interested in just the attachment of sperm to the zona. So I know at this point that obviously sperm can attach. I haven't examined the penetration of zona or the complicated events that occur later.

DR. BLAQUIER: Today, more and more labs are using the human zona pellucida either to predict fertility or as a functional assay of sperm capabilities, and, depending on what they are presenting, people using material from cadavers will recover oocytes in very different states of maturation. Do you have any information on the ability of human zona pellucida to bind all sites of human sperm when the oocytes are at different stages of maturation?

DR. SACCO: No. I don't have any information on that, but the people working with the hemizona assay may.

DR. ALEXANDER: I will present some material tomorrow concerning that, but I would also like to ask you a question. At the American Fertility Society meeting in San Francisco, November 1987, there was a presentation by a Korean group in which immature oocytes from ovaries were cultured in human follicular fluid. They found that after the eggs were cultured for 48 hr, the eggs could be penetrated and fertilized by spermatozoa and actually produce offspring, even though the same oocytes would have taken at least 10 days to mature in vivo. Do you have any information as to whether mature follicular fluid helps the maturation not only of the egg itself but also of the zona pellucida?

DR. SACCO: Studies involving the addition of follicular fluid have become very popular recently. As such, I think we may get some interesting information in the near future out of these experiments. There are many claims that the addition of follicular fluid has an effect on sperm capacitation, sperm acrosome reaction, and so forth and that it significantly increases the fertilizability of sperm. I don't know if there is some type of effect on the zona pellucida, but it is an area that many researchers are beginning to investigate.

20

Glycosylation and Maturation of the Mammalian Zona Pellucida

Therese M. Timmons, Sheri M. Skinner, and Bonnie S. Dunbar

The mammalian oocyte is encased during the early stages of ovarian follicular development by a unique glycoprotein structure termed the *zona pellucida* (ZP). The synthesis of the individual ZP glycoproteins and their subsequent assembly to form the matrix are complex processes that are not yet clearly understood. The initial stages of ZP assembly coincide with the differentiation and proliferation of the granulosa cells [Dunbar et al., 1989b; Wolgemuth et al., 1984], which are ultimately responsible for the production of steroids in collaboration with the surrounding thecal cells. The formation of a mature ZP matrix is estimated to take days or weeks, depending on the species involved [Dunbar et al., 1989b]. Both the granulosa cells and the oocyte itself have been implicated as the site of ZP glycoprotein synthesis in various species [Wolgemuth et al., 1984; Bleil and Wassarman, 1980; Philpott et al., 1987], and this topic is still the focus of considerable controversy.

Unlike the testis, the ovary is not an immunologically sequestered organ, and all cell types in the ovary are exposed to the full range of serum components, including antibodies. Consequently, antibodies against ZP glycoproteins may play a role in disease-related infertility such as that associated with premature ovarian failure. Clinical reports indicate that antibodies to ovarian antigens, including those of the ZP, may be responsible for a significant proportion of these cases and for the associated infertility problems [Damewood et al., 1986; Mignot et al., 1989; Bousquet et al., 1982]. In addition, the suitability

Gamete Interaction: Prospects for Immunocontraception, pages 277–292

of ZP glycoproteins for a contraceptive vaccine in various mammalian species is being actively studied by numerous researchers [Dunbar et al., 1989a; Skinner et al., 1984; Sacco et al., 1981; Henderson et al., 1987a,b]. The challenge facing these investigators is to isolate and characterize a particular epitope that, when injected into the host, will elicit an immune response that results in complete infertility in the absence of any deleterious side effects and that does not interfere with other normal ovarian functions.

In light of these studies in immunoreproduction, it is important to understand the events surrounding the synthesis and assembly of the mammalian ZP and the functions of its constituent glycoproteins in fertilization and normal ovarian development. This information will help to identify potential causes of infertility and to target specific ovarian antigens that could be used in a safe and effective contraceptive vaccine.

MORPHOLOGICAL ANALYSIS OF THE COMPONENTS OF THE MAMMALIAN ZP

Although the ZP appears to be fairly amorphous under the light microscope, other techniques reveal the presence of layers and differentiated regions within the matrix. Electron microscopy has shown all mammalian ZP to have a lattice-like outer surface and a smoother inner surface [Dudkiewicz et al., 1976; Jackowski and Dumont, 1979; Phillips and Shalgi, 1980]. Distinct layers are visible in electron micrographs of the ZP matrix of nonrodent species [Hope, 1965; Konecny, 1959], implying a regular arrangement of the matrix components. This layered appearance can be enhanced through the use of certain histochemical staining procedures [Baranska et al., 1975; Wolgemuth and Gavin, 1981] and by the binding of a monoclonal antibody that recognizes a carbohydrate determinant present in the ZP (see below).

A series of histochemical stains has also been employed to differentiate the ZP of atretic follicles from those of normal growing follicles [Centola, 1982], even before degenerative changes can be detected morphologically. Following treatment of paraffin-embedded sections of porcine ovaries with Shorr's S3 and hematoxylin stain, the ZP of healthy follicles is stained uniformly green. In contrast, the ZP of follicles in any stage of degeneration that is microscopically detectable is stained a bright orange. However, the ZP of some follicles that appear normal and the ZP of many primary follicles are also stained orange completely or partially by this procedure, indicating their ultimate destiny as atretic follicles. Although the chemical basis for the color change is not understood, alterations in the carbohydrate moieties of the ZP would be detected by such a staining regimen. Biochemical analysis of this phenomenon will give new insight into the molecular events underlying follicular development and the process of atresia.

The asymmetric distribution of various carbohydrate structures within the ZP matrix is further demonstrated by the binding patterns of plant lectins having a wide range of specificities. Nicholson et al. [1975] have presented evidence that the outer regions of the mouse, rat, and hamster ZP bind wheat-germ agglutinin (WGA; N-acetyl-D-glucosamine and sialic acid residues) and *Ricinus communis I* agglutinin (RCA[I]; β-D-galactose and α-D-galactose residues). In contrast, Dunbar et al. [1980] demonstrated WGA binding in the inner regions of the porcine and bovine ZP, and RCA(I) binding in the outer ZP surfaces. Concanavalin A (α-D-glucose and α-D-mannose residues) was localized uniformly throughout the ZP matrix of all five of these mammalian species. Additional lectins have been used as probes in various species [Nicholson et al., 1975; Dunbar et al., 1980; Watanabe et al., 1981], and the collective results indicate that the ZP carbohydrate moieties exhibit marked species differences in distribution within the matrix structure.

GLYCOPROTEIN COMPONENTS OF THE MAMMALIAN ZP

The individual glycoprotein components of the ZP number between three and five, depending on the species examined [Dunbar et al., 1981; Sacco et al., 1981]. They are resolved by two-dimensional polyacrylamide gel electrophoresis (PAGE) into "families" with a common polypeptide backbone, each of which exhibits extensive charge and molecular weight heterogeneity. This microheterogeneity is due to the presence of highly charged oligosaccharide side chains, and this complex structure has given rise to a confusing and inconsistent nomenclature [Timmons and Dunbar, 1988]. With a system based on the molecular weight of the least glycosylated members of a particular family, the porcine ZP glycoproteins can be identified as ZP1 (82K), ZP2 (61K), ZP3 (55Kα), and ZP3β (55Kβ). An alternate method, being used especially for the rabbit ZP (see below), names the glycoproteins on the basis of their apparent molecular weights after partial deglycosylation by endo-β-galactosidase (EBGD): 55K (EBGD), 75K (EBGD), and 85K (EBGD).

It should be noted that fully glycosylated ZP glycoproteins from the mouse can be resolved by one-dimensional nonreducing PAGE into three major bands, presumably because the specific post-translational modifications present do not introduce the same degree of molecular weight heterogeneity as do those of other mammalian species [Sacco et al., 1981].

CHARACTERIZATION OF CARBOHYDRATE ANTIGENS ASSOCIATED WITH THE ZONA PELLUCIDA

The binding of lectins, as mentioned above, has been widely used to study oligosaccharides present on individual glycoprotein and glycolipid molecules and those accessible on cell surfaces. However, lectin specificities are too broad to allow the detection of a particular carbohydrate structure or to rule out its presence with any confidence. An antibody generated against a given carbohydrate antigen affords a much more specific structural probe.

It is clear from the numerous reports characterizing antibodies against the ZP that the major ZP antigens consist of either an amino acid sequence or a particular conformation rather than a carbohydrate structure alone [Drell et al., 1984; Maresh and Dunbar, 1987; Timmons et al., 1987; Sacco et al., 1981]. However, a monoclonal antibody (PS1) that recognizes a carbohydrate moiety found in the ZP of several mammalian species has been generated through the use of a porcine ZP glycoprotein immunogen excised from a silver-stained polyacrylamide gel [Drell and Dunbar, 1984; Timmons et al., 1990a]. Although the immunogen was a single spot from a two-dimensional polyacrylamide gel, the antibody reacts with the most completely glycosylated members of three porcine ZP glycoproteins resolved by two-dimensional PAGE in the presence of reducing agents. According to the nomenclature described above, these are ZP1 (82K), ZP2 (61K), and ZP3α (55K). PS1 also recognizes at least one of the ZP glycoproteins of several other mammalian species, including rabbit, cat, dog, and baboon (Fig. 2). Preliminary investigations into the biochemical structure of the epitope have demonstrated that it is carried on an N-linked rather than an O-linked carbohydrate chain in the pig, because PS1 binding to ZP glycoproteins in immunoblots is destroyed by prior treatment of the glycoproteins with endo-β-N-acetylglucosaminidase F (endo F).

PS1 antibody binding is also sensitive to treatment of the glycoproteins with EBGD, an enzyme specific for the degradation of lactosaminoglycans (LAG) [Fukuda and Matsumura, 1976]. The carbohydrate content of porcine ZP glycoproteins has been reported, and each contains approximately equimolar amounts of galactose and N-acetyl glucosamine [Dunbar et al., 1980; Hedrick and Wardrip,

1987]. These repeating Gal-β-1–4GlcNAc-β-1–3 carbohydrate structures are commonly found as part of glycolipids and glycoproteins
on cell surfaces and are known to function in cell adhesion and
cell–cell interaction in several systems [Macek and Shur, 1988; Dutt et
al., 1987; Fukuda, 1985; Hakomori, 1981]. In fact, studies by Brown
and Jones [1987] have shown that all the major porcine ZP glycoproteins are involved in binding of boar sperm to the ZP surface, perhaps via the LAG structures. Berger et al. [1989] have confirmed that
sperm binding to the pig oocyte ZP is mediated by carbohydrate and
involves multiple ZP glycoproteins. Consequently, it is of interest to
note that the monoclonal antibody PS1 or its Fab fragments inhibits
the binding of porcine sperm to porcine ZP, whereas other monoclonals developed in this laboratory directed against protein epitopes
have no effect on sperm/ZP interaction (Timmons et al., 1990b].

These studies collectively demonstrate that the PS1 antigen is
present on an N-linked oligosaccharide associated with the surface of
the porcine ZP, involved in the initial stages of sperm–ZP binding.
Detailed biochemical analysis of its structure will help to elucidate
the mechanism by which homologous sperm–ZP attachment, binding, and penetration occur during the process of mammalian fertilization.

Carbohydrate analysis of the mouse ZP glycoproteins indicates
that all three glycoproteins contain asparagine-linked complex-type
oligosaccharides, and at least two also contain serine–threonine-
linked carbohdyrates [Wassarman, 1988]. A specific class of O-linked
oligosaccharides on the ZP3 molecule (83K) containing an α-linked
galactose residue at the nonreducing terminus functions as the primary initial attachment site for sperm [Bleil and Wassarman, 1988],
possibly through the action of galactosyltransferase activity residing
on the sperm surface [Shur and Hall, 1982].

Additional evidence from the hamster [Ahuja, 1985] supports the
conclusion that the initial recognition and binding between sperm
and ZP is mediated by high-affinity sperm lectins and complementary ZP glycoconjugates [O'Rand, 1988]. However, this initial attachment is not entirely species specific and must be stabilized by further
secondary contacts between the sperm surface and the ZP if the
fertilization process is to proceed. These species-specific contacts are
provided by regions of the ZP proteins that vary among species
(Timmons, Cook, and Dunbar, in preparation).

All glycoproteins reported thus far to carry polylactosaminoglycans are membrane anchored, with the exception of secretory glycoproteins such as erythropoietin [Sasaki et al., 1987] and α1-acid glycoprotein [Yoshima et al., 1981], which contain only one or two

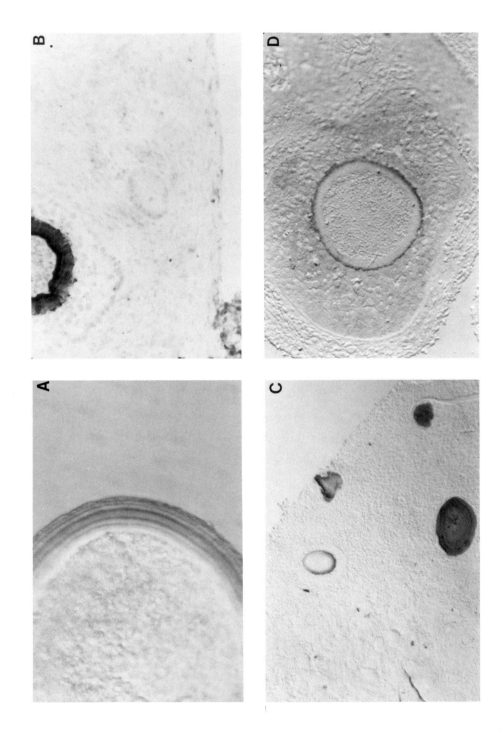

N-acetylactosamine repeat units. Based on carbohydrate analysis and on the magnitude of the decrease in apparent molecular weight as measured by one-dimensional SDS-PAGE after EBGD treatment (Fig. 2), ZP glycoproteins contain numerous repeat units per molecule. Therefore, they represent another class of molecules carrying LAG structures: nonmembrane-bound extracellular matrix constituents containing large LAG chains. Polylactosaminoglycans also carry important cell surface determinants such as the ABO blood group and specific embryonal antigens, and these carbohydrate structures can exhibit striking changes during development and cellular differentiation [Fukuda, 1985]. By analogy, dramatic changes in the polyactosaminoglycan structures of the ZP involved in extracellular matrix interactions with the oocyte and granulosa cells might be expected during follicular development.

DEGLYCOSYLATION OF ZP GLYCOPROTEINS

Because of the high degree of post-translational modification of mammalian ZP components, it is impossible to resolve them by one-dimensional SDS-PAGE and often difficult to do so even with two-dimensional PAGE. Both chemical and enzymatic methods of deglycosylation are useful in reducing the microheterogeneity and enabling clean separation of the remaining ZP protein cores by one-dimensional PAGE.

Information on the ZP oligosaccharides from several species is now available [Yurewicz et al., 1987; Hedrick and Wardrip, 1987; Salzmann et al., 1983]. Precise oligosaccharide structures are not yet known, but most of the ZP constituent glycoproteins carry both N- and O-linked sugars [Yurewicz et al., 1987; Florman and Wassarman, 1985; Timmons et al. 1990a]. Trifluoromethane sulfonic acid

---

Fig. 1.   Immunocytochemical localization of antibodies to the zona pellucida (ZP), illustrating distinct morphological regions within the mammalian ZP. The tissues were processed using established techniques, and antibodies were visualized (B, C, and D) with the peroxidase/diaminobenzidine system [Dunbar et al., 1989c]. **A:** Monoclonal antibody directed against a carbohydrate antigen present in the mammalian ZP is discretely localized in layers within the porcine ZP structure. **B:** Rabbit antiserum generated against total solubilized porcine ZP is localized in a uniform diffuse pattern throughout the rabbit ZP matrix. **C:** Sheep antiserum generated against total solubilized rabbit ZP is visualized with varying intensities in different regions of the rabbit ZP matrix. **D:** Dog antiserum generated against total solubilized porcine ZP is specifically localized in the outer layer of the dog ZP.

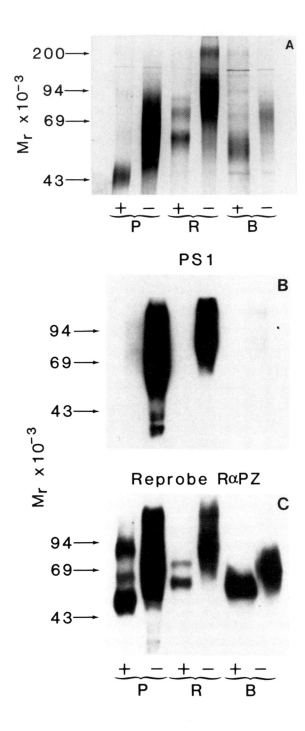

will completely remove both types of carbohydrate chains, leaving only the galactose residue still linked to the serine or threonine residue in the protein backbone [Karp et al., 1982]. A variety of glycosidases are effective in removing carbohydrate moieties from the ZP glycoproteins [Timmons et al., 1990a; Wassarman, 1988], including both exo- and endoglycosidases. EBGD has proved especially useful because the ZP components of all species examined contain LAG structures. If the reaction is allowed to go to completion, the partially deglycosylated glycoproteins that still contain the high mannose core carbohydrates and other non-LAG structures can be easily and reproducibly resolved by one-dimensional PAGE (Fig. 2).

DIFFERENTIAL EXPRESSION OF ZP GLYCOPROTEINS DURING FOLLICULAR DEVELOPMENT

Identification of the specific cell type(s) that synthesize the ZP and understanding the details of its assembly during follicular development are active areas of reproductive research. Numerous investigators have suggested that the oocyte [Bousquet et al., 1981], the granulosa cells [Chiquoine, 1960], or both [Wolgemuth et al., 1984] are involved in the production of the ZP matrix in various nonrodent species. Other studies in the mouse have shown that the oocyte alone is capable of synthesizing the ZP proteins [Bleil and Wassarman, 1980]. These investigations, however, were radiolabeling stud-

---

Fig. 2.   Electrophoretic separation of zona pellucida (ZP) glycoproteins from several mammalian species. ZP from pig (P), rabbit (R), and baboon (B) were isolated and solubilized by established methods [Dunbar et al., 1980]. The ZP glycoproteins were partially deglycosylated by endo-β-galactosidase [Fukuda and Matsumura, 1976; Yurewicz et al., 1987], separated by one-dimensional SDS-PAGE [Laemmli, 1970], and either silver stained (Timmons, Cook, and Dunbar, in preparation) or electroblotted onto polyvinylidine difluoride membrane [Matsudaira, 1987]. The membrane was probed with antibodies and visualized with ^{125}I-protein A by standard protocols [Dunbar, 1988]. **Lanes 1, 2;** Pig ZP glycoproteins; **lanes 3, 4;** rabbit ZP glycoproteins; **lanes 5, 6;** baboon ZP glycoproteins. The samples in lanes 2, 4, and 6 were treated prior to electrophoresis with endo-β-galactosidase (EBGD). **A:** Silver-stained one-dimensional SDS-polyacrylamide gel, illustrating the molecular weight heterogeneity characteristic of mammalian ZP glycoproteins (lanes 2, 4, and 6), which is reduced after EBGD treatment (lanes 1, 3, and 5). **B:** Immunoblot of A, probed with monoclonal antibody PS1. Note the absence of antibody binding by ZP glycoproteins treated with EBGD (lanes 1, 3, and 5). **C:** Immunoblot of A, probed with polyclonal rabbit antiserum generated against total pig ZP. The antibodies recognize protein epitope(s) present in all three species.

ies conducted over a 24 hr period, which is not sufficient time to follow the entire synthesis and assembly period.

Antibodies to total ZP proteins were used in initial studies in the rabbit, which demonstrated localization of ZP antigens in the oocyte and later in the granulosa cells. However, the antigens were visualized only in the inner layer of granulosa cells, those intimately associated with the oocyte. No ZP antigens were identified in the large growing or antral follicles [Dunbar and Wolgemuth, 1983]. These early studies have been repeated with different antibodies generated in sheep against proteins 55K (EBGD) and 75K (EBGD) of the rabbit ZP. Immunocytochemical localization of these antibodies in rabbit ovary demonstrates a differential expression of these two ZP glycoproteins during normal in vivo follicular growth and development [Dunbar et al., 1989b]. The rabbit 75K (EBGD) is produced very early in follicular development, but the 55K (EBGD) component is not expressed until the follicles are in the initial stages of growth in the young rabbit ovary.

Investigations into the site of ZP synthesis have recently been extended to include the development of primary granulosa cell culture [Maresh et al., 1990]. Early-stage granulosa cells isolated from primary follicles from sexually immature (6-week-old) rabbits are grown on poly-D-lysine or EHS basement membrane biomatrix substrata in a serum-free, hormonally defined medium to facilitate the analysis of proteins synthesized and secreted under various conditions. ELISA assays and immunoblots of one- and two-dimensional PAGE separations of secreted proteins, processed using monoclonal and polyclonal antibodies, demonstrate expression of ZP proteins by granulosa cells in vitro in the absence of oocytes. Furthermore, the synthesis of two specific ZP proteins was markedly affected by the substrate used for cell culture: 55K (EBGD) is secreted by cells grown on either EHS biomatrix or poly-D-lysine, but a greater amount of 75K (EBGD) is secreted by cells grown on poly-D-lysine. However, the apparent molecular weights of these antigens are approximately 170 and 180 kd, as determined by SDS-PAGE, as compared with the 90–120 kd range observed for the glycoproteins isolated from mature rabbit ZP (Dunbar et al., 1981]. Therefore, it is likely that proper post-translational modification has not occurred or that the ZP antigens produced by the granulosa cells in culture are normally selectively proteolyzed to their mature forms. The interaction of the granulosa cells with the oocyte or other ovarian cells may be necessary for the complete processing of the ZP glycoproteins.

ROLE OF ANTIBODIES IN FOLLICULAR DEVELOPMENT AND INFERTILITY

The interaction of cell surface components with the appropriate extracellular matrix molecules is responsible for numerous aspects of cellular differentiation and development in many systems [Reid and Jefferson, 1984]. The importance of the extracellular matrix has been recently established in the maintenance of Sertoli–germ cell interactions [Hadley et al., 1985]. Reports confirm that antibodies to the ZP can inhibit both the attachment of sperm to the ZP surface and the penetration of the ZP matrix during fertilization [Dunbar and Wolgemuth, 1984; Henderson et al., 1987a]. However, these antibodies may have effects on the ovary unrelated to their inhibition of sperm–ZP interaction, whether the antibodies are associated with an autoimmune disease or with the administration of an anti-ZP immunocontraceptive, because of their interaction with ZP proteins as they are secreted by the granulosa cells and/or oocyte. This would prevent the ZP matrix from establishing its normal contacts with the cells of the developing follicle.

As a result, the large antral follicles that secrete steroids do not form, and all oocytes are recruited to grow while their follicle cells differentiate. These oocytes are, in turn, destroyed as they begin to synthesize the ZP, causing the total depletion of germ cells and follicles [Dunbar, 1990]. This results in infertility, but with the side effects arising from the lack of steroid-producing follicle cells.

In view of the differential expression of the two rabbit ZP glycoproteins observed during follicular development (see above), antibodies to different ZP components will exert their influence on ovarian development and function at different times and with different results. Knowledge of the synthesis and functions of each ZP glycoprotein will enable the design of an effective immunocontraceptive while enhancing our understanding of normal ovarian development.

REFERENCES

Ahuja KK (1985): Inhibitors of glycoprotein biosynthesis block fertilization in the hamster. Gamete Res 11:179.

Baranska W, Konwinski M, Kuwaja M (1975): Fine structure of the zona pellucida of unfertilized egg cells and embryos. J Exp Zool 192:193.

Berger T, Davis A, Wardrip NJ, Hedrick JL (1989): Sperm binding to the pig zona pellucida and inhibition of binding by solubilized components of the zona pellucida. J Reprod Fertil 86:559.

Bleil JD, Wassarman PM (1980): Synthesis of zona pellucida proteins by denuded and follicle-enclosed mouse oocytes during culture in vitro. Proc Natl Acad Sci USA 77:1029.

Bleil JD, Wassarman PM (1988): Galactose at the nonreducing terminus of O-linked oligosaccharides of mouse egg zona pellucida glycoprotein ZP3 is essential for the glycoprotein's sperm receptor activity. Proc Natl Acad Sci USA 85:6778.

Bousquet D, Jacques S, Roberts KD, Chapdelaine A, Bleau G (1982): Zona pellucida antibodies in a group of women with idiopathic infertility. Am J Reprod Immunol 2:73.

Bousquet D, Leveille MC, Roberts KD, Chapdelaine A, Bleau G (1981): The cellular origin of the zona pellucida antigen in the human and hamster. J Exp Zool 215:215.

Brown CR, Jones R (1987): Binding of zona pellucida proteins to a boar sperm polypeptide of Mr 53,000 and identification of zona moieties involved. Development 99:333.

Centola GM (1982): Light microscopic observations of alterations in staining of the zona pellucida of porcine follicular oocytes: Possible early indication of atresia. Gamete Res 6:293.

Chiquoine AD (1960): The development of the zona pellucida of the mammalian ovum. Am J Anat 106:149.

Damewood MD, Zacur HA, Hoffman GJ, Rock JA (1986): Circulating antiovarian antibodies in premature ovarian failure. Obstet Gynecol 68:850.

Drell DW, Dunbar BS (1984): Monoclonal antibodies to rabbit and pig zonae pellucidae distinguish species-specific and shared antigenic determinants. Biol Reprod 30:445.

Drell DW, Wood DM, Bundman D, Dunbar BS (1984): Immunological comparison of antibodies to porcine zonae pellucidae in rats and rabbits. Biol Reprod 30:435.

Dudkiewicz AB, Shivers CA, Williams WL (1976): Ultrastructure of hamster zona pellucida treated with zona-precipitation antibody. Biol Reprod 14:175.

Dunbar BS (1988): Two-Dimensional Electrophoresis and Immunological Techniques. New York: Plenum Press.

Dunbar BS (1989): Ovarian antigens and infertility. Am J Reprod Immunol 21:28.

Dunbar BS, Liu C, Sammons DW (1981): Identification of the three major proteins of porcine and rabbit zonae pellucidae by high-resolution two-dimensional gel electrophoresis: Comparison with follicular fluid, sera and ovarian cell proteins. Biol Reprod 24:1111.

Dunbar BS, Lo C, Powell J, Stevens VC (1989a): Use of a peptide adjuvant for the immunization of baboons with denatured and deglycosylated pig zona pellucida glycoproteins. Fertil Steril 52:311.

Dunbar BS, Maresh GA, Washenik KJ (1989b): Ovarian development and the formation of the mammalian zona pellucida. In Dietl J (ed): The Mammalian Egg Coat: Structure and Function. New York: Springer-Verlag, p 38.

Dunbar BS, Wardrip NJ, Hedrick JL (1980): Isolation, physicochemical properties and the macromolecular composition of the zona pellucida from porcine oocytes. Biochemistry 19:356.

Dunbar BS, Washenik KJ, Skinner SM (1989c): Strategies for preparation and use of monoclonal and polyclonal antibodies. In Hughes MR, Schrader WT, O'Malley BW (eds): Hormone Action and Molecular Endocrinology, 13th ed. Houston: Houston Biological Associates.

Dunbar BS, Wolgemuth DJ (1984): Structure and function of the mammalian zona pellucida, a unique extracellular matrix. In Satir B (ed): Modern Cell Biology, Volume 3. New York: Alan R. Liss, p 77.

Dutt A, Tang J-P, Carson DD (1987): Lactosaminoglycans are involved in uterine epithelial cell adhesion in vitro. Dev Biol 119:27.

Florman HM, Wassarman PM (1985): O-linked oligosaccharides of mouse egg ZP3 account for its sperm receptor activity. Cell 41:313.

Fukuda M (1985): Cell surface glycoconjugates as onco-differentiation markers in hematopoietic cells. Biochem Biophys Acta 780:119.

Fukuda MN, Matsumura TE (1976): Purification and characterization of endo-beta-galactosidase from *Escherichia freundii* induced by hog gastric mucin. J Biol Chem 256:3900.

Hadley MA, Byers SW, Suarez-Quan CA, Kleinman HH, Dym M (1985): Extracellular matrix regulates Sertoli cell differentiation, testicular cord formation, and germ cell development in vitro. J Cell Biol 101:1511.

Hakomori S (1981): Glycosphingolipids in cellular interaction, differentiation, and oncogenesis. Annu Rev Biochem 50:733.

Hedrick JL, Wardrip NJ (1987): On the macromolecular composition of the zona pellucida from porcine oocytes. Dev Biol 121:478.

Henderson CJ, Braude P, Aitken RJ (1987a): Polyclonal antibodies to a 32-KDa deglycosylated polypeptide from porcine zonae pellucidae will prevent human gamete interaction in vitro. Gamete Res 18:251.

Henderson CJ, Hulme MJ, Aitken RJ (1987b): Analysis of the biological properties of antibodies raised against intact and deglycosylated porcine zonae pellucidae. Gamete Res 16:323.

Hope J (1965): The fine structure of the developing follicle of the rhesus ovary. J Ultrastruct Res 12:592.

Jackowski S, Dumont JN (1979): Surface alterations of the mouse zona pellucida and ovum following in vitro fertilization: Correlation with cell cycle. Biol Reprod 20:150.

Karp DR, Atkinson JP, Shreffler DC (1982): Genetic variation in glycosylation of the fourth component of murine complement. J Biol Chem 257:7330.

Konecny M (1959): Etude histochemique de la zone pellucide des ovules de chatle. C R Soc Biol (Paris) 153:893.

Laemmli UK (1970): Cleavage of structural proteins during the assembly of the head of bacteriophage T4. Nature 227:680.

Macek MB, Shur BD (1988): Protein–carbohydrate complementarity in mammalian gamete recognition. Gamete Res 20:93.

Maresh GA, Dunbar BS (1987): Antigenic comparison of five species of mammalian zonae pellucidae. J Exp Zool 244:299.

Maresh GA, Timmons TM, Dunbar BS (1990): Effects of extracellular matrix on the expression of specific ovarian proteins. Biol Reprod (in press).

Matsudaira P (1987): Sequence from picomole quantities of proteins electroblotted onto polyvinylidine difluoride. J Biol Chem 262:10035.

Mignot MH, Schoemaker J, Kleingeld M, Rao BR, Drexhage HA (1989): Premature ovarian failure. I: The association with autoimmunity. Eur J Gynecol Reprod Biol 30:59.

Nicholson GL, Yanagimachi R, Yanagimachi H (1975): Ultrastructural localization of lectin-binding sites on the zonae pellucidae and plasma membranes of mammalian eggs. J Cell Biol 66:263.

O'Rand MG (1988): Sperm–egg recognition and barriers to interspecies fertilization. Gamete Res 19:315.

Phillips DM, Shalgi RM (1980): Surface properties of the zona pellucida. J Exp Zool 213:1.

Philpott CC, Ringuette MJ, Dean J (1987): Oocyte-specific expression and developmental regulation of ZP3, the sperm receptor of the mouse zona pellucida. Dev Biol 121:568.

Reid LM, Jefferson DM (1984): Cell culture studies using extracts of extracellular matrix to study growth and differentiation in mammalian cells. In Mathur J (ed): Mammalian Cell Culture. New York: Plenum Press, p 239.

Sacco AG, Yurewicz EC, Subramanian MG, deMayo FJ (1981): Zona pellucida composition: Species cross reactivity and contraceptive potential of antiserum to a purified pig zona antigen (PPZA). Biol Reprod 25:997.

Salzmann GS, Greve JM, Roller RJ, Wassarman PM (1983): Biosynthesis of the sperm receptor during oogenesis in the mouse. EMBO J 2:1451.

Sasaki H, Bothner B, Dell A, Fukuda M (1987): Carbohydrate structure of erythropoietin expressed in Chinese hamster ovary cells by a human erythropoietin cDNA. J Biol Chem 262:12059.

Shur BD, Hall NG (1982): A role for mouse sperm surface galactosyltransferase in sperm binding to the egg zona pellucida. J Cell Biol 95:574.

Skinner SM, Mills T, Kirchick HJ, Dunbar BS (1984): Immunization with zona pellucida proteins results in abnormal ovarian follicular differentiation and inhibition of gonadotropin-induced steroid secretion. Endocrinology 115(b):2418.

Timmons TM, Dunbar BS (1988): Antigens of mammalian zona pellucida. In Mathur S, Fredericks CM (eds): Perspectives in Immunoreproduction: Conception and Contraception. New York: Hemisphere Publishing Corporation, p 242.

Timmons TM, Kimura H, Lo C, Dunbar BS (1990a): Characterization of a carbohydrate antigen involved in the structure and function of mammalian zona pellucida glycoproteins. Submitted.

Timmons TM, Kimura H, Washenik K, Ou R, Lo C, Dunbar BS (1990b): Involvement of a carbohydrate antigen in mammalian sperm/ZP interaction. Submitted.

Timmons TM, Maresh GA, Bundman DS, Dunbar BS (1987): Use of specific monoclonal and polyclonal antibodies to define distinct antigens of the porcine zonae pellucidae. Biol Reprod 36:1275.

Wassarman PM (1988): Zona pellucida glycoproteins. Annu Rev Biochem 57:415.

Watanabe M, Muramatsu T, Shirne H, Ugai K (1981): Discrete distribution of binding sites for *Dolichos biflorus* agglutinin (DBA) and for peanut agglutinin (PNA) in mouse organ tissues. J Histochem Cytochem 29:779.

Wolgemuth DJ, Celenza J, Bundman DS, Dunbar BS (1984): Formation of the rabbit zona pellucida and its relationship to ovarian follicular development. Dev Biol 106:1.

Wolgemuth DJ, Gavin BJ (1981): Ultrastructural and biochemical characterization of gene expression in follicular oocytes in neonatal and prepubertal rats. In Byskov AG (ed): Proceedings of the Fifth Workshop on Development and Function of the Reproductive Organs. Amsterdam: Excerpta Medica, p 289.

Yoshima H, Matsumoto A, Mizuochi T, Kawasaki T, Kobata A (1981): Comparative study of the carbohydrate moieties of rat and human plasma alpha(1)-acid glycoproteins. J Biol Chem 256:8476.

Yurewicz EC, Sacco AG, Subramanian MG (1987): Structural characterization of the $Mr =$ 55,000 antigen (ZP3) of porcine oocyte zona pellucida. J Biol Chem 262:564.

DISCUSSION

DR. WAITES: I would like to inquire about the data you presented on the secretion of zona pellucida antigens by the granulosa cells that seemed to demonstrate that there was an increased secretion of follicle-stimulating hormone. Is this true?

DR. DUNBAR: The data were not standardized for total protein content. They were equivalent gels from top to bottom, and we normalized the protein. There is a dramatic increase in the effect on matrices but not on epicytes. As a matter of fact, we have not seen any effect on epicytes. We have been following inhibin in several culture studies. We find that inhibin is not properly glycosylated, depending on which matrix you put it, an indication that the whole glycosylation process occurs on these matrices. At a recent Cell Biology meeting there were a lot of papers showing this. So I think these complex extracellar matrices are going to be very important in signaling for proper glycosylation.

DR. AITKEN: Do the antibodies against the recombinant peptides have any biological activity?

DR. DUNBAR: We are in the process of conducting that experiment.

DR. HECHT: In the one-dimensional gels of deglycosylated proteins that you presented, the bands were quite broad. Have these proteins been subjected to any other treatment?

DR. DUNBAR: We used trifluoromethane sulfonic acid, but even with enzymes it is very difficult to deglycosylate these proteins completely. For example, on two-dimensional gels very little glyco marking is seen, but there is still some residual glycosylation, sufficient to produce heterogeneity. That is not to say that there may not be some other modifications that we have not yet pinpointed.

DR. HERR: You suggested in the conclusion of your discussion that immunization of baboons may have potential in your zona vaccine development program. A few years ago, you were suggesting that total ablation of the oocytes would occur after injection in this species. Has your view on this changed?

DR. DUNBAR: We must keep in mind that we are looking at a very complex system. There are distinct antigens that are formed at different stages of development, and the time at which they occur is different in different species. What we did initially, through the CONRAD program, was to pick epitope-selected antibodies from our early clones. We used these antibodies to stain follicles of different stages, and where we saw staining of a multilayered or very-late stage follicle we knew that those antigens were of most interest. Immunization with these antigens would be unlikely to inhibit the early stages of oocyte maturation.

DR. HERR: Can you identify those antigens that are involved in early ablation?

DR. DUNBAR: We can in the rabbit. But, if you look at the different proteins of different species and try to relate one to the other in the different species, they are not always the same protein. As such, I do not foresee identifying those antigens until we have the sequences of all of these different species-specific proteins and have matched them up. What has really been fascinating is that all of the internal sequences are very distinct except that they have similar properties: For example, they are very hydrophobic and low in protein content. Yet it is conceivable that, when we examine the antigens, we will have to be very careful to identify and select those parts of the molecule that will be in the different species. This is where we are at present. Clearly, it is going to be by determining the sequence in each species, and ultimately in the human, that we will finally be able to pinpoint the immunogenic determinants.

21

Evaluation of Glycosylated and Deglycosylated Porcine Zona Antigens for Contraceptive Efficacy In Vivo and In Vitro

R.J. Aitken, M. Paterson, P. Braude, and
P. Thillai Koothan

The concept of using the zona pellucida as the target for a contraceptive vaccine stems from studies carried out more than 15 years ago by Shivers et al. [1972]. These investigators discovered that an antiserum raised against aqueous extracts of hamster ovarian tissue was able to block the fertilization of hamster ova in vitro. It was subsequently established that the primary source of ovary-specific antigens was the zona pellucida in a variety of species, including laboratory rodents [Sacco and Shivers, 1973; Oikawa and Yanagimachi, 1975], domestic animals [Shivers, 1974], and man [Sacco, 1977]. Antibodies raised against cumulus-free mouse ova [Tsunoda, 1977] and isolated mouse zonae pellucidae [Tsunoda and Chang, 1978; Henderson et al., 1988] were consequently examined for their ability to block fertilization in vitro and were found to be extremely effective [Tsunoda, 1977; Tsunoda and Chang, 1978].

The mechanism by which antizona antibodies inhibit fertilization in vitro appears to involve the occlusion of sperm-receptor sites on the zona pellucida either by a process of steric hindrance [Aitken et al., 1982] or by direct interaction [Sacco et al., 1984]. In our experience, the steric hindrance mechanism appears to predominate, particularly in heterologous systems in which the zona antigens used to

Gamete Interaction: Prospects for Immunocontraception, pages 293–311
© 1990 Wiley-Liss, Inc.

induce antibody formation and the zonae pellucidae being targeted in the in vitro fertilization system are from different species [Henderson et al., 1988]. In such circumstances polyclonal antibodies capable of inhibiting sperm binding to the zona pellucida are characterized by their capacity to induce the formation of an immunoprecipitate on the outer surface of the zona by cross-linking superficially located antigenic determinants. If the cross-linking activity of such antibodies is destroyed by the preparation of univalent (Fab) antibody fragments, then immunoprecipitate formation is prevented and the antibody's capacity to suppress sperm–zona interaction is lost [Aitken et al., 1982]. Similarly, if isolated zona fragments are coated with polyclonal antizona antibodies, there is a unilateral suppression of sperm binding to the outer surface of the zona pellucida, where the immunoprecipitate is located [Aitken and Richardson, 1981].

The presence of unique antigenic determinants on the outermost surface of the zona pellucida appears to be associated with the presence of a high concentration of carbohydrate residues in this location, as indicated by the asymmetrical binding of lectins [Oikawa et al., 1973, 1975]. The presence of a carbohydrate-rich zone on the external zona surface is related to the fact that the sperm-receptor sites are composed of carbohydrate and, specifically, can be localized to the O-linked oligosaccharide side chains of one of the major zona glycoproteins [Florman and Wassarman, 1985; Florman et al., 1984]. Chemical removal of these oligosaccharides completely destroys the ability of the mouse zona glycoprotein ZP3 to serve as a sperm receptor, while the free carbohydrate side chains exhibit sperm "receptor" activity, at the nanogram level, in competition assays [Wassarman, 1988].

The fact that antibodies directed against this superficially located domain will suppress sperm–zona interaction by steric hindrance in heterologous systems is of central importance to our strategy for developing a contraceptive vaccine because this is the mechanism by which antibodies directed against the porcine zona pellucida disrupt the fertilization of human ova in vitro [Trounson et al., 1980]. The contraceptive potential of vaccines based on cross-reactive porcine zona antigens has been further supported by active immunization experiments involving a number of different primate species [Sacco et al., 1983; Gulyas et al., 1983; Henderson et al., 1988].

Of key importance to the further development of an antizona vaccine is elucidation of the role played by carbohydrate residues in defining those porcine zona epitopes with potential as contraceptive immunogens. Data have already been obtained indicating that chemical deglycosylation of porcine ZP3 leads to changes in the antigenic properties of this glycoprotein complex that may have a bearing on its ability to induce the formation of antibodies capable of disrupting sperm–zona interaction in the human [Sacco et al., 1986]. Full evaluation of the biological potency of such deglycosylated porcine zona peptides is of direct relevance to contraceptive vaccine development, because it will indicate the potential value of engineered vaccines based on synthetic or recombinant peptide molecules. Because the sperm binding sites on the human zona pellucida are both highly specific [Bedford, 1977] and, in all probability, resident in the carbohydrate side chains of the zona glycoproteins, our hope would be that cross-reactive peptide-encoded antigens could be identified that exhibit sufficient abundance and spatial proximity to the human sperm-binding sites for antibodies against them to occlude the latter by steric hindrance [Henderson et al., 1987b]. Alternatively, less superficially orientated, peptide-encoded determinants may be of value if they can induce the formation of antibodies, which, by their cross-linking activity, could render the zona pellucida impenetrable by spermatozoa [East et al., 1985]. In the studies reported in this chapter, we have addressed this area of research by investigating the contraceptive efficacy of deglycosylated porcine zona peptides in vivo and in vitro.

PREPARATION OF DEGLYCOSYLATED ANTIGENS

The porcine zona pellucida is known to contain three major glycoprotein families that we have identified as ZP1, ZP2, and ZP3 in order of decreasing average molecular mass [Henderson et al., 1987b], in keeping with the nomenclature of Sacco et al. [1981]. These glycoproteins and their isomers span the molecular mass range from approximately 20,000 to 125,000 and exhibit isoelectric points of pH 4–8.5. The marked microheterogeneity that is exhibited by these glycoprotein chains appears to be associated with the differential glycosylation of the peptide cores [Hedrick and Wardrip, 1981] and has made the purification of the constituent glycoproteins extremely difficult.

To remove this heterogeneity, chemical deglycosylation has been carried out using the trifluoromethane sulfonic acid (TFMS) and anisole method of Karp et al. [1982]. The porcine zona glycoproteins were found to be rich in carbohydrate residues, particularly N-acetylglucosamine, which made up 59% of the total carbohydrate pool. Removal of the carbohydrate side chains with TFMS generated five backbone peptides with relative molecular masses of approximately

66, 52, 36, 32, and 16 kd with the bands at 32 and 36 kd, representing the core peptides of ZP3, predominating [Henderson et al., 1987b]. Related studies by Sacco et al. [1986] also resolved two core peptides in the backbone of ZP3 with similar relative molecular masses of 38 and 35 kd. Both these authors and ourselves [Henderson et al., 1987b] observed a slight reduction in relative molecular mass when this peptide doublet was resolved under nonreducing conditions. Reduction of the deglycosylated zona peptides was also necessary to observe the 16 kd component, the appearance of which is associated with a diminution in the intensity of the 32 kd band. These results have led us to speculate that under nonreducing conditions the 32 kd band is composed of two entities, one a 32 kd monomer and the other a dimer formed of two 16 kd monomers.

Two-dimensional electrophoresis of the deglycosylated zona peptides revealed some residual charge heterogeneity on the part of the 32 kd component. The reason for this heterogeneity is not known; it does not appear to be due to the presence of residual N-acetylglucosamine N-linked to asparagine, but may reflect chemical derivatization of the polypeptide chain by sulfation, phosphorylation, or carbamylation.

This residual heterogeneity has not, however, prevented the purification of the four major zona core peptides to homogeneity on one-dimensional polyacrylamide gels with electroelution procedures [Henderson et al., 1987a]. These purified, deglycosylated zona peptides have been used to raise polyclonal antibodies that have, in turn, been assessed for their ability to interfere with sperm–zona interaction in vitro and in vivo.

ANTIBODY INDUCTION

Injection of unfractionated deglycosylated zona peptides into rabbits resulted in the formation of antibodies that bound ^{125}I-labeled ZP tracer and adhered to human or porcine zonae pellucidae, resulting in immunoprecipitate formation at the zona surface and the disruption of sperm–zona binding [Sacco et al., 1986; Henderson et al., 1987b]. Immunoblots with polyclonal antisera raised against the deglycosylated zona peptides indicated that the antibodies generated could interact with the three major glycoprotein chains and all of the core peptides [Henderson et al., 1987a]. In contrast, when antisera raised against heat-solubilized, glycosylated zonae pellucidae, in either rabbits or marmosets, was examined in immunoblotting experiments for cross-reactivity against the resolved deglycosylated core peptides, strong reactions were noted with the 66, 52, and 36 kd components, but labeling of the 32 and 16 kd molecules was either weak or absent [Henderson et al., 1987b].

Polyclonal antibodies raised against the individual, purified, deglycosylated peptides were found to exhibit strong cross-reactivity with both the deglycosylated and the native glycoprotein chains, indicating the presence of many shared epitopes between the various zona constituents [Henderson et al., 1987a; Dunbar et al., 1989].

Immunofluorescence studies demonstrated that antibodies against the 32 and 66 kd peptides bound predominantly to the outer surface of the zona pellucida, leading to immunoprecipitate formation similar to that previously observed with antibodies raised against unfractionated, intact, and deglycosylated zona antigens. In contrast, the antisera raised against the 52 and 36 kd deglycosylated peptides bound throughout the depth of the zona with no tendency to concentrate on the outer surface.

Assessment of these antisera against the zona core peptides for their ability to disrupt sperm–zona interaction in the human indicated that, although they all possessed some disruptive activity, the most profound inhibition was observed with the anti-32 kd preparations that suppressed sperm binding by around 95%. This suppressive activity was in keeping with the capacity of the anti-32 kd antibodies to bind to antigenic determinants on the zona surface and induce the formation of an immunoprecipitate. Although anti-66 kd antibodies also showed a tendency to localize at the zona surface, they were without significant biological activity presumably because of an inadequate spatial proximity between the cross-reactive antigenic determinants on the human zona pellucida and the sperm-binding sites.

INFLUENCE OF GLYCOSYLATION ON CONTRACEPTIVE ACTIVITY IN VIVO

In view of the apparent ability of the deglycosylated 32 kd zona peptide (DGZP 32) to induce the formation of antibodies with biological activity in a human sperm-binding assay, it was considered relevant to assess the contraceptive potential of this peptide in an active immunization study using a primate model, the common marmoset. In the first series of experiments animals were vaccinated according to the immunization schedule laid out in Table 1. The three control animals, receiving adjuvant alone, showed no adverse reaction to the treatment, and all conceived after the introduction of fertile males, giving birth at 149, 164, and 160 days, respectively, from the day when the mating studies were commenced (Fig. 1).

TABLE 1. Immunization Schedule for Marmosets in Group 1[a]

Injection	Time	Treatment	Control
Primary	Day 0	100 μg DGZP-32 250 μg MDP 1 Part alum 2 Parts peanut oil	As treatment, but replacing DGZP with saline
First booster	2 Months	100 μg DGZP-32 250 μg MDP 1 Part alum 2 Parts NUFA	As treatment, but replacing DGZP with saline
Second booster	5 Months	100 μg DGZP-32 1 Part alum 2 Parts NUFA	As treatment, but replacing DGZP with saline
Mating	6 Months		

[a]DGZP, deglycosylated zona peptide; NUFA, nonulcerative Freund's adjuvant. MDP, muramyl dipeptide.

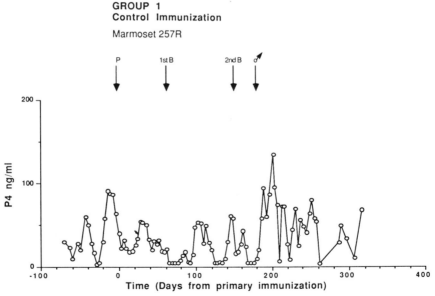

GROUP 1
Control Immunization
Marmoset 257R

Fig. 1.   Plasma progesterone profiles of a control marmoset injected according to the schedule given in Table 1. B, booster; P, primary.

Three of the four immunized animals developed a poor antibody response, which stabilized at a titer of less than 1:320 at the point when the males were introduced. All of these animals rapidly conceived and ultimately gave birth 172, 177, and 208 days from the

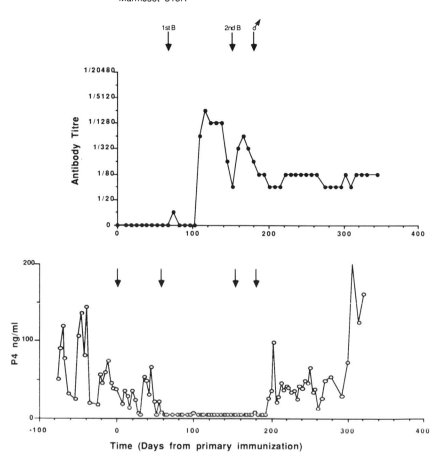

Fig. 2.　Antibody titer and plasma progesterone values for an animal immunized with the 32 kd deglycosylated porcine peptide. Note the disruption of normal ovarian cyclicity following the induction of immunity and the subsequent onset of pregnancy. B, booster.

commencement of the mating trials. In all three of these animals the induction of immunity was associated with a reversible disruption of normal ovarian cyclicity (Fig. 2).

The poor immunogenicity of the 32 kd peptide observed in these studies might have been anticipated from our earlier work with polyclonal antisera against the wild-type peptides. The disruption of ovarian cyclicity was less expected, however, and appeared to be temporally related to the induction of immunity. Although studies in other species, notably the rabbit, have suggested that induction of immunity against the zona pellucida may be associated with the disruption of normal follicular development [Skinner et al., 1984], we have not previously observed such disruption when marmosets were actively immunized with glycosylated porcine zona antigens, absorbed onto alum [Henderson et al., 1988]. It is difficult to attribute this disruption of cyclicity to an adjuvant effect, as has been observed in other studies [Sacco et al., 1987], because no disruption of ovarian function was observed in the adjuvant-only controls. It is also diffi-cult to ascribe this side effect directly to the presence of antizona antibodies, because the fourth immunized animal in this group de-veloped the highest antibody titers of all and yet exhibited no dis-turbance of ovarian cyclicity. Instead, this animal has experienced an uninterrupted series of normal ovarian cycles for more than 12 months since the beginning of the immunization schedule and throughout this period has remained infertile. This particular mar-moset has recently been boosted in order to assess the long-term consequences of inducing immunity against the 32 kd peptide (Fig. 3).

In an attempt to improve antibody titers, a second group of seven animals (four treated, three controls) were immunized according to the modified protocol given in Table 2, in which nonulcerative Freund's adjuvant (NUFA) and bacillus Calmette-Guérin (BCG) were used to enhance the immune response to the 32 kd peptide and an additional month was interposed between the first and second in-jections. The three control animals again showed no disruption of ovarian function following the administration of adjuvant alone, and they all rapidly conceived following the introduction of a male. One of the immunized animals, in which the antibody titer plateaued at 1:640, also conceived and gave birth to a singleton 169 days after commencement of the mating trials. The remaining three immunized animals in this group have remained infertile for 7 months, in asso-ciation with antibody titers that have been sustained at around 1:1,280. All three of these animals have now received booster injec-tions to prolong their infertility. Measurement of plasma pro-gesterone levels in these animals has again revealed sporadic, minor disruptions of the normal ovulatory pattern, which appeared to co-incide with the administration of antigen, but rapidly reverted to normal (Fig. 4).

To compare the responses, side effects, and contraceptive efficacy achieved by administration of the deglycosylated 32 kd porcine zona antigen with the results obtained with fully glycosylated ZP3, we

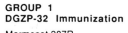

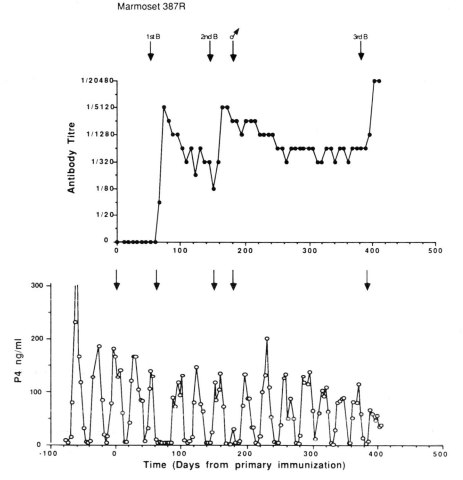

Fig. 3. Antibody titer and plasma progesterone values for an animal immunized with the 32 kd deglycosylated porcine zona peptide. Note normal ovarian cyclicity despite the presence of antibody titers of sufficient intensity to induce long-term infertility. B, booster.

have purified the latter and immunized a cohort of five additional marmosets. Two of these animals were immunized with the adjuvant mixture [6-0-stearoyl-muramyl dipeptide (MDP), alum, and peanut oil] used for the primary injection in group 1 (Table 1), with 100 μg ZP3 replacing DGZP 32, while the remaining three received the same amount of ZP3 in the BCG, NUFA used for group 2. Re-

TABLE 2. Immunization Schedule for Marmosets in Group 2[a]

Injection	Time	Treatment	Control
Primary	Day 0	100 μg DGZP-32 20 μl BCG 1 Part alum 2 Parts NUFA	As treatment, but replacing DGZP with saline
First booster	3 Months	100 μg DGZP-32 1 Part alum 2 Parts NUFA	As treatment, but replacing DGZP with saline
Second booster	6 Months	100 μg DGZP-32 1 Part alum 2 Parts NUFA	As treatment, but replacing DGZP with saline

[a]DGZP, deglycosylated zona peptide; BCG, bacillus Calmette-Guérin; NUFA, nonulcerative Freund's adjuvant.

gardless of the adjuvant composition, a difference between the ZP3 and DGZP 32–treated animals was immediately apparent, with the primary injection of glycosylated antigen inducing an immediate antibody response (Figs. 5, 6) that has remained elevated for 200 days without the necessity for booster injections. The titers recorded in those animals given a primary injection of ZP3 with BCG and NUFA plateaued at 1:20,480, whereas those marmosets receiving ZP3 in MDP and peanut oil stabilized at the significantly lower titer of 1:1,280. In contrast, the primary administration of DGZP 32 was associated with a weak antibody response or no response at all (Figs. 2, 4).

To date only one of the five marmosets immunized against ZP3 has shown any disruption of ovarian cyclicity (Fig. 6) in the form of a period of anovulation that lasted 100 days and then spontaneously reverted to normal. Such disruption of ovarian function has now been observed in a wide variety of primate species following the induction of immunity against a variety of porcine zona antigens, including ZP3. For example, in a recent study of actively immunized baboons [Dunbar et al., 1989] the formation of anti-ZP3 antibodies was associated with decreased levels of plasma estradiol and, in some animals, anovulation. These authors also immunized a cohort of baboons against a deglycosylated 80 kd porcine zona peptide that appears to be equivalent to the 66 kd molecule identified in our own studies. No overt disruption of ovarian cyclicity was observed following the induction of immunity against this peptide, although histological analysis of the ovaries removed from these animals revealed numerous abnormalities, including an apparent increase in the rate of follicular atresia and a paucity of developing follicles. This

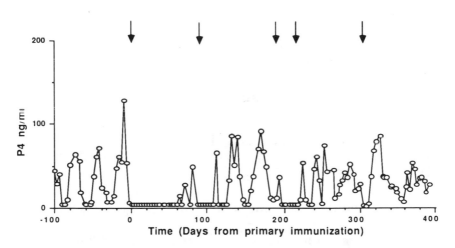

GROUP 2
DGZP-32 Immunization

Marmoset 369R

Fig. 4. Antibody titer and plasma progesterone values for an animal immunized with the 32 kd deglycosylated porcine zona peptide (group 2). Note temporary impairment of normal ovarian cyclicity following the primary and first and second booster injections.

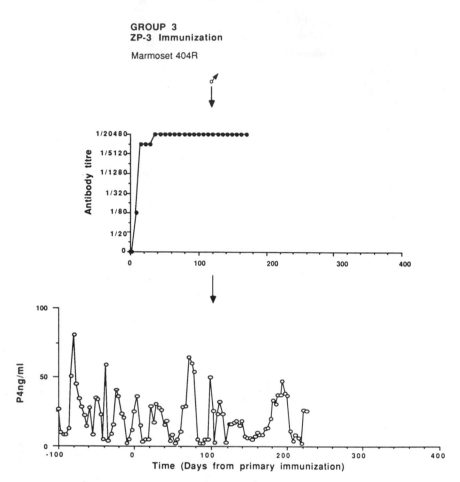

Fig. 5.   Antibody titers and plasma progesterone levels in a marmoset immunized with ZP-3 in a BCG:NUFA adjuvant. Note the rapid rise in antibody titers and the normal patterns of ovarian cyclicity.

study did not, however, include control animals injected with adjuvant alone.

Previous studies [Aitken et al., 1984; Sacco et al., 1987] have suggested that the administration of adjuvants alone, particularly Freund's complete adjuvant, may be capable of disrupting ovarian function. However, we doubt whether the ovarian dysfunction observed in our most recent studies can be attributed to a simple adjuvant effect, because none of the control animals given adjuvant alone exhibited any abnormalities of ovarian function and all conceived rapidly after the introduction of the male. Similarly, it is dif-

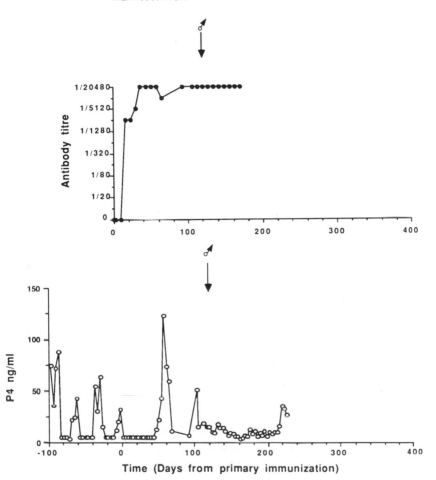

Fig. 6. Antibody titers and progesterone levels in a marmoset immunized against ZP3 using a BCG-NUFA adjuvant mixture. Note temporary disruption of ovarian function after the induction of immunity. (N.B. This animal also exhibited transient acyclicity prior to immunization.)

ficult to ascribe such disruptions directly to the presence of antizona antibodies, because there appears to be no correlation between antibody titer and the occurrence of anovulation. A majority of the ZP3–immunized animals are currently cycling normally despite antibody titers of more than 1:20,000, while the marmosets immunized against DGZP 32 in groups 1 and 2 were exhibiting evidence of abnormal ovarian function in the presence of antibody titers that were either very low or, as in Figure 4, undetectable. The disruptions that we do see tend to be short lived and temporally related to the administration of antigen rather than to the evolution of antizona antibody titers. Sacco et al. [1987] also reported that the disruption of ovarian function in squirrel monkeys immunized against ZP3 was severe only in the short term and that normal cyclicity appeared to have been re-established after 10–15 months.

INFLUENCE OF GLYCOSYLATION ON CONTRACEPTIVE ACTIVITY IN VITRO

To obtain further information on the relative importance of the carbohydrate side chains of the zona glycoproteins in the development of contraceptive immunogens, we compared antibodies directed against DGZP 32 and ZP3 for their ability to disrupt the fertilization of viable human ova in vitro. This project involved the incubation of viable human ova, still within their cumulus masses, for a period of 3 hr with purified polyclonal IgG from rabbits, which had been actively immunized with a variety of porcine zona antigens. After this brief period of exposure to the anti-ZP antibodies, the cumulus masses were washed three times and transferred to a population of human spermatozoa at a concentration of 2–5 × 10^5/ ml. After a further 20 hr incubation period, the ova were stripped of any residual corona cells and assessed for the presence of pronuclei. Each individual experiment included a control incubation incorporating purified IgG from nonimmunized rabbits.

The fertilization rate for the control incubations was 74% (20/27), in contrast to the complete suppression of fertilization observed with antibodies against unfractionated ZP or purified ZP3. Dose–response studies with the anti-ZP3 antibody indicated a progressive increase in contraceptive efficacy as the concentration of antibody in the medium was increased, giving fertilization rates (n) that ranged from 80% (5) to 0% (12) with antibody titers of 1:320 and 1:3,413, respectively. In contrast, antibodies raised against unfractionated deglycosylated porcine zona antigens, including all five major core peptides, could only suppress the fertilization of human ova to a level of 33%, even at a titer of 1:3,413. Similarly, antibodies against DGZP 32 were ineffective in suppressing the fertilization of human ova over a range of antibody concentrations up to a maximum of 1:3,413, at which point the fertilization rate was still 67% (12).

CONCLUSIONS

The results obtained in the in vivo and in vitro experiments described in this chapter clearly emphasize the importance of the carbohydrate side chains of the zona glycoproteins in determining the immunogenicity and contraceptive efficacy of individual epitopes. The differences in immunogenicity were clearly apparent in the active immunization studies in which the administration of a single 100 μg dose of ZP3 was adequate to generate high titers of antizona antibody that have been sustained for more than 200 days. Equivalent primary administrations of the purified 32 kd core peptide from ZP3, in the same adjuvant, generated an antibody response that was either weak or undetectable.

When antibodies against ZP3 and ZPDG 32 were employed at equivalent titers in a human in vitro fertilization system, only the former were found to be effective in completely suppressing sperm–egg interaction. Although antibodies against unfractionated deglycosylated zona peptides or the purified 32 kd component clearly interact with the isolated human zona pellucida, inducing immunoprecipitate formation on the outer zona surface and suppressing the level of sperm–zona binding by 95% [Henderson, et al., 1987a], this activity apparently is still not sufficient to suppress the fertilization of human ova in vitro.

Although this result is of clear interest in terms of contraceptive development, it should be borne in mind that it demonstrates a relative rather than an absolute lack of efficacy on the part of antibodies raised against the zona core peptides compared with their glycosylated counterparts. In vitro, the duration of exposure to antizona antibody is clearly limited compared with the in vivo situation, while the number of spermatozoa used to effect fertilization $(2-5 \times 10^5/\text{ml})$ is unphysiological in relation to the number that the ovum is likely to encounter following natural insemination. Because active immunization with the 32 kd peptide certainly does have a reversible contraceptive effect in vivo, the deglycosylated zona peptides should not be completely overlooked in terms of contraceptive development, particularly if the immunogenicity of the molecule were improved by incorporation of a T-cell helper sequence. Nevertheless, the results obtained in these studies indicate that emphasis should now be placed on elucidating the biochemical composition of the carbohydrate side chains of the zona glycoproteins and determining the way in which these structures define the antigenicity and sperm-binding properties of these molecules.

A second area of research that clearly requires attention is the disruption of ovarian function that occasionally accompanies the induction of immunity against the zona pellucida. This side effect does not, in our most recent experiments at least, appear to be directly related to the use of adjuvants or to the titer of antizona antibodies. The mechanism by which such disruption is manifest is clearly a high priority for research, and the possibility that different mechanisms are responsible for the short-term, reversible effects described by Sacco et al. [1987] and by ourselves and the long-term, irreversible damage to the growing follicle population detected by Skinner et al. [1984] should be considered. With a knowledge of the mechanisms involved, it should be possible to engineer vaccines with which the disturbance of ovarian function is minimized or eliminated and our objective of a prolonged yet reversible suppression of fertility, without adverse side effects, is realized.

ACKNOWLEDGMENTS

These studies were supported by CONRAD and by the Medical Research Council of the United Kingdom. All studies involving human in vitro fertilization were approved by the Voluntary Licensing Authority of the United Kingdom.

REFERENCES

Aitken RJ, Holmes Richardson DW, Hulme MJ (1982): Properties of intact and univalent (Fab) antibodies raised against insolated, solubilized mouse zonae. J Reprod Fertil 66: 327–334.

Aitken RJ, Richardson DW (1981): Mechanism of sperm-binding inhibition by anti-zona antisera. Gamete Res 4:41–47.

Aitken RJ, Richardson DW, Hulme M (1984): Immunological interference with the properties of the zona pellucida. In Crighton DB (ed): Immunological Aspects of Reproduction in Mammals. London: Butterworths, pp 305–326.

Bedford JM (1977): Sperm/egg interaction: The specificity of human spermatozoa. Anat Rec 188:477–488.

Dunbar BS, Lo C, Powell J, Stevens VC (1989): Use of a synthetic peptide adjuvant for the immunization of baboons with denatured and deglycosylated pig zona pellucida glycoproteins. Fertil Steril 52:311–318.

East I, Gulyas BJ, Dean J (1985): Monoclonal antibodies to the murine zona pellucida protein with sperm receptor activity: Effects on fertilization and early development. Devl Biol 109:268–273.

Florman HM, Bechtol CB, Wassarman PM (1984): Enzymatic dissection of the functions of the mouse egg's receptor for sperm. Devl Biol 106:243–255.

Florman HM, Wassarman PM (1985): O-linked oligosaccharides of mouse egg ZP3 account for its sperm receptor activity. Cell 41:313–324.

Gulyas BJ, Gwatkin RBL, Yuan LC (1983): Active immunisation of cynomolgus monkeys (*Macaca fascicularis*) with porcine zonae pellucidae. Gamete Res 4:299–307.

Hedrick JL, Wardrip NJ (1981): Microheterogeneity of zona glycoproteins is due to carbohydrate, abstracted. J Cell Biol 91:77a.

Henderson CJ, Braude P, Aitken RJ (1987a): Polyclonal antibodies to a 32 k Da deglycosylated polypeptide from the porcine zona pellucida will prevent human gamete interaction in vitro. Gamete Res 18:251–265.

Henderson CJ, Hulme MJ, Aitken RJ (1987b): Analysis of the biological properties of antibodies raised against intact and deglycosylated porcine zonae pellucidae. Gamete Res 16:323–341.

Henderson CJ, Hulme MJ, Aitken RJ (1988): Contraceptive potential of antibodies to the zona pellucida. J Reprod Fertil 83:325–343.

Karp DR, Atkinson JP, Shreffler DC (1982): Genetic variation in glycosylation of fourth component of murine complement. J Biol Chem 257:7330–7335.

Oikawa T, Nicolson GL, Yanagimachi R (1975): Trypsin-mediated modification of the zona pellucida glycopeptide structure of hamster eggs. J Reprod Fertil 43:133–136.

Oikawa T, Yanagimachi R (1975): Block of hamster fertilization by anti-ovary antibody. J Reprod Fertil 45:487–494.

Oikawa T, Yanagimachi R, Nicolson GL (1973): Wheat germ agglutinin blocks mammalian fertilization. Nature 241:256–259.

Sacco AG (1977): Antigenicity of the human zona pellucida. Biol Reprod 16:164–173.

Sacco AG, Pierce DL, Subramanian, MG Yurewicz EC, Dukelow WR (1987): Ovaries remain functional in squirrel monkeys (*Saimiri sciureus*) immunized with porcine zona pellucida 55,000 macromolecule. Biol Reprod 36:481–490.

Sacco AG, Shivers CA (1973): Localization of tissue-specific antigens in the rabbit ovary, oviduct and uterus by the fluorescent antibody technique. J Reprod Fertil 32:415–420.

Sacco AG, Subramanian MG, Yurewicz EC (1984): Association of sperm receptor activity with a purified pig zona antigen (PPZA). J Reprod Immunol 6:89–103.

Sacco AG, Subramanian MG, Yurewicz EC, De Mayo FJ, Dukelow WR (1983): Heteroimmunization of squirrel monkeys (*Saimiri sciureus*) with a purified porcine zona antigen (PPZA): Immune response and biologic activity of antiserum. Fertil Steril 29:350–358.

Sacco AG, Yurewicz EC, Subramanian MG, De Mayo FJ (1981): Zona pellucida composition: Species cross-reactivity and contraceptive potential of antiserum to a purified pig zona antigen (PPZA): Biol Reprod 25:997–1008.

Sacco AG, Yurewicz EC, Subramanian MG (1986): Carbohydrates influence the immunogenic and antigenic characteristics of the ZP3 macromolecule (Mr 55,000) of pig zonae pellucidae. J Reprod Fertil 76:575–586.

Shivers CA, Dudkiewicz AB, Franklin LE, Fussel EN (1972): Inhibition of sperm–egg interaction by specific antibody. Science 178:1211–1213.

Skinner SM, Mills T, Kirchick HJ, Dunbar BS (1984): Immunization with zona pellucida proteins results in abnormal ovarian follicular differentiation and inhibition of gonado-trophin induced steroid secretion. Endocrinology 115:2428–2432.

Trounson AO, Shivers CA, McMaster R, Lopata A (1980): Inhibition of sperm binding and fertilization of human ova by antibody to porcine zona pellucida and human sera. Arch Androl 4:29–35.

Tsunoda Y (1977): Inhibitory effect of anti-mouse egg serum on fertilization in vitro and in vivo in the mouse. J Reprod Fertil 50:353–355.

Tsunoda Y, Chang ML (1978): Effect of antisera against eggs and zonae pellucidae on fertilization and development of mouse eggs in vivo and in culture. J Reprod Fertil 54:233–237.

Wassarman PM (1988): The zona pellucida: A coat of many colours. BioEssays 6:161–166.

DISCUSSION

DR. ISOJIMA: What amino acid sequence did you get from that porcine ZP3 protein, and what deglycosylated molecule did you get for porcine ZP4 that is 23 kd? We obtained a 16 kd molecule as the deglycosylated form of ZP4 and analyzed the amino acid sequence of it. We also obtained two monoclonal antibodies against the 16 kd molecule and proved that one of the monoclonal antibodies, 5H4, blocked 70% sperm binding to zona pellucida in human by in vitro fertilization.

DR. AITKEN: We have done end-terminal sequencing of the 32 and 36 kd peptides. The end-terminal sequence from the 36 kd peptide was the same as that published by Dr. Sacco for his larger molecular weight subunit in ZP3. The end terminus of the 32 kd peptide was end-terminal blocked. I believe that Dr. Sacco reported that it was something like 84% or 85% end-terminal blocked. Our approach was to take Sacco's published end-terminal sequence, synthesize the peptide based on that sequence, link it to keyhole limpet hemocya-nin, and make an antibody against it. Then we performed a Western blot and found that the antibody cross-reacted with the 32 kd pep-tide. So, I am certain that our two peptides were the same as the ones that Dr. Sacco reported.

DR. GUPTA: I have a question regarding long-term effects. You have some noncomplementary effects, especially when you immu-nize with nonulcerating adjuvant. You suggest that it may be be-cause of the long-term effect of the immunization. In my opinion, there may be a qualitative change in the antibodies after immunization with alum and MDP or nonulcerating Freund's adjuvant. We have observed that, when you immunize marmoset monkeys with glycosylated ZP3 using alum or MDP, there are no effects on ovulation. This is in spite of the fact that these animals have been immunized for more than 1 year and the antibody titers are high. We have also found that the follicles of the animals that were immunized with complete Freund's adjuvant were degenerated. So, perhaps one has to look at the qualitative change in the antibody that is being produced.

DR. AITKEN: I can sympathize with that. We have carried out many studies using alum as the adjuvant, while repeatedly boosting the animals to maintain antibody titers. With alum, we didn't see any disruption of ovarian function, but I am not yet sure whether this was because we used alum, as you are suggesting, or whether we simply did not carry out those experiments for long enough. Most lasted from 12 to 18 months, and then we stopped boosting. As soon as the alum boosting was withdrawn, the antibody titers declined and the fertility of the animals returned. So you may be right. It may be an adjuvant-dependent effect, or it may be something caused by long-term exposure to those antizona antibodies.

DR. CHIN: Have you examined the extent of the glycosylation for the various zona proteins?

DR. AITKEN: No, we have not done that for the resolved glycoproteins. The whole porcine zona pellucida is about 40% carbohydrate, but we haven't worked out the extent of glycosylation of the individual peptides or glycoproteins. You can still see some nonglycosylated core peptides in two-dimensional Western blots of wild-type glycoprotein, so the core peptides are not entirely glycosylated. It is a very difficult study to do because the degree of glycosylation is changing with the development of the oocytes, and we are collecting hundreds of thousands of zona pellucidae from ovaries with no reference to the stage of development of the follicles. This may account for some of the heterogeneity that we have observed.

DR. CHIN: Does the type of glycosylation actually affect the types of antibodies that are produced, compared with the deglycosylated material? Is the heterogeneity that you have demonstrated caused by the antibodies reacting with different carbohydrate molecules?

DR. AITKEN: We don't see any obvious differences in two-dimensional Western blots. When we compare antibodies against ZP3 with antibodies against some of the core peptides, we see a considerable amount of sharing of epitopes. All three glycoprotein chains seem to be darkly stained.

22

Zona Pellucida: Target for a Contraceptive Vaccine

Jurrien Dean and Sarah E. Millar

The mammalian zona pellucida has been recognized as a candidate target for a contraceptive vaccine since the early 1970s. The zona pellucida is unique to the ovary, where it forms an extracellular matrix surrounding growing oocytes. It is highly immunogenic, and it is known that passive administration of antizona pellucida antibodies results in long-term, reversible contraception. However, active vaccination with heterologous purified zona pellucida components that induce antizona antibodies has resulted in widespread ovarian histopathology and abnormal ovarian function [for review, see Henderson et al., 1988]. Although partially purified zona preparations and the use of Freund's adjuvant may have exacerbated these adverse effects, the data suggest that there are properties intrinsic to the zona proteins that evoke a cytotoxic response in ovarian tissue.

Most vaccines are developed to protect against an exogenous infectious agent. Thus their design maximizes humoral (antibody or B-cell response) and cellular (T-cell response) reactions. The latter provides T-cell helper function (to maximize the antibody response) as well as T-cell-mediated cytotoxicity. The design of a zona pellucida–based contraceptive vaccine, however, requires the elicitation of antizona pellucida antibodies that result in effective contraception without ovarian cytotoxicity. Thus it may be important to separate the B-cell response that must be directed against the zona protein and the T-cell response that may cause cytotoxicity in ovarian tissue. We have investigated a contraceptive strategy based on vaccination with a zona pellucida peptide containing a B-cell epitope coupled to a carrier protein that provides T-cell epitopes to maximize the im-

Gamete Interaction: Prospects for Immunocontraception, pages 313–326

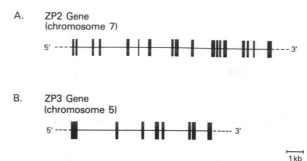

Fig. 1. Mouse zona pellucida genes. Each mouse gene is found in single copy in the mouse genome. **A:** ZP2 contains 18 exons (45–190 bp) in a transcription unit of 12.1 kbp linked to the Tyr locus on chromsome 7. **B:** ZP3 contains eight exons (92–338 bp) in a transcription unit of 8.6 kbp linked to the Gus locus on chromosome 5.

mune response [Millar et al., 1989]. Because the genes that code for zona pellucida proteins are conserved among mammals [Ringuette et al., 1986], this strategy, which involves the vaccination with self zona pellucida peptides, may be applicable to other mammalian species.

MOLECULAR BIOLOGY OF THE MOUSE ZONA PELLUCIDA

The mouse ovary contains thousands of resting oocytes (average diameter of 15 μm) that have entered into the prophase of the first meiotic division. Throughout the reproductive life of the animal, cohorts of these oocytes are recruited into a 2 week growth phase that is followed by proliferation of surrounding granulosa cells to form mature follicles. Subsequently, oocytes undergo meiotic maturation and are ovulated in preparation for fertilization in the oviduct [Bachvarova, 1985].

The zona pellucida is synthesized by oocytes during their growth phase and is secreted to form an extracellular matrix that surrounds the oocyte, the ovulated egg, and the preimplantation embryo. The zona pellucida mediates species-specific events at fertilization, provides a major block to polyspermy, and protects the growing embryo as it passes down the oviduct prior to implantation [Yanagimachi, 1988; Wassarman, 1988]. The mouse zona pellucida is composed of three sulfated glycoproteins designated ZP1, ZP2, and ZP3 [Bleil and Wassarman, 1980a; Shimizu et al., 1983], and specific biological functions have been attributed to each [Wassarman, 1988].

Recently, the single-copy genes that code for mouse ZP2 and ZP3 have been isolated (Fig. 1). Gene ZP2 is located 11.3 cM distal to the

Tyr locus on chromosome 7, where its 18 exons (45–190 bp) encompass a 12.1 kbp transcription unit. Gene ZP3 contains eight exons (92–338 bp) in an 8.6 kbp transcription unit located 9.2 cM distal to the Gus locus on chromosome 5 [Kinloch et al., 1988; Chamberlin and Dean, 1989; Liang et al., 1990; Lunsford et al., 1990]. The zona genes are conserved among eutherian mammals, all of which have a zona pellucida, but they are not detected by Southern hybridization in lower eukaryotic species with the exception of chickens [Ringuette et al., 1986, 1988].

The mouse ZP2 and ZP3 genes are transcribed uniquely in oocytes. Although not detectable in resting oocytes, the ZP2 and ZP3 transcripts accumulate rapidly in growing oocytes and represent 1% and 0.4%, respectively, of poly(A$^+$) RNA in 50 μm diameter oocytes. There are no detectable zona transcripts in the surrounding granulosa cells [Philpott et al., 1987; Liang et al., 1990]. During meiotic maturation and subsequent ovulation, both zona transcripts appear to be deadenylated and degraded to less than 5% of their peak levels [Liang et al., 1990]. Zona pellucida protein synthesis closely follows the abundance of zona transcripts during oogenesis, and there is no detectable zona protein synthesis in ovulated eggs [Bleil and Wassarman, 1980b; Shimizu et al., 1983]. The zona pellucida proteins secreted during oogenesis form a stable extracellular matrix [Shimizu et al., 1983] that persists and is biologically active during preimplantation development.

The nucleic acid sequences of full-length ZP2 and ZP3 cDNAs have been used to deduce the structure of the zona pellucida gene transcripts and their protein products (Fig. 2). The 2,201 nucleotide (nt) ZP2 mRNA includes very short, untranslated regions of 30 and 32 nt at the 5′ and 3′ ends, respectively. It contains a single open reading frame that codes for a polypeptide chain of 713 amino acids, the first 34 of which represent a signal peptide that directs the secretion of this extracellular matrix protein. The secreted ZP2 protein has a predicted core molecular weight of 80,217 daltons and contains seven potential N-linked glycosylation sites (Asn-X-Ser/Thr) and 108 serines and threonines that represent potential O-linked glycosylation sites [Liang et al., 1990]. The ZP3 mRNA is 1,317 nt long and, like ZP2, has very short 5′ (29 nt) and 3′ (16 nt) untranslated regions. There is a single open reading frame encoding a 424 amino acid protein with a predicted molecular weight of 46,307 daltons. After cleavage of a 22 amino acid signal peptide, the secreted ZP3 protein has six potential N-linked glycosylation sites, 72 potential O-linked glycosylation sites, and a core molecular weight of 43,943 daltons [Ringuette et al., 1988]. Following post-translational modifications,

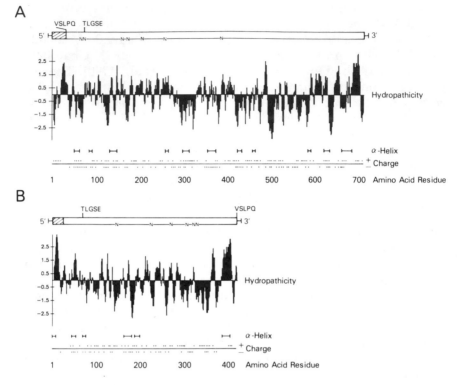

Fig. 2.   Mouse zona pellucida mRNAs and proteins. The sequences of ZP2 and ZP3 are novel and unrelated one to another (except for 2 five amino acid identities indicated by the single amino acid code). Each protein has an N-terminal signal peptide (▨). **A:** ZP2 mRNA is 2.2 kb (minus its polyA tail) with a single open reading frame encoding 713 amino acids and contains seven potential N-linked glycosylation sites (N) and 117 threonines/serines that are potential O-linked glycosylation sites. **B:** ZP3 mRNA is 1.3 kb (minus its polyA tail) with a single open reading frame encoding 424 amino acids and contains six potential N-linked glycosylation sites (N) and 74 threonines/serines. Hydropathicity [Kyte and Doolittle, 1982], α-helical content [Garnier et al., 1978], and charge distribution of each protein is plotted beneath the corresponding open reading frame.

the mature, extracellular ZP2 and ZP3 sulfated glycoproteins have masses of 120,000–140,000 and 83,000 daltons, respectively [Bleil and Wassarman, 1980a; Shimizu et al., 1983]. The two zona pellucida transcripts and resultant proteins are unrelated to sequences present in the Genetic Sequence Data Bank and the National Biomedical Research Foundation Protein Data Bank, and, when compared with one another, there is nothing to suggest a common genetic ancestry. However, the proteins share 2 five amino acid identities (VSLPQ and TLGSE, Fig. 2), and both contain a very hydrophobic region near their carboxyl termini [Liang et al., 1990; Ringuette et al., 1988]. These motifs may play a role in directing the secretion of the zona proteins or in their interactions as they form the supramolecular structure of the zona pellucida matrix.

CONTRACEPTIVE EFFECTS OF ANTIZONA MONOCLONAL ANTIBODIES

Monoclonal antibodies (IgG) specific to ZP2 and ZP3 have been derived from spleen cells isolated from male rats immunized with intact mouse zonae pellucidae [East and Dean, 1984; East et al., 1985]. When administered to female mice, these antibodies localize uniquely to the ovary, where they coat the zonae pellucidae surrounding growing oocytes [East et al., 1984a,b, 1985]. The antibody binding persists after ovulation, and the presence of either anti-ZP2 or anti-ZP3 antibodies precludes fertilization in vitro and in vivo. Contraception lasts for more than 14 estrous cycles after the administration of 250 μg of antizona pellucida monoclonal antibody. Fertility resumes as the antizona antibody titers decline to levels at which they no longer bind effectively to intraovarian zonae pellucidae. Subsequently, when resting oocytes are recruited into the growth phase and form a zona pellucida, no antibodies bind to their zonae. When ovulated, these eggs can be fertilized and develop normally. The antizona pellucida monoclonal antibodies cause neither ovarian histopathology nor abnormal oocyte growth in the immunized females and, if administered after fertilization, have no adverse effect on normal development. These antimouse zona pellucida antibodies do not cross-react with mammalian zonae from species other than rodents [East et al., 1984a, 1985]. The recent cloning of the zona genes has allowed the characterization of the primary structure of the zona pellucida proteins. These data have suggested alternative contraceptive strategies based on active immunization with zona proteins or peptides.

VACCINATION WITH A ZONA PELLUCIDA PEPTIDE

Because of the adverse effects associated with immunization with purified zona proteins that include both B- and T-cell epitopes [Henderson et al., 1988], we devised a vaccination strategy based on immunization with zona pellucida peptides that contain B-cell epitopes. Rather than employ predictive algorithms [e.g., Hopp and Woods, 1981] or strategies involving the synthesis of multiple peptides [Geysen et al., 1984; Houghten, 1985], we have made use of the specificity of one of the aforementioned monoclonal antibodies to define a B-cell epitope on mouse ZP3. The ZP3 cDNA was randomly fragmented and cloned into the λgt11 expression vector, and the resultant epitope library [Mehra et al., 1986] was screened with a monoclonal specific to ZP3 [East et al., 1985]. Eight clones were isolated that expressed ZP3 peptide–β-galactosidase fusion proteins recognized by the anti-ZP3 monoclonal antibody. The nucleic acid sequence of the ZP3 cDNA inserts (Fig. 3A) contained a common 24 nucleic acid sequence encoding seven amino acids (Fig. 3B). This small peptide sequence must contain the ZP3 B-cell epitope recognized by the anti-ZP3 monoclonal antibody [Millar et al., 1989]. The epitope lies adjacent to the most hydrophilic portion of ZP3 and partially overlaps a sequence predicted to form an amphipathic α-helix (Fig. 3C), a structure associated with some T-cell epitopes [Margalit et al., 1987; Rothbard and Taylor, 1988].

A 16 amino acid peptide (NH$_2$-Cys Ser Asn Ser Ser Ser Ser Gln *Phe Gln Ile His Gly Pro Arg* Gln-COOH) from ZP3 containing the seven amino acid B-cell epitope (italicized) was coupled to keyhole limpet hemocyanin (KLH) and used with Freund's adjuvant to vaccinate 16 female mice at intervals of 10–16 days. A plateau level of antizona pellucida antibodies was obtained after three immunizations (Fig. 4) despite additional immunizations over a period of 3 months. The antisera cross-reacted with ZP3 on Western blots and reacted with native zonae pellucidae in frozen ovarian sections. Mice immunized with KLH alone in Freund's adjuvant had no detectable antizona pellucida antibodies [Millar et al., 1989].

After the 3 month immunization period, 12 of the experimental animals (vaccinated with the ZP3 peptide–KLH conjugate) were mated with fertile males (Fig. 5). Three experimental animals (group 1) gave birth to litters within 1 month (as did all of the control KLH-immunized animals) and had, as a group, the lowest average initial antizona pellucida antibody titer (Fig. 5, insert). Nine (75%) experimental animals were infertile for 4 to 10 months. Three of these animals (group 2) gave birth to litters after 4 to 6 months and initially had an intermediate average titer that dropped significantly at the time of delivery. The remaining six animals (group 3) were infertile for the entire 10 months and had the highest average initial titer of antizona pellucida antibodies (Fig. 5). Thus there appears to be an association with the concentration of antizona antibodies and the ability to induce and reverse anti-ZP3–associated contraception [Millar et al., 1989].

This zona pellucida–based vaccine did not appear to affect long-term reproductive function adversely. Four immunized (but not

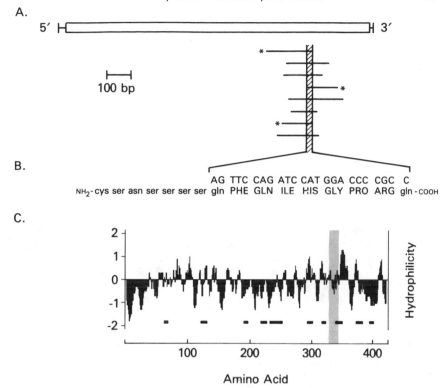

Fig. 3. Zona pellucida peptide vaccine. **A:** Eight recombinant λgt11 clones were isolated from a ZP3 epitope library based on the expression of a β-galactosidase/ZP3 fusion protein recognized by an anti-ZP3 monoclonal antibody. The ZP3 cDNA inserts from these clones are aligned on the ZP3 mRNA, and the hatched bar indicates the sequences in common. Three clones (asterisks) define the 5′ and 3′ ends of the epitope. **B:** The DNA sequence of the overlapping region among the eight positive clones and the corresponding amino acid sequence are shown in capital letters. The longer, 16 amino acid peptide was used for immunization. **C:** Hydrophilicity [Hopp and Woods, 1981] of the ZP3 protein. Horizontal filled-in bars beneath the hydrophilicity plot indicate amphipathic α-helical segments [Margalit et al., 1987]. The speckled vertical bar represents the 16 amino acid peptide shown in B that was used to immunize experimental animals. (Reproduced from Millar et al., 1989, with permission of the publisher.)

mated) females had normal ovarian histology, and, as noted above, the contraceptive effect was reversible, at least in some of the animals. Thus the design of a zona pellucida contraceptive containing B-cell, but not T-cell, zona pellucida epitopes may be able to circumvent previously reported ovarian histopathology and reproductive abnormalities that occurred after immunization with zona proteins. The average litter sizes of both the control, KLH-only immunized

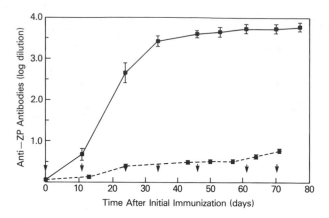

Fig. 4.   Peptide vaccinated mice produce antizona antibodies. Sixteen animals were immunized with 100 µg of ZP3 peptide–keyhole limpet hemocyanin (KLH) conjugate (squares) or KLH alone (circles) using Freund's adjuvant. Antibody titers for each animal were measured by ELISA, and the mean value for the log of the dilution for each time point was calculated (bars represent the standard error). The days on which booster injections were administered are indicated by arrows. (Reproduced from Millar et al., 1989, with permission of the publisher.)

animals (five pups), and the ZP3 peptide–KLH animals that reversed (three pups) were lower than nonimmunized animals (10 pups). The decreases in litter sizes of the experimental animals may be due to the effect of intraperitoneal administration of Freund's adjuvant on fecundity as well as the persistent low levels of antizona antibodies that were observed even in those animals in which the contraceptive effect was reversed [Millar et al., 1989].

CONCLUSIONS

The success of immunization with a zona pellucida peptide from the same species depends on the production of high concentrations of antizona antibodies despite the fact that the zona peptide is a self-antigen. Our studies indicate that B lymphocytes capable of recognizing ZP3 epitopes have escaped the induction of immune tolerance that occurs early in development and involves the functional inactivation of B cells and the deletion of T cells that recognize self-antigens [Pullen et al., 1989; Nossal, 1988]. Having mounted an immunological response against the ZP3 peptide–KLH conjugate, however, it does not appear that the immune system continues to be stimulated by the endogenous ZP3 protein. The 16 amino acid ZP3 peptide portion of the immunogen contains a B-cell epitope but may not include T-cell epitopes (which are provided by the KLH moiety)

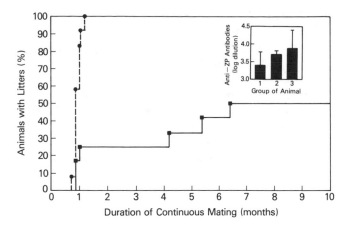

Fig. 5. Long-term contraception in vaccinated mice. Two weeks after the last immunization, experimental (injected with ZP3 peptide–keyhole limpet hemocyanin [KLH]) and control (injected with KLH) female mice were individually and continuously caged with fertile males at a ratio of 1:1. The percentage of females that gave birth to a litter is plotted as a function of the duration of continuous mating for experimental (squares) and control (circles) animals. The inserted bar graph shows the average titers (log dilution) of antibodies to zonae pellucidae at the beginning of the mating period for three groups of experimental mice: group 1, animals (N = 3) that gave birth within 1 month; group 2, animals (N = 3) that gave birth between 4 and 7 months; and group 3, animals (N = 6) that did not give birth to litters during the 10 month study. (Reproduced from Millar et al., 1989, with permission of the publisher.)

that stimulate helper T-cell functions. Thus the endogenous ZP3 protein that contains the same ZP3 peptide but not the T-cell epitopes of the carrier protein cannot itself stimulate the proliferation of helper T cells primed by the ZP3 peptide–KLH conjugate.

This dissociation of zona pellucida B- and T-cell epitopes may also be important for the successful development of a contraceptive vaccine based on the zona pellucida that does not result in abnormal ovarian function. The monoclonal antibody used to define the peptide containing the mouse B-cell epitope does not cross-react with nonrodent mammals [East et al., 1985]. Thus it is not anticipated that this particular vaccine will be useful in other species. However, the zona pellucida genes are conserved among mammals [Ringuette et al., 1986], and the homologous genes can be readily isolated. For example, the human homolog of ZP3 has been identified, and its DNA sequence is more than 80% conserved [Chamberlin and Dean, 1990]. Thus the strategy of developing a contraceptive vaccine by immunizing with a self-zona pellucida peptide can be tested in any mammal from which the zona genes have been isolated.

The application of this contraceptive vaccine approach to other mammalian species remains to be determined. While our studies support the feasibility of a contraceptive vaccine based on a zona pellucida protein, additional studies are needed to optimize the presentation of zona epitopes to the immune systems of mammalian species. Because the immunological response of the host can vary considerably among individuals of a given species [Berzofsky, 1985; Getzoff et al., 1988], we are now exploring the potential of vaccinating animals with a "cocktail" of different B-cell epitopes (self) of zona proteins to obtain 100% infertility in outbred populations of experimental animals.

REFERENCES

Bachvarova R (1985): Gene expression during oogenesis and oocyte development in mammals. In Browder LW (ed): Developmental Biology: A Comprehensive Synthesis, Vol I. New York: Plenum Press, pp 453–425.

Berzofsky JA (1985): Intrinsic and extrinsic factors in protein antigenic structure. Science 229:932–940.

Bleil JD, Wassarman PM (1980a): Structure and function of the zona pellucida: Identification and characterization of the proteins of the mouse oocyte's zona pellucida. Dev Biol 76:185–202.

Bleil JD, Wassarman PM (1980b): Synthesis of zona pellucida proteins by denuded and follicle-enclosed mouse oocytes during culture in vitro. Proc Natl Acad Sci USA 77:1029–1033.

Chamberlin ME, Dean J (1989): Genomic organization of a sex specific gene: The primary sperm receptor of the mouse zona pellucida. Dev Biol 131:207–214.

Chamberlin ME, Dean J (1990): Characterization of a gene unique to mammals: Zona pellucida 3. Proc Natl Acad Sci USA 87:6014–6018.

East IJ, Dean J (1984): Monoclonal antibodies as probes of the distribution of ZP2, the major sulfated glycoprotein of the murine zona pellucida. J Cell Biol 98:795–800.

East IJ, Gulyas B, Dean J (1985): Monoclonal antibodies to the murine zona pellucida protein with sperm receptor activity: Effects on fertilization and early development. Dev Biol 109:268–273.

East IJ, Mattison DR, Dean J (1984a): Monoclonal antibodies to the major protein of the murine zona pellucida: Effects on fertilization and early development. Dev Biol 104:49–56.

East IJ, Keenan AM, Larson SM, Dean J (1984b): Scintigraphy of normal mouse ovaries with monoclonal antibodies to ZP2, the major zona pellucida protein. Science 235:938–941.

Garnier J, Osguthorpe DJ, Robson B (1978): Analysis of the accuracy and implications of simple methods for predicting the secondary structure of globular proteins. J Mol Biol 120:97–120.

Getzoff ED, Tainer JA, Learner RA, Geysen HM (1988): The chemistry and mechanism of antibody binding to protein antigens. Adv Immunol 43:1–98.

Geysen HM, Meloen RH, Barteling SJ (1984): Use of peptide synthesis to probe viral antigens for epitopes to a resolution of a single amino acid. Proc Natl Acad Sci USA 81:3998–4002.

Henderson CJ, Hulme MJ, Aitken RJ (1988): Contraceptive potential of antibodies to the zona pellucida. J Reprod Fertil 83:325–343.

Hopp TP, Woods KR (1981): Prediction of protein antigenic determinants from amino acid sequences. Proc Natl Acad Sci USA 78:3824–3828.

Houghten RA (1985): General method for the rapid solid-phase synthesis of large numbers of peptides: Specificity of antigen-antibody interaction at the level of individual amino acids. Proc Natl Acad Sci USA 82:5131–5135.

Kinloch RA, Roller RJ, Fimiani CM, Wassarman DA, Wassarman PM (1988): Primary structure of the mouse sperm receptor polypeptide determined by genomic cloning. Proc Natl Acad Sci USA 85:6409–6413.

Kyte J, Doolittle RF (1982): A simple method for displaying the hydropathic character of a protein. J Mol Biol 157:105–132.

Liang L-F, Chamow SM, Dean J (1990): Oocyte-specific expression of mouse Zp2: Developmental regulation of the zona pellucida gene family. Mol Cell Biol 10:1507–1515.

Lunsford RD, Jenkins N, Kozak C, Silan C, Liang L-F, Copeland NG, Dean J (1990): Genomic mapping of mouse ZP2 and Zp-3: Two oocyte-specific genes encoding zona pellucida proteins. Genomics 6:184–187.

Margalit H, Spouge JL, Cornette JL, Cease KB, Delisi C, Berzofsky JA (1987): Prediction of immunodominant helper T cell antigenic sites from the primary sequence. J Immunol 138:2213–2229.

Mehra V, Sweetser D, Young RA (1986): Efficient mapping of protein antigenic determinants. Proc Natl Acad Sci USA 83:7013–7017.

Millar SE, Chamow SM, Baur AW, Oliver C, Robey F, Dean J (1989): Vaccination with a synthetic zona pellucida peptide produces long-term contraception in female mice. Science 246:935–938.

Nossal GP (1988): Cellular mechanisms in B lymphocyte activation and tolerance. J Immunol 141(Suppl 7):S21–24.

Philpott CC, Ringuette MJ, Dean J (1987): Oocyte-specific expression and developmental regulation of ZP3, the sperm receptor of the mouse zona pellucida. Dev Biol 121:568–575.

Pullen AM, Kappler JW, Marrack P (1989): Tolerance to self antigens shapes the T-cell repertoire. Immunol Rev 107:125–139.

Ringuette MJ, Chamberlin ME, Baur AW, Sobieski DA, Dean J (1988): Molecular analysis of cDNA coding for ZP3, a sperm binding protein of the mouse zona pellucida. Dev Biol 127:287–295.

Ringuette MJ, Sobieski DA, Chamow SM, Dean J (1986): Oocyte-specific gene expression: Molecular characterization of a cDNA coding for ZP3, the sperm receptor of the mouse zona pellucida. Proc Natl Acad Sci USA 83:4341–4345.

Rothbard JB, Taylor WR (1988): A sequence pattern common to T cell epitopes. EMBO J 7:93–100.

Shimizu S, Tsuji M, Dean J (1983): In vitro biosynthesis of three sulfated glycoproteins of murine zonae pellucidae by oocytes grown in follicle culture. J Biol Chem 258:5858–5863.

Wassarman PM (1988): Zona pellucida glycoproteins. Annu Rev Biochem 57:415–442.

Yanagimachi R (1988): Mammalian fertilization. In Knobil E, Neil J (eds): The Physiology of Reproduction. New York: Raven Press, pp 135–185.

DISCUSSION

DR. DUNBAR: My question concerns your immunization studies. Do you know how you are breaking immune tolerance when this cannot be accomplished in a lot of other animals, such as the rabbit? Even if you extensively immunize rabbits with total rabbit zona, together with adjuvants, it seems impossible to generate an autoimmune response.

DR. DEAN: I think that that is a very interesting question and raises a number of additional points. One is, why are you able to get antizona antibodies to begin with? Another is, why don't you continue to get an immune response in the presence of the endogenous protein? We don't know the answer to these questions. Clearly, our studies indicate that the mouse B cells are capable of being stimulated to make antibodies that bind to the zona. That's true not only in the vaccinia studies but also in our peptide studies. As to why they aren't normally activated, I do not know. You are aware, I am sure, that you can take 3-day-old mice and thymectomize them, and they will make antizona antibodies, among others. So the clone is clearly there. It seems to be a question of activation.

DR. CHIN: This brings up the subject of autoimmune tolerance. If you inject with native zona proteins, do you get an autoimmune response in the mouse?

DR. DEAN: We've never done that. In the early studies by Ralph Gwatkin, hamster zona were used to immunize mice, and antizona antibodies were produced. Yet, when he immunized mice with mouse zona, a very low antibody titer was produced, so he was really not able to analyze whether autoimmunity had been elicited.

We are trying to immunize against an endogenous protein, and it may be important to separate the epitopes that stimulate B cells to make the antibodies from those that may stimulate T cells that might be involved in the ovarian toxicity. If we can separate these two epitopes and use just one of them, it may be possible to generate an effective contraceptive vaccine without toxicity.

DR. CHIN: You mentioned that there was a single ZP1 gene, and yet you localized it to two chromosomes. Could you explain this?

DR. DEAN: When isolated zona are separated on SDS gel, three bands are seen, ZP1, ZP2, and ZP3. If the ZP1 band is isolated and reduced, its molecular weight drops. Thus it is thought to be made up of a dimer. The question that has never really been resolved at the protein level is whether it is a homo- or heterodimer. We have a putative ZP1 clone that localizes to two different chromosomal localizations in the mouse genome. One possible explanation is that ZP1 is a heterodimer and we have found both sites, but this is still speculation.

DR. CHIN: The second question concerns your animal group. Clearly, you don't have enough animals to really have statistical significance in which to analyze, but some of the animals had very high titers. Could you comment on how those animals with high antibody titers were able to conceive?

DR. DEAN: I don't know. We were surprised to see the variation in the antibody titers. I would point out, though, that these studies were designed basically to ask if an antibody response can be generated with a small peptide. I think that we have answered that question. I would also point out that these studies were carried out in an outbred population of mice. Presumably they had different haplotypes, and some would be high responders and some low responders to any given polypeptide. That could account for the variation in antibody titers. However, we cannot yet answer the question of why a relatively high antibody titer did not have a contraceptive effect.

DR. HERR: You showed results of in situ hybridization experiments resolving the issue of whether granulosa cells or oocytes are synthesizing these proteins and showed that ZP3 is coming from the oocyte. Have you carried out similar studies with ZP2?

DR. DEAN: Our observations are that both ZP2 and ZP3 are transcribed only in oocytes.

DR. PRIMAKOFF: What is your explanation for suggesting that the toxicity problems in the ovary are caused by a T-cell response?

DR. DEAN: I didn't mean to suggest that. I think that it is clearly one possibility. It is also possible that a complement-mediated or some other immune response is responsible. However, there is a real possibility that these events are T-cell mediated, and this is why we are trying to design peptides that will have B-cell epitopes but not T-cell epitopes.

DR. PRIMAKOFF: In the group of four or five mice that remained infertile through the duration of the study, did their antibody titers fall below the level at which other immunized mice became fertile? And if so, did they regain fertility?

DR. DEAN: Their antibody titers were definitely falling, but they had not become as low as the mice that regained fertility. The study was terminated because our control animals, after extensive immunizations and mating programs, were becoming infertile. Thus we did not feel that they could be used for valid comparison anymore.

General Discussion

DR. DUNBAR: The first item that I would like to raise during this general discussion of zona pellucida antigens is that long-term studies are very important.

DR. AITKEN: I agree that previously we have not seen any disruption of ovarian function. But as I mentioned before, our experiments were extended for 12 or 18 months, largely because we were using alum as the adjuvant. This required repeated injection of antigen every 6 weeks. When we stopped immunizations, the fertility of the animals returned. We are now using the muramyl dipeptide and peanut oil adjuvants and are obtaining antibody titers that remain elevated for much longer periods of time. Now, after more than 18 months of immunity, we are starting to see some lessening of ovarian function. Thus I agree that this is a very key area. Clearly we are going to have a look at the long-term effects of inducing immunity against zona pellucida glycoproteins.

DR. TALWAR: I would like to hear some discussion on the problem of ovarian damage resulting from immunization against the zona proteins. First, may I inquire about the discrepancy in results in the marmoset monkeys that were immunized in vivo with the deglycosylated ZP-3? They were rendered infertile without any effect on ovulation, and the marmoset antibodies were able to block the attachment of sperm to the zona in your human in vitro fertilization system. However, in your subsequent assays of marmoset fertilization in vitro, the antibodies raised to deglycosylated ZP-3 did not prevent fertilization. How do you interpret this? Could it be that the marmoset is the wrong model to extrapolate to humans? If not, where is the gap in these two observations?

DR. AITKEN: Concerning the difference between the in vitro and in vivo model, I don't think that I could conclude from the in vitro fertilization studies that the deglycosylated peptide has no contraceptive activity. It is just extremely weak relative to the glycosylated peptide. In the active immunization model, the zona pellucida is being exposed to the presence of antizona antibody for the entire duration of folliculogenesis. In the in vitro situation, the egg is exposed to antibody for a very short time, a 3 hour incubation. Second,

Gamete Interaction: Prospects for Immunocontraception, pages 327–331
© 1990 Wiley-Liss, Inc.

the test of fertilization in vitro is much more stringent than the in vivo test simply because of the numbers of spermatozoa used. In a human in vitro fertilization (IVF) attempt, the egg is exposed to something on the order of 200,000 to 500,000 sperm per milliliter. Thus the inhibition of sperm binding has to be, in my view, 100%; otherwise, fertilization will occur. I think the use of the salt-stored zona has been misleading in this respect. We thought we had a complete antifertility effect when we were seeing 95% or so suppression of sperm binding, but in IVF just one sperm bound to the zona seems to be compatible with fertilization. As such, I don't think it can be concluded from the in vitro experiments that antibodies to the deglycosylated peptides are totally without activity. It is just that in relation to those raised to the glycosylated peptides, these antibodies are less able to suppress fertilization.

DR. TALWAR: Is it the titer or quality of antibodies that is more important?

DR. AITKEN: It is not so much the titer. The titers we were employing were the same. I think it is the nature of the target antigen. As I demonstrated in the immunocytochemical studies, when antibody is made against the glycosylated native peptide, most of the antibody targets are to the outermost surface of the zona pellucida. This is the region that is very rich in carbohdyrate and where the sperm-binding sites are located. With antibodies raised against the core peptide, the distribution of binding is much more uniform.

DR. TALWAR: Why does the ovarian damage occur? For instance, most of these antibodies localize on the zona. Although there are some antibodies that cross-react with granulosa cells, the majority of the antibodies that we have seen to date are focused on the zona and not on any other structure in the ovaries. So, why does ovarian damage occur? Is it atresia caused by lack of nutrition to the oocytes and the disappearance of the follicles in the presence of persistently high antibody titers, or is there a cell-mediated immunity component? I think that this is an important issue and would like to elicit some comments from those researchers who are currently working in this area.

DR. AITKEN: Although T-cell infiltration into the ovary occurs under these circumstances, I don't think that what occurs is cell-mediated damage. My guess is that the core peptides, as we have seen with the in situ hybridizations, are made by the oocyte. After that, the proteins are produced, maybe even after they are secreted from the oocyte. Then there are further modifications to the structure of the zona pellucida. A very interesting study by Matt Kauffman concerning this issue was published in a recent edition of *Gamete Research.* He showed that, during folliculogenesis, the carbohydrate structure of the zona pellucida, particularly on the outermost surface, changes. I think this is a result of modifications in the zona structure induced by corona cells or cumulus cells. Perhaps when antibodies are made against the carbohydrate determinants on the outer surface of the zona pellucida, particularly those determinants that are being modified by the corona cells or cumulus cells, some cross-reactivity with these cells is likely, for example, cross-reactivity with galactosyltransferases, which these cells are secreting. But cross-reaction is not inevitable, because, as was shown previously, there are carbohydrate determinant antigens that induce the formation of antibodies that react with the zona pellucida structure only and not with any other neighboring cells. Thus it seems feasible to identify carbohydrate determinant epitopes that will not be associated with ovarian dysfunction, and this is the task that now lies before us.

DR. TALWAR: Is it necessary for antibodies to react with other cells or is the antifertility effect caused solely by antibodies completely encircling the oocyte? Zona formation starts in the primordial follicles; thus a high antibody titer would restrict the growth of oocytes, leading to atresia.

DR. AITKEN: It is possible that the cross-reactivity with the cumulus cells, or with those epitopes that cross-react with the cumulus or corona cells, is necessary to achieve the contraceptive effect. However, I think the data suggest that this is not the case.

DR. TALWAR: What is one to be careful of in order to avoid ovarian damage? Should the epitopes or the determinants be restrictive enough not to have cross-reacting antibodies with other cells in the ovaries? And even if the antibodies are only reacting with the zona, but completely binding to it, would they not lead to damage to the oocytes? For example, if the oocyte is completely sealed off, there will be no nutrition for the oocyte and the follicle to grow. Thus, it may die. Therefore, is it not inherent in the proposition that, if we have a high enough and long enough immune response, there will be atresia of the follicles? Or, can we just target antibody somewhere without restricting the growth of the follicles, and would there then be damage to the ovaries?

DR. AITKEN: In my opinion, ovarian damage is not an inevitable consequence of inducing immunity against the zona pellucida. For example, consider the studies that we carried out some time ago actively immunizing rats with mouse zona pellucida antigens. In those animals, we found that we could induce long-term infertility; sterility, in fact, if we raised the titers high enough. And there was never any sign of disruption of ovarian function in that model.

DR. SEHGAL: I think the sum total effect on the ovary is dependent on the species, the adjuvant, and the type of antigen used. We still have rhesus monkeys that were immunized 3 to 4 years ago with a single dose of whole zona pellucida and complete Freund's adjuvant (CFA). They are totally infertile, and they exhibit ovarian atrophy. In fact, an elevated follicle-stimulating hormone level suggested that there was no negative feedback from the ovary. In rabbit studies, we used, in addition to CFA, alum, glutaraldehyde, and porcine zona. In those studies we were able to intercept pregnancy, but there was a profound effect on ovarian function and ovarian morphology with all three of these adjuvants. The third point I wish to make is that we have used deglycosylated zona proteins, but we have not separated out the peptides in any way. This cocktail of the deglycosylated proteins is able to elicit antibodies in rabbits that will prevent fertilization. Thus a specific peptide may be ineffective, but, if the whole cocktail of the deglycosylated proteins is used, it is quite effective. Also, we have found that the whole zona molecule is not capable of evoking any degree of immune response, but the peptide is able to produce antibodies in the same species. This phenomenon is very interesting and has yet to be explained. The last comment I wish to make is that the zona proteins do not appear to exhibit any T-cell epitopes, as we have observed granuloma formation and no inflammation in rabbits killed at different time intervals after immunization.

DR. DUNBAR: A paper was published recently by Cherrie Mahi-Brown and Yanagimachi. They showed, by electron micrographs, a possible mechanism of action on the early oocyte caused by antibody accumulating between the granulosa cells and the oocyte. We have carried out passive immunization experiments and found that the antibodies will interfere with the oocyte cumulus cell junction. I think that if you interfere with the oocyte and the follicular cells, which are the essential unit of follicular growth, serious problems will arise. This is why we have been looking for a very late-stage, in fact, ultra-late-stage, antigen. Even if this antigen is produced by the granulosa, if the differentiation of follicular cells and their steroidogenic capabilities is already underway, then the severe effects that we see when all the primordial follicles are involved may not occur. The strategy is clear, but it may take a long time and much patience to dissect out the correct antigens.

DR. MITCHISON: Another system in which these questions have been asked concerns autoimmunity to pancreatic islets. There is a model of diabetes that uses trans-genes to obtain a T-cell infiltration into a small organ of this sort. One of the more exciting possibilities raised by Dr. Dean's approach is the potential for introducing into the ovarian follicle something like the gamma-interferon genes, for example, which are known to be effective in generating local autoimmunity in pancreatic islet beta cells by local infiltration. It would be very nice to be able to make an exact comparison between follicles and islets.

DR. ANDRADA: I would like to address the problem that was raised by Dr. Talwar concerning the action of zona pellucida antibodies on the ovaries. I was not surprised that he obtained the results he did when he used CFA, because this will induce an autoimmune disease in many organs. This may suggest a need for controls, for example, immunizations without CFA or with CFA, but without the antigen, to see what would happen.

DR. SEHGAL: If you give CFA alone, nothing happens. If you give whole zona alone, as we have tried in rabbits and monkeys, nothing happens. Peptides can evoke antibody response, but whole zona proteins are not effective.

23

Studies With Clinically Defined Sera From Fertile and Infertile Patients: An Overview

Tage Hjort

About 10 years ago, the Steering Committee of the WHO Task Force on Vaccines for Fertility Regulation began a study on clinically defined sera from fertile and infertile patients. The study was completed about 5 years ago with the publication of a series of papers describing the study and analyzing the results. However, with the results that have appeared more recently in this field, there are new lessons to be learned. This chapter reviews the study and, in addition, offers an opportunity to reassess the philosophy of the project.

The aim of the study was "to investigate the experiments of nature in which naturally occurring immunity to reproductive tract antigens is associated with infertility." In other words, the task was to find certain immune responses consistently associated with infertility and to use the sera from patients with such responses for identification of corresponding antigens, antigens that one could assume would be suitable candidates for birth control vaccine development. Thus strict clinical criteria were set up for several relevant categories of individuals to be tested for antibodies. Primarily males and females from couples with unexplained infertility and various control groups such as fertile males and females, pregnant females, and postpartum females were selected. The WHO Reference Bank for Reproductive Immunology, established at the University of Aarhus, served as a collection point for collaborating centers from around the world. Large serum samples (50–200 ml) together with clinical information

Gamete Interaction: Prospects for Immunocontraception, pages 333–344

from individuals fulfilling the criteria for one of the categories were received. Small coded samples of the sera were distributed to laboratories to test for antibodies to sperm, zona pellucida, trophoblast, and trophoblast products. Fourteen clinical departments in nearly as many countries cooperated in the collection of a total of 329 serum samples, and 20 laboratories tested the sera and returned the results to the Reference Bank for decoding and analysis.

The study was planned at a time when it could be foreseen that the then new hybridoma technique might lead to the recognition of many new reproductive tract antigens, some of which might also turn out to be suitable candidates for vaccines. The justification for a study involving so much time and effort from so many investigators might therefore be questioned. However, using antigens for vaccine development that are natural auto- and isoantigens should, a priori, have certain advantages, because (1) they are known to stimulate immune responses in humans, (2) studies of patients with naturally occurring immunity could provide guidance with regard to antibody levels necessary to achieve efficacy, and (3) the nature and degree of any side effects in humans could be evaluated before immunization experiments were begun. These aspects in themselves might justify the study, but at the same time the simultaneous study of antibodies to a broad spectrum of reproductive tract antigens in well-characterized groups of individuals would provide useful insight into the role of immune responses in infertility.

To make the study meaningful, one condition should be fulfilled: when the immunological reaction leading to infertility does not take place in the blood but in the genital tract, as with reactions with sperm and zona pellucida, the antibodies detected in serum should represent the antibodies in the genital tract in a rather exact way. Several observations during recent years have shown that this may not always be the case (see below).

PROBLEMS ENCOUNTERED

The study did not proceed without problems. Even though information gathered from clinical departments during the planning stage had indicated that the collection of sera should not cause problems, it turned out that the large serum volumes requested (50–200 ml) were considered unacceptable in several countries. Also, the strict criteria led to difficulties in finding donors for some of the categories. In particular, the project suffered because so few fertile males and females were recruited. Not many couples met the criteria (two living children and no abortions, the most recent child conceived within the previous 2 years, desire for conception interval less than 2 years), and such individuals were rarely seen in clinical departments.

Serum samples were kept at −70°C and usually distributed frozen. However, for practical reasons some laboratories received lyophilized samples, and it caused some concern that precipitation occurred during reconstitution of some of these samples. The two kinds of samples were therefore compared [Bronson et al., 1985] by means of the sensitive immunobead-binding test for antisperm antibodies, and no major discrepancies were observed for either IgG or IgA antibodies. Only tail-tip-directed antibodies of the IgM class were found more commonly with frozen than with lyophilized sera. Furthermore, the reactivity in the sperm agglutination and immobilization tests had been checked before distribution from the Reference Bank and found to be the same in both frozen and lyophilized sera.

RESULTS

Antibody Reactivity Against Trophoblast and Trophoblast Products

An ELISA technique was used to test 195 female sera for antibodies to deoxycholate-solubilized syncytiotrophoblast plasma membranes isolated from human term placental villous tissue. Only a few of the sera showed any reactivity. Two samples, one from a woman with unexplained infertility and one from the postpartum group, revealed significantly detectable antibody, and five sera were characterized as weakly positive. All sera also were tested by radioimmunoassays for antibodies reactive with the carboxyterminal peptide of the β-subunit of human chorionic gonadotropin (hCG) and for antibodies to the pregnancy glycoprotein SP1. No positive reactions were recorded. Thus immune reactions to trophoblast that caused infertility were not identified [Johnson et al., 1985].

Antibody Reactivity With Porcine Zona Pellucida

When the study was launched, the existence of true zona-specific antibodies in humans was still questioned, even though several clinical studies on antizona antibodies as a cause of infertility had been published. Nevertheless, this was an attractive field, because cross-reactivity between human and porcine zona had been demonstrated [Sacco, 1977]. Porcine zona material, which can be obtained in large quantities, could be used for detection of antibodies in human sera

TABLE 1. Antizona Pellucida Reactivities Recorded in
Three Different Techniques

Clinical categories	Immuno-fluorescence technique		Passive hemagglu-tination reaction		^{131}I-protein A radio-immuno-binding assay	
	No. positive/ No. tested	Percent positive	No. positive/ No. tested	Percent positive	No. positive/ No. tested	Percent positive
Females						
Unexpl. infertility	6 / 34	18	2 / 83	2.4	3 / 21	14
Prim. amenorrhea	0 / 2		1 / 2	(50)	0 / 1	
Female controls	3[a] / 41	7	2[b] / 92	2.2	0 / 17	0
Males			0 / 130	0	10[c] / 51	20

[a]Two pregnant, one virgin.
[b]One pregnant, one postpartum.
[c]Three unexplained infertility, six vasectomized, one aspermatogenesis.

and might also serve as a suitable candidate for a vaccine. The early studies, using immunofluorescence technique with porcine zona-coated eggs, had revealed a high incidence of positive reactions with sera from infertile females [Shivers and Dunbar, 1977] but also with sera from various control groups, including males [Sacco and Moghissi, 1979]. Obviously, there was a problem with the specificity of the reactions, and it appeared that absorption of sera with pig erythrocytes before testing could remove the antizona activity in most cases [Mori et al., 1978]. Therefore, in the present study it was requested that sera be absorbed with pig erythrocytes before being scored as positive.

Testing for antibodies to zona pellucida was performed in five laboratories, each laboratory using its special technique [Mori et al., 1985]. In one case, only coded female sera were delivered. Two of the laboratories using the same purified porcine zona antigen in a radio-immunoassay and a passive hemagglutination technique, respectively, recorded totally negative results. A likely explanation could be that the autoimmunogenic epitopes were not present in the antigen preparation.

The results of three studies in which zona-reactive antibodies were detected are summarized in Table 1. For simplicity, several of the female categories were included within "female controls," i.e., fertile females, virgins, and pregnant, postpartum, and postmenopausal women. As in previous studies, use of immunofluorescence techniques revealed rather high incidences of positive reactions, even after absorption of the sera with pig erythrocytes. Passive hemagglutination with bovine erythrocytes coated with purified porcine zona material seemed to provide the most specific reaction, with only negative results found with male sera and only a few positive reactions with female sera. The strongest reaction (titer of 32) was recorded with one of the only two serum samples from patients with primary amenorrhea. The protein A radioimmunobinding assay revealed positive reactions only among patients with unexplained infertility and, surprisingly, among infertile and vasectomized males. The purified zona preparation used in this test consisted of five glycoproteins, and it was suggested that one or more of these might cross-react with a component in sperm; indeed, an important aspect that needs further investigation.

Although zona-reactive antibodies were demonstrated in three of the five tests, the results were difficult to evaluate because different sera were recorded positive with the different tests, possibly because of differences in the antigen preparations used. Furthermore, all the reactivities were rather weak, so it was not difficult to choose particular sera that could be used to identify and isolate a special zona antigen for a vaccine candidate.

Antibody Reactivity With Sperm

Antibodies reactive with sperm components are commonly found in human sera. This was clearly demonstrated by immunoblotting technique with an SDS–β-mercaptoethanol–urea extract of washed and dithiothreitol-treated sperm [Lehmann et al., 1985]. When the sera were tested at 1:100 dilution, nearly one-half of the sera, from fertile as well as infertile individuals, showed reactivity with at least one antigenic band (81 of 197 female sera and 55 of 127 male sera). A total of 15 different antigenic determinants with molecular weights (MW) from 13,700 to 150,000 were identified by the sera. Antibodies to a single antigenic determinant with MW of about 14,000 were found significantly more frequently in sera from males with unexplained infertility than in the other categories, but the reactivity was not correlated with the occurrence of sperm antibodies detectable in other tests (e.g., sperm agglutinins).

Therefore, the problem was not to find sperm antibodies, but to identify those associated with infertility. In this context, antibodies to the sperm-specific lactate dehydrogenase LDH-C_4 were of special interest, because, in immunization experiments with mice, rats, and baboons, high levels of anti-LDH-C_4 have been found to interfere

with female fertility and also because LDH-C_4 is the best-character-
ized sperm antigen. The sera were tested for anti-LDH-C_4 in a liquid-
phase radioimmunoassay [Shelton and Goldberg, 1985]. Because antibodies to LDH-C_4 from one species cross-react with LDH-C_4 from
all other species, purified and radiolabeled mouse LDH-C_4 was used.
The normal level in the test system was defined by the sera from
fertile males and females, and levels that were ≥ 2 S.D. above the
mean of the combined fertile groups were designated as "elevated
values." Such values were recorded in 20% of the vasectomized
males, in 11% of females with unexplained infertility, and in 9% of
the infertile males. However, several of these patients showed only
marginally elevated values. A few positive reactions also were recorded in other categories, and, surprisingly, the highest value was
observed with serum from a virgin, a finding for which the clinical
information did not offer any explanation. Anti-LDH-C_4 activity was
not correlated with the results of any of the other antisperm antibody
tests, although some coincidences were seen. In particular, it was
noted that one of the two sera from females with unexplained infertility with a relatively strong reactivity in the conventional antisperm
antibody tests also showed a relatively high level of anti-LDH-C_4.

The fact that the normal level was defined on the basis of relatively
few fertile controls compared with the number of infertile patients,
and the generally weak reactivities recorded, made it difficult to
evaluate the significance of the results. Nevertheless, it can be concluded that the trend of the results was in support of LDH-C_4 as a
candidate for a contraceptive vaccine.

Immune responses to sperm membrane antigens have been
known for quite many years to be associated with infertility. This has
been most convincingly demonstrated for male infertility [Rümke et
al., 1974]. Many laboratories have been working with techniques for
detection of antibodies to sperm membrane antigens, so it was easy
to recruit laboratories for this study. Several laboratories carried out
the common agglutination tests (gelatin agglutination and tray agglutination) and complement-dependent immobilization tests. Fur-
tunately, more recently developed techniques also were included: a
spermocytotoxicity test, passive hemagglutination reaction, indirect
immunobead-binding test, ELISA in various modifications, and a
[125]I-protein A–radioimmunobinding assay. With so many tests the
results can only be briefly summarized.

The results obtained with the various tests (except ELISA) for three
of the male categories are listed in Table 2 [Bronson et al., 1985]. In
spite of two workshops arranged by the WHO Task Force in an
attempt to standardize some of the techniques [Rose et al., 1976;

TABLE 2. Antibody Reactivities in Male Sera by Conventional Techniques and Immunobead-Binding[a]

Technique and laboratory	Fertile		Unexplained Infertility		Vasectomized	
	p/t	Percent positive	p/t	Percent positive	p/t	Percent positive
Gelatin agglutination						
Lab. 4	0/26	0	10/82	12	2/15	13
Tray agglutination						
Lab. 4	0/26	0	7/82	9	4/15	27
Lab. 6	0/20	0	8/71	11	3/15	20
Lab. 11	2/25	8	6/82	7	5/15	33
Lab. 16	0/26	0	2/82	2	3/15	20
Sperm immobilization						
Lab. 4	0/26	0	8/82	10	5/15	33
Lab. 6	0/20	0	0/71	0	3/15	20
Lab. 11	2/25	8	2/82	2	0/15	0
Spermocytotoxicity						
Lab. 10	0/26	0	6/82	7	0/15	0
Passive hemagglutinin						
Lab. 10	2/26	8	2/82	2	0/15	0
Immunobead binding						
Lab. 1: IgG	2/26	8	17/80	21	9/15	60
IgM	0/26	0	3/80	4	1/15	7
IgA	0/26	0	3/80	4	6/15	40

[a]p/t, No. of significant reactions/No. of sera tested.

WHO Reference Bank for Reproductive Immunology, 1977], there were considerable differences in the technical set-ups and sensitivities of basically similar tests. In the various agglutination and spermocytotoxicity tests, only titers ≥ 32 were considered significant, except in one laboratory that used smaller volumes of serum relative to the sperm suspension and, therefore, considered reactions significant even with undiluted serum. Taking these conditions into consideration, the results were quite clear-cut. In the small group of fertile men three of the four laboratories performing sperm agglutination and immobilization tests had negative results. It should be noted that the laboratory recording positive results in fertile men also had some disagreement between results with sera included in the collection as duplicates. In agreement with previous results in the literature, about 10% of the men with unexplained infertility had significant levels of sperm agglutinins. One laboratory, using different optical conditions for recording reactions, apparently detected only head-to-head agglutinins and, therefore, found fewer positive reactions. As expected, higher incidences were found in the vasectomized group even though the sera were obtained rather early after vasectomy (6–12 months). The immunobead-binding test seemed the most sensitive, with somewhat higher incidences for IgG antibodies in all categories. In addition to the general agreement in antibody incidences, these tests also showed mutually good correlation. Thus, with very few exceptions, all sera recorded positive in sperm immobilization (the least sensitive test) were also positive in sperm agglutination, and sera with sperm agglutinins revealed positive immunobead-binding (the most sensitive test).

The results with the spermocytotoxicity test and the passive hemagglutination reaction did not fit into this pattern. These techniques were not correlated with any other technique; nor were they mutually correlated. Thus, to avoid confusion in this area, it should be kept in mind that these techniques [Mathur et al., 1981] must involve other antigen–antibody systems than the "classic" tests.

Previous studies employing the agglutination and immobilization tests on female sera have given divergent results, but in the present study all laboratories recorded only scarce and weak activities. Again, the IgG immunobead-binding test revealed the highest number of positive reactions: 10 of 83 infertile women but also 2 of 21 fertile controls. Otherwise, mainly low titers (4–8) in the tray agglutination test were recorded, often with disagreement between the different laboratories, and positive reactions occurred as frequently in the control groups as in the infertile group. Only two sera from women with unexplained infertility were positive in most of the tests performed and gave stronger reactions than sera from the other categories. Thus immune infertility caused by the presence of antisperm antibodies could seriously be considered in only two patients.

ELISA would, for several reasons, be a convenient and attractive technique for detection of antisperm antibodies. Thus seven laboratories tested eight different ELISA procedures [Mettler et al., 1985]. As antigen in the ELISA test, whole sperm (five techniques), a sperm membrane autolysate, the supernatant after ultracentrifugation of homogenized sperm, or a lithiumdiiodosalicylate extract of sperm was used. Again, the results were difficult to interpret. The agreement between duplicates was generally not as good as in the conventional tests, and, although several of the techniques revealed the highest incidences of positive reactions in the infertile groups (e.g., 7–26% for women), different sera were recorded positive in the different tests. Thus there was no correlation between any of the ELISA tests, and only one technique (the only one that used suspended sperm and F[ab']$_2$ of affinity-isolated antigen-specific antibody) showed fair correlation with the conventional techniques. It should be noted that the ELISA with extract of homogenized sperm detected only seven positive sera, all from patients with unexplained infertility (six females, one male). Also the ^{125}I-protein A–radioimmunobinding assay, using polystyrene beads coated with detergent-solubilized sperm antigen, gave few positive reactions, but 7 of the 10 positive sera were from infertile or vasectomized patients [Czuppon, 1985].

Thus immune responses of a certain magnitude, directed against the sperm membrane antigens involved in sperm agglutination and immobilization, and possibly the responses detected in one of the ELISA techniques, fulfilled the criterion of being consistently associated with infertility. These antigens may, therefore, be considered candidates for a sperm vaccine. However, none of the sera reacting with these antigens were particularly potent; thus they would probably be poor reagents for the isolation and characterization of these antigen(s).

CONCLUSIONS AND REFLECTIONS

With regard to the identification of antigens to be used for vaccine development, the results were disappointing. As the results from the different laboratories became available, the study unavoidably became a comparison of techniques, thereby clearly illustrating the technical problems of this field. The results with sperm were particularly unexpected, and it became evident that the new techniques (e.g., ELISA tests) were not ready for clinical use. In contrast, some of the classic techniques, which are often viewed with skepticism, appeared to be fairly reproducible and clinically most relevant.

In retrospect, one can speculate whether the chosen approach with a single serum sample from a large number of individuals was optimal for identifying candidates for contraceptive vaccine development. A different approach was used when a group of vasovasostomized men were studied in our laboratory over several years [Meinertz et al., 1989]. This was also a clinically well-defined group, as the men had all previously proven their fertility, had been vasectomized, and subsequently after some years had a vasovasostomy. At the time of vasovasostomy sperm agglutinins were determined in serum and seminal plasma, and in the follow-up study the men were asked to answer a questionnaire and deliver a serum and semen sample to be tested for free sperm agglutinins and sperm-bound antibodies by means of the MAR test. For an evaluation of the return of fertility, only those men were included who had answered the questionnaire, delivered serum and semen samples, had motile sperm in the ejaculate, had tried to induce conception, and had an apparently healthy fertile partner. Only the results for some of the more illustrative subgroups are reviewed. Among men with a negative MAR test, the conception rate was 67% (10/15); with IgG on all sperm but no IgA, 85% (11/13) had induced conception; with both IgG and IgA on all sperm, the conception rate dropped to 22% (5/23); and among those in the latter group who had serum titers $\geq$256, none had induced conception (0/10). Only one man with a pure IgG response had a similarly high serum titer; he was fertile. These results underline the importance of IgA antisperm antibodies, as also has been indicated in several previous studies of infertile patients [e.g., Hendry et al., 1982]. Therefore, a sperm vaccine based on sperm membrane antigens would probably not be sufficient if only a certain level of IgG antibodies develop in serum, but the vaccine should also induce the same degree of local immunity as seen in naturally occurring immune infertility.

The vasovasostomy study differs in several ways in its design from the WHO study. Instead of recording the fertility status and immunological findings at a given time in a large number of individuals, most of whom have none of the relevant antibodies, we followed a group known to have a high incidence of antibodies to sperm, and antibodies in the genital tract were included in the study. This offered a better opportunity to distinguish between different degrees of immune response and to compare the fertility of groups characterized by certain immunological parameters (antibody levels in serum and in the genital tract, Ig class of the antibodies, and so forth), thereby providing information essential for the evaluation of an antigen as a candidate for a vaccine.

In planning future studies the experiences from this comprehensive WHO study should be kept in mind. It would seem more productive to concentrate on a single group of antigens so that the number of clinical categories of individuals can be limited, to plan detailed protocols for laboratory tests, to limit the number of participating laboratories, to study antibody levels both in serum and in the genital tract, and to follow the individuals over a longer period of time. Such a study might give final answers to some of the questions we have been facing for many years.

REFERENCES

Bronson R, Cooper G, Hjort T, Ing R, Jones WR, Wang SX, Mathur S, Williamson HO, Rust PF, Fudenberg HH, Mettler L, Czuppon AB, Sudo N (1985): Anti-sperm antibodies, detected by agglutination, immobilization, microcytotoxicity and immunobead-binding assays. J Reprod Immunol 8:279–299.

Czuppon AB (1985): Detection of anti-spermatozoal antibodies by a ^{125}I-protein-A radioimmunobinding assay. J Reprod Immunol 8:313–319.

Hendry WF, Stedronska J, Lake RA (1982): Mixed erythrocyte–spermatozoa antiglobulin reaction (MAR test) for IgA anti-sperm antibodies in subfertile males. Fertil Steril 37: 108–112.

Johnson PM, Cheng HM, Stevens VC, Matangkasombut P (1985): Antibody reactivity against trophoblast and trophoblast products. J Reprod Immunol 8:347–352.

Lehmann D, Temminck B, Da Rugna D, Leibundgut B, Muller H (1985): Blot-immunobinding test for the detection of anti-sperm antibodies. J Reprod Immunol 8:329–336.

Mathur B, Williamson HO, Derrick FC, Madyasta PR, Melchers JT, Holtz L, Baker ER, Smith CL, Fudenberg HH (1981): A new microassay for spermocytotoxic antibody: Comparison with passive hemagglutination assay for antisperm antibodies in couples with unexplained infertility. J Immunol 126:905–909.

Meinertz H, Linnet L, Fogh-Andersen P, Hjort T (1989): Antisperm antibodies and fertility after vasovasostomy: A follow-up study on 216 men. J Reprod Immunol 15(Suppl):60.

Mettler L, Czuppon AB, Alexander N, D'Almeida M, Haas Jr GG, Hjort T, Moller Jensen J, Ing R, Jones WR, Wang SX, Witkin SS, Bongiovanni AM (1985): Antibodies to spermatozoa and seminal plasma antigens detected by various enzyme-linked immunosorbent (ELISA) assays. J Reprod Immunol 8:301–312.

Mori T, Kamada M, Hasebe H, Irahara M, Shivers A, Czuppon AB, Mettler L, Mathur S, Dunbar BS (1985): Antibody reactivity with porcine zona pellucida. J Reprod Immunol 8:337–345.

Mori T, Nishimoto T, Kitagawa M, Noda Y, Nishimura T, Oikawa T (1978): Possible presence of autoantibodies to zona pellucida in infertile women. Experientia 34:797–799.

Rose NR, Hjort T, Rümke Ph, Harper MJK, Vyazov O (1976): Techniques for the detection of iso- and auto-antibodies to human spermatozoa. Clin Exp Immunol 23:175–199.

Rümke Ph, van Amstel N, Messer EN, Bezemer PD (1974): Prognosis of fertility of men with sperm agglutinins in serum. Fertil Steril 25:393–398.

Sacco AG (1977): Antigenic cross-reactivity between human and pig zona pellucida. Biol Reprod 16:164–173.

Sacco AG, Moghissi KS (1979): Anti-zona pellucida activity in human sera. Fertil Steril 31:503–506.

Shelton J, Goldberg E (1985): Serum antibodies to LDH-D$_4$. J Reprod Immunol 8:321–327.

Shivers CA, Dunbar BS (1977): Autoantibodies to zona pellucida: A possible cause for infertility in women. Science 197:1082–1084.

WHO Reference Bank for Reproductive Immunology (1977): Auto- and iso- antibodies to antigens of the human reproductive system. Clin Exp Immunol 30:173–180.

DISCUSSION

DR. SEHGAL: I have a comment concerning our experience measuring antisperm antibodies. We have used whole sperm and glutaraldehyde-fixed ELISA plates, and they seemed to work quite well. We also observed antizona antibodies in the sera of infertile women. The positive indexes were about 7–8%, but the titers were very low. As such, it seems this is not an important antibody as far as infertility is concerned. Concerning the antibodies raised to porcine zona, we did Western blots with human spermatozoa and found three to four bands and they appeared to be peptides. In fact, we submitted this paper for publication and it was returned for reasons that are known to the referees. I think that there was some cross-reactivity, but whether to carbohydrates or peptides is not clear.

DR. TALWAR: In those subjects who had evidence of immunological factors related to infertility, were there any other types of clinical abnormalities noted?

DR. HJORT: We have detailed clinical information on these patients and they apparently had no other autoimmune diseases.

DR. TALWAR: Because in most cases it would be the autoantigens that you would have detected, this data would seem very valuable.

DR. GOLDBERG: Can you tell me if the virgin with the high activity against LDH-C_4 was also positive in any of the other tests?

DR. HJORT: This was a very puzzling situation. Although there could be some cross-reacting antigen somewhere, we looked very carefully into the history and found nothing.

24

Characterization of Spermatozoa Antigens by Monoclonal and Polyclonal Antibodies

Satish K. Gupta and Nancy J. Alexander

The search for sperm antigens pertinent to contraceptive vaccine development often involves the use of serum from patients with putative immunologic infertility or monoclonal antisperm antibodies. With both of these approaches, an important technique in the initial assessment of antigen characteristics is immunoblotting to define molecular weight. The antigen preparation used for such blotting techniques is an essential consideration; yet numerous preparations (pooled-washed or swim-up sperm) and extraction procedures such as sodium dodecyl sulfate (SDS) [Naaby-Hansen and Bjerrum, 1985], sodium deoxycholate (DOC) [Hald et al., 1987; Naz et al., 1986], lithium 3,5-diiodosalicylate (LIS) [Naz et al., 1986], and octylphenoxypolyethoxyethanol (NP-40) [Herr and Eddy, 1980] are commonly used. Different human sperm extracts prepared from thrice-washed and swim-up sperm with different solubilizing agents separated by SDS-polyacrylamide gel electrophoresis (SDS-PAGE) have been compared. Sperm prepared by the swim-up method seem the most appropriate and constant for defining sperm antigens. Mouse monoclonal antisperm antibodies and polyclonal autoantibodies present in vasectomized men were used to characterize spermatozoa antigen preparations. Not all monoclonals reacted with both thrice-washed and swim-up sperm antigen, again pointing to the significance of a better-defined antigen preparation when determining fertility-associated antigens. Employing sera obtained from

Gamete Interaction: Prospects for Immunocontraception, pages 345–357
© 1990 Wiley-Liss, Inc.

vasectomized subjects who underwent vasovasostomy, attempts have been made to identify antigens associated with infertility. Although serum samples from infertile men with a vasovasostomy always reacted with sperm antigens by immunoblot, no particular antigen was found to be associated with infertility.

STANDARDIZATION OF SPERMATOZOA ANTIGEN PREPARATION EMPLOYED FOR ANTIGEN CHARACTERIZATION

Since sperm antigens are prepared in many ways, we considered it important to standardize antigen preparation. Semen ejaculates obtained from normal male donors or from men attending an infertility clinic (The Jones Institute for Reproductive Medicine, Norfolk) were allowed to liquify at room temperature. Sperm were collected by centrifugation at 400g for 15 min, washed three times in Tris-buffered saline (TBS; 10 mM Tris, 145 mM NaCl, pH 7.4), pooled from several donors, and stored at $-70°C$ before use (thrice-washed sperm). Alternately, after liquefaction, 2 ml of semen were carefully placed beneath BWW medium [Biggers et al., 1971], and motile sperm were allowed to swim up for a 60 min incubation period at 37°C. Motile sperm in BWW medium were pooled, counted with a Cell Soft Automated Semen Analyzer (CRYO Resources Ltd., New York, NY), washed three times in TBS, and stored at $-70°C$ (swim-up sperm).

To compare the efficacy of extraction procedures, antigens were extracted from the same pool of thrice-washed sperm by the LIS, DOC, NP-40, 3-[(3-cholamidopropyl)dimethylammonio]-1-propane sulfonate (CHAPS), and dithiothrietol (DTT) methods. The solubilized components were analyzed by SDS-PAGE with a 10% separating gel and silver stained. Extracts prepared by LIS, DOC, CHAPS, and 0.3% NP-40 had almost identical profiles [Gupta et al., 1990a]. The profile obtained by the DTT method was different from those of LIS, DOC, CHAPS, and NP-40 extracts as evidenced by the absence of high-molecular-weight bands of 150 and 200 kd. The DTT method consistently resulted in the lack of the 150 and 200 kd bands, perhaps because of the action of sonication and/or the treatment with DTT. This extraction procedure, however, does retain relevant antigens, because these antigens will induce preferential lymphocyte adherence inhibition in vasectomized men compared with intact controls [Anderson et al., 1982].

When different pools of swim-up sperm were compared, it was observed that their protein profiles were much more similar than

TABLE 1. Reactivity in ELISA of 10 Monoclonal Antibodies With Swim-Up and Ca²⁺ Ionophore-Treated Human Sperm

| Monoclonal antibody | Isotype | S.D. units[a] | |
		Swim-up	Ca^{2+} treated
MA-42	IgG$_1$	8.5	1.4
MA-43	IgG$_1$	3.0	4.7
MA-44	IgG$_1$	9.2	2.8
MA-45	IgG$_1$	4.6	6.5
MA-46	IgG$_1$	11.2	3.5
MA-47	IgG$_1$	10.2	3.2
MA-48	IgG$_1$	10.1	3.7
MA-49	IgG$_1$	8.6	8.2
MA-50	IgG$_1$	2.8	6.3
MA-51	IgG$_{2a}$	10.9	1.6

[a]Standard deviation unit calculated by subtracting control sample mean (X_c) from test sample mean (X_t) and then dividing by standard deviation of control (SD_c); ($X_t - X_c$)/SD_c.

those of different pools of thrice-washed sperm. We suggest that swim-up sperm preparations provide a more repeatable and relevant sperm antigen profile. With swim-up preparation, only the living motile sperm likely to be associated with fertilization are collected for extraction. It was also observed that, by immunoblot, a panel of 12 monoclonal antibodies gave different reactivity patterns with antigen extracted from swim-up as compared with those from thrice-washed sperm [Gupta et al., 1990a]. Antigens extracted from only swim-up sperm were used for further characterization of spermatozoa antigens by monoclonal as well as polyclonal antibodies.

STUDIES WITH MONOCLONAL ANTIBODIES

Ten hybrid cell clones secreting monoclonal antisperm antibodies were developed [Gupta and Talwar, 1980]; 9 of 10 antibodies were of the IgG$_1$ type and one (MA-51) was of the IgG$_{2a}$ type (Table 1). Reactivity of the monoclonal antibodies was tested in ELISA with swim-up and CA^{2+} ionophore–treated human sperm (Table 1). Seven out of 10 monoclonals showed strong (>5 S.D. units) reactivity with swim-up sperm, whereas three showed a weak reaction (<5 S.D. units but >2 S.D. units). Monoclonals MA-42, MA-44, MA-46, MA-47, MA-48, and MA-51 showed reactivity of lower order with Ca^{2+} ionophore–treated (postcapacitated) sperm as compared with swim-up sperm. However, three monoclonals, MA-43, MA-45, and MA-50, showed higher reactivity with Ca^{2+} ionophore–treated sperm in contrast to swim-up sperm. Monoclonal MA-49 reacted equally with both types of sperm preparation [Gupta et al., 1990b]. The differential reactivity of monoclonal antibodies with swim-up sperm as compared with Ca^{2+} ionophore–treated (capacitated) sperm in ELISA may be due to reorganization of surface antigens during capacitation. Indeed, Saxena et al. [1986] observed shifts of sperm surface antigens as revealed by immunofluorescence during in vitro capacitation. Monoclonal antibody MA-49, which reacted equally well with capacitated and noncapacitated sperm, must react with antigen(s) that are not altered by capacitation.

Specificity of the 10 monoclonal antibodies was investigated in ELISA with human white blood cells (WBC), human red blood cells (RBC), human platelets, Raji cells, mouse sperm, monkey sperm, and human seminal plasma. With the exception of MA-49, none of the monoclonal antibodies reacted with platelets, mouse sperm, WBC, RBC, and Raji cells. MA-49 recognizes a 68 kd antigen (possibly albumin) in addition to 14 and 20 kd antigens in immunoblot and reacts with WBC, RBC, and Raji cells. All 10 monoclonal antibodies reacted with human seminal plasma, suggesting that these antibodies have been generated against the spermatozoa coating antigens. Such antibodies may affect fertility. For example, one human–mouse heterohybridoma (MCA H6-3C4) reacts with human seminal plasma and secretes high-titer sperm immobilization (SI) and sperm agglutination (SA) antibodies similar to those found in infertile patients [Isojima et al., 1987]. This monoclonal recognizes an antigenic epitope with a Gal-Gluc-Nac structure and a sialic acid at the terminal region of the carbohydrate chain [Isojima, 1988]. Monoclonals to sperm antigens developed in our laboratory often are directed toward carbohydrate moities [Kurpisz et al., 1990].

Four of the 10 monoclonal antibodies described above, MA-42, MA-44, MA-47, and MA-50, caused sperm agglutination with a mixed pattern. The monoclonal antibodies MA-42, MA-44, and MA-47 reacted more by ELISA to swim-up rather than Ca^{2+} ionophore–treated sperm, suggesting the presence of antigens that cause agglutination being located on the outer plasma membrane. MA-50, however, reacted more to Ca^{2+} ionophore–treated sperm even though it caused sperm agglutination. This finding indicates that the site of reaction for MA-51 is not the outer plasma membrane but must be the other sites on the sperm surface.

Monoclonal antibodies MA-42, MA-44, MA-46, MA-47, MA-48, MA-49, and MA-50 recognized, by immunoblot, antigens having apparent molecular weights of 14 and 20 kd (Table 2). In addition to the 14 and 20 kd antigens, MA-49 also recognized a 68 kd antigen.

TABLE 2. Apparent Molecular Weights of Antigens Recognized by MCAs in Immunoblot Using NP-40 Extract of Human Sperm and Human Seminal Plasma

Monoclonal antibody	Apparent molecular weight (kd)	
	NP-40 extract	Seminal plasma
MA-42	14, 20	14, 17, 18, 20, 22
MA-43	>200	0
MA-44	14, 20	14, 17, 18, 20, 22, 25, 26, 28
MA-45	70, 72, >200	38, 70, 72, >200
MA-46	14, 20	14, 17, 18, 20, 22, 25, 26, 28
MA-47	14, 20	14, 15, 16, 17, 18
MA-48	14, 20	14, 18, 19, 23, 24, 25
MA-49	14, 20, 68	14, 18, 19, 23, 24, 25, 30, 32, 33, 35, 37, 38, 65
MA-50	>200	0
MA-51	14, 20	14, 15, 17, 20

MA-45 recognized 70, 72, and >200 kd antigens. Monoclonal antibodies MA-43 and MA-50 recognized antigens >200 kd. All MCAs except MA-43 and MA-50 showed multiple bands with human seminal plasma, demonstrating that these monoclonals are to coating antigens (Table 2). Monoclonal antibodies MA-46 and MA-50 were effective in preventing the attachment of precapacitated human sperm to zona denuded hamster oocytes (Table 3). The reasons for other monoclonal antibodies having the same immunoreactivity pattern in immunoblot while differing in their functional properties is worth exploring. One explanation may be that 14, 20, and 200 kd antigens on spermatozoa are complex in nature. To isolate and analyze these antigens in two-dimensional SDS-PAGE followed by immunoblotting would be of interest.

STUDIES WITH POLYCLONAL ANTIBODIES

Vasectomy in men, to a variable degree, leads to the development of autoantibodies against spermatozoa [Zappi et al., 1970; Tung, 1975]. We have attempted to identify sperm autoantigens responsible for generating autoantibodies after vasectomy by means of immunoblotting. We have correlated the immunoblot results with SA and SI activities. Furthermore, attempts were made to identify spermatozoa autoantigens associated with infertility by employing pre- and postvasovasostomy serum samples.

TABLE 3. Reactivity of Antispermatozoa
Monoclonal Antibodies in the Hamster
Oocyte Penetration Test

Monoclonal antibodies	Percent penetration
MA-42	80
MA-43	60
MA-44	50
MA-45	10
MA-46	0
MA-47	10
MA-48	50
MA-49	40
MA-50	0
MA-51	10

SPERM AUTOANTIGENS RECOGNIZED BY SERA FROM VASECTOMIZED MEN

Of the 40 vasectomy serum samples, 28 were positive in the SA assay with a titer of ≥40, and 21 had immobilization values over 3.5. Of these 28 serum samples, 22 (78.6%) were also positive by immunoblot (Table 4). The autoantigens recognized by vasectomy serum samples were 65 (36%), 52 (10.7%), 50 (78.6%), 42 (21.4%), 40 (36%), 37 (64%), 28 (43%), 26 (29%), and 23 (3.6%), kd. In contrast, of the 12 vasectomy serum samples that were negative by the SA (antibody titer of ≤10) and SI tests, only three reacted (one with 50, 28, and 23 kd antigens; one with a 50 kd antigen; and one with a 40 kd autoantigen). Serum samples obtained from prepubertal children and from nonvasectomized subjects were used as controls. None of the 10 serum samples obtained from nonvasectomized individuals showed any specific reaction except to a 55 kd antigen that was also recognized by the majority of sera of vasectomized subjects. Moreover, none of the 15 prepubertal serum samples revealed any specific binding with sperm antigens by immunoblot.

In a study by Naaby-Hansen and Bjerrum [1985], five antigens with molecular weights of 120, 78, 64, 41, and 32 kd under reduced conditions were recognized by infertile sera; the 120, 41, and 32 kd antigens could be correlated to the agglutinating activity of the reactive sera. Six serum samples in our studies, in spite of being positive in sperm agglutination assay, did not react in immunoblot. This may be due to the complicated interactions of agglutination in which antibodies of differing specificities and affinities (low as well as high) can contribute to a positive reaction. Moreover, conformational

TABLE 4. Binding Pattern in Western Immunoblot of
Immunoglobulins From 28 Sera Obtained From
Vasectomized Men[a]

Serum sample No.	Titer in		Antigens recognized by immunoblot (kd)								
	SA	SI	65	52	50	42	40	37	28	26	23
1	+80	∝	+	+	+	−	+	+	+	+	−
2	+40	∝	−	−	+	−	+	+	+	+	−
3	±40	12.4	−	−	+	−	−	−	−	−	−
4	±80	∝	−	−	+	−	−	−	−	−	−
5	±40	∝	+	−	+	−	−	−	−	−	−
6	±40	∝	−	−	−	−	−	−	−	−	−
7	±40	∝	+	−	+	−	−	+	+	+	−
8	+640	∝	+	−	+	+	+	+	+	+	−
9	±40	∝	−	−	+	−	−	+	−	−	−
10	±40	1.6	−	−	+	−	−	+	−	−	−
11	±40	6.6	−	−	+	−	+	+	−	−	−
12	+80	∝	−	−	+	−	−	+	−	−	−
13	+40	1.54	−	−	+	−	−	+	−	−	−
14	+40	∝	−	−	−	−	−	−	−	−	−
15	+40	∝	+	−	+	−	−	+	+	−	−
16	±40	∝	−	−	+	−	−	+	+	−	−
17	±40	1.86	−	−	−	−	−	−	−	−	−
18	+160	1.94	+	−	+	+	+	+	+	+	−
19	+40	15.5	−	−	−	−	−	−	−	−	−
20	±40	1.25	+	−	+	+	+	+	+	−	−
21	+40	∝	−	−	+	−	−	+	−	−	+
22	+40	1.8	+	−	+	+	+	+	+	−	−
23	+40	3.8	−	−	−	−	−	−	−	−	−
24	±40	1.26	−	−	−	−	−	−	−	−	−
25	+40	5	−	−	+	−	+	−	−	−	−
26	±40	26	+	+	+	+	+	+	+	+	−
27	+40	∝	−	−	+	−	−	−	−	−	−
28	+40	89	+	+	+	+	−	+	+	+	−

[a]SA, sperm agglutination assay; SI, sperm immobilization test.

epitopes recognized by the antibodies may be lost after SDS treatment and thus not detectable in immunoblotting. In the Naaby-
Hansen and Bjerrum [1985] study, IgM antibodies, unlike the IgG
antibodies, failed to show any specific pattern; IgM antibodies from
both normal and infertile subjects showed identical sperm-binding
reactions. Spermatozoa autoantigens recognized by serum samples

from vasectomized men in our study, e.g., 65, 42, and 40 kd, may be comparable to the 64 and 41 kd autoantigens reported by Naaby-Hansen and Bjerrum [1985]. None of the vasectomized sera in our study reacted with high-molecular-weight autoantigens. We suggest that our results may be due to the fact that motile sperm rather than washed sperm were employed to extract proteins.

Three out of 12 vasectomy serum samples negative in the sperm agglutination assay reacted by immunoblot. The autoantigens recognized by these sera were the same as those recognized by vasectomized sera positive in the sperm agglutination assay; thus no major antigen can be associated with sperm agglutination or immobilization. However, sera from nonvasectomized men and from prepubertal children did not give any specific reaction in immunoblot, which is contrary to the observations by Hald et al. [1987]. Again, this discrepancy may be due to the fact that we used motile sperm in contrast to thrice-washed sperm for preparation of our antigen extract.

The autoantigens revealed by immunoblot do not exhibit absolute correlation with antisperm antibody titers in SA or SI assays. Moreover, the pattern of autoantigens recognized has no association with SA or SI activities. Serum samples negative for SA or SI but having positive reactivity in immunoblot indicate that the antisperm antibodies may be reacting to internal antigens of spermatozoa as compared with external antigens.

Some vasectomized men, in spite of successful vasovasostomies, remain infertile [Lee and McLaughlin, 1980]. The continued presence of circulating antispermatozoa antibodies has been postulated as the cause of such subfertility. Serum samples obtained before and after vasovasostomy from an additional 31 men were used to characterize sperm autoantigens by Western immunoblot. Sperm counts after vasovasostomy and the ability to impregnate the spouse were recorded (Table 5). Twenty-one of 31 (67.7%) men after vasovasostomy caused a pregnancy. Pre- and postoperative serum samples from 9 of these 21 (47.6%) men did not react with sperm antigens by immunoblot. Ten subjects after vasovasostomy failed to impregnate their partner. Seven of these subjects had successful vasovasostomies as indicated by normal sperm count and motility. Out of these 10, all (100%) reacted in immunoblot. Thus, based on information from these seven men, after vasovasostomy there appears to be a negative association with immunoblot results and the return of fertility.

Pre- or postvasovasostomy sera samples of 26 out of 31 men tested in the present study revealed similar immunoblot patterns. Only in five cases could a shift in the pattern be observed following vasova-

TABLE 5. Binding Pattern in Immunoblot of Immunoglobulins From Pre- and Postvasovasostomy Serum Samples Obtained From 31 Men and Ability to Impregnate the Female Partner Following Reconstructive Surgery[a]

Subject No.	Serum sample	Serum titer		Time (count/motility)[b]	Pregnancy[c]	Antigens recognized by immunoblot (kd)
		SI	SA			
1	Pre	2.1	+ 40	29; 93/50	Yes, 40	—
	Post (24)	1.8	± 320			—
2	Pre	1.2	—	14; 13/60	Yes, 16	—
	Post (6)	2.0	+ 160			—
3	Pre	∞	± 160	16; 24/50	Yes	—
	Post (12)	1.2	+ 10			—
4	Pre	∞	± 160	3; 24/35	Yes, 5	—
	Post (12)	4.7	+ 80			—
5	Pre	0.9	—	12; 69/180	Yes, 12	—
	Post (8)	2.4	± 40			—
6	Pre	1.1	0	9; 60/60	Yes, 9	—
	Post (4)	2.0	0			—
7	Pre	1.5	+ 40	4; 58/60	Yes, 4	—
	Post (12)	1.4	± 10			—
8	Pre	1.2	+ 10	5; 68/60	Yes, 5	—
	Post (15)	1.1	± 10			—
9	Pre	1.14	—	12; 87/56	Yes, 12	—
	Post (12)	2.38	± 160			
10	Pre	0.92	—	5; 9/40	Yes, 6	70, 65
	Post (12)	1.08	—			70, 65
11	Pre	1.06	—	6; 114/60	Yes, 6	65
	Post (0)	1.1				65
12	Pre	0.92	+ 20	7; 55/60	Yes, 8	70
	Post (6)	0.89	± 20			70
13	Pre	8.22	+ 20	3; 65/70	Yes, 4	65
	Post (4)	1.17	—			65
14	Pre	0.96	—	9; 162/60	Yes, 9	70, 65
	Post (8)	1.37	+ 10			70, 65
15	Pre	1.5	—	7; 25/60	Yes, 8	70, 58, 25, 23
	Post (4)	1.28	—			70, 58, 25, 23
16	Pre	1.4	—	4; 48/40	Yes, 4	65
	Post (4)	0.92	—			65
17	Pre	1.12	± 40	6; 60/50	Yes, 6	65
	Post (9)	2.45	± 20			65
18	Pre	6.2	+ 40	6; 15/60	Yes, 6	58, 35, 30, 28
	Post (6)	∞	± 160			—

(*continued*)

TABLE 5. (Continued)

Subject No.	Serum sample	Serum titer		Time (count/motility)[b]	Pregnancy[c]	Antigens recognized by immunoblot (kd)
		SI	SA			
19	Pre	1.9	+ 40	13; 9/40	Yes, 12	—
	Post (13)	1.2	+ 80			25
20	Pre	—	—	4; 12/25	Yes, 6	—
	Post (4)	0.96	—			65
21	Pre	1.4	+ 20	6; 15/60	Yes, 6	65
	Post (5)	1.02	± 20			70, 65
22	Pre	24.7	± 40	8; 54/30	No	58, 35, 30, 28
	Post (8)	3.9	+ 20			58, 35, 30, 28
23	Pre	2.3	± 320	12; 16/40	No	58, 35, 30, 28
	Post (11)	2.9	+ 80			58, 35, 30, 28
24	Pre	∞	± 80	12; 39/40	No	65
	Post (16)	3.2	± 40			65
25	Pre	∞	+ 80	12; 7/30	No	65
	Post (12)	2.6	+ 40			65
26	Pre	5.5	± 80	9; 28/70	No	65
	Post (24)	1.7	80			65
27	Pre	68	160	12; <1/0	No	65, 25
	Post (9)	∞	± 80			65, 25
28	Pre	2.32	± 320	12; 16/40	No	65
	Post (11)	2.92	+ 80			65
29	Pre	1.3	+ 40	12; 38/40	No	58
	Post (12)	4.4	± 40			58
30	Pre	1.49	—	10; 22/0	No	65, 35, 30, 14
	Post (10)	1.40	—			65, 35, 30, 14
31	Pre	∞	+ 40	12; 6/2	No	70, 65
	Post (12)	∞	± 80			70

[a]Pre, prevasovasostomy; post, postvasovasostomy (month after vasovasostomy); SI, sperm immobilization test; SA, sperm agglutination test.
[b]Time (month) after vasovasostomy; sperm count (10⁶/ml)/percent motility.

^{b}Time (month) after vasovasostomy; sperm count (10^6/ml)/percent motility.
[c]Pregnancy, month after vasovasostomy.

sostomy. In one case, the prevasovasostomy serum sample recognized 55, 35, 30, and 28 kd autoantigens and was negative following vasovasostomy, and in a second case reactivity with 65 kd band disappeared. In three cases, an additional autoantigen was recognized (one subject to a 70 kd antigen, a second subject to a 65 kd antigen, and a third subject to a 25 kd antigen) following vasovasostomy.

Autoantigens recognized by serum samples from men who successfully impregnated their partners following vasovasostomy were similar to those recognized by men who failed to impregnate their partners. Thus no unique spermatozoa autoantigens were associated with infertility.

CONCLUDING COMMENTS

To characterize spermatozoa antigens associated with fertility, an important consideration should be given to the sperm preparation employed. We suggest that swim-up sperm rather than thrice-washed sperm are far more appropriate for these studies. To avoid batch-to-batch variations, a large pool must be collected before any experiments are begun. Monoclonal antibodies are useful in delineating the spermatozoa antigens involved in the regulation of fertility. For example, monoclonal antibodies MA-46 and MA-50 block the attachment of sperm to zona denuded hamster oocytes and should be further studied.

Serum samples of vasectomized men positive for SA and SI activities were often positive (78.6%) in immunoblot, whereas only 25% of those vasectomy serum samples that were negative for SA and SI reacted by immunoblot. Some of the vasectomized men (30%), despite a successful vasovasostomy based on motile sperm return, did not show a return of fertility. Pre- and postvasovasostomy serum samples from 47.6% of the men who demonstrated return of fertility did not react by immunoblot. However, at least in a small sample, pre- and postvasovasostomy serum samples from 100% of the men who failed to impregnate their partner were positive in immunoblot. No particular autoantigen revealed by immunoblotting was associated with infertility. The autoantigens revealed by immunoblot did not exhibit an absolute correlation with SA and SI activities, but a negative association with immunoblot results and return of fertility was observed.

REFERENCES

Anderson DJ, Alexander NJ, Fulgham DL, Vandenbark AA, Burger DR (1982): Immunity to tumor-associated antigens in vasectomized men. JNCI 69:551–555.

Biggers JD, Whitten WK, Whittingham DG (1971): The culture of mouse embryos in vitro. In Daniel JC Jr (ed): Methods in Mammalian Embryology. San Francisco: W.H. Freeman, pp 86–116.

Gupta SK, Fulgham DL, Alexander NJ (1990a): Sperm preparation affects reactivity of mononclonal antibodies. J Reprod Immunol (in press).

Gupta SK, Fulgham DL, Alexander NJ (1990b): Characteristics of monoclonal antibodies reactive with human sperm and seminal plasma. Indian J Exp Biol 28:501–507.

Gupta SK, Talwar GP (1980): Development of hybridomas secreting anti-human chorionic gonadotropin antibodies. Indian J Exp Biol 18:1361–1365.

Hald J, Naaby-Hansen S, Egense J, Hjort T, Bjerrum OJ (1987): Auto-antibodies against spermatozoal antigens detected by immunoblotting and agglutination: A longitudinal study of vasectomized males. J Reprod Immunol 10:15–26.

Herr JC, Eddy EM (1980): Detection of mouse sperm antigens by a surface labeling and immunoprecipitation approach. Biol Reprod 22:1263–1274.

Isojima S (1988): Recent advances in defining human seminal plasma antigens using monoclonal antibodies. Am J Reprod Immunol 17:150–155.

Isojima S, Kameda K, Tsuji Y, Shisgeta M, Ikeda Y, Koyama K (1987): Establishment and characterization of a human hybridoma secreting monoclonal antibody with high titers of sperm immobilizing and agglutinating activities against human seminal plasma. J Reprod Immunol 10:67–78.

Kurpisz M, Clark GF, Mahony MC, Anderson TL, Alexander NJ (1990): Mouse monoclonal antibodies against human sperm: Evidence for immunodominant glycosylated antigenic sites. Clin Exp Immunol (in press).

Lee L, Mclaughlin MC (1980): Vasovasostomy: A comparison of macroscopic and microscopic techniques at one institution. Fertil Steril 33:54–55.

Naaby-Hansen S, Bjerrum OJ (1985): Auto- and iso-antigens of spermatozoa detected by immunoblotting with human sera after SDS-PAGE. J Reprod Immunol 7:41–57.

Naz RK, Phillips TM, Rosenblum BB (1986): Characterization of the fertilization antigen for the development of a contraceptive vaccine. Proc Natl Acad Sci USA 83:5713–5717.

Saxena N, Peterson AN, Sharif S, Saxena NK, Russel LD (1986): Changes in the organization of surface antigens during in vitro capacitation of boar spermatozoa as detected by monoclonal antibodies. J Reprod Fertil 78:601–614.

Tung KSK (1975): Human sperm antigens and antisperm antibody studies on vasectomy patients. Clin Exp Immunol 20:93–104.

Zappi E, Ahmed U, Davis J, Shulman S (1970): Immunologic consequences of vasectomy. Fed Proc 29:374.

DISCUSSION

DR. ANDERSON: Did you examine the seminal plasma from vasectomized men?

DR. GUPTA: We have used the seminal plasma from both vasectomized and nonvasectomized men, and we did not find any difference in either case. I am aware of studies that show that some antigens are lost on vasectomy, but we did not find any signficant difference in the two categories.

DR. ANDERSON: You reported that vasectomized men have antibodies against seminal plasma antigens. Presumably, they would be directed against products of accessory organs that are not immunologically privileged. Why did we not see autoimmune problems in the accessory glands of these men?

DR. GUPTA: We have observed autoantibodies against seminal plasma components in the vasectomized individual. I do not know the relevance, if any, of these autoantibodies to cause autoimmune disease.

DR. HECHT: Why are your monoclonals recognizing such a large subset of different-sized proteins?

DR. GUPTA: The different components in the seminal plasma proteins may have a common determinant to which the monoclonal antibody is directed. It is not surprising that a monoclonal antibody, or even a polyclonal antibody, raised against a given antigen can give multiple bands.

DR. THAU: Where did the different sperm pools come from?

DR. GUPTA: These pools of sperm came either from the donors who came from the Infertility Clinic or from normal men. We make up pools with a certain percentage of normal sperm, in terms of motility and sperm count, and then we pool them. Once we have sperm from at least 5 to 10 individuals in a given pool, we begin the extraction procedure.

DR. THAU: Did you compare the swim-up sperm with the thrice-washed sperm in the same pools?

DR. GUPTA: No. The swim-up pool of sperm is collected separately. When we began work on the swim-up pool, we collected semen from 10 individuals to make the swim-up pool. We then collected semen from another 10 individuals, and made another pool. Thus the swim-up pool is different from the nonswim-up pool. The three different swim-up pools that I demonstrated were made at different times.

25

Development of Heterohybridomas to Define Human Sperm-Coating Antigens

Shinzo Isojima, Kinu Kameda, Koji Koyama, Iglika Batova, and Yoshiyuki Tsuji

There are many kinds of antigens on the surface of sperm and also many kinds of antibodies against these antigens in the sera of women. We can divide them roughly into two categories, namely, sperm membrane intrinsic antigens and sperm-coating antigens (SCA) from the human seminal plasma (HSP) [Isojima et al., 1968, 1972]. Our group has been more concerned with SCA, because they are already soluble and easier to purify. Even among SCA, there are many antigenic molecules that may contain several epitopes. Therefore, the identification of antigenic epitopes and purification of antigenic molecules may be difficult using polyclonal antibodies against sperm. For these reasons, we attempted to establish hybridoma cell lines to HSP that secrete monoclonal antibodies (mAbs) with sperm-immobilizing (SI) or sperm-agglutinating (SA) activities and to use the mAbs for purification of sperm antigen with immunoaffinity chromatography.

ESTABLISHMENT OF RAT–MOUSE HETEROHYBRIDOMA AGAINST HUMAN SEMINAL PLASMA ANTIGEN

In 1980, we succeeded in establishing rat–mouse heterohybridoma to HSP that secreted mAb 1C4 (IgM) with strong SI activity [Shigeta et al., 1980]. Rat spleen cells immunized to HSP and mouse myeloma

Gamete Interaction: Prospects for Immunocontraception, pages 359–375
© 1990 Wiley-Liss, Inc.

cells (P3U1) were successfully fused in the presence of PEG-1500, and the hybridoma 1C4 was established. The supernatant from the hybridoma 1C4 culture medium gave a positive SI value (SIV = 2.0) [Isojima et al., 1968] to 160-fold dilution, and 1.1 μg/ml of immunoglobulin from the supernatant gave SIV-2.8. mAb 1C4 (prot. 18.8 mg/ml) reacted with HSP (prot. 30 mg/ml) and also with human milk protein (prot. 60 mg/ml) by immunodiffusion. Both precipitin lines were completely fused; therefore, an antigen corresponding to mAb 1C4 must be a common antigen between HSP and human milk protein. The precipitin line between mAb 1C4 and HSP fused with a precipitin line between the mAb and HSP-No. 7 antigen (Ferrisplan) by immunoelectrophoresis. Therefore, an antigen corresponding to mAb 1C4 could be the HSP-No. 7 antigen (Ferrisplan), an iron-containing molecule that is also found in human milk.

The purification of the antigenic molecule corresponding to mAb 1C4 in HSP was performed by using immunoaffinity chromatography (CNBr-activated Sepharose 4B) on bound mAb γ-globulin and the antigen (molecular weight 15 kd) was successfully purified 196 times to become more effective in neutralizing SI activities than the original HSP protein [Isojima et al., 1982]. But this purified antigen of HSP was a common antigen with human milk and would not be a good candidate for contraceptive vaccine. In 1979, Bechtol et al. succeeded in producing a mouse mAb that recognized different antigens of spermatogenesis; our mAb 1C4 was the first mAb expressing strong human SI activity.

PRODUCTION OF HSP-SPECIFIC MONOCLONAL ANTIBODIES WITH STRONG SI ACTIVITIES

As a second step, we attempted to produce mAbs with SI or SA activities specific to HSP antigens. Mice were immunized with HSP (for hybridoma 2C6) or with ejaculated sperm (for hybridomas 2E5 and 2B6), and the spleen cells from the immunized mice and mouse myeloma cells (P3U1 or NS-1) were fused in the presence of PEG-1000. After HAT selection, the supernatants of culture media were examined for immunoglobulin production and SI or SA activities. The fused cell lines with the strongest SI activities were cloned, and the hybridomas 2C6, 2E5, and 2B6 were established [Isojima et al., 1986]. mAb 2C6 was IgM and expressed 800 SI_{50} (quantitative 50% sperm immobilization unit) as SI activity and 1:100 dilutions as SA activity in the supernatant of culture medium (14 μg/ml). mAbs 2E5 and 2B6 were IgG_3 and expressed 1,000 and 300 SI_{50} as SI activities and 1:1,000 and 1:300 dilutions as SA activities in each supernatant of culture medium, respectively. These mAbs were HSP specific, because their SI activities were completely absorbed with HSP but could not be absorbed with a sufficient amount of human milk protein or extrects of human liver or kidney. mAb 2C6 also had a blocking effect on sperm binding to human zona pellucida, besides SI and SA activities.

Many mAbs against human sperm [Lee et al., 1982a; Wolf et al., 1983; Isahakia and Alexander, 1984; Naz et al., 1984], hamster sperm [Moore and Hartman, 1984], rabbit sperm [O'Rand et al., 1984], and guinea pig sperm [Primakoff et al., 1988a] were produced, and the characteristics of antigens corresponding to these mAbs were studied. But our studies were concerned with the mAbs against human SCA in HSP.

SUCCESSFUL ESTABLISHMENT OF HUMAN–MOUSE HETEROHYBRIDOMA TO HSP

In 1986, we reported three human mouse heterohybridomas (H2-3H1, H3-1B12, and H3-1B5) that secreted SA mAb in the culture media [Kyurkchiev et al., 1986]. mAb H3-1B5 showed SI activity in addition. Hybridomas H2-3H1 and H3-1B12 lost antibody (Ab) production after 40 days of culture, and H3-1B5 maintained Ab production for 90 days. These heterohybridomas were established by the following procedure. Peripheral blood lymphocytes (PBL) from sterile women with high titers of SI Abs were taken and preincubated with washed human sperm and pokeweed mitogen (PWM) for 3 days before fusion with mouse myeloma cells NS-1 or SP2/0 in the presence of PEG-1000. The supernatants of culture media were examined for human Ig production and also for SI and SA activities after HAT selection. SI-positive cell lines that produced SA Abs were cloned by the limiting dilution method. Hybridoma H3-1B5 also produced SI mAbs besides SA Ab.

ESTABLISHMENT OF THE STABLE HUMAN–MOUSE HETEROHYBRIDOMA H6-3C4

The SA and SI activities of human mAbs previously obtained were very weak, and no hybridoma could survive more than 3 months. Therefore, we attempted to establish a more stable human hybridoma, and finally succeeded. The establishment of hybridoma H6-3C4 [Isojima et al., 1987] was performed as described previously, but in 1987 Ikeda also used a cloning procedure with a semisolid

TABLE 1. Stability of Hybridoma H6-3C4

Months after cell fusion	Concentration of IgM (μg/ml)	Sperm immobilization (SI$_{50}$ unit)	Sperm agglutination (dilution)
2	1.5	5,000	1:1,600
4	N.D.[a]	8,400	N.D.
6	2.1	6,900	1:3,200
8	2.0	5,900	1:3,200
15	1.5	4,500	1:2,000
18	N.D.	6,300	1:4,000
21	N.D.	4,000	1:2,000
25	N.D.	3,500	1:2,000
28	N.D.	5,000	N.D.
36	N.D.	4,500	1:2,000

[a]N.D., not determined.

medium after HAT selection and established the same cell clone as obtained by liquid culture. Hybridoma H6-3C4 was established from the PBL of a sterile woman (36 years old) with 46 SI$_{50}$ [Isojima and Koyama, 1976] as SI activity. The mAb secreted from the hybridoma was human IgM, λ and had extremely high titers of 5,000 SI$_{50}$ as SI activity and 1:1,600 dilutions as SA activity in the culture medium. This hydridoma H6-3C4 secreted the same level of antibody titers as at the beginning of culture for almost 4 years (Table 1).

Human sperm could absorb the SI activity of mAb H6-3C4 in a dose-dependent manner, but sperm from other species, except the boar, did not. The absorbing ability of boar sperm was approximately one-twentieth that of human sperm. After absorption, the SI activity of the mAb dropped in parallel with SA activity. The antibody activities of mAb H6-3C4 were retained after absorption with various human organ extracts and biological fluids, including human lymphocytes and erythrocytes, but they were lost by absorption with human azoospermic semen and fluids of the seminal vesicle. The binding of ^{125}I-mAb H6-3C4 to sperm was completely inhibited by mAb H6-3C4 and partially inhibited by the serum of the patient from whom the lymphocytes were used to establish hybridoma H6-3C4. Similar binding inhibitions were observed by adding our mouse mAb 2C6, 2E5, and 2B6 to the reaction system. Therefore, the antigenic epitope corresponding to mAb H6-3C4 seems to be similar to that in mAbs 2C6, 2E5, and 2B6 (Table 2).

Chromosome analysis showed that hybridoma H6-3C4 cells contains two types of chromosome, an acrocentric type from mice and a

TABLE 2. Results of Competitive Binding Inhibition Assay With ^{125}I-labeled mAb H6-3C4 by mAbs 2C6, 2E5, 2B6, and H6-3C4

mAbs	Percent inhibition[a]
H6-3C4	97.8
2C6	76.0
2E5	96.7
2B6	76.1
1C4	3.7

[a]Inhibition on sperm binding of [125]I mAb H6-3C4 with various mAbs.

metacentric type from humans. At least seven human chromosomes, including chromosome numbers 5, 9, 11, 12, 14, 17, and 22, were identified by Q-band staining. Immunofluorescent staining with mAb H6-3C4 showed that human ejaculated sperm were distinctively stained on their surface. The ejaculated sperm were generally stained on their entire surface.

In 1985, Herr et al. reported the successful establishment of human–mouse heterohybridomas that produced sperm binding Abs using PBL from vasectomized patients whose blood lymphocytes were taken 6 to 9 months after vasectomies. Their human–mouse hybridomas secreted IgM (κ or λ), but there is no information available concerning the biological activity of the mAb for sperm. In 1987, Kurpisz et al. also reported the successful production of human mAbs against human sperm from the hybridoma, which was established by Epstein-Barr virus (EBV) transformation of a patient's lymphocytes and microfusion with the UC726-6 lymphoblastoid cell partner. The mAbs obtained by these procedures expressed SI and SA activities.

CHARACTERISTICS OF ANTIGENIC MOLECULES CORRESPONDING TO EACH MAB

1 HSP was first treated with trypsin and applied on Sephacryl S-300. The major fraction obtained was used as partially purified HSP (P-HSP). When P-HSP was passed through the RCA-120 Agarose column, the obtained P-HSP fraction lost the antigenicity to inhibit the binding of mAbs H6-3C4, 2C6, 2E5, and 2B6 to sperm, but the fraction eluted by adding 0.1 M lactose solution in the column showed antigenicity by ELISA assay. From these experiments, the antigenic molecules corresponding to these mAbs were assumed to be

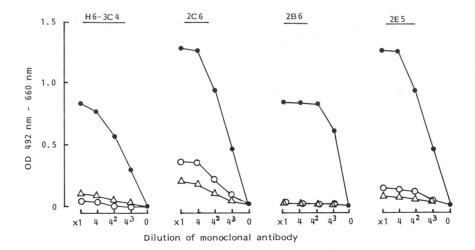

Fig. 1.   Reactivity of SI mAbs H6-3C4, 2C6, 2B6, and 2E5 to spermatozoa treated with trifluoromethane sulfonic acid (TFMS) and periodate. ●, Nontreated spermatozoa; ○, TFMS-treated spermatozoa; △, periodate-treated spermatozoa.

composed of a carbohydrate chain including a Gal–GlcNAc structure.

2   Binding inhibition between mAbs and sperm by the lectin wheat germ agglutinin (WGA) was examined by ELISA assay, and it was proved that the binding of mAb H6-3C4 to sperm was inhibited by WGA. Therefore, the existence of galactose or sialic acid in the carbohydrate moiety of antigen corresponding to mAb H6-3C4 was considered.

3   ELISA assays coated with trifluoromethane sulfonic acid (TFMS)-treated sperm showed that the bindings of mAb H6-3C4, 2C6, 2E5, and 2B6 to treated sperm were drastically damaged. Similar phenomena were also shown when the periodic acid–treated sperm were coated for the ELISA inhibition assay. Figure 1 shows the reactivities of these mAbs to sperm that were treated with TFMS or periodic acid. These experiments suggested that the antigenic epitopes of sperm-coating antigens, corresponding to mAbs H6-3C4, 2C6, 2E5, and 2B6 contained a carbohydrate structure.

4   Absorption effects of HSP on SI activities of mAbs H6-3C4 and 2C6 were examined before and after treatment of HSP with TFMS [Edge et al., 1981]. The TFMS treatment of HSP was performed by precipitating HSP by saturation with

$(NH_4)_2SO_4$ followed by dialysis and treatment of the dialized solution (10 mg/ml) with TFMS for 3 hr at 4°C. The absorption effect of HSP on the SI activity of mAb H6-3C4 was completely destroyed after TFMS treatment, but that of mAb 2C6 was retained to some degree although it was drastically damaged. From these results, the antigenic epitope corresponding to mAb H6-3C4 seems to be composed of carbohydrate and that to mAb 2C6 may be composed of carbohydrate and peptide.

5   Absorption effects of sperm on SI activities of mAbs H6-3C4 and 2C6 were also examined before and after treatment of sperm with periodate [Shapiro and Erickson, 1981]. The washed ejaculated sperm were treated with 10 mM $NaIO_4$ in PBS for 10, 30, 90 min and were used for absorption of mAbs H6-3C4 and 2C6. The absorption effect of sperm on the SI activity of mAb 2C6 was drastically destroyed after treatment of sperm with periodate, but that of mAb H6-3C4 was much less diminished. The carbohydrate structure of the antigen to mAb H6-3C4 may resist periodate treatment like type 2 neolactosamine, but the carbohydrate moiety of the antigen to mAb 2C6 may be sensitive to periodate treatment, like type 1 neolactosamine.

LOCALIZATION OF ANTIGENIC EPITOPES CORRESPONDING TO MAB

Paraffin-embedded sections of various human tissues (surgical specimens) were used for staining with mAbs by the avidin–biotin complex (ABC) method [Hsu et al., 1981]. Table 3 summarizes the results of the staining patterns produced by various mAbs. mAbs H6-3C4, 2C6, and 2B6 did not stain testicular tissue. Among the male accessory glands, mAb H6-3C4 stained the glandular epithelium of caudal epididymis, sperm in the caudal epididymal duct, and the surface of the seminal vesicle. mAb 2C6 stained the glandular epithelium of caput, corpus, and caudal epididymis, and mAbs 2E5 and 2B6 stained the glandular epithelium of corpus and caudal epididymis. Conversely, mAb 1C4 stained spermatozoa, spermatid in the testis, and epithelium of the seminal vesicle, but did not stain any part of the epithelium in epididymis.

Of somatic tissues besides male accessory organs, the distal tubules of kidney was the most important tissue that contained antigenic molecules, including epitopes corresponding to all mAbs (H6-

TABLE 3. Localization of Antigen Epitopes in Tissues Corresponding to mAbs

Human tissues	H6-3C4 human–mouse IgM (λ)	2C6 mouse IgM	2E5 mouse IgG	2B6 mouse IgG	1C4 rat–mouse IgM
Testis					
Spermatogonia	−	−	−	−	−
Spermatid	−	−	−	−	+
Spermatozoa	−	−	−	−	+
Epididymis					
Caput	−	+	−	−	−
Corpus	−	+	+	+	−
Cauda	+	+	+	+	−
Seminal vesicle					
Surface of epithelium	+	−	−	−	+
Prostate	−	−	−	−	+
Ejaculated sperm	+	+	+	+	+
Kidney					
Distal tubule	+	+	+	±	+
Proximal tubule	−	±	+	±	−
Mammary gland	−	−	−	−	+
Lung	+	−	N.T.[a]	−	+
Skin epidermis	+	−	N.T.	−	+
Fundus of stomach	+	±	N.T.	±	+

[a]N.T., not tested.

3C4, 2C6, 2E5, 2B6, 1C4). The duct of the salivary gland also contained antigenic epitopes corresponding to these mAbs. It is interesting that there is no HSP-specific or sperm-specific antigenic epitope relevant to SI Abs.

The antigenic epitope corresponding to mAb H6-3C4 (human mAb) existed in the distal tubules of kidney, alveolar cells of lung, epithelial cells of skin, salivary gland, and placental villi. The sterile woman from whom peripheral blood lymphocytes were drawn to establish the hybridoma H6-3C4 possessed the same SI Ab as mAb H6-3C4. However, this woman is healthy and exhibits no pathological findings by regular medical examinations, except that she is still sterile. Therefore, the existence of a certain antigenic epitope in somatic tissue may not be necessarily harmful for the body, though the antibody against its antigenic epitope is circulating in the blood stream.

CHEMICAL STRUCTURE OF ANTIGENIC EPITOPE CORRESPONDING TO MAB H6-3C4

The identification of antigenic epitopes on sperm that correspond to SI and SA Abs raised in sterile women is important to study. Several investigations [Lee et al., 1982b; Lehman et al., 1985; Naaby-Hansen and Bjerrum, 1985] reported immunoblot assays using radiolabeled λ-globulin of antisperm-positive patients' sera after SDS-PAGE of solubilized human sperm. These results showed that several sperm-binding Abs to various molecules in sperm extracts were present in women's sera but do not identify the biologically relevant antigenic epitopes corresponding to antisperm Abs in women's sera. Human mAb H6-3C4 was the ideal Ab for identifying a biologically relevant antigenic epitope in sperm-coating antigens, because it possesses a very high titer of SI and SA activities. Recently, in collaboration with Hakomori's research group [Tsuji et al., 1988], we disclosed the chemical structure of the antigenic epitope corresponding to mAb H6-3C4. Several glycolipids obtained from blood group O erythrocytes, human placenta, or human sperm and characterized as a lacto-series type 2 chain were stained with mAb H6-3C4 by thin-layer chromatography (TLC) immunostaining, which was performed on high-performance TLC (HPTLC) according to a modified method [Kannagi et al., 1982, 1983a] of a procedure originally described by Magnani et al. [1980]. As the major positive bands, lactonorhexaosylceramide (nLc_6) and lactonoroctaosylceramide (nLc_8) were characterized as neutral glycolipids; 2→3 sialylnorhexaosylceramide ($V1^3NeuAcnLc_6$), 2→6 sialylnorhexaosylceramide ($V1^6NeuAcnLc_6$), 2→3 sialylnoroctaosylceramide ($VIII^3NeuAcnLc_8$), and 2→6 sialylnoroctaosylceramide ($VIII^3NeuAcnLc8$) were characterized as gangliosides. Solid-phase RIA of various glycolipids was also performed on 96-well flexible vinyl plastic plates [Kannagi et al., 1983b], and it was shown that 2→6 sialylnorhexaosylceramide, 2→3 sialylnoroctaosylceramide, and norhexaosylceramide reacted with mAb H6-3C4. Therefore, mAb H6-3C4 reacted with glycolipids having a long unbranched type 2 chain, regardless of substitution with sialic acid at the terminal region, but did not react with those having a branched or shorter type 2 chain. This specificity is similar to that of anti-i antibody. Anti-i antibody reacted only to norhexaosylceramide; it did not react to the same structure substituted with sialic acid at the terminal region. mAb H6-3C4 is a very interesting and peculiar antibody, because it reacted to unbranched repetitive neolactosamine regardless of substitution with sialic acid at the terminal region. Table 4 shows the reactivities of mAb H6-3C4 to various glycolipids.

TABLE 4. Glicolipids Reacted With mAb H6-3C4

i(n Hex)	Galβ1→4GlcNAcβ1→3Galβ1→4GlcNAc
	β1→3Galβ1→4Glc→Cer (lactonorhexaosylceramide)
2.3 S-i	NeuAc2→3Galβ1→4GlcNAcβ1→3Galβ1
	→4GlcNAcβ1→3Galβ1→4Glc→Cer
	(2→3 sialyllactonorhexaosylceramide)
2.6 S-i	NeuAc2→6Galβ1→4GlcNAcβ1→3Gal
	β1→4GlcNAcβ1→3Galβ1→4Glc→Cer
	(2→6 sialyllactonorhexaosylceramide)
i(n Oct)	Galβ1→4GlcNAcβ1→3Galβ1→4
	GlcNAcβ1→3Galβ1→4GlcNAcβ1→3Galβ1→4 Glc→Cer
	(lactonoroctaosylceramide)

CLONING OF H6-3C4 PRODUCING GENES (μ AND λ GENES) AND CLASS SWITCHING OF MAB FROM IGM (λ) TO IGG$_1$ (λ)

To stabilize the gene coding for antibody molecules to HSP, the cloning of human chromosomes carrying Ig genes from the human–mouse heterohybridoma H6-3C4 was attempted, because the human chromosome carrying Ig genes in the heterohybridoma often may be deleted from the hybridoma over a long period of cell culture [Komori et al., 1988]. The class switching of mAb H6-3C4 IgM(λ) to IgG$_1$(λ) was essential, because the Ig class of SI Abs raised in most women was found in our recent studies to be IgG$_1$. Fourteen SI-positive sera from sterile women with unknown cause did not competitively inhibit the binding of mAb H6-3C4 to sperm except a donor serum from whom PBL were drawn to make the hybridoma H6-3C4 and another patient's serum. The reason could be that IgM of mAb H6-3C4 possessed stronger affinity to bind sperm than the antibodies of IgG class or that most women recognized different antigenic epitopes of HSP from that corresponding to mAb H6-3C4. The other important reason to make a class-switch IgG$_1$ of mAb H6-3C4 was that the SI Abs secreted to the cervical mucus might be IgG. The rearranged human immunoglobulin μ and λ genes from the human–mouse heterohybridoma H6-3C4, which produced a human mAb to HSP, were isolated. The V region gene of the clone H6-3C4 μ heavy-chain gene was joined to the human Cγ11 region gene, which had been cloned from the human plasma cell leukemia line ARH-77 [Kudo et al., 1985]. The reconstructed genes contained a human heavy-chain enhancer region DNA in J–C intron as a heavy-chain gene-expression-control element. The clone H6-3C4 λ light-chain gene was also joined to the human heavy-chain-enhancer region DNA as a light-chain gene-expression-control element.

This novel heavy-chain gene was integrated into the PSV2gpt vector and transfected into mouse myeloma cell line X63Ag8.653 by protoplast fusion. The resultant stable transformants, which produced human γ heavy chain, then were transfected with the λ chain gene derived from the hybridoma H6-3C4 by electroporation. The stable transformants obtained after selection produced human Ig molecules (γ, λ) that showed human SI activity. The Ig from the stable transformants were assessed by immunoblotting of the proteins in the culture supernatants. After the SDS-PAGE of the culture supernatants, the human Ig molecules with a molecular weight of 160 kd under nonreducing conditions and the 54 kd band of human γ chain and 25 kd band of human λ chain under reducing conditions were observed. The SI activities of the culture supernatants of the transformants were 10–20 SI_{50} units compared with 5,000 SI_{50} units of parental hybridoma. The amount of mAb IgG secreted from the transformants was about 0.2–0.5 μg/ml, whereas the parental hybridoma H6-3C4 secreted 5 to 10 times higher numbers of mAbs.

MONOCLONAL ANTIBODIES TO THE PEPTIDE MOLECULES OF SPERM SURFACE ANTIGENS

Mab 3B2-F7

BALB/c mice were immunized with washed ejaculated human sperm, including SCA, and the spleen cells of immunized mice were fused with mouse myeloma cells P3U1 in the presence of PEG-4000. To select hybridomas secreting mAb to the peptide portion of HSP, the glycosylated HSP was prepared as coating antigens for ELISA. Deglycosylation of HSP with TFMS was performed by the method of Edge et al. [1981]. The TFMS-treated HSP was then treated with neuraminidase, β-N-acetylglycosaminidase, α-N-acetylglycosaminidase, and β-galactosidase. Endoglycosidase D and glycopeptidase A were also used in treatments. As the last step, N-glycanase (Gnzyme) was applied for digestion of TFMS-treated HSP. By TFMS treatment for 8 hr, no low-molecular-weight material stainable by Coomassie blue and periodic Shiff was detected by SDS-PAGE. With ELISA that was coated with a deglycosylated HSP, the supernatants of 11 hybridomas were distinctly positive, and a hybridoma named 3B2-F7 secreting mAb having SI activity was selected after several clonings. To clarify the characteristics of the antigen epitope corresponding to mAb 3B2-F7, the deglycosylated HSP was treated with pronase, protease from bovine pancreas, subtilopeptidase A, and protease of *Streptomyces griseus*. The antigenicity corresponding to the mAb was almost completely destroyed by these enzymes and also partly by trypsin and V8 protease. The antigen epitope corresponding to mAb 3B2-F7 was proved to be an approximately 36 kd molecule as shown by Western blotting after SDS-PAGE. The localization of antigenic epitope corresponding to the mAb in various tissues was examined by ABC staining, and clear staining of the epithelium of human epididymis and sperm in the lumen of caudal epididymis and some staining of testis were observed. As for somatic tissues, the Langerhans islands of pancreas and epithelial cells of distal tubules of the kidney were distinctly stained, and connective tissue was faintly stained. The sperm binding and penetration to human zona pellucida were strikingly blocked when the mAb was added to the IVF system.

Mab 3B10

CBA/n mice, known to be a strain with poor antibody production against carbohydrate antigens, were used for immunization. They were immunized with homogenized washed sperm membrane fragments, and the lymphocytes of immunized mice were fused with mouse myeloma NS-1 cells in the presence of PGE-4000. The hybridomas were selected for secreting antibodies to react with deglycosylated HSP after HAT selection. A hybridoma secreting mAb that showed the strongest reaction with deglycosylated HSP was cloned, and mAb 3B-10 was obtained. The mAb did not show SI and SA activities but indicated a clear blocking effect on sperm binding to human zonae pellucidae. The antigenic epitope was identified in 15 kd molecules of HSP by SDS-PAGE and Western blot procedures. ABC staining indicated that the antigenic epitope was distributed in the testis, epididymis, prostate, connective tissues and trophoblastic tissue of placenta. The mAb did not stain fresh sperm but did stain fixed sperm. Therefore, it could be speculated that the antigenic epitope of peptide might be a sperm membrane intrinsic peptide that is distributed in the germ cells in testis, epithelial cells of epididymis, prostate, and trophoblast cells and connective tissues.

CONCLUSIONS

SI Abs raised in sterile women were found to be polyclonal antibodies against several kinds of sperm antigen, including SCA; thus the production of mAbs was essential to identify and purify an antigen corresponding to each SI Ab.

1   mAb 1C4 with strong SI activity was produced from a rat–mouse heterohybridoma to HSP and characterized as a glycoprotein. The corresponding antigen purified 196 times was identified as HSP No. 7 antigen (Ferrisplan), which shared antigenicity with human milk protein and was found to exist in the spermatocytes, spermatid, and spermatozoa in the testicular tissue and also in the epithelial cells of the seminal vesicle.

2   Mouse mAbs 2C6, 2E5, and 2B6, specific to HSP, possessed strong SI and SA activities; the antigenic epitopes to these mAbs were identified as being composed of carbohydrate moieties including a Gal-GlucNAc structure. mAb 2C6 also inhibited sperm binding to human zona pellucida. The corresponding antigenic epitopes to these mAbs did not exist in the testicular tissue, but appeared in the epithelia of caput, corpus, and caudal epididymis.

3   Human SI mAb H6-3C4 (IgM[λ]) was successfully produced from the human–mouse heterohybridoma that was established by fusing PBL from a sterile woman possessing 45 SI_{50} as SI activity and mouse myeloma cells, after preincubation with washed sperm and PWM. Hybridoma H6-3C4 was very stable and continued to secrete extremely high titers of mAb, 5,000 SI_{50} as SI activity, 1:1,600 dilutions as SA activity for 4 years. The antigenic epitope corresponding to the mAb H6-3C4 was not present in the testis, but existed in the epithelial cells of caudal epididymis and the surface of cells in the seminal vesicle.

4   The chemical structure of the antigenic epitopes to mAb H6-3C4 was identified as unbranched repetitive type 2 neolactosamine regardless of substitution with sialic acid at the terminal region (i blood group antigen and sialyl i blood group antigen).

5   The antigenic epitopes of HSP corresponding to SI mAbs 2C6, 2E5, and 2B6 obtained in our laboratory were composed of carbohydrate structures.

6   Cloning of human chromosomes carrying Ig gene was performed from the hybridoma H6-3C4, and the class switching of mAb H6-3C4 IgM(λ) to IgG_1(λ) was also attempted. Stable transformants were obtained to produce human Ig molecules (γ, λ) that showed human SI activity.

7   There are two mAbs against peptide antigens of sperm surface components, including sperm-coating antigens. mAb 3B2-F7, with weak SI activity, blocked sperm binding to human zonae pellucidae. mAb 3B-10 did not have any SI or SA activities but blocked sperm binding to human zonae pellucidae. The antigenic epitopes corresponding to mAbs 3B2-F7 and 3B-10 existed in germinal cells of testis, epithelial cells of epididymis, and connective tissues.

ACKNOWLEDGMENTS

We are grateful to Dr. S. Hakomori and Dr. T. Watanabe for their kind advice and collaborations. We thank Miss N. Kashiwagi for her kind assistance.

REFERENCES

Bechtol KB, Brown SC, Kennett RH (1979): Recognition of differentiation antigens of spermatogenesis in the mouse by using antibodies from spleen cell–myeloma hybrids after syngeneic immunization. Proc Natl Acad Sci USA 76:363–367.

Edge SB, Faltynek CR, Hof L, Reichert LE Jr, Weber P (1981): Deglycosylation of glycoproteins by trifluoromethanesulfonic acid. Anal Biochem 118:131–137.

Herr JC, Flowler JE, Jr, Howards SS, Sigman M, Sutherland WM, Koons DJ (1985): Human antisperm monoclonal antibodies constructed postvasectomy. Biol Reprod 32:695–711.

Hsu SM, Raine L, Fanger H 91981): A comparative study of the peroxidase-antiperoxidase method and an avidin–biotin complex method for studying polypeptide hormones with radio immunoassay antibodies. Am J Clin Pathol 75:734–738.

Ikeda Y (1987): Establishment of human monoclonal sperm immobilizing antibody by semi-solid culture method. Adv Obstet Gynecol (Jpn) 39:251–259.

Isahakia M, Alexander NJ (1984): Interspecies cross-reactivity of monoclonal antibodies directed against human sperm antigens. Biol Reprod 30:1015–1026.

Isojima S, Kameda K, Tsuji Y, Shigeta M, Ikeda Y, Koyama K (1987); Establishment and characterization of a human hybridoma secreting monoclonal antibody with high titers of sperm immobilizing and agglutinating activities against human seminal plasma. J Reprod Immunol 10:67–78.

Isojima S, Koyama K (1976): Quantitative estimation of sperm immobilizing antibody in the sera of women with sterility of unknown etiology: The 50% sperm immobilization unit (SI_{50}). Excerpta Medica Int Congr Ser 370:11–14.

Isojima S, Koyama K, Fujiwara N (1982): Purification of human seminal plasma No. 7 antigen by immunoaffinity chromatography on bound monoclonal antibody. Clin Exp Immunol 49:449–456.

Isojima S, Koyama K, Shigeta M, Tsuji Y, Kyurkchiev SD, Kameda K, Kubota K (1986): Antibodies to spermatozoa relevant to infertility and purification of the corresponding antigens. In Ludwig H, Thomsen K (eds): Gynecology and Obstetrics. Berlin: Springer-Verlag, pp 717–721.

Isojima S, Li TS, Ashitaka Y (1968): Immunologic analysis of sperm-immobilizing factor found in sera of women with unexplained infertility. Am J Obstet Gynecol 101:677–683.

Isojima S, Tsuchiya K, Koyama K, Tanaka C, Naka O, Adachi H (1972): Further studies on sperm-immobilizing antibody found in sera of unexplained cases of sterility in women. Am J Obstet Gynecol 112:199–207.

Kannagi R, Levery SB, Ishigami F, Hakomori S, Shevinsky LH, Knowles BB, Solter D (1983a): New globoseries glycophospholipids in human teratocarcinoma reactive with the monoclonal antibody directed to a developmentally regulated antigen, stage specific embryonic antigen3. J Biol Chem 258:8934–8942.

Kannagi R, Nudelman E, Levery SB, Hakomori S (1982); A series of human erythrocyte glycosphingolipids reacting to the monoclonal antibody directed to a developmentally regulated antigen, SSEA-1. J Biol Chem 257:14865–14874.

Kannagi R, Stroup R, Cochran NA, Urdal DL, Young Jr WW, Hakomori S (1983b): Factors affecting expression of glycolipid tumor antigens. Influence of ceramide composition and coexisting glycolipid on the antigenicity of gliotraosylceramide in murine lymphoma cells. Cancer Res 43:4997–5005.

Komori S, Yamasaki N, Shigeta M, Isojima S, Watanabe T (1988): Production of heavy-chain class-switch variants of human monoclonal antibody by recombinant DNA technology. Clin Exp Immunol 71:508–516.

Kudo A, Ishihara T, Nishimura Y, Watanabe T (1985): A cloned human immunoglobulin heavy chain gene with a novel direct-repeat sequence in 5′ flanking region. Gene 33:181–189.

Kurpisz M, Simon LL, Alexander NJ (1987): EBV transformation and microfusion as the potential source of human monoclonal anti-sperm antibodies. Am J Reprod Immunol Microbiol 15:61–65.

Kyurkchiev SD, Shigeta M, Koyama K, Isojima S (1986): A human–mouse hybridoma producing monoclonal antibody against human sperm coating antigen. Immunology 57:489–492.

Lee C, Huang Y-S, Huang C-H, Hu PC, Menge AC (1982a): Monoclonal antibodies to human sperm antigens. J Reprod Immunol 4:173–181.

Lee CY, Huang YS, Hu PC, Gomel V, Menge AC (1982b): Analysis of sperm antigens by sodium dodecyl sulfate gel/protein blot radioimmunobinding method. Anal Biochem 123:14–22.

Lehman D, Temminck B, Da Rugna D, Leibundgut B, Muller H (1985): Blot-immunobinding test for the detection of anti-sperm antibodies. J Reprod Immunol 8:329–336.

Magnani JL, Smith DF, Ginsburg V (1980): Detection of gangliosides that bind cholera toxin. Direct binding of ^{125}I-labeled toxin to thin-layer chromatograms. Anal Biochem 109:399–402.

Moore HDM, Hartman TD (1984): Localization by monoclonal antibodies of various surface antigens of hamster spermatozoa and the effect of antibody on fertilization in vitro. J Reprod Fertil 70:175–183.

Naaby-Hansen S, Bjerrum OJ (1985): Auto- and iso-antigens of human spermatozoa detected by immunoblotting with human sera after SDS-PAGE. J Reprod Immunol 7:41–57.

Naz RK, Alexander NJ, Isahakia M, Hamilton MS (1984): Monoclonal antibody to a human germ cell membrane glycoprotein that inhibits fertilization. Science 225:342–344.

O'Rand MG, Irons GP, Porter JP (1984): Monoclonal antibodies to rabbit sperm autoantigens. I. Inhibition of in vitro fertilization and localization on the egg. Biol Reprod 30:721–729.

Primakoff P, Cowan A, Hyatt H, Tredick-Kline J, Myles DG (1988a): Purification of the guinea pig sperm PH-20 antigen and detection of a site-specific endoproteolytic activity in sperm preparations that cleaves PH-20 into two disulfide-linked fragments. Biol Reprod 38:921–934.

Primakoff P, Lathrop W, Woolman L, Cowan A, Myles D (1988b): Fully effective contraception in male and female guinea pigs immunized with the sperm protein PH-20. Nature 335:543–546.

Shapiro M, Erickson RP (1981): Evidence that the serological determinant of H-Y antigens is carbohydrate. Nature 290:503–505.

Shigeta M, Watanabe T, Murayama S, Koyama K, Isojima S (1980): Sperm-immobilizing monoclonal antibody to human seminal plasma antigens. Clin Exp Immunol 42:458–462.

Tsuji Y, Clausen H, Nudelman E, Kaizu T, Hakomori S, Isojima S (1988): Human sperm carbohydrate antigens defined by an antisperm human monoclonal antibody derived from an infertile woman bearing antisperm antibodies in her serum. J Exp Med 168:343–356.

Wolf DP, Sokoloski JE, Dandekar P, Bechtol KB (1983): Characterization of human sperm surface antigens with monoclonal antibodies. Biol Reprod 29:713–723.

DISCUSSION

DR. HECHT: With your H6-3C4 antibody, did it cross-react with any adult tissues?

DR. ISOJIMA: We found an antigen epitope corresponding to mAb H6-3C4 in epithelial cells of the distal tubules of the kidney, on the surface of alveolar cells, and in the basal cells of skin when sensitive ABC staining was used. We also evaluated the blood type I antigen of H, A, and B antigens. If fucose is bound to the terminal galactose of the i structure, it will be blood type H substance. When another GalNAc or galactose is bound to the H type substance, it will be a blood type A or type B substance. Usually red blood cells of the newborn contain a large amount of i antigen, but, in the adult, i antigen in red blood cells is transferred completely to I antigen (branched neolactosamine). Therefore, it's presence may not be surprising; a negligible amount of i antigen is preserved in some somatic tissues. Antibody to i or sialyl i antigens in an adult woman were not harmful to somatic tissues.

DR. DACHEUX: There is a monoclonal antibody obtained in France against trophoblast cells that recognizes capacitated human sperm. So, it seems that trophoblasts have a common antigen with sperm, although I don't know why.

DR. ISOJIMA: As indicated in my presentation, the sialyl i and sialyl I antigens that were coating antigens of live sperm were present on the surface of the human trophoblast. These antigens were still partly preserved even after capacitation and an ionophore-induced acrosome reaction. We have mAbs to trophoblast that immobilize or agglutinate live sperm.

DR. HERR: Do you know the mass of the number of peptides that might be bearing these structures, either in seminal plasma or extracted from sperm? For example, have you done a Western blot with the monoclonal antibody and sperm extracts of seminal vesicle material?

DR. ISOJIMA: You mean the peptide portion carrying the epitopes corresponding to mAb H6-3C4?

DR. HERR: Yes. How many bands are observed by Western blot?

DR. ISOJIMA: When SDS-PAGE was performed with azoospermic semen, antigen epitopes to mAb H6-3C4 were identified as five to six bands between 15 and 25 kd by Western blot, but there was no distinct band except a 17 kd faint band by protein staining. Therefore, our experimental results are not conclusive as to whether the molecules carrying epitopes to mAb H6-3C4 contain a small amount of core peptide or only glycolipid. According to ABC staining with mAb H6-3C4, the epithelial layer in seminal vesicle was stained. Semen from vasectomized men still retained some absorptive capability for SI activity with mAb H6-3C4. Therefore, the antigenic epitopes corresponding to mAb H6-3C4 are mainly secreted from the caudal epididymis, but some could possibly be secreted from the seminal vesicle. We have not yet examined the seminal vesicle extract by Western blot using mAb H6-3C4.

26

Development of Human–Human Antisperm Monoclonal Antibodies

Maciej Kurpisz

The monoclonal antibody technology developed by Kohler and Milstein [1975] provided a tremendous tool for modern immunology generating hybridoma cell lines producing antibodies to given antigenic specificities. This possibility triggered other methods of identification and chemical analysis of the molecules recognized by these antibodies. As a consequence, the high specificity and affinity of the antibodies thus obtained made it possible to recognize molecules and furthered the understanding of their biological role. High-affinity monoclonal antibodies became the critical factor and/or indicator of a wide range of biological tests, significantly increasing the sensitivity of detection of antigenic substances. The basic role of these antibodies remained the same, i.e., the most precise immunological tool for identification of antigen. Thus the monoclonal antibody became essential in all situations in which the correct identification of molecule(s) or cell(s) was of fundamental importance. This role, however, was to be shortly revised when it became clear that the complexity of monoclonal antibody reactions and the reliability of their specificity occurred only in well-defined circumstances.

To understand the interaction of a monoclonal antibody with a given antigen is in the first instance to be able to evaluate its activity to a variety of other substances, i.e., to exclude or to confirm its cross-reactivity.

A significant number of studies had to be done to establish the similarities of surface structures of unrelated cell types. This unfortunately was even more clear while studying the structures of trans-

Gamete Interaction: Prospects for Immunocontraception, pages 377–400
© 1990 Wiley-Liss, Inc.

formed malignant cells, embryonal cell lines, and germ cells. When the monoclonal antibodies in most cases failed to differentiate between these families of cell types, the limitations of contemporary hybridoma technology became evident and the prospective goal of diagnosis and treatment of malignant processes by humoral factors became difficult to achieve. The vast majority of candidate antigens of the reproductive system for targets of immunological attack (alternative means of contraception) were excluded from further studies on the basis of their cross-reactivity. Furthermore, as in the case of the studies of tumor-specific markers, there are serious doubts as to whether we currently possess highly specific monoclonal antibodies to germ cells. Thus the situation after two decades of intensive monoclonal antibodies studies leads us to the conclusion that we overexplored extensively used systems of monoclonal antibody production in rodents without developing satisfactory alternatives. We have therefore to accept the consequences and limitations of genetically coded immunological responses of rodents to antigen. This species predisposition to mount immunological responses against certain privileged structures led us to define the immunodominant epitopes. It seems very probable that the repertoire of mouse humoral response is limited in its spontaneous form, and random trials to obtain new families of specific monoclonal antibodies have a very low chance of success [James, 1987; Kurpisz et al., 1989]. Therefore, another model for generation of monoclonal antibodies (besides rodents) may be potentially very didactic and useful.

The alternative model of generation of antibody-producing cell lines is human hybridomas that can be obtained through the immortalization of antibody-secreting B cells of naturally sensitized human subjects. Human monoclonal antibodies, besides being the alternatives for mouse hybridomas, have also several other advantages.

1   Human monoclonal antibodies may recognize private-specific components of human organisms and/or cells other than those thus far identified by murine antibodies. Antigen purification and epitope mapping by human monoclonal antibodies has been achieved for bacterial [Atlaw et al., 1985], viral (HIV) [Banapour et al., 1987], or parasite organisms (*Plasmodium falciparum* [Schmidt-Ulrich et al., 1986]). Thus we have some reason to hope for human tumor- and/ or germ-specific monoclonal antibodies.

2   Human hybridomas would be a good model for comparative (to rodents) studies of humoral immune response toward particular antigens. They would eventually confirm

obvious differences in the mounting of immunological responses based on genetic differences between the species or alternatively could confirm the universality of certain immunodominant components in mammals for antibody induction. This information could answer questions of immunodominant cross-reactive structures of human sperm [Wunderlich et al., 1981; Kurpisz et al., 1989].

3   Human monoclonal antibodies cannot be replaced by other agents in the study of initiation and onset of autoimmune reactions and disease in human subjects, the role of natural autoantibodies in humans, identification of main families of autoantigens of different autoimmunological syndromes at different phases of autoaggression, and so forth, including the study of reproductive system antigens participating in autoimmune orchitis or natural antisperm antibodies in the female reproductive tract.

4   A big hope of monoclonal antibodies is their therapeutic value to human subjects. Contrary to mouse monoclonals, human ones can be repeateably used without threat of harmful sensitization of the recipient. In addition, although the development of therapeutically effective human antitumor antibodies has been thus far disappointing, there is a hope that human monoclonal antibodies may inhibit disadvantageous reactions at transplantation [Pistillo et al., 1985]. There is also a quite justified expectation for the prospective application of human monoclonal antibodies for passive immunization, for example, for short-term immunocontraception.

Human monoclonal antibodies can be obtained using different approaches: 1) classic fusion of human B cells with a human parental cell line; 2) immortalization of antibody-producing cells using Epstein-Barr virus (EBV) or alternative transforming agents; 3) combination of EBV transformation (preselection of antibody-producing cells) and subsequent fusion; 4) construction of heterohybridomas by fusion of human B cells with mouse myeloma cell lines; and 5) genetic engineering by a) "humanization" of mouse monoclonal antibodies by association of constant heavy chain of human immunoglobulin to mouse variable region (transfectoma), b) construction of heterohybridoma by introduction of human genes coding for variable regions of immunoglobulin into mouse myeloma cell line, and c) transfection of human myeloma cell line with DNA of antibody-secreting cells.

HUMAN–HUMAN HYBRIDOMA AS THE SOURCE OF HUMAN MONOCLONAL ANTIBODIES

The first reports of human–human hybridomas, in 1980 [Croce et al., 1980; Olsson and Kaplan, 1980], described production of human monoclonal antibodies against 2,4-dinitrophenyl-hapten (DNP) and measles virus. The technology was quickly extended to a variety of other antigens [for review, see James and Bell, 1987]. Our attempts to obtain human antisperm monoclonal antibodies by fusing B lymphocytes from vasectomized individuals with a human lymphoblastoid fusion partner did not, however, provide high-affinity antibodies [Kurpisz et al., 1987].

The major problems of existing human–human hybridoma technology are 1) slow growth of human hybridomas, 2) low hybridization frequency, 3) low cloning efficiency, 4) mixed Ig production (spontaneous secretion of immunoglobulins by majority of fusion partner cell lines), and 5) low Ig production. Disadvantageous parameters of parental cell lines used as fusion partners greatly contribute to the above-mentioned inefficiency. The characteristics of the available human parental cell lines are presented in Table 1. Attempts to increase fusion frequency and stability of human hybridomas are possible since the introduction of human tetraploid fusion partners. Other sources suggest the importance of particular cell types taken from lymphoid tissue for human hybridomas [for review, see James and Bell, 1987]. Similarly, it seems that lymphoid cells from spleen, tonsils, or lymph nodes as in mice make better fusion partners than peripheral blood lymphocytes, although the latter for practical and ethical considerations will continue to be the main source for human monoclonal antibody production in the foreseeable future.

THE EBV TRANSFORMATION AS THE SOURCE OF HUMAN MONOCLONAL ANTIBODIES

The Epstein-Barr discovery is associated with two findings, i.e., the description of endemic lymphoma among children in Africa by Burkitt [1962] and the subsequent identification of the virus in cultures of lymphoma cells by Epstein [Epstein et al., 1964]. EBV was the fifth human herpesvirus to be discovered. It was soon found that in vitro EBV infects only primate lymphocytes of the immunoglobulin-producing or B-lymphocyte series [Henle et al., 1967]. The C3d receptor (complement receptor type 2) serves as the surface structure binding for EBV [Weis et al., 1986]. After infection with EBV, lym-

TABLE 1. Main Types of Currently Used Human Fusion Partners

Original cell type	Cell line	No. of clones per 10^7 cells	Percent hybrids per 100 wells	References
Human myeloma	SK0-007 RPMI-8226	1.5	38	Olsson and Kaplan [1980]
		—	—	Matsuoko et al. [1967] Pickering and Gelder [1982]
Human leukemia	LICR-LON-HMy2	7.0	17	Edwards et al. [1982]
Human lymphoblastoid	GM-1500 GM-4672	— 1.0	— —	Croce et al. [1980] Shoenfeld et al. [1982]
	GK-5	—	—	Dwyer et al. [1983]
	UC-729/HF-2	—	46	Glassy et al. [1983] Levy et al. [1983]
	UC-729-6	12.0	51	Glassy et al. [1983]
	LTR228	—	—	Larrick et al. [1983] Levy et al. [1983]
	H35.1.1	—	—	Choivazzi et al. [1982]
Human B cell lymphoma	RH-L4	—		Olsson et al. [1983]
Human–human tetraploid	KR-12 = KR4+RPMI-8226			Kozbor et al. [1984]
Mouse myeloma	NS-1	50.0	80	Levy and Dilley [1978] Abrams et al. 1983]

phocytes express at least one new antigen, called EBV nuclear antigen (EBNA) [Pope et al., 1971]. EBV stimulates DNA synthesis in infected cells about 20 hr after EBNA synthesis begins, i.e., approximately 24–36 hr after exposure to virus [Einhorn and Ernberg, 1978], while the DNA synthesized during transformation is predominantly cellular [Gerber and Hoyer, 1971]. It is believed that the transformation that occurs about 72 hr after inoculation involves the integration of the EBV genome into the host genome [Strominger and Thorley-Lawson, 1979].

Shortly after EBV identification, Epstein and Barr reported the first successful attempts to establish continuous lymphoblastoid cell lines

[Epstein and Barr, 1964] by use of the virus. More than a decade passed before it was realized that EBV can cause polyclonal activation and immortalization of antibody-producing human B cells [Rosen et al., 1977].

Steinitz and coworkers [1977] were the first to recognize that this capability could be used to establish permanent cell lines to produce human antibodies of predetermined specificity. Varieties of human monoclonal antibodies were soon obtained using this approach [for review, see James and Bell, 1987]. Among others, EBV-transformed B lymphocytes synthesizing human antisperm antibodies have been generated [Winger et al., 1983; Kurpisz et al., 1987]. In the first attempt [Winger et al., 1983], EBV transformation was undertaken on a purified B-lymphocyte population (depletion of T cells was performed using the rosette technique with sheep red blood cells [SRBC] pretreated with 2-amino-ethylisothiouronium bromide hydrobromide with subsequent Percoll separation of rosetting from nonrosetting cells). Then, the enrichment of antigen-specific cells was performed using the method of B-cell adherence on coated sea urchin sperm [Winger et al., 1983], known as the panning technique. Finally, a number of EBV-transformed cell lines producing antisperm antibodies detected by enzyme-linked immunosorbent assay (ELISA) and immunofluorescence were generated. The resultant antibodies represented both the IgM and IgG classes and reacted to sea urchin, mouse, boar, and human sperm.

In our hands, we obtained successful EBV transformation of human cell lines producing antisperm antibodies using as well purified B-lymphocyte subpopulations as mononuclear cell suspensions (Tables 2, and 3). Vasectomized individuals sensitized to their own sperm donated peripheral blood for these experiments.

As was seen in these experiments, the mononuclear leukocyte suspensions can be used with EBV infection to produce antisperm antibodies in limiting dilution culture conditions without T-cell depletion. After 2 weeks, the number of positive wells for antisperm antibody production was even higher than that obtained in a similar experiment for B cells (Table 2). A week later, however, a dramatic decrease in the number of positive wells was observed (Table 3), and percentages of EBV-infected mononuclear leukocytes positive for antisperm antibody production approximated those obtained with purified B lymphocytes. Interestingly, the presence of cyclosporin A alone in the limiting dilution culture did not increase the number of wells with antisperm antibodies. These two observations (comparative number of antisperm antibody producers in culture of EBV-infected mononuclear leukocytes or EBV-transformed B lymphocytes

TABLE 2. EBV Infection of B Lymphocytes and Antisperm Antibody Production

Treatment before infection[a]	Percent antibody-positive cultures			
	1 week[b]	2 weeks	3 weeks	6 weeks
None	2.1	2.9	1.9	1.0
Stimulation with 5 μg/ml DTT sperm extract	2.1	2.9	N.D.	1.7
Stimulation with 10 μg/ml DDT sperm extract	5.2	5.0	N.D.	0.6

[a]Human lymphocytes were T-cell depleted (T cells were removed by rosette formation with neuraminidase-treated SRBC followed by Ficoll-Hypaque gradient separation), infected immediately with EBV, and placed in limiting dilution cultures (10^1 to 10^5 cells/well) with irradiated umbilical cord lymphocytes or cultured for 72 hr with DTT extract of sperm (sperm pellet was treated with 0.4 mM dithiothreitol and then sonicated) before fractionation, infection, and plating.
[b]Time of screening after infection using whole sperm as the target in the ELISA.

TABLE 3. EBV Transformation of Mononuclear Cell Suspension and Antisperm Antibody Production: Effect of Cyclosporin A and Feeder Cells on Transformation

Cyclosporin A[a]	Cord blood lymphocytes[a]	Percent antibody-positive cultures		
		1 week[b]	2 weeks	3 weeks
−	−	2.1	7.5	1.5
−	+	1.9	1.2	0.8
+	−	1.9	4.6	0.8
+	+	4.2	4.6	1.7

[a]Mononuclear cells were exposed to EBV and then placed in limiting dilution cultures with or without 2 μg/ml cyclosporin A with or without irradiated cord blood lymphocytes.
[b]Limiting dilution cultures were screened 1, 2, and 3 weeks following infection using a whole-sperm ELISA.

and lack of advantageous effect of cyclosporin A in culture) seem to challenge the hypothesis of cyclosporin A control over the T-suppressor cell-negative effect on EBNA-positive cells [Bird et al., 1981]. In fact, it has been shown recently that cyclosporin A inhibits the development of mature single positive ($CD4^+8^-$ or $CD4^-8^+$) T cells without affecting the $CD4^-8^-$ TCR-positive cells (TCR—T cell receptor) and may have induced autoimmunological reactions [Jenkins et al., 1988].

The EBV transformation may be potentially the simplest way of obtaining human monoclonal antibodies, but the number of antibody-producing cells decreases with the time of culture; furthermore, there were only a few wells repeatedly positive for antisperm antibody production. Thus after several years of experience with this technique we list the main disadvantages of this methodology:

1   The low stability of EBV-transformed antibody-producing cell lines
2   The low level of immunoglobulin production (<1 μg/ml)
3   The rapid decrease of antibody production with time (especially for IgG)
4   Difficulties in cloning

To overcome these problems, alternative methods of B-cell transformation or fusion of EBV-infected B cell line with available cell partners must be explored.

Recently, two other methods of lymphocyte transformation became available. One of them is a variation of EBV infection [Stevenson et al., 1986], which can also be used by B-cell precursors. In this method, the lymphoblastoid cell line is established by transfection of lymphocytes with purified viral DNA of B95-8 (EB) strain enclosed in fusogenic Sendai virus envelope (RSVE) and subsequent exposure of the cells to EBV from a P3HR-1 cell line (HR-1–nontransforming EB strain). The cell line thus obtained is positive for EBV DNA (incomplete genome) but does not express EBNA. The other approach was the successful transfection of human peripheral blood lymphocytes with DNA from mouse cytoplasts (from the L929 cell line) [Abken et al., 1988]. The transfection induced proliferation of lymphocytes and the formation of B- and T-cell-derived cell lines with unlimited growth potential. The cell lines that can be grown in serum-containing media as well as in chemically defined serum-free media have a nearly normal human karyotype and do not express the malignant phenotype. Whether these forms of cell transformation will provide better stability and higher immunoglobulin production of antibody-producing cells remains to be evaluated.

HUMAN MONOCLONAL ANTIBODY PRODUCTION BY EBV TRANSFORMATION OF HUMAN LYMPHOCYTES FOLLOWED BY FUSION WITH IMMORTAL PARTNER LINES

Kozbor and coworkers [1982] successfully combined the techniques of transformation and cell fusion to produce hybridomas secreting antibodies directed against tetanus toxoid. Thus produced human hybridomas resulted in enhanced stability and antibody secretion, as well as in increased rates of hybrid recovery when com-

TABLE 4. Activity of Human–Human Antisperm Monoclonal
Antibodies: Sperm Agglutination and Sperm
Immobilization Assays

Techniques used for immortalization	Antibody source	Sperm immobilization	Sperm agglutination
Parent myeloma (negative control)	Supernatant concentrate[a]	Negative	Negative
Microfusion of EBV-infected B cells with lymphoblastoid cells	Superantant concentrate[a]	>1/64	1/80
Microfusion of EBV-infected B cells with lymphoblastoid cells	Supernatant concentrate[a]	>1/64	1/40
Fusion of peripheral blood B cells with lymphoblastoid cells	Ascites fluid culture super-natant	>1/64 >1/8	1/2,560 1/10

[a]10 ×- $(NH_4)_2SO_4$ concentrate of culture supernatant.

pared with the use of untransformed lymphocytes [for reviews, see Roder et al., 1985, Larrick et al., 1985]. Since then, with this technique a variety of antibodies have been produced to different antigens [for reviews, see Crawford, 1985; Larrick et al., 1985; Roder et al., 1985; James and Bell, 1987]. We modified this method to obtain human monoclonal antisperm antibodies [Kurpisz et al., 1987]. The activities of produced antisperm antibodies were tested in sperm functional assays (Table 4).

To improve chances of fusion of preselected EBV-infected antibody-producing cells with immortal cell partners, we introduced a microfusion technique that took place in the original microplate well positive for antibody production. Another possibility to improve the fusion outcome would be to apply a recently developed electrofusion method. Ultrashort pulses of electricity can make the cell membranes fuse [Zimmerman, 1982]. This technique has also been used to produce hybridomas [Bischoff et al., 1982; Vienken et al., 1983; Vienken and Zimmerman, 1985] and with some success for human hybridomas [Bischoff et al., 1982]. Since it was reported [Vienken and Zimmerman, 1985] with murine cells that electrofusion gave approximately one hybrid from 3×10^4 lymphocytes (yields comparable with the best results obtained with PEG [polyethylene glycol]), the electrofusion technique became a very interesting alternative to explore.

A better hybridization frequency is obtained with fusion of EBV-infected cells with immortal cell partners rather than those obtained from peripheral blood lymphocytes. For example, the hybridization frequency of lymphoblastoid cells with KR-4 was 1×10^{-5} whereas for nontransformed lymphocytes, only 4×10^{-7} [Kozbor et al., 1982]. Also the values obtained for human monoclonal antisperm antibodies in sperm functional tests are clearly better (Table 4) when obtained with the EBV-hybridoma approach.

Overall, there are several advantages of the EBV hybridoma technique over the other discussed methods of human monoclonal antibodies production. It 1) preselects antibody-producing cells prior to fusion; 2) provides relatively high fusion frequences (1 for 10^{-5}); 3) provides relatively high levels of immunoglobulin production (up to 100 μg/ml); and 4) provides the chance for longer maintenance of antibody production (although frequent recloning is sometimes necessary). However, there are also some disadvantages: 1) human monoclonal antibodies derived by the EBV hybridoma method are predominantly of IgM class; 2) the majority of currently used human fusion cell partners are immunoglobulin secretors (e.g., the widely used KR-4 line interferes with specific antibody production, secreting its own IgG-k); and 3) the in vivo use of products produced by EBV-transformed cells may be hazardous because of the presence of virus or transforming DNA. These disadvantages of the EBV hybridoma technique can in fact be overcome. The simplest way to produce human EBV hybridomas secreting IgG antibodies would be earlier preselection of EBV-infected antibody-producing cells according to the class of immunoglobulin [Cole et al., 1984]. In blood donors with few positive cells, however, that approach may not be relevant. Rather, the possibility of a spontaneous switch of immunoglobulin class that occurs in vitro with the frequency of one variant among 10^5–10^7 cells could be explored. The two approaches that can be successfully used for switched clone selection are fluorescence-activated cell sorting and sib selection [Aguila et al., 1986]. The sib selection technique applies ELISA for detection of immunoglobulin class. Detection of the spontaneous switch of immunoglobulin class out of relatively high numbers of microcultures with an initial cell concentration of 1,000 cells per well can be accomplished. In case of detection of an IgG class variant, the cell concentration may be gradually lowered, replating interesting wells at a concentration of 100 cells per well, then 10 cells per well, and then cloning. The obtained specific human monoclonal antibodies have to be additionally purified, separating them from spontaneously secreting antibodies. This can be easily done if the class or subclass of specific antibody is different from the one secreted by the fusion partner. In other cases, nonsecreting fusion partner lines, e.g., HFB 1 (human myeloma) [Hunter et al., 1982] or RH-L4 [Olsson et al., 1983], could be used. Alternatively, tetraploid immortal cell lines (described in another section) are available. The concern about the potential hazard of EBV particles produced in antibodies from the EBV hybridoma technique was overcome in a clinical experiment in which Watson and coworkers [1983] devised a chamber for human hybridoma in vivo growth. This chamber was implanted subcutaneously into the abdominal wall of a patient with an advanced malignant glioma. Human hybridoma cells producing antibodies that react with malignant gliomas [Sikora et al., 1982] and derived initially from this particular patient's lymphocytes, were placed in this chamber. The hybridoma cells expressed EBNA, but did not secrete the virus.

Thus, although we successfully challenged the existing disadvantages of EBV hybridoma technology, this technique, like the other alternatives for human monoclonal antibody production, does not solve the two basic problems with all human hybridoma systems: 1) the lack of adequate numbers of antigen-specific B cells and, 2) the low affinity of human MAbs.

STRATEGIES TO IMPROVE CURRENTLY EXISTING HUMAN HYBRIDOMA TECHNOLOGY FOR LOW SENSITIZED HUMAN SUBJECTS

In Vivo Immunization

Although practical and ethical considerations have hampered human monoclonal antibody development, human lymphocytes immune to a range of target antigens after active in vivo challenge have been obtained [for review, see James and Bell, 1987]. These include bacterial, viral, parasite, blood group (rhesus D), and even some tumor antigens, e.g., vaccination with irradiated cultured melanoma cells [Irie et al., 1979]. Undoubtedly, this procedure increases the number of antigen-specific cells and antibody affinity. However, the same ethical reasons do not allow stimulation of individuals with autoimmune syndromes that could lead to increased pre-existing auto- (or iso-) sensitization (sperm-sensitized individuals should be classified to this category).

In Vitro Immunization

In an effort to circumvent the problem of obtaining suitable immune lymphocytes from donors, increasing attention is being de-

TABLE 5. Human Monoclonal Antibodies Produced by the In Vitro Immunization[a]

Antigen	Lymphoid tissue	Additional in vitro conditions	Dose (µg/ml)	References
Cells				
SRBC	PBL tonsil	PWM, AB serum	0.1[b]	Strike et al. [1984]
Allogeneic	Spleen	B- and T-cell fractionation, T-cell irradiation, PWM, irradiated allogeneic stimulators	1:1	Hulette et al. [1987]
Peptides/proteins				
Tetanus toxoid	Spleen, tonsil	Mixture adherent and non-adherent cells, conditioned media, AB serum	0.6	Ho et al. [1985] Ho [1987]
Acid phosphatase	Spleen	PWM, then T-cell depleted	0.1	Yamaura et al. [1985]
Haptens				
Azophenylarso- nate	Spleen, tonsil	T-cell-depleted, PWM, and T-cell-irradiated feeder	1–10	Wasserman et al. [1986]
DNP, sperm whale myoglobin	Spleen	T-cell-depleted, LPS, MDP, PHA, *Staphylococcus aureus* Cowan I	1–10	Bieber and Teng [1987]
Tumor antigens				
Melanoma p97	PBL	T-cell-depleted, Leu- OMe treatment	1.0	Borrebaeck et al. [1988]

[a]DNP, dinitrophenyl; PBL, peripheral blood lymphocytes; PWM, pokeweed mitogen; LPS, lipopolysaccharide; MDP, muramyl dipeptide, PHA, phytohemagglutinin, Leu-OMe, L-leucin methyl ester.
[b]Percent (v/v) suspension of SRBC (sheep red blood cells).

voted to in vitro methods of sensitization and amplification of specific B-cell responses. Examples of these procedures are illustrated in Table 5.

A variety of techniques have been used in addition to the main scheme of in vitro antigenic sensitization. This indicates that there is no universal scheme for such procedures. Moreover, the parallel in vitro immunization of human peripheral blood lymphocytes (PBLs)

TABLE 6. Effect of In Vitro Lymphocyte Stimulation on Antisperm Antibody Production by EBV-Infected Cells[a]

		Percent of cultures positive for antibody reacting in an ELISA against	
Exp.	In vitro stimulation before infection	Whole sperm	DTT extract of sperm
1	None; 10 μg/ml DTT sperm extract for	2.9	0.6
	72 hours	5.0	3.3
2	None; 10 μg/ml DTT sperm extract for	4.4	2.0
	10 days	1.3	2.8

[a]Human lymphocytes were T-cell depleted by sheep red blood cell rosette formation followed by Ficoll-Hypaque gradient separation and placed in limiting dilution cultures with irradiated umbilical cord lymphocytes. Dithiothreitol (DTT) extract was prepared by adding 0.4 mM of DTT to the sperm pellet with subsequent sonication.

and human splenocytes against the same antigens, e.g., tetanus toxoid [Ho, 1987] or DNP [Bieber and Teng, 1987], generally confirmed the superior performance of the latter. The splenocytes (which, as indicated earlier, have better fusion frequencies) cannot be realistically considered as candidates for in vitro manipulation from sperm-sensitized individuals.

There is, however, one encouraging exception in respect to in vitro sensitization of human peripheral blood lymphocytes, i.e., the in vitro immunization against melanoma antigen with prior application of the lysomotropic agent Leu-OMe [Borrebaeck et al., 1988]. L-amino acid esters have the ability to diffuse freely into the lysosomes of human monocytes, macrophages, and cytolytic cells [Goldman and Kaplan, 1973; Shau and Golub, 1985]. When the lysosome-rich subpopulations of human peripheral blood lymphocytes were removed by treatment with the Leu-OMe, the remaining cells responded vigorously to antigen challenge in vitro.

Our attempts at in vitro lymphocyte sensitization to sperm are presented in Table 6. Although previously stimulated peripheral blood lymphocytes acquire better fusion abilities and antigen-specific sensitization [Smith and Teng, 1987], this may not be universally true, e.g., B lymphocytes prior to EBV infection. Stimulated lymphocytes are transformed with very low efficiency [Henderson et al., 1977]. Furthermore (Table 6), the 10-day stimulation with the sperm antigens (meant to be applied as long as it is necessary for back transformation of blast cells to the small lymphocyte stage) did not effectively improve the frequency of antisperm antibody-producing clones. The 3 days of stimulation with sperm extract, however, improved the frequency of positive wells for antisperm antibody production (Tables 2, 6). We therefore confirm earlier results [Ho, 1987] indicating that, with some antigens, the in vitro stimulation may enrich a population of specific B lymphocytes. This is not, however, a general phenomenon [Burnett et al., 1985]. Unfortunately, the affinity of antibodies secreted after stimulation with sperm extract B cells was not improved (unpublished data).

Cytokine Growth Factors

Additional procedures with a variety of conditioned media, mitogenic-induced cytokines, and so forth, have been used to improve human monoclonal antibody production (Table 5). In some reports, growth factors have been used to enhance fusion frequency, B-cell sensitization, or level of antibody production [Bieber and Teng, 1987; Ho, 1987; Smith and Teng, 1987]. The conflicting results may be due to the low purity of the cytokines and/or to a relatively poor knowledge of their influence on immunoglobulin secretion [McCormack and Cunningham, 1988; Snapper and Paul, 1988; Stevens et al., 1988]. It has been known, for example, that the T_H cell lines induce the secretion of IgM and IgG_3 [Stevens et al., 1988] by IL-3 and granulocyte–monocyte colony-stimulating factor (GM-CSF) production. Furthermore T_{H1} (HDK-1) produces interleukin-2 (IL-2) and γ-interferon (γ-IFN) thus enhancing antigen-specific IgG_{2a} production, whereas, with the T_{H2} cell line (T-286), the IL-4 (BSF-1, B-cell-stimulatory factor) and IL-5 enhance IgG_1 and IgA secretion [Stevens et al., 1988]. γ-IFN stimulates IgG_{2a} isotype and inhibits the production of IgG_3, IgG_1, IgG_{2b}, and IgE, whereas IL-4 promotes switching to IgG_1 and IgE but markedly inhibits IgM, IgG_3, IgG_{2a}, and IgG_{2b} production [Snapper and Paul, 1988]. Furthermore, the ILs act as reciprocal regulatory agents. In our hands, use of ILs did not improve the switching frequency of our IgM-producing human–human hybridoma (antisperm antibodies) to IgG class, and they did not significantly increase IgG production by our EBV-infected antisperm antibody-producing cell lines (unpublished data). There was, however a successful attempt to promote IgM secretion by our human–human antisperm hybridoma with IL-2 (Fig. 1).

The activity of our supernatants was related to immunoglobulin concentration (RIA results obtained from a standard curve of coated μ heavy chains). After addition of IL-2 to the culture, immunoglobulin levels up to 25 μg/ml were achieved (about 10-fold higher than that produced by untreated hybridomas). This observation con-

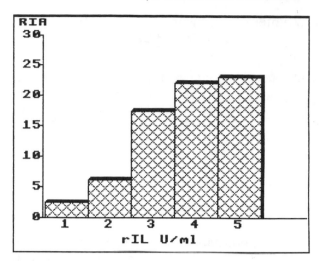

Fig. 1. Histogram showing the effect of increased recombinant IL-2 (rIL-2) concentrations on sperm-binding activity of human–human hybridoma culture supernatants (cpm × 10^{-2}) determined by radioimmunoassay (RIA). The bars indicate 1, background control value; 2, no rIL-2; 3, 50 U/ml rIL-2; 4, 500 U/ml rIL-2; 5, 1,000 U/ml rIL-2. Values represent the average of several independent determinations.

firmed similar results obtained with other IgM-producing human–human hybridomas [McCormack and Cunningham, 1988].

Feeder Cells

The action of cytokines used to enhance secretion of certain immunoglobulin isotypes can be greatly enhanced by feeder layers [for review, James and Bell, 1987]. The main cell types used to maintain human–human hybridoma growth or EBV-infected cell lines are presented in Table 7.

We have found a superior performance of cord blood lymphocytes for human–human hybridoma growth or EBV-infected cell lines [Kurpisz et al., 1987], confirming earlier reports [Stein et al., 1983; Stein and Sigal, 1983]. Xenogeneic mouse feeder cells can also be used with some success especially by combining thymocytes with cells from the peritoneal exudate (unpublished data). The possible synergism between cytokine addition and feeder cell type, however, remains to be evaluated.

SCID–hu mice

The use of SCID mice for human–human hybridoma technology is intriguing. These mice have a severe combined immunodeficiency

TABLE 7. Maintenance of Human–Human Hybrid Growth and
EBV-Infected Cell Lines

Cell system used	Main cell types
Allogeneic (autologous)	Cord blood lymphocytes, peripheral blood leukocytes, peripheral blood T cells, peripheral blood monocytes, lymphoblastoid cell lines
Embryonic (allogeneic)	Fibroblasts, lung fibroblasts, kidney, lung, amnion, melanoma
Xenogeneic	Mouse thymocytes, splenocytes, peritoneal exudate

and are unable to mount an effective cellular or humoral response [McCune et al., 1988]. Thus they can be reconstituted with different human cell types and/or tissues. Some data also suggest [McCune et al., 1988] that SCID mice can support human B-cell differentiation, although this may reflect the survival of transplanted mature B cells that then differentiate into plasma cells. Evidence for differentiation of mature human B cells in SCID mice in response to immunization with tetanus toxoid was described by others [Mosier et al., 1988]. If this is so, it should also be possible to introduce the immortalized EBV-infected antibody-producing cell lines to SCID mice. Because in situ hybridoma cell growth appears to be superior to other types of cultures, we would expect to obtain a substantial increased level of immunoglobulin production with perhaps even enhanced affinity.

HETEROMYELOMAS AS AN ALTERNATIVE SOURCE OF HUMAN ANTIBODY PRODUCTION

The problems of fusing lymphocytes with human partners has encouraged several groups to fuse with mouse myelomas instead [Wunderlich et al., 1981; Astaldi et al., 1982]. A variety of human monoclonal antibodies have been produced using this technique [for review, see James and Bell, 1987], taking advantage of better fusion frequency and better immunoglobulin production than human–human hybridomas. This method became especially popular for human monoclonal antisperm antibody production [Herr et al., 1985; Kyurkchiev et al., 1986; Isojima et al., 1987; Tsuji et al., 1988]. Most reports, however, detected sperm coating rather than integral sperm antigens [Kyurkchiev et al., 1986; Isojima et al., Tsuji et al., 1988]. However, one such monoclonal antibody [Isojima et al., 1987; Tsuji

TABLE 8. Interspecies Hybrids Used as the Fusion Partners for Human Monoclonal Antibody Production

Fusion partner	Original line	Cell type	Secreted Ig	References
SHM-D3	U266 × 63-Ag-8.653	m/h hybrid myeloma	Nonsecretor	Teng et al. [1983]
SBC-H20	B cell × SP2/08 A2	m/h hybrid myeloma	Nonsecretor	Foung et al. [1985]
3 HL	SHM-D3 × B lymphoma	m/h/h hybrid myeloma	IgM (λ)	Teng et al. [1985]
HM-5	P3-X63-Ag8; UI × h lymphocyte × h lymphocyte	m/h/h hybrid myeloma	Nonsecretor	Ichimori et al. [1985]

m, mouse; h, human.

et al., 1988] has allowed the molecular characterization of a recognized epitope. There are two main disadvantages of heteromyeloma systems.

1 Loss of human chromosomes from such hybrids often occurs. Individual mouse–human hybrids show considerable karyotypic heterogeneity [Lane and Fauci, 1983], and frequent recloning is apparently necessary to minimize karyotypic drift and maintain human antibody secretion. The reported instability of heteromyelomas may also be overcome by using recently established interspecies hybrids as fusion partners (Table 8).

2 Post-translational modification of human monoclonal antibodies made in interspecies hybridoma cells could render them immunogenic and, therefore, less useful than human monoclonal antibodies produced from an entirely human cell.

GENETIC ENGINEERING

Humanization of Mouse Monoclonals

Morrison and coworkers [1984] have engineered chimeric immunoglobulin chains, consisting of the binding sites (V) of the mouse myeloma protein combined with the constant region (C) of human immunoglobulin. Chimeric light- and heavy-chain genes were con-

structed, inserted into plasmid vectors, and then sequentially transfected into mouse myeloma cells. Furthermore, the affinity/specific-
ity as well as the isotype can be changed by site-directed mutagenesis
[Roberts et al., 1987].

Genetic Construction of Heterohybridomas

Recently, genes coding for the variable regions of a human antitetanus antibody were cloned and expressed in the mouse myeloma
cell line SP 2/0 along with promoter and enhancer sequences [Gillies
et al., 1983]. The resultant stable transfected myeloma cell line secretes much greater amounts of antibody than the original hetero-
hybrid, and antibodies obtained apparently exhibit unchanged biological properties. This technology has also been explored to obtain
antibodies against sperm [Komori et al., 1988]. In this approach, a
genetic switch from the antibody isotype IgM to IgG was applied.

Genetic Construction of Human–Human Hybridomas

Current methods include 1) transfection of specific antibody-secreting B-cell lines with tumor-cell-derived DNA and 2) the transfection of permanent myeloma cell lines with DNA from antibody-
secreting cell lines [Strelkauskas et al., 1987] to obtain human–human
hybridomas. Construction of analogous systems to produce human
antisperm antibodies should only be a matter of time.

FINAL REMARKS

The exploitation of human monoclonal antibody technology is still
in its early stage, although the amount of fundamental information
about B-cell proliferation, differentiation, and transformation is extensive. It also provides a model for the study of the control of
antibody gene expression and the relationship between antibody
structure and function. Perhaps with the application of human
monoclonal antibody production to medical treatment, we will learn
more about diagnosis and immunological therapy, as well as immunocontraception.

REFERENCES

Abken H, Butzler C, Willecke K (1988): Immortalization of human lymphocytes by transfection with DNA from mouse L929 cytoplasts. Proc Natl Acad Sci USA 85:468–472.

Abrams PG, Knost JA, Clarke G, Wilburn S, Oldham RK, Foon KA (1983): Determination of the optimal human cell lines for development of human hybridomas. J Immunol 131: 1201.

Aguila HL, Pollock RR, Spira G, Schraff MD (1986): The production of more useful monoclonal antibodies. Immunol Today 7:380–383.

Astaldi GCB, Wright EP, Willems C, Zeijlemaker WP, Janssen MC (1982): Increase of hybridoma formation by human lymphocytes after stimulation in vitro: Effect of antigen, endothelial cells and PWM. J Immunol 128:2539.

Atlaw T, Kozbor F, Roder JC (1985): Human monoclonal antibodies against *Mycobacterium leprae*. Infect Immun 49:104.

Banapour B, Rosenthal K, Rabin L, Sharma V, Young L, Fernandez J, Engleman E, McGrath M, Reys G, Lifson J (1987): Characterisation and epitope mapping of a human monoclonal antibody reactive with the envelope glycoprotein of human immunodeficiency virus. J Immunol 139:4027.

Bieber M, Teng NHH (1987): In vitro sensitization for the production of human monoclonal antibodies. In Strelkauskas AJ (ed): Human Hybridomas: Diagnostic and Therapeutic Applications. New York: Marcel Dekker, pp 39–46.

Bird AG, McLachan SM, Britten S (1981): Cyclosporin A promotes the spontaneous outgrowth in vitro of Epstein-Barr virus induced B cell lines. Nature 289:300.

Bischoff R, Eisert RM, Schedel J, Vienken J, Zimmerman U (1982): Human hybridoma cells produced by electro-fusion. FEBS Lett 147:64.

Borrebaeck CAK, Danielsson L, Moller SA (1988): Human monoclonal antibodies produced by primary in vitro immunization of peripheral blood lymphocytes. Proc Natl Acad Sci USA 85:3995–3999.

Burkitt DP (1962): A tumor safari in East and Central Africa. Br J Cancer 16:379–386.

Burnett KG, Leund JP, Martinis J (1985): Human monoclonal antibodies to defined antigens. In Engleman EG, Foung SKH, Larrick J, Raubitschek AA (eds): Human Hybridomas and Monoclonal Antibodies. New York: Plenum press.

Choirazzi N, Wasserman RL, Kinkel HG (1982): Use of Epstein-Barr virus–transformed B-cell lines for the generation of immunoglobulin-producing human B-cell hybridomas. J Exp Med 156:930.

Cole SP, Campling BG, Louwan IH, Kozbor D, Roder JC (1984): A strategy for the production of human monoclonal antibodies reactive with lung tumor cell lines. Cancer Res 44:2750–2754.

Crawford DH (1985): Production of human monoclonal antibodies using Epstein–Barr virus. In Engleman EG, Foung SKH, Larrick J, Raubitschek AA (eds): Human Hybridomas and Monoclonal Antibodies. New York: Plenum Press.

Croce CM, Linnenbach A, Hall W, Steplewski Z, Koprowski H (1980): Production of human hybridomas secreting antibodies to measles virus. Nature 288:488.

Dwyer DS, Bradley RJ, Urguhart CK, Kearny JF (1983): Naturally occurring anti-idiotypic antibodies in myasthenia gravis patients. Nature 301:611.

Edwards PAW, Smith CM, Neville AM, O'Hare MJ (1982): A human–human hybridoma system based on fast-growing mutant of the ARH-77 plasma cell leukemia-derived line. Eur J Immunol 12:641.

Einhorn L, Ernberg I (1978): Induction of EBNA precedes the first cellular S-phase after EBV infection of human lymphocytes. Int J Cancer 21:157–160.

Epstein MA, Achong BG, Barr Y (1964): Virus particles in cultured lymphoblasts from Burkitt's lymphoma. Lancet 1:702–703.

Epstein MA, Barr YM (1964): Cultivation in vitro of human lymphoblasts from Burkitt's malignant lymphoma. Lancet 1:252–253.

Foung SKH, Perkins S, Arvin A, Lifson J, Mohagheghpour N, Fishwild D, Grumet FC, Engleman EG (1985): Production of human monoclonal antibodies using a human mouse fusion partner. In Engleman EG, Foung SKH, Larrick J, Raubitschek A (eds): Human Hybridomas and Monoclonal Antibodies. New York: Plenum Press, p 135.

Gerber P, Hoyer B (1971): Induction of cellular DNA synthesis in human leukocytes by Epstein-Barr virus. Nature 231:46–47.

Gillies SD, Morrison SL, Oi VT, Tonegawa S (1983): A tissue specific transcription enhancer element is located in the major intron of a rearranged immunoglobulin heavy chain gene. Cell 33:717.

Glassy MC, Handley HH, Hagiwara H, Royston I (1983): UC 729-6, a human lymphoblastoid B-cell line useful for generating antibody-secreting human–human hybridomas. Proc Natl Acad Sci USA 80:6327–6331.

Goldman R, Kaplan A (1973): Rupture of rat liver lysosomes mediated by L-amino esters. Biochim Biophys Acta 318:205–216.

Henle W, Diehl V, Kohn G, zur Hausen H, Henle G (1967): Herpes-type virus and chromosome marker in normal leukocytes after growth with irradiated Burkitt cells. Science 157:1064–1065.

Henderson E, Robinson J, Frank A, Miller G (1977): Epstein-Barr virus transformation of lymphocytes separated by size or exposed to bromodeoxyuridine and light. Virology, 82:196–205.

Herr JC, Fowler JE, Howards SS, Sigman M, Sutherland WM, Koons DJ (1985): Human antisperm monoclonal antibodies constructed postvasectomy. Biol Reprod 32:695–711.

Ho M-K (1987): Production of human monoclonal antibodies by in vitro immunisation. In Strelkauskas AJ (ed): Human Hybridomas: Diagnostic and Therapeutic Applications. New York: Marcel Dekker, pp 23–38.

Ho M-K, Rand N, Murray J, Kato K, Rabin H (1985): In vitro immunisation of human lymphocytes. 1. Production of human monoclonal antibodies against bombesin and tetanus toxoid. J Immunol 135:3831–3838.

Hulette CM, Effros RB, Walford RL (1987): Immunization of normal human splenocytes in vitro to produce human monoclonal antibodies to cellular antigens. Tissue Antigen 30:25–33.

Hunter KW Jr, Fisher GW, Hemming VG, Wilson SR (1982): Anti-bacterial activity of a human monoclonal antibody to *Haemophilus influenzae* type B capsular polysaccharide. Lancet 2:798.

Ichimori Y, Sasano K, Itoh H, Hitotsumachi S, Kimura Y, Kaneko K, Kida M, Tsukamoto K (1985): Establishment of hybridomas secreting human monoclonal antibodies against tetanus toxoid and hepatitis B virus surface antigen. Biochem Biophys Res Commun 129:26–33.

Irie RF, Giullano AE, Morton DL (1979): Oncofetal antigen: Tumor-associated fetal antigen immunogenic in man. JNCI 73:367.

Isojima S, Kameda K, Tsuji Y, Shigeta M, Ikeda Y, Koyama K (1987): Establishment and characterization of human hybridoma secreting monoclonal antibody with high titers of sperm immobilizing and agglutinating activity against human seminal plasma. J Reprod Immunol 10:67–75.

James K (1988): Human monoclonal technology—Are its achievements, challenges, and potential appreciated? Scand J Immunol 65:257–260.

James K, Bell GT (1987): Human monoclonal antibody production. J Immunol Methods 100:5–40.

Jenkens MK, Schwartz RH, Pardoll DM (1988): Effects of cyclosporine A on T cell development and clonal deletion. Science 241:1655–1657.

Kohler G, Milstein C (1975): Continuous cultures of fused cells secreting antibody of predefined specificity. Nature 256:495.

Komori S, Yamasaki N, Shigeta M, Watanabe T, Isojima S (1988): Sperm immobilizing human monoclonal antibody from transformants established by the method of recombinant DNA. Presented at the 9th European Immunology Congress, Rome.

Kozbor D, Lagarde AE, Roder JC (1982): Human hybridomas constructed with antigen-specific Epstein-Barr virus-transformed cell lines. Proc Natl Acad Sci USA 79:6651–6655.

Kozbor D, Triputi P, Roder JC, Croce CM (1984): A human hybrid myeloma for production of human monoclonal antibodies. J Immunol Methods 133:3001.

Kurpisz M, Clarke GF, Mahoney M, Anderson TL, Alexander NJ (1989): Mouse monoclonal antibodies to immunodominant glycosylated antigenic sites. Clin Exp Immunol 78:250–255.

Kurpisz M, Simon LL, Alexander NJ (1987): EBV transformation and microfusion as the potential source of human monoclonal antibodies. Am J Reprod Immunol Microbiol 15: 61–65.

Kyurkchiev SD, Shigeta M, Koyama S, Isojima S (1986): A human–mouse hybridoma producing monoclonal antibody against human sperm coating antigen. Immunology 57: 489–492.

Lane HC, Fauci AS (1983): Establishment of human–human and human–mouse B cell hybrid and their use in the study of B cell activation. In Hayes BF, Eisenbarth GS (eds): Monoclonal Antibodies: Probes for the Study of Autoimmunity and Immunodeficiency. New York: Academic Press.

Larrick J, Raubitschek AA, Dyer B, Hart GS, Lippman D, Hohnsen D, Wang M, Weintraub H (1985): In vitro expansion of human B-cells for the production of human monoclonal antibodies. In Engleman EG, Foung SKH, Larrick J, Raubitschek AA (eds): Human Hybridomas and Monoclonal Antibodies. New York: Plenum Press.

Larrick JW, Truitt KE, Raubitschek AA, Senyk G, Wang J (1983): Characterization of human hybridomas secreting antibody to tetanus toxoid. Proc Natl Acad Sci USA 80:6376.

Levy R, Dilley J (1978): Rescue of immunoglobulin secretion from human neoplastic lymphoid cells by somatic cell hybridization. Proc Natl Acad Sci USA 76:2411.

Levy JA, Viroloinen V, Defeudi V (1968): Human lymphoblastoid lines from lymph node and spleen. Cancer 22:517.

Matsuoko Y, Moore GE, Yagi Y, Pressman D (1967): Production of free light chains of immunoglobulin by hematopoietic cell line derived from a patient with multiple myeloma. Proc Soc Exp Biol Med 125:1246.

McCormack JM, Cunningham MW (1988): Recombinant human interleukin 2 (rIL-2) enhancement of antibody production by human–human hybridomas. Cell Immunol 115: 325–333.

McCune JM, Namikawa R, Kaneshima H, Shultz LD, Lieberman M, Weissman IL (1988): The SCID-hu mice: Murine model for the analysis of human hematolymphoid differentiation and function. Science 241:1632–1639.

Morrison SL, Johnson MJ, Herzenberg LA, Oi VT (1984): Chimeric human antibody molecules: Mouse antigen-binding domains with human constant region domains. Proc Natl Acad Sci USA 81:6851.

Mosier DE, Gulizia RJ, Baird SM, Wilson DB (1988): Transfer of a functional human immune system to mice with severe combined immunodeficiency. Nature 335:257–259.

Olsson L, Kaplan L (1980): Human–human hybridomas producing monoclonal antibodies of predefined specificity. Proc Natl Acad Sci USA 77:5429–5431.

Olsson L, Kronstrom H, Cambon-De Mouzon A, Honsik C, Brodin T, Jacobsen B (1983): Antibody producing human–human hybridomas. I. Technical aspects. J Immunol Methods 61:17.

Pickering JW, Gelder FB (1982): A human myeloma cell line that does not express immunoglobulin but yields a high frequency of antibody-secreting hybridomas. J Immunol 129:406.

Pistillo MP, Mazzoleni O, Tanigaka N, Hammerling U, Longo A, Frumento G, Ferrara GB (1985): Human anti-HLA monoclonal antibodies: Production, characterization and application. Hum Immunol 21:265.

Pope JH, Scott W, Reedman BM, Water MK (1971): EB virus as a biologically active agent. In Nakahara W, Nishioka K, Hirayama T, Ito Y (eds): Recent Advances in Human Tumor Virology and Immunology. Tokyo: University of Tokyo Press, pp 177–188.

Roder JC, Kozbor D, Cole SPC, Atlaw T, Campling BC, McGarry RC (1985): The Epstein-Barr virus–hybridoma technique. In Engleman EG, Foung SKH, Larrick J, Raubitschek AA (eds): Human Hybridomas and Monoclonal Antibodies. New York: Plenum Press.

Roberts S, Cheetham JC, Rees AR (1987): Generation of an antibody with enhanced affinity and specificity for its antigen by protein engineering. Nature 328:731–734.

Rosen A, Gergely P, Jondal M, Klein G, Britton S (1977): Polyclonal Ig production after Epstein-Barr virus infection of human lymphocytes in vitro. Nature 267:52.

Schmidt-Ulrich R, Brown J, Whittle H, Lin P (1986): The human–human hybridomas secreting monoclonal antibodies to the MW 195,000 *Plasmodium falciparum* blood stage antigen. J Exp Med 163:179.

Shau H, Golub S (1985): Depletion of NK cells with the lysomotropic agent L-leucine methyl ester and the in vitro generation of NK activity from NK precursor cells. J Immunol 134:1136–1141.

Shoenfeld Y, Hsn-Lin SC, Gabriels J, Silberstein LE, Furie BC, Furie B, Stollar BD, Schwartz RS (1982): Production of autoantibodies by human–human hybridomas. J Clin Invest 70:205.

Sikora K, Alderson T, Phillips J, Watson JV (1982): Human hybridomas from malignant gliomas. Lancet 1:11.

Smith LH, Teng NNH (1987): Applications of human monoclonal antibodies in oncology. In Strelkauskas AJ (ed): Human Hybridomas: Diagnostic and Therapeutic Applications. New York: Marcel Dekker, pp 121–158.

Snapper CM, Paul WE (1988): Interferon gamma and B cell stimulatory factor-1 reciprocally regulate Ig isotype production. Science 236:944–947.

Stein LD, Ledgley CJ, Sigal NH (1983): Patterns of isotype commitment in human B cells: Limiting dilution analysis of Epstein-Barr virus–infected cells. J Immunol 130:1640–1645.

Stein LD, Sigal NH (1983): Limiting dilution analysis of Epstein-Barr virus–induced immunoglobulin production. Cell Immunol 79:309–319.

Steinitz M, Klein G, Koskimies S, Makela O (1977): EB virus–induced B lymphocyte cell lines producing specific antibody. Nature 269:420–423.

Stevens TL, Bossie A, Sanders VM, Fernandez-Botia R, Coffman RL, Mosmann TR, Vitetta ES (1988): Regulation of antibody isotype secretion by subsets of antigen-specific helper T cells. Nature 334:255–258.

Stevenson M, Volsky B, Hendeskog M, Volsky DJ (1986): Immortalization of human T lymphocytes after transfection of Epstein-Barr virus DNA. Science 233:980–984.

Strelkauskas AJ, Taylor CL, Smith MR, Bear PD (1987): Transfection of human cells: An alternative method for establishment of human hybrid clones. In Strelkauskas AJ (ed): Human Hybridomas: Diagnostic and Therapeutic Applications. New York: Marcel Dekker, pp 95–117.

Strike LE, Devens BH, Lundak RL (1984): Production of human–human hybridomas secreting antibody to sheep erythrocytes after in vitro immunisation. J Immunol 132: 1798–1803.

Strominger J, Thorley-Lawson D (1979): Early events in transformation of human lymphocytes by the virus. In Epstein MA, Achong BG (eds): The Epstein-Barr Virus. Berlin: Springer-Verlag, pp 185–204.

Teng NNH, Kaplan HS, Herbert JM, Moore C, Douglas H, Wunderlich A, Braude AJ **(1985):** Protection against Gram negative bacteremia and endotoxinemia with human monoclonal IgM antibodies. Proc Natl Acad Sci USA 82:1790.

Teng NNH, Lam KS, Riera FC, Kaplan HS (1983): Construction and testing of mouse–human heteromyelomas for human monoclonal antibody production. Proc Natl Acad Sci USA 80:7308–7312.

Tsuji T, Clausen H, Nudelman E, Kaizu T, Hakomori S-I, Isojima S (1988): Human sperm carbohydrate antigens defined by an antisperm human monoclonal antibody derived from an infertile woman bearing antisperm antibodies in her serum. J Exp Med 168:343–356.

Vienken J, Zimmerman U (1985): An improved electrofusion technique for production of mouse hybridoma cells. FEBS Lett 182:278.

Vienken J, Zimmerman U, Fouchard M, Zagury D (1983): Electrofusion of myeloma cells on the single cell level: Fusion under sterile conditions without proteolytic enzyme treatment. FEBS Lett 163:54.

Wasserman RL, Budens RD, Thaxton ES (1986): In vitro stimulation prior to fusion generates antigen-binding human–human hybridomas. J Immunol Methods 93:275–283.

Watson JV, Alderson T, Sikora K, Phillipps J (1983): Subcutaneous culture chamber for continuous infusion of monoclonal antibodies. Lancet 1:99.

Weis JJ, Richards SA, Smith JA, Fearon DT (1986): Purification of the B lymphocyte receptor for the C3d fragment of complement and the Epstein-Barr virus by monoclonal antibody affinity chromatography, and assessment of its functional capacities. J Immunol Methods 92:79–87.

Winger L, Winger C, Shastry P, Russell A, Longenecker M (1983): Efficient generation in vitro, from human peripheral blood cells, of monoclonal Epstein-Barr virus transformants producing specific antibody to a variety of antigens without prior deliberate immunization. Proc Natl Acad Sci USA 80:4484–4488.

Wunderlich D, Teramoto YA, Alford C, Schlom J (1981): The use of lymphocytes from axillary lymph nodes of mastectomy patients to generate human monoclonal antibodies. Eur J Clin Oncol 17:719.

Yamaura N, Makino M, Walsh LJ, Bruce AW, Choe B-K (1985): Production of monoclonal antibodies against prostatic acid phosphatase by in vitro immunisation of human spleen cells. J Immunol Methods 84:105.

Zimmerman U (1982): Electric field–mediated fusion and related electrical phenomena. Biochim Biophys Acta 694:227.

27

Anti-Idiotypic Antibodies as Immunizing Antigens for Immunocontraception

Christopher P. Carron

Immunocontraception represents an attractive mode of fertility regulation because of its potential for safety, reversibility, efficacy, low-cost wide usage, and global acceptability. Rapid progress in understanding the immune system and availability of a impressive array of tools for the production of synthetic and recombinant proteins provides a strong foundation for the development of a molecular or subunit vaccine.

In most cases to date, vaccines for human and animal health have been composed of whole organisms, viruses, or bacteria capable of inducing high levels of immunity over long periods of time. Although immunization with whole sperm and sperm extracts can induce infertility in experimental models, such preparations could not be used as vaccine for many reasons [for discussion, see Naz, 1988]. Studies by Goldberg and colleagues [reviewed in Goldberg, 1987] and more recent work by Primakoff et al. [1988] demonstrate that immunization with a single purified native sperm antigen can induce effective and reversible infertility and underscore the feasibility of developing a contraceptive vaccine that targets sperm-specific antigens and prefertilization events.

However, practical limitations exist with respect to the utilization of native sperm proteins as contraceptive vaccine components, and, therefore, it will be necessary to design an immunocontraceptive, using one or more recombinant sperm proteins or synthetic peptides derived from these proteins, that mimics protective epitopes to a degree sufficient for induction of protective immunity. One of the

Gamete Interaction: Prospects for Immunocontraception, pages 401–414

limitations of the use of synthetic peptides or recombinant antigen as a vaccine is the potential for expressed protein or peptide to represent epitopes lacking conformational similarity to native antigen epitopes. Vaccines composed of anti-idiotypic antibodies that mimic sites on proteins and carbohydrates represent a new approach to the stimulation of protective immunity and provide an alternative for the production of conformational B-cell antigens.

NETWORK THEORY

Jerne's network theory [Jerne, 1974] defines the immune system as a dynamic interactive network of idiotypes (Id) and complementary anti-idiotypes (anti-Id) on antibodies and B- and T-lymphocyte antigen receptors. The regulation of B-lymphocyte response via an interactive Id network is generally accepted. *Id* refers to the collective set of epitopes or antigenic determinants that define the variable region (V) of a given antibody (Ig) or cellular antigen receptor. Epitopes in the V region of Ig or antigen receptor are frequently referred to as *idiotopes*. The complementary determining regions (CDR) of the V_L and V_H domains of antibody molecules and B-lymphocyte receptors determine both antibody specificity and Id. Antibodies directed against idiotypic determinants are called *anti-idiotypic antibodies*. Mutual recognition and interaction of idiotypes and complementary anti-idiotypes on free molecules and cellular receptors of B lymphocytes controls the levels of specific immune reactants and represents the conceptual basis for Id network regulation of B-lymphocyte responses of the immune system.

The basis for an idiotypic network involving T lymphocytes is less clear. T-lymphocyte Id have been discussed in two different contexts. From one point of view, it is considered that T and B lymphocytes share Id. This idea is supported by serological and cellular studies demonstrating cross-reactivities between antibody V regions and T-cell receptors with similar specificity for antigen indicating that T- and B-cell receptors share idiotypic determinants [Ramseier and Lindenmann, 1972; Binz and Wigzell, 1977; Cosenza et al., 1977; Janeway, 1980; Cone, 1981]. Several lines of evidence argue against the idea that T cells express B-cell-like immunoglobulin Id [discussed in Fitch, 1988]. In many cases, information interpreted as showing T-lymphocyte expression of immunoglobulin Id comes from observations using complex and incompletely characterized antigen and lymphoid cell test systems. Furthermore, it is now clear that B- and T-cell antigen receptors utilize distinctly different genes [Mak and Yanagi, 1984; Davis, 1985; Hood et al., 1985]. However, it would be unwise to ignore the evidence supporting B and T cell sharing of Id. Exclusion of gene sharing by T and B lymphocytes does not rule out the possibility that conformational complementarity at the structural level (not at the genetic or molecular level) of the B- and T-cell antigen receptor provides the basis for the observed idiotypic cross-reactivity [McNamara et al., 1984a]. Moreover, it is likely that other mechanisms may be discovered to explain Id sharing. The hypothesis that B and T lymphocytes share Id remains attractive in providing a means for functionally distinct cells to utilize a common recognition process.

From a second point of view T cells have been considered to express Id in a manner analogous to, but quite distinct from, B cell Id. In this case, T cell Id can be defined as the set of epitopes displayed by the variable region of the T-cell antigen receptor; antiserum reactive with a given T-cell Id would not be expected to react with any B-cell Id. There is no doubt that B cells can recognize T-cell Id as target antigen (e.g., see Staerz et al., 1985] and that antibodies specific for T-cell Id can modulate T-cell antigen recognition and function [Acha-Orbea et al., 1988; Urban et al., 1988; Owhashi and Heber-Katz, 1988; discussed in Fitch, 1988]. From this point of view, it is more clear how T and B lymphocytes may be interconnected functionally in a regulatory network involving Id and anti-Id.

PUTATIVE B- AND T-CELL ANTI-Id IN THE IMMUNE NETWORK

Bona [1988] suggests that the immune system of each individual contains the anti-Id clones described here.

1 B cells that recognize the Id of the Ig receptor of other B cells are referred to as *B-cell-defined anti-Id*. This class of anti-Id offers an alternative to traditional vaccines composed of live attenuated organisms or subunit vaccines where protective immunity is mainly dependent on neutralizing antibodies. The induction of antisperm antibodies by immunization with B-cell-defined anti-Id reagents represents a powerful alternative to antigen-driven immune responses.

2 B cells that produce antibodies specific for Id determinants of the T-cell receptor, referred to as *T-cell-defined anti-Id*, represent a class of anti-Id with increasing importance for immune intervention in autoimmune disease. T-cell-defined anti-Id have been used effectively for immune intervention in murine experimental autoimmune encephalomyelitis

(EAE). In mice, T cells mediating EAE exhibit limited usage of T-cell receptor (TCR) V genes, and the majority share the same V_B8 segment [Acha-Orbea et al., 1988; Urban et al., 1988]. Passive immunization with the V_B8-specific monoclonal anti-Id resulted in prevention and reversal of EAE [Staerz et al., 1985; Acha-Orbea et al., 1988; Urban et al., 1988; see also Owhashi and Heber-Katz, 1988]. Restricted usage of T-cell receptor V genes in autoimmune disease raises possibilities for anti-Id immunotherapy.

3   T-cell clones bearing an antigen receptor recognizing Id determinants of the immunoglobulin receptor of B-cell clones are referred to as *Id-specific T cells*. This class of anti-Id has been identified in various T-cell subsets such as suppressor [Bona and Paul, 1979], helper [Bottomly and Mosier, 1979], and effector T cells [Sherr et al., 1981; Jayarman and Bellone, 1982; Binz and Wigzell, 1978].

4   T cells have been described that recognize the Id of the antigen receptor of other T cells. This type of anti-Id T cell has been described in experimental systems such as in animals with graft-versus-host immunity [Kimura and Wilson, 1984] or immunity against allografts [Lancaster et al., 1985].

B-CELL-DEFINED ANTI-Id ANTIBODIES

The potential for the use of B-cell-defined anti-Id antibodies as vaccines is the focus of this chapter. The following terms are used [a more complete discussion of terminology and concepts related to B-cell-defined anti-Id can be found in several review articles: Bona and Kohler, 1984; Kohler et al., 1985; Bona et al., 1986].

The term *Ab1* refers to the first antibody in the immunization scheme. Ab1 can be either a monoclonal or polyclonal antibody that recognizes bacterial, viral, or sperm antigen. Anti-Id antibodies recognize Id determinants that lie within the variable region of Ab1. The terms *anti-Id* and *Ab2* are used interchangeably. *Ab2* represents the second antibody in the immunization scheme, and *Ab3* refers to the antibodies produced in response to immunization with Ab2.

B-cell-defined anti-Id antibodies have been categorized based on immunochemical and functional properties and are discussed below [Bona and Kohler, 1984]. Ab2α anti-Id are specific for idiotopes associated with framework determinants of Ab1. Ab2α binding to Ab1 does not alter antigen binding by Ab1. In contrast, Ab2γ anti-Id recognize antigen combining site associated idiotopes of Ab1 and can inhibit binding of antigen to Ab1. The binding of Ab2α and Ab2γ to

Ab1 can have similar effects, possibly because the binding of either category of Ab2 to B-cell antigen receptor could activate signal transduction pathways and the induction or suppression of specific antibody. Ab2β represent a category of anti-Id antibodies that are said to bear the "internal image" of the antigen and mimic the native antigen epitope recognized by Ab1. Native antigen inhibits Ab2β binding to Ab1. The most straightforward approach to the identification of Ab2β appears to be provided by in vitro screening for inhibition of binding of Ab1 to Ab2 by the reference antigen followed by in vivo assessment of the induction of an antigen-specific immune response following immunization with Ab2 in multiples species [Hildegund et al., 1988].

USE OF ANTI-Id ANTIBODIES AS VACCINES

There are several examples that support the concept that anti-Id antibodies can mimic various biologically active substances such as hormones [Sege and Peterson, 1978a], vitamins [Sege and Peterson, 1978b], and receptor ligands [Wassermann et al., 1982; Schreiber et al., 1980; Marasco et al., 1982; Pain et al., 1988; Vaux et al., 1988]. In 1981, Nisonoff and Lamoyi and Roitt et al. suggested that anti-Id might be exploited as a new type of vaccine for the production of protective immunity. Since then, a number of investigators have demonstrated the potential of anti-Id to induce immunity to parasites, bacteria, viruses, and transformed cells; representative examples are discussed below, and a more complete listing is presented in Table 1.

Sacks et al. [1982] first reported anti-Id–induced protective immunity in mice infected with *Trypanosoma rhodesiense*. Anti-Id was produced against *Trypanosoma*-specific neutralizing mouse monoclonal antibody. Immunization with anti-Id protected mice against subsequent infection with parasite. Interestingly, protection by anti-Id was strain specific. Moreover, anti-Id failed to induce detectable antigen-binding activity in the absence of immunization with antigen. These results underscore the observation that antigen-binding activity can be a minor component of the response to Ab2 and that subsequent immunization with antigen is necessary to demonstrate that antigen-specific clones were primed by anti-Id [Sacks and Sher, 1983].

Kennedy and coworkers [1983, 1984, 1986] demonstrated that anti-Id could be useful as vaccine against hepatitis B virus. Hepatitis B surface antigen (HBsAg) is the envelope material of hepatitis B virus (HBV). Human antibodies to HBsAg share a common idiotype with antibodies against HBsAg produced in mice and a variety of other

TABLE 1. Use of Anti-Id as Vaccine

Antigen system	Anti-Id	Immune Response	References
Parasites			
Trypanosoma surface glycoprotein	Xenogeneic, polyclonal	Induced neutralizing antibodies and protective immunity in mice; genetically restricted	Sacks et al. [1982]; Sacks and Sher [1983]
Schistosoma mansoni	Monoclonal	Induction of cytotoxic antibodies	Grzych et al. [1985]
Bacteria			
Streptococcus pneumonia	Monoclonal	Induced neutralizing antibodies and protective immunity	McNamara et al. [1984b]
Escherichia coli	Monoclonal	Induced neutralizing antibodies and protective immunity in neonates	Stein and Soderstrom [1984]
Viruses			
Hepatitis B virus	Xenogeneic, polyclonal	Prior injection with anti-Id enhanced response to immunization with native antigen; anti-Id alone induced virus neutralizing antibodies	Kennedy et al. [1983, 1984, 1986]
Rabies virus	Xenogeneic, polyclonal	Induction of neutralizing antibodies	Reagan et al. [1983]
Poliovirus type II	Monoclonal	Induction of neutralizing antibodies, no protection	UytdeHaag and Osterhaus [1985]
Tobacco mosaic virus	Xenogeneic, polyclonal	Stimulation of silent B cell clones	Francotte and Urbain [1984]
Reovirus type III	Syngeneic, monoclonal	Induction of neutralizing antibodies; inducation of DTH cytolytic T cells; binds to virus receptor	Sharpe et al. [1984]
Tumors			
SV-40 sarcoma	Xenogeneic, polyclonal	Partial inhibition of tumor growth	Kennedy et al. [1985]
Melanoma	Xenogeneic, polyclonal	Induction of T cells that mediate DTH; induced antigen-binding Ab3	Nepom et al. [1984]

species. Rabbit anti-Id antibodies prepared against the common idiotope of HBsAg-specific antibodies were used to induce Ab2 antibodies in mice [Kennedy et al., 1983, 1984]. Antibodies to HBsAg
could be induced solely by injecting mice with rabbit anti-Id antibodies. Moreover, prior injection of anti-Id antibodies increased the response when the mice were subsequently injected with HBsAg,
demonstrating that anti-Id could prime the immune response to
HBsAg [Kennedy et al., 1983, 1984]. Immunization with anti-Id induced anti-HBsAg antibodies (Ab3) that expressed the common interspecies Id and recognized the immunogenic determinant of the
HBsAg shared by naturally occurring anti-HBsAg. Kennedy and coworkers [1986] showed subsequently that the rabbit anti-Id elicited a
protective antibody response to HBsAg in immunized chimpanzees.

McNamara et al. [1984b] used a monoclonal anti-Id to immunize
mice against lethal infection with Streptococcus pneumonia. Antibodies that bind to phosphorylcholine (PC), a bacterial wall component, protect mice against lethal infection with *Streptococcus*. A monoclonal anti-Id (termed 4C11) was prepared against the binding site of
the PC-specific antibody and conjugated to KLH. Mice immunized
with the 4C11–KLH conjugate developed high titer antibody to PC.
4C11–KLH significantly increased the resistance of mice to lethal
challenge with bacteria. The LD_{50} for mice primed with PC and 4C11
coupled to carrier was 100 times greater than that for nonimmunized
control mice, indicating that an anti-Id vaccine can be as effective in
providing protection as the conventional vaccine based on nominal
antigen.

IDIOTOPE VACCINE FOR IMMUNOCONTRACEPTION

We have been interested in utilizing anti-Id as immune response
modifiers and antigen surrogates for the manipulation of immunity
to sperm antigens and immunocontraception. Immunization with
anti-Id that mimics protective sperm antigen epitopes represents an
alternative strategy for induction of immunity to sperm and immunologic contraception. We are testing this approach in a model system of antibody-mediated inhibition of fertilization.

The mouse monoclonal antisperm antibodies M42.15 mAb and
M29.6 mAb recognize distinct mouse sperm antigens, prevent mouse
fertilization in vitro and in vivo [Saling et al., 1985, 1986; Saling and
Lakoski, 1985; Saling and Weibel, 1985; Saling, 1986] and have been
used as Ab1 for the induction of anti-Id. In initial studies, rabbit
anti-Id to the Id of M29.6 mAb and of M42.15 mAb were developed
and used as immunogen [Carron et al., 1988]. These anti-Id compet-

itively inhibited M42.15 and M29.6 mAb binding to mouse sperm, and anti-Id M42 prevented M42.15 mAb inhibition of fertilization [Carron et al., 1989a]; these results suggest that the anti-Id preparations possessed subpopulations directed against idiotopes similar or adjacent to the antigen-binding site of the mAb. Immunization of outbred female mice with Ab2 induced anti-(anti-Id) (Ab3) that shared properties with M29.6 mAb and with M42.15 mAb, but lacked antigen-binding activity.

These results parallel the majority of cases in which specific antigen-binding antibody has been found to be a minor component in the response to immunization with polyclonal Ab2. The anti-(anti-Id) response (Ab3) to immunization with Ab2 is complex and varies with the type of Ab2 used for immunization. Ab3 antibodies induced by immunization with Ab2 could, as discussed by Sachs et al. [1981] and others [Sacks and Sher, 1983; Sacks, 1985; Bluestone et al., 1986], include antibodies that 1) react with idiotopes expressed on the anti-Id and have no serological or genetic relationship with the starting Ab1 and 2) have structural similarities to the original idiotype in that they share idiotopes with Ab1 (referred to as *Id'*). The Id' subset of the Ab3 population may or may not bind antigen. In many cases, antigen-binding idiotype-bearing antibody has been found to be a minor component in the response to Ab2, and immunization with nominal antigen was necessary to reveal that specific idiotype-bearing antigen-specific clones were primed by anti-Id [Urbain et al., 1977; Wikler et al., 1979; Bluestone et al., 1981; Bona et al., 1981; Sacks and Sher, 1983].

Anti-Id antibodies obtained by immunization across xenogeneic barriers are heterogeneous with respect to specificity and function [Bona and Kohler, 1984]. Because of the intrinsic heterogeneity of polyclonal anti-Id, we subsequently produced monoclonal anti-Id against M42.15 mAb [Carron et al., 1989a,b]. Two monoclonal anti-Id antibodies to M42.15 mAb, designated *anti-Id 6E8* and *anti-Id 7D2*, were identified that inhibited completely M42.15 mAb binding to sperm. Moreover, soluble M42.15 antigen, isolated from mouse caudal sperm, inhibited anti-Id 6E8 and anti-Id 7D2 binding to M42.15 mAb. These and additional data suggest that anti-Id 6E8 and anti-Id 7D2 recognize overlapping, but probably not identical, sites on M42.15 mAb. Anti-Id 6E8 and anti-Id 7D2 recognize private idiotopes of M42.15 mAb, requiring the association of M42.15 mAb V_H and V_L. Together, these results suggest that anti-Id 6E8 and anti-Id 7D2 recognize three-dimensional idiotopes within or near the antigen combining site of M42.15 mAb.

Immunization of Balb/c female mice with anti-Id 6E8 and anti-Id

7D2 induced Id-positive Ab3. Antigen-binding activity in the sera of immune mice was measured by ELISA using solid-phase M42.15 antigen isolated from mouse testes as target. Balb/c mice immunized with anti-Id 6E8 contained Ab3 with M42.15 antigen-binding activity. Taken together, these results demonstrate the feasibility of inducing antisperm antibodies by immunization with anti-Id antibodies and provide a basis for an idiotope vaccine for contraception.

Given the potential for the generation of virtually unlimited quantities of recombinant proteins and synthetic peptides, it is unlikely that anti-Id will replace strategies based on the production of subunit or molecular vaccines. Rather, the use of B-cell-defined anti-Id represents an alternative and complementary tactic for the induction of protective immunity dependent on neutralizing antibodies. It is not difficult to envision an immunocontraceptive vaccine resulting from a merging of molecular biology and anti-Id technologies.

ACKNOWLEDGMENTS

Support for this project was provided the A.W. Mellon Foundation and by the National Institutes of Health.

REFERENCES

Acha-Orbea H, Mitchel DJ, Timmermann L, Wraith DC, Tausch GS, Waldor MK, Zamvil SS, McDevitt HO, Steinman L (1988): Limited heterogeneity of T cell receptors from lymphocytes mediating autoimmune encephalomyelitis allows specific immune intervention. Cell 54:263–273.

Binz H, Wigzell H (1977): Antigen-binding idiotypic T- lymphocyte receptors. Contemp Top Immunobiol 7:113–277.

Binz H, Wigzell H (1978): Induction of specific immune unresponsiveness with purified mixed leucocyte culture-activated T-lymphoblasts as autoimmunogen. III. Proof for the existence of autoantiidiotypic killer T cells and transfer of suppression to normal syngeneic recipients by T or B lymphocytes. J Exp Med 147:63.

Bluestone JA, Epstein SL, Ozato K, Sharrow SO, Sachs DH (1981): Anti-idiotypes to monoclonal anti-H-2 antibodies. II. Expression of anti-H-2K^k idiotypes on antibodies induced by anti-idiotype or H-2K^k antigen. J Exp Med 154:1305–1318.

Bluestone JA, Oberdan L, Epstein SL, Sachs DH (1986): Idiotypic manipulation of immune response to transplantation antigens. Immunol Rev 90:5–27.

Bona CA (1988): Anti-idiotypes. In Bona CA (ed): Biological Application of Anti-Idiotypes. Boca Raton, FL. CRC Press Inc., Vol 1, pp 1–12.

Bona CA, Heber-Katz E, Paul WE (1981): Idiotype-anti-idiotype regulation: Immunization with a levan-binding myeloma protein leads to the appearance of auto anti-anti-idiotype antibodies and to the activation of silent clones. J Exp Med 153:951–967.

Bona CA, Kang C-Y, Kohler H, Monestier M (1986): Epibody: The image of the network created by a single antibody. Immunol Rev 90:115–127.

Bona C, Kohler H (1984): Anti-idiotypic antibodies and internal images. In Venter JC, Fraser CM, Lindstrom J (eds): Receptor Biochemistry and Methodology. New York: Alan R Liss, Vol IV, pp 141–149.

Bona C, Paul WE (1979): Cellular basis of expression of idiotypes. I. Suppressor cells specific for MOPC460 idiotype regulate the expression of cells secreting anti-trinitrophenylantibodies bearing 460 idiotype. J Exp Med 144:592–XX.

Bottomly K, Mosier DE (1979): Mice whose B cells cannot produce the T15 idiotype also lack an antigen-specific helper T cell required for T15 expression. J Exp Med 150:1399.

Carron CP, Jarvis HW, Saling PM (1988): Characterization of antibodies to idiotypic determinants of monoclonal anti-sperm antibodies. Biol Reprod 38:1093–1103.

Carron CP, Mathias A, Saling PM (1989a): Anti-idiotype antibodies prevent antibody binding to mouse sperm and antibody mediated inhibition of fertilization. Biol Reprod 41:153–162.

Carron CP, Mathias A, Saling PM (1989b): Monoclonal anti- idiotype antibodies: Induction and modulation of the immune response to sperm antigen. Am J Reprod Immunol 19:74a.

Cone R (1981): Molecular basis for T lymphocyte recognition of antigens. Prog Allergy 29:182.

Cosenza H, Julius M, Augustin A (1977): Idiotypes as variable region markers: Analogies between receptors to phosphorylcholine-specific T and B lymphocytes. Annu Rev Immunol 3:3–33.

Davis M (1985): Molecular genetics of the T cell-receptor beta chain. Annu Rev Immunol 3:537.

Fitch FW (1988): Antibodies specific for the T-cell receptor. In Bona CA (ed): Biological Application of Anti-Idiotypes. Boca Raton, FL. CRC Press, Inc., pp 137–151.

Francotte M, Urbain J (1984): Induction of anti-tobacco mosaic virus antibodies in mice by rabbit antiidiotypic antibodies. J Exp Med 160:1485–1494.

Goldberg E (1987): LDH-C$_4$ as the model sperm antigen for a contraceptive vaccine. In Talwar GP (ed): Progress in Vaccinology, Vol 1: Contraception Research for Today and the Nineties. New York: Springer-Verlag, pp 277–283.

Grzych JM, Capron M, Lambert PH, Dissous C, Torres S, Capron A (1985): An anti-idiotype vaccine against experimental schistosomiasis. Nature 316:74–76.

Hildegund C, Ertl, Bona A (1988): Criteria to define anti-idiotypic antibodies carrying the internal image of an antigen. Vaccine 6:80–84.

Hood L, Kronenberg M, Hunkapiller T (1985): T cell antigen receptors and the immunoglobulin supergene family. Cell 40:225.

Janeway C (1980): Idiotypes, T-cell receptors, and T–B cooperation. Contemp Top Immunobiol 9:171.

Jayarman S, Bellone CJ (1982): Hapten-specific responses to phenyltrimethyl amino hapten. III. Mice whose delayed-type hypersensitivity responses cannot be abrogated by the presence of anti-Idiotypic suppressor T cells lack a critical modulatory T cell function. J Exp Med 155:1810.

Jerne NK (1974): Towards a network theory of the immune system. Ann Immunol (Paris) 125C:373–389.

Kennedy RC, Adler-Storthz K, Henkel RD, Sanchez Y, Melnick JL, Dreesman GR (1983): Immune response to hepatitis B surface antigen: Enhancement by prior injection of antibodies to the idiotype. Science 221:853–855.

Kennedy RC, Dreesman GR, Butel JS, Landford RE (1985): Suppression of in vivo tumor formation induced by Simian virus 40 transformed cells in mice receiving anti-idiotypic antibodies. J Exp Med 161:1431.

Kennedy RC, Eichberg JW, Lanford RE, Dreesman GR (1986): Anti-idiotypic antibody vaccine for type B viral hepatitis in chimpanzees. Science 232:220–223.

Kennedy RC, Melnick JL, Dreesman GR (1984): Antibody to hepatitis B virus induced by injecting antibodies to the idiotype. Science 223:930–931.

Kimura H, Wilson DB (1984): Antiidiotypic cytotoxic T cells in rats with graft-versus-host disease Nature 308:463.

Kohler H, Muller S, Bona C (1985): Internal antigen and immune network Proc Soc Exp Biol Med 178:189–195.

Lancaster F, Chui YL, Batchelor JR (1985): Antiidiotypic T cells suppress rejection of renal allografts in rats. Nature 315:336.

Mak T, Yanagi Y (1984): Genes encoding the human T cell antigen receptor. Immunol Rev 81:221.

Marasco WA, Becker EL (1982): Antiidiotype as antibody against formyl peptide chemotaxis receptor of the neutrophil. J Immunol 128:963.

McNamara M, Gleason K, Kohler H (1984a): T-cell helper circuits Immunol Rev 79:87–104.

McNamara MK, Ward RE, Kohler H (1984b): Monoclonal idiotype vaccine against *Streptococcus pneumoniae* infection. Science 226:1325–1326.

Naz RK (1988): The fertilization antigen (FA-1): Applications in immunocontraception and infertility in humans. Am J Reprod Immunol 166:21–27.

Nepom GJ, Nelson KA, Holbecck SL, Hellstrom J, Hellstrom VI (1984): Induction of immunity to a human tumor marker by in vivo administration of anti-idiotypic antibodies in mice. Proc Natl Acad Sci USA 81:2864.

Nisonoff A, Lamoyi E (1981): Implications of the presence of an internal image of the antigen in anti-idiotypic antibodies: Possible application to vaccine production. Clin Immunol Immunopathol 21:397–406.

Owhashi M, Heber-Katz E (1988): Protection from experimental allergic encephalomyelitis conferred by a monoclonal antibody directed against shared idiotype on rat T cell receptors specific for myelin basic protein. J Exp Med 168:2153–2164.

Pain D, Kanwar YS, Blobel G (1988): Identification of a receptor for protein import into chloroplasts and its localization to envelope contact zones. Nature 331:232–237.

Primakoff P, Lathrop W, Woolman L, Cowan A, Myles D (1988): Fully effective contraception in male and female guinea pigs immunized with the sperm protein PH-20. Nature 335:543.

Ramseier H, Lindenmann J (1972): Aliotypic antibodies. Transplant Rev 10:57–96.

Reagan KJ, Wunner WH, Wiktor TJ, Koprowski H (1983): Anti-idiotypic antibodies induce neutralizing antibodies to rabies virus glycoprotein. J Virol 48:660–666.

Roit IM, Male DK, Guarnotta G, De Carvalho LP, Cooke A, Hay FC, Lydyard PM, Thanavala Y, Ivanyi J (1981): Idiotypic networks and their possible exploitation for manipulation of the immune response. Lancet 1:1041.

Sachs DH, El-Gamil M, Miller G (1981): Genetic control of the immune response to staphylococcal nuclease. X. Effects of in vivo administration of anti-idiotypic antibodies. Eur J Immunol 11:509–516.

Sacks DL (1985): Molecular mimicry of parasite antigens using anti-idiotypic antibodies. Curr Top Microbiol Immunol 119:45–55.

Sacks DL, Esser KM, Sher A (1982): Immunization of mice against African trypanosomiasis using anti-idiotypic antibodies. J Exp Med 155:1108–1119.

Sacks DL, Sher A (1983): Evidence that anti-idiotype induced immunity to experimental African trypanosomiasis is genetically restricted and required recognition of combining site-related idiotopes. J Immunol 131:1511–1515.

Saling PM (1986): Mouse sperm antigens that participate in fertilization. IV. A monoclonal antibody prevents zona penetration by inhibition of the acrosome reaction. Dev Biol 117:511.

Saling PM, Irons G, Waibel R (1985): Mouse sperm antigens that participate in fertilization. I. Inhibition of sperm fusion with the egg plasma membrane using monoclonal antibodies. Biol Reprod 33:515.

Saling PM, Lakoski KA (1985): Mouse sperm antigens that participate in fertilization. II. Inhibition of sperm penetration through the zona pellucida using monoclonal antibodies. Biol Reprod 33:527.

Saling PM, Waibel R (1985): Mouse sperm antigens that participate in fertilization. III. Passive immunization with a single monoclonal antisperm antibody inhibits pregnancy and fertilization in vivo. Biol Reprod 33:537.

Saling PM, Morton PC, Waibel R (1986): Contraceptive effect of two anti-sperm monoclonal antibodies, administered singly and in combination, in the mouse. In Talwar GP (ed): Immunological Approaches to Contraception and Promotion of Fertility. New York: Plenum Publishing Co., Inc., p 191.

Schreiber AB, Conrand PO, Andre C, Vray B, Stossberg AD (1980): Anti-alprenelol anti-Id antibodies bind to beta-adrenergic receptors and modulate catecholamine-sensitive adenylate cyclase. Proc Natl Acad Sci USA 77:7385.

Sege K, Peterson PA (1978a): Use of anti-idiotypic antibodies as cell surface receptor probes. Proc Natl Acad Sci USA 75:2443–2447.

Sege K, Peterson PA (1978b): Anti-idiotypic antibodies against anti-vitamin A transport protein react with prealbumin. Nature 272:167–168.

Sharpe AH, Gaulton GN, McDade KK, Fields BB, Green MI (1984): Syngeneic monoclonal antiidiotype can induce cellular immunity to reovirus. J Exp Med 160:1195.

Sherr DH, Ju ST, Dorf ME (1981): Hapten-specific T-cell responses to 4-hydroxy-3-nitrophenyl acetyl. XII. Fine specificity of antiidiotypic suppressor T cells (Ts2). J Exp Med 154:539.

Staerz UD, Rammensee H-G, Bendetto JD, Bevan BJ (1985): Characterization of a murine monoclonal antibody specific for an allotypic determinant on T cell antigen receptor. J Immunol 134:3994.

Stein KE, Soderstrom T (1984): Neonatal administration of idiotype or anti-idiotype primes for protection against *Escherichia coli* K13 infection in mice. J Immunol 134:1225–1229.

Urban JL, Kumar V, Kono DH, Gomex C, Horvath SJ, Clayton J, Ando DG, Sercarz EE, Hood L (1988): Restricted use of T cell receptor V genes in murine autoimmune encephalomyelitis raises possibilities for antibody therapy. Cell 54:577–592.

Urbain J, Wikler M, Franssen JD, Collignon C (1977): Idiotypic regulation of the immune system by the induction of antibodies against anti-idiotypic antibodies. Proc Natl Acad Sci USA 74:5126–5130.

UytdeHaag FGCM, Osterhaus ADME (1985): Induction of neutralizing antibody in mice against poliovirus type II with monoclonal anti-idiotype antibody. J Immunol 134:1225.

Vaux DJ, Helenius A, Mellman I (1988): Spike-nucleocapsid interaction in Semliki Forest virus reconstructed using network antibodies. Nature 336:36–42.

Wassermann NH, Penn AS, Freimuth PI, Treptow N, Wentzel S, Cleveland WL, Erlanger BF (1982): Antiidiotypic route to anti-acetylcholine receptor antibodies and experimental myasthenia gravis. Proc Natl Acad Sci USA 77:4810.

Wikler M, Franssen J-D, Collignon C, Leo O, Mariame B, Van de Walle P, DeGroote D, Urbain J (1979): Idiotypic regulation of the immune system: Common idiotypic specificities between idiotypes and antibodies raised against anti-idiotypic antibodies in rabbits. J Exp Med 150:184–195.

DISCUSSION

DR. TALWAR: The anti-idiotypic approach is especially interesting for the carbohydrate type of antigens, which appear to be very important in the sperm interactions. The main problem that many investigators have found is the lack of predictability in the response. Have you had this experience, or are you only demonstrating the approach that works?

DR. CARRON: Yes, I am demonstrating the one that works. We tried for some time with polyclonal rabbit antibodies and were not successful at inducing antigen-binding activity. As far as the results that I have demonstrated today, they clearly represent the properties of the limited number of monoclonal antibodies. The problem is predictability. We massaged the situation a bit by using a totally syngeneic system. So, consequently, we were able to make it work possibly by using a syngeneic versus an outbred model.

General Discussion

DR. HERR: In attempting to construct the hybridomas in the human, we are limited by the availability of suitable fusion immunized cells and by the opportunity to fuse them with the various fusion partners, be they human lymphoblastoid cells or the construction heterohybridomas. An intense epdidymitis may occur after vasectomy, and a number of granulomas may form at various sites. In fact, if a vasectomized man met an untimely death, and if we could obtain the epididymis, it might provide a better set of cells to construct fusions that might yield more suitable antibodies. I simply raise that kind of paradigm as a potential source of tissues that might give us a better number of fusions.

DR. HJORT: Regarding the issue of sperm-immobilizing antibodies in human serum and why they were so common in Japan, Dr. Isojima said that we didn't find these antibodies. That is not true. In several of the sera from Japan we found antibodies. It is easier to find female sera antibodies in Japan than in almost any other country, and I wonder if there is any explanation for this. In my own country, we very rarely see immobilizing antibody levels, and, when we do, they are in people from Turkey and other Islamic countries. Thus I wonder if there are some traditions in different populations that expose women in different ways to sperm antigens.

DR. ISOJIMA: I have to say that there were many discrepant results between my laboratory and other laboratories in sperm immobilization assays for the WHO Sera Bank. Many other laboratories reported that our monoclonal antibody 2C6 was negative in sperm immobilization, though it possessed a very strong immobilizing activity. In contrast, we also found that several immobilization-positive sera from the WHO Bank were negative in our assay system. Therefore, standardization of assay technique must be done before you can say the ratio of immobilization-positive sera among Japanese women is higher than among those in other countries. We always use more than 200 CH_{50} titers of guinea pig sera as complement, because complement is a very important factor for the sensitivity of the sperm-immobilization test. If the commercial preparations of complement are used, the results of the test might not be reliable. The anti-

Gamete Interaction: Prospects for Immunocontraception, pages 415–418
© 1990 Wiley-Liss, Inc.

complementary factor in the human seminal plasma always consumed less than one CH_{50} in our assay system, and we use enough titer of complement for as much as 10 CH_{50} of guinea pig sera. Human sera contain usually one-fifth of CH_{50} on average compared with guinea pig sera; thus we should not use human serum as a complement source if we expect sensitive results.

DR. ALEXANDER: Dr. Hjort mentioned that different cultures might account for the formation of antisperm antibodies. For example, there is some information that homosexual men are much more likely to have antisperm antibodies. In addition, work in our laboratory reveals that women with genital tract infections are much more likely to have antisperm antibodies.

DR. MITCHISON: Dr. Isojima raised the issue of specificity. It sounded like another heterophil antibody like the one that led the retrovirologists astray a few years ago, when they were looking for naturally occurring antibodies to various rhinoviruses that are glycosylated. They thought that this was evidence of immunization, and it was not. Those are antibodies that were probably generated against the bacterial flora. That doesn't mean that they are devoid of interest, but it does mean that they are poor vaccine candidates, especially because these carbohydrate determinates are present beyond our capacity to manipulate them. We know how to handle protein antigens, but we don't know how to handle carbohydrate antigens. By and large, they are IgM antibody, although some belong to this rather mysterious group of products of CD5 or Ly-1B cells, which seem to be driven through the network rather than through antigenic simulation. Somehow or other, they don't seem to be the most inaccessible part of the B-cell spectrum. My next concern is the issue of affinity selection, not using antibodies of proteins that might be of use as vaccine candidates, for example, the C3b protein itself, or its ligand One could imagine that the zona receptors could be cloned directly by affinity selection. I am very impressed by the progress that Brian Seed has made in picking out Fc receptors by affinity selection rather than by using antibodies.

DR. SUTCLIFFE: Brain Seed's experiments were very nice, because they simply asked, can we turn something in a COS cell that will allow a COS cell to interact with fixed Fc regions? It turned out to be an Fc receptor. Some of my colleagues in the Department of Genetics are thinking of cloning neuropeptide receptors that perhaps could be used as an activity receptor. The main thing is to get a system with sufficient receptors expressed on the surface, because that will help to drive the kinetics toward immobilization. I think it's going to be a question of getting the mathematics of the dissection constants right so that one can actually select the cells at the end of the day.

DR. GOLDBERG: It seems to me that there is still a great deal of emphasis on generating more and more antibodies to different sperm antigens. I just wonder if our emphasis is misplaced. It is clear, for example, that while it is possible to generate antibodies against sperm, these antibodies, whether they are made or are naturally occurring, are against weak antigens. If that were not the case, women would become very actively immunized against sperm antigens, whether surface antigens or not. We really have to get back to the basic question of the nature of the antigens. While heroic methods have been attempted in the past to isolate membrane proteins and to extract sperm, I think that you have to define the problem more precisely and utilize the modern methods that are available.

DR. ISOJIMA: With regard to Mitchison's question concerning the carbohydrate moiety, I also speculate that there may be some similarities of carbohydrate antigens between human sperm and bacteria or virus, but there is no proof of whether sperm-immobilizing antibodies were generated by bacterial or viral infections. When we published a paper concerning the carbohydrate epitope of sperm-coating antigen corresponding to human sperm-immobilizing monoclonal antibody H6-3C4 in *The Journal of Experimental Medicine*, another paper that identified a very similar carbohydrate structure of *Neisseria gonorrhea* as our antigen epitope appeared in the same journal, but the structure was not exactly the same as ours. In contrast, clinically we could see many possible occasions for women to be sensitized against sperm. When we perform laparoscopy in women, we can find many motile spermatozoa and also many macrophages in the peritoneal cavity. Therefore, we can speculate that macrophages possibly pick up the sperm in the peritoneal cavity and then transfer their antigenic information to immunocompetent lymphocytes. We cannot neglect the fact that most women positive for sperm-immobilizing antibodies raised antibodies against sperm-coating carbohydrate epitopes, and they were healthy except they were infertile. So far, I have never seen fertilization-blocking antibodies in our in vitro fertilization and embryo transfer experiences in women. Clarke in Australia reported some fertilization-blocking antibodies in sterile women, but I am not sure, because no other people examined those sera. So far, we don't know if women with unexplained sterility have fertilization-blocking antibodies in their sera, but it is very important to examine this in the future.

DR. SEHGAL: I just wanted to make a comment about the incidence of sperm-immobilizing antibodies in Indian patients. We recently conducted a number of surveys and found that these antibodies are not uncommon in the Indian population. Frequently, high titers were found in the sera of women who were infertile. Second, as a listener over the past several days, I feel that every speaker is armed with a favorite antigen. Short peptides have problems of cross-reactivity, as we have learned from the human chorionic gonadotropin experience. I am wondering why we left out conformational antigens altogether?

28

Molecular Biological Approaches for Antigen Production

William W. Chin

One of the major goals of the worldwide effort in immunocontraception is the isolation and characterization of sperm, zona pellucida, and other antigens that may be appropriate targets for immunologic intervention. An immunocontraceptive program of this type requires large quantities of scarce target proteins that are difficult to obtain by traditional biochemical techniques. Fortunately, molecular biology and recombinant DNA techniques have permitted the production of target antigens in bulk. The objective of this chapter is to review the molecular biological approaches for antigen production.

RECOMBINANT SPERM AND ZONA ANTIGENS

The production of recombinant antigens representing sperm, zona pellucida, and other proteins would be advantageous for a number of reasons. From a cellular point of view, expression of these proteins, usually membrane antigens, would allow further definition of their roles in physiology. In addition, the effects of authentic antigens on cell function could be assessed. At the biochemical level, molecular biology would allow analysis of structure–function relationships of specific antigens. The effects of mutant antigens either as extracellular proteins or as surface antigens may also be evaluated. Finally, on the immunologic level, antibodies to these proteins could, theoretically, interfere with sperm–egg interactions and thus lead to contraception. On the one hand, antibodies could be produced against synthetic oligopeptides corresponding to deduced

Gamete Interaction: Prospects for Immunocontraception, pages 419–433
© 1990 Wiley-Liss, Inc.

amino acid sequences of a given antigen such that nonauthentic proteins or peptide fragments derived thereof may be sufficient to induce immunologic responses. On the other hand, the use of authentic antigens may be necessary if various modifications, including protein folding, subunit interactions, or other post-translational modifications, are critical to induce a particular immunologic response.

Other applications of molecular genetics and recombinant antigens might include the use of mutant proteins as inhibitors of sperm–egg interactions. Thus the full understanding of the biochemical, biologic, and immunologic characteristics of specific antigens may not be restricted to their use in immunocontraception. It is possible that inhibitors, as peptide fragments, mutant peptides, or partially modified proteins, may serve as partial agonists or antagonists of natural action. Last, while proteins may be used in combination with adjuvants and appropriate sustained-release delivery systems to promote an immune response, it is likely that genetic engineering will permit the introduction of genes encoding appropriate antigens into live attenuated viruses such as vaccinia or poliovirus.

Nature of Specific Antigens

One of the most important considerations in a discussion of antigen production is an understanding of the nature of a specific antigen. In particular, does the antigen have a *simple* structure, that is, a single polypeptide backbone that does not undergo further folding or intra- and intermolecular covalent bond formation, or modification of constituent amino acids? Or, is the antigen *complex*, that is, does the protein backbone consist of amino acids that are glycosylated, phosphorylated, sulfated, acetylated, and so forth? Or must the polypeptide precursor undergo proteolytic cleavage, folding, or subunit interactions to yield the biologically and perhaps immunologically active component. The production of a simple peptide can be performed by either prokaryotic or eukaryotic host cells, as discussed below. However, the production of complex molecules often requires eukaryotic cells with a focus on mammalian cells.

Molecular Cloning of cDNAs and Genes Encoding Specific Antigens

Another aspect of the issue of large-scale production of specific antigens is the molecular cloning of cDNAs and genes encoding sperm, zona pellucida, and other antigens. The ability to isolate these genetic elements is absolutely crucial to allow large production of their encoded proteins, and there are a number of approaches that one may take to obtain such cDNAs and genes [Sambrook et al., 1989]. First, a biochemical approach may be taken. This involves the isolation, purification, and characterization of a specific antigen. Thereafter, peptide mapping and amino acid sequencing will provide information from which the nucleotide sequence can be deduced and oligodeoxyribonucleotide probes produced for screening of cDNA libraries. Second, an immunologic approach may be followed in which antibodies directed against a specific antigen, either polyclonal or monoclonal, are used to screen expression cDNA libraries in either bacterial or mammalian cell hosts. Third, a functional approach may be employed to select cDNAs expressed in specific cells by assaying for the presence or absence of biological activity. Finally, if a particular sperm or zona pellucida protein results from differential expression either in response to specific factors or in a developmental stage, then subtraction or differential hybridization cDNA cloning techniques may be used for identifying antigens.

FLOW OF GENETIC INFORMATION

Before one considers the detailed approaches to production of a specific antigen, it is essential to review the basic flow of genetic information that is shown in Figure 1. A particular antigen is encoded by a gene. This gene is transcribed in the nucleus to produce a precursor RNA [Maniatis et al., 1987]. This precursor or heteronuclear RNA is rapidly modified via RNA processing to yield a messenger RNA (mRNA) that is quickly transported from the nucleus to the cytoplasm, where it interacts with the protein synthetic machinery [Nevins, 1983; Padgett et al., 1986]. After translation of the mRNA, a precursor protein is synthesized. This new molecule can be further modified by undergoing a number of post-translational processing steps, including protein folding, site-specific proteolytic cleavages, glycosylation, phosphorylation, sulfation, disulfide linkage formation, as well as possible oligomerization in the case of complex proteins involving subunit–subunit interactions. The resultant mature protein may then be either secreted or retained intracellularly depending on its established fate. In the case of most sperm and ovum antigens to be considered for contraceptive vaccine development, these proteins are located at the cell surface as membrane proteins.

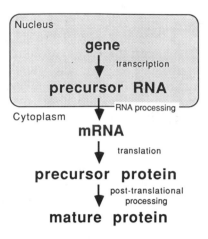

Fig. 1. Flow of genetic information. Information encoded in a gene is transformed into a precursor RNA via the process of *transcription* in the nucleus. This molecule then undergoes rapid modification via *RNA processing* to produce a messenger RNA (mRNA), which is transported into the cytoplasm. The information in the mRNA is transformed into a precursor protein via the process of *translation*. This precursor protein then undergoes post-translational processing to yield the mature protein that may be secreted or retained intracellularly. The post-translational processes include proteolytic cleavage, protein folding, subunit–subunit interactions, glycosylation, phosphorylation, and acetylation.

GENERAL PROTEIN EXPRESSION

The key concept in the use of molecular genetics to produce recombinant antigens in large quantities is that recombinant DNAs, when introduced in a given host cell, can be used as a template for the increased production of transcripts encoding a particular antigen and subsequent translation and processing to yield mature protein. In essence, the introduced genetic material is considered "self" by the host cell, and thus the exogenous gene commandeers the host cell to produce proteins as if it were its own (Fig. 2). Factors that need to be considered when using this approach are requirements for complex polypeptides, level of expression, stability of protein, and location of protein within or without the cell. Indeed, intracellular protein may be more difficult to isolate and to purify from a mixture of cellular proteins than from protein that is secreted into the extracellular space. In the presence of serum-free culture media, in the case of a mammalian host cell, such secreted proteins can easily be isolated and purified.

As stated above, one of the most important initial questions to ask in the process of antigen expression is whether an authentic molecule is required, that is, whether it is simple or complex, and hence

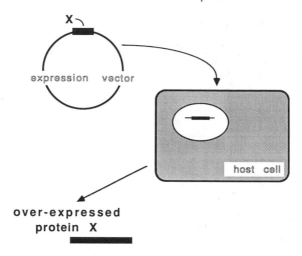

Fig. 2. Overexpression of foreign proteins using recombinant DNA techniques. This schematic diagram depicts the introduction of an expression vector bearing a cDNA encoding protein X into a host cell that is then commandeered to overproduce protein X as either a secreted form (as shown) or an intracellular form.

whether the protein alone would be sufficient. If only the expression of antigenic domains is required, then expression of peptide fragments or production of synthetic oligopeptides may suffice. Unfortunately, because synthetic oligopeptides are still expensive to produce, peptide fragments remain the immunogen of choice. Of note, many of the proteins on which we will focus are membrane-spanning proteins and thus will generally possess leader peptides (15 to 20 amino acid hydrophobic NH_2-terminal sequences found typically in precursors of proteins destined for secretion or membrane location) as well as membrane-spanning domains. Thus their precursors are likely to be relatively lipophilic and be either located in the membrane or stored as packets within granules, possibly awaiting secretion.

There are two major components to protein expression using recombinant DNA techniques. The first is the *expression vector* (Fig. 3). A prototypical expression vector possesses a transcriptional unit cloned into a plasmid pBR322-derivative vector. The plasmid pBR322 derivatives allow for insertion of foreign DNA into a vector that can autonomously replicate because of the presence of an origin of replication (ori), while an ampicillin-resistance gene (amp^r) permits the selection of successfully transfected bacteria [Lindenmaier et al., 1982]. In addition, these prokaryotic sequences contain sufficient

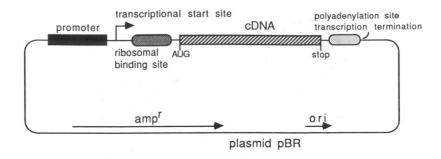

Fig. 3. A generalized expression vector. The key elements in an expression
vector are shown. The cDNA encodes the precursor polypeptide from the initiation codon, AUG (Met), to the stop codon. The ribosomal binding site or
Shine-Delgarno sequence is critical for efficient translation mediated via improved binding of ribosomal RNA subunits. In addition, a polyadenylation site/
transcription termination signal at the 3' end of the transcriptional unit determines the end of transcription by the RNA polymerase. Last, a promoter is
necessary to determine the level of activity of the transcriptional unit as well as
the transcriptional start site. The promoter is generally specific for a particular
host cell. High levels of protein production are generally dependent on highly
active promoter elements. This transcriptional unit is placed into a plasmid
pBR322 vector that also includes an ampicillin-resistance gene (amp^r) in order to
select for recombinant DNAs and an origin of replication (ori) to allow autono-
mous replication of the recombinant DNA in specific bacteria.

unique restriction enzyme sites to facilitate the construction of appropriate recombinant DNAs but lack certain "poison" sequences
that would normally limit duplication and thus allow efficient replication in eukaryotic host cells.

The transcriptional unit consists of structural and regulatory regions. The structural region consists, in general, of a complementary
DNA that encodes the entire polypeptide precursor. In addition,
there are signals that increase the efficiency of translation of its
mRNA, including the presence of a ribosomal binding or Shine-
Delgarno site (procaryote—binding to the 3' end of the 16S ribosomal
RNA) [Gold et al., 1981; Coleman et al., 1985; Marquis et al., 1986;
Kaufman et al., 1987] as well as a polyadenylation site (AAUAAA
located 10–30 nucleotides upstream of the site of polyadenylation)/
transcription termination signal [a GU- or U-rich region downstream
of the site) present at the 3' end of the gene [Birnstiel et al., 1985].
The regulatory region consists of a promoter that is a site of RNA
polymerase binding and includes a TATA box (25–30 bp upstream of
the start of transcription) and upstream elements (within 100–200
bp). This site increases the level of transcription of the structural
gene as well as determines the precise point of initiation of the RNA

HOST CELLS

	procaryotes *E. coli*	lower eucaryotes *yeast* *insect cells*	higher eucaryotes *mammalian cells*
Advantages	1. large amounts 2. inexpensive	1. good production 2. secretion (yeast) 3. some PT processing	1. complex PT processing

Disadvantages	1. no complex PT
	   processing
	2. some proteins
	   unstable
	3. intracellular,
	   in general
			1. expensive
			2. low yield

Fig. 4. Host cells. The advantages and disadvantages of a number of host cells including procaryotes (*E. coli*), lower eukaryotes (yeast, insect cells), and higher eukaryotes (mammalian cells) for recombinant protein expression.

transcript (transcriptional start site). This vector when introduced into an appropriate host cell will utilize the host RNA transcriptional machinery to produce multiple copies of the structural gene acting as a template.

The second is the choice of *host cells*. Figure 4 indicates the advantages and disadvantages of various host cells. The most common prokaryotic host cell is *Escherichia coli*. Because of its short doubling time, this bacterium can be expected to produce large amounts of proteins with low cost. However, the disadvantages are that it cannot accomplish complex post-translational processing, often produces unstable proteins, and retains them intracellularly. The use of lower eukaryotic hosts, yeast, and insect cells has the advantage of good production rates and some post-translational processing. In the case of yeast, proteins can be secreted into the media, whereas in insect cells, particularly the baculovirus system [Luckow and Summers, 1988], recombinant proteins may be packed into dense molecular forms within the cell. Finally, with higher eukaryotes, mammalian cells may be used to express proteins that require complex post-translation processing. The major disadvantages of the use of mammalian cells are relative low yield even in the presence of high level expression vectors and increased expense because of media costs.

Once proteins are expressed either as simple or complex polypeptides, they will require further amplification, isolation, and purification [Shatzman and Rosenberg, 1987]. These steps involve classic

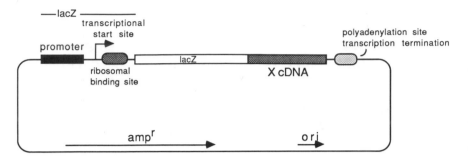

Fig. 5.   Overexpression of a fusion protein in *E. coli*. A lacZ promoter controls the transcription of a lacZ/X recombinant DNA encoding a β-galactosidase/protein X fusion protein. A large part of lacZ and protein X are located at the NH₂-terminal and COOH-terminal ends of the fusion protein, respectively. Polyadenylation site/transcriptional termination signals are required as shown. This transcriptional unit is located in a pBR-based vector that includes the ampicillin-resistance gene (ampʳ) and the origin of replication (ori).

biochemical techniques that are described extensively in relevant publications and will not be discussed further in this chapter.

PROKARYOTIC GENE EXPRESSION

Expression in prokaryotes is generally straightforward. The major decision is the choice of a number of highly inducible systems or strong promoters that are active in specific bacteria [de Boer et al., 1983; Hall et al., 1983; Shatzman et al., 1983]. Figure 5 shows an example of the use of the β-galactosidase (lacZ) gene in *E. coli*, a gene that is normally under constitutive negative regulation by a repressor protein [Hall et al., 1983]. However, the binding of repressor protein with isopropylthio-β-D-galactoside can interrupt this repression, thus allowing increased transcription. This is a particularly active endogenous gene in *E. coli*. If an antigen is not required in its full-length, authentic state, a fusion protein may be sufficient for the specific needs. In particular, a portion of an antigen may be combined at the COOH-terminal end of an NH₂-terminal fragment of β-galactosidase, which is expressed as the combined fusion protein. The fusion protein may be detected functionally, because β-galactosidase activity is retained in the NH₂-terminal fragment of the enzyme. Then, large amounts of the fusion protein can be expressed and isolated by SDS polyacrylamide gel electrophoresis. The purified protein can be used directly as an immunogen. Other inducible prokaryotic promoters include trpE, trp-lac, bacteriophage λpₗ, and bacteriophage T7.

If an authentic protein is desired, then other approaches may be necessary. The use of strong bacterial promoters along with a good ribosomal binding site and AUG (initiator methionine) may be used to increase transcription of the adjacent cDNA encoding the authentic protein. In this approach, as much as 1–30% of the total cell protein may be synthesized. However, inasmuch as an incorrect folding and instability of proteins within this system is a common problem, it may be more efficient to produce a precursor protein that is more stable. Once expressed, the precursor may then be further cleaved extracellularly using chemicals such as cyanogen bromide or enzymes such as factor Xa. Furthermore, foreign proteins may be engineered to be secreted from the bacterium into the periplasmic space, thus possibly improving their stability [Talmadge et al., 1980; Kikuchi et al., 1981].

Once these proteins are synthesized, levels of cloned gene product may be assessed by using traditional biochemical techniques, such as SDS polyacrylamide gel electrophoresis, to assay for either stained or newly synthesized labeled proteins. Other approaches include Western blot assays and ELISA, which focus on the immunologic characteristics of a particular antigen. Also, the biological activity, if present, may be determined.

Levels of expression in bacteria may be modulated via mutagenesis to increase translational initiation. Another approach is to develop mutant strains that may permit increased transcription by decreasing transcription termination or by altering RNA metabolism. The location of proteins in a fusion protein may variably stabilize mRNA and increase translation efficiency. Alterations of the kinetics of the transfection and the nature of the construct by moving various control elements relative to one another, increasing copy number by changing inducers, or using other approaches could theoretically increase yield. Finally, improvements in protein purification will also result in larger yield. In particular, inclusion bodies produced in bacteria that contain recombinant DNA protein products in concentrated form may facilitate protein purification approaches.

EUKARYOTIC GENE PROTEIN EXPRESSION

As shown in Figure 6, the vectors utilized for expression in these cell systems are very similar to those used in prokaryotic systems. The only difference is the use of a promoter that may be expressed only in eukaryotic cells and accompanied by an enhancer element. Enhancers are generally position- and orientation-independent cis-DNA elements that bind trans-acting proteins that may be expressed only in specific cell types or tissues. They, by unknown mechanisms,

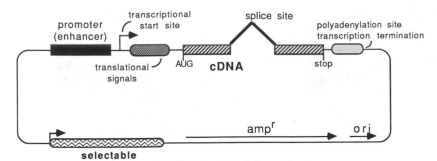

selectable
marker gene :DHFR, dihydrofolate reductase
Tn5/Tn605, aminoglycoside 3' phosphotransferase
TK, thymidine kinase
gpt, xanthine-guanine phosphoribosyl transferase
ADA, adenosine deaminase

Fig. 6. A mammalian expression vector. A strong promoter, assisted by appropriate enhancer sequences appropriate for a specific host cell, controls the activity of the transcriptional unit. Translational and polyadenylation site/transcription termination signals are included, along with an intron with appropriate splice donor and acceptor sites within the cDNA to improve RNA processing and stability. A selectable marker gene is present to select cells that have integrated this expression vector. Examples of such marker genes are shown. The copy number of some selectable marker genes may be amplified by drug treatment. Again, as shown in Figures 3 and 5, this expression vector is based on pBR, which includes the ampicillin resistance gene (amp^r) and the origin of replication (ori).

increase the activity of RNA polymerase II and hence the transcriptional rate [Dynan and Tjian, 1985]. In addition, these yeast and mammalian expression vectors may also possess intron splice donor and acceptor sites within the cDNA. The presence of introns that require splicing appears to increase the activity of many transcriptional units and the stability of its encoded mRNA [Charnay et al., 1984]; Gruss et al., 1979]. Last, the presence of a selectable marker enables selection of mammalian cells that have integrated various expression vectors [Colbere-Garapin et al., 1981; Kaufman and Sharp, 1982; Kaufman et al., 1986; Mulligan and Berg, 1980]. They include 1) thymidine kinase, 2) dihydrofolate reductase, 3) ornithine decarboxylase, 4) aminoglycoside phosphotransferase, 5) xanthine-guanine phosphoribosyl transferase, and 6) adenosine deaminase. Furthermore, certain selectable markers allow for increases in copy number of the particular vector. For instance, the use of the dihydrofolate reductase (DHFR) gene in dfhr⁻ cell lines and in the presence of methotrexate can increase the copy number of the vectors 50- to 100-fold [Schimke, 1984].

The promoter sequences are usually derived from viruses such as simian virus 40 (SV40) [Elder et al., 1981], adenovirus (Ad) [Berkner, 1988], vaccinia [Fuerst et al., 1987], human cytomegalovirus (CMV), Rous sarcoma virus (RSV), mouse mammary tumor virus (MMTV), and so forth. Alternatively, strong housekeeping gene promoters derived from genes such as metallothionein [Karin et al., 1983] may also be used. In addition, enhancers from these viruses and viral promoters may be utilized. Polyadenylation and termination transcription sites may be obtained from an SV40 gene. Finally, splicing signals can be obtained either from SV40 or immunoglobulin systems.

SV40-promoter containing vectors are generally amplified many fold in cells expressing T antigen (i.e., COS cells). Other viruses that have been used are the Epstein-Barr virus (EBV) [Lupton and Levine, 1985] and the bovine papilloma virus (BPV) [Law et al., 1983]. Both of these can produce recombinant DNAs in low copy numbers in mammalian host cells as they replicate episomally. The particular promoter and transcriptional start site used can be either natural, that is, the promoter normally associated with a given gene, or it can be provided by the vector, that is, the virus or housekeeping gene promoter and its associated transcriptional start site.

In general, foreign protein expression in eukaryotes requires stable transfection of host cells involving integration of exogenous genomes into that of the recipient. In addition, each host cell, although usually capable of most post-translational processing steps, may perform the modifications slightly differently. Thus Chinese hamster ovary cells are capable of greater terminal sialylation of N-linked carbohydrate moieties than certain fibroblast cell lines such as CV-1 or 3T3. Transfection approaches have been described elsewhere [Sambrook et al., 1989], and all involve the introduction of foreign DNA into mammalian cells by plasma membrane perturbation via the uptake of macromolecular complexes, or detergent or electrical disruption.

OTHER APPROACHES

The use of DNA viruses (vaccinia or herpes), RNA viruses (polio and TD70), and bacterial vectors such as bacillus Calmette-Guérin (BCG) hold promise for future expression of proteins in viruses and bacteria without going through the laborious task of purifying and isolating protein antigens [Bloom 1989]. Unfortunately, the state of the art of these approaches is still quite young, and problems such as pathogenicity need to be resolved before such methods can be considered for widespread use.

Finally, two other approaches, utilizing transgenic animals, may be applied to the production of large quantities of recombinant antigens [Pavirani et al., 1989]. The first is the production of *trans-hybridomas*. This approach involves the controlled expression of cDNAs encoding a specific antigen by B-cell regulatory DNA sequences in lymphoid cells of transgenic mice. A potential promoter includes the mouse Ig heavy-chain enhancer adjacent to the mouse Igκ promoter and an associated sequence encoding the Igκ signal sequence present in the first intron of its gene. The cDNA encoding the foreign antigen is placed directly 3' of this signal sequence. Transgenic mice are generated in the standard fashion, and the transgenes expressing the protein are identified. Spleen cells from such progeny are fused to myelomas cells to form trans-hybridomas. These cells then can be grown as cell lines that actively produce and secrete the foreign antigen.

The other approach is called *trans-immortalization*. The key concept here is the production of tumors of the lymphoid system by the introduction of an oncogene in tandem with the cDNA encoding the foreign antigen, both under control of immunoglobulin promoters. In this fashion, lymphoid tumors are produced that can make large quantities of both the oncogene product and the foreign antigen. Thus, in these two novel approaches, large quantities of foreign antigen can be produced.

SUMMARY

In this chapter we have considered the use of recombinant DNA techniques to produce large quantities of specific antigens. It is important to determine whether the antigen of interest is simple or complex in structure. In addition, it is critical to establish the projected use of a given antigen. In particular, is the antigen to be used for immunization purposes only or also in biochemical and biological characterizations? In the former case, authentic or nonauthentic polypeptides may be used. Thus a peptide fragment or a synthetic oligopeptide may serve as the immunogen. In the latter case, only an authentic protein may be employed. The answers to these two questions will determine the most appropriate vectors and host cells to be used. A prokaryotic host cell may be used for the production of simple antigens in large quantities with low cost. However, numerous eukaryotic proteins are poorly expressed because of either problems in protein folding leading to intracellular instability or low level expression. The use of eukaryotic host cells is critical for the production of complex antigens that require extensive post-translational modifications, including extensive folding, proteolytic cleavages, glycosylation, phosphorylation, subunit–subunit interaction, and so forth.

Another major issue is the ability of this technology to maximize expression via in vitro mutagenesis. Finally, the use of newer techniques such as trans-hybridomas, trans-immortalization, and live attenuated viruses carrying the genes encoding specific antigens lie at the vanguard of approaches in immunocontraception.

REFERENCES

Berkner KL (1988). Development of adenovirus vectors for the expression of heterologous genes. BioTechniques 6:616.

Birnstiel ML, Busslinger M, Strub K (1985): Transcription termination and 3' processing: The end is in site! Cell 41:349.

Bloom BR (1989): Vaccines for the third world. Nature 342:115.

Charnay P, Treisman R, Mellon P, Chao M, Axel R, Maniatis T (1984): Differences in human α- and β-globin gene expression in mouse erthroleukemia cells: The role of intragenic sequences. Cell 38:251.

Colbere-Garapin F, Horodniceanu F, Kourilsky P, Garapin A-C (1981): A new dominant hybrid selective marker for higher eucaryotic cells. J Mol Biol 150:1.

Coleman J, Inouye M, Nakamura K (1985): Mutations upstream of the ribosome-binding site affect translational efficiency. J Mol Biol 181:139.

de Boer HA, Comstock LJ, Vasser M (1983): The tac promoter: A functional hybrid derived from the trp and lac promoters. Proc Natl Acad Sci USA 80:21.

Dynan WS, Tjian R (1985): Control of eucaryotic messenger RNA synthesis by sequence-specific DNA-binding proteins. Nature 316:774.

Elder JT, Spritz RA, Weissman SM (1981): Simian virus 40 as a eucaryotic cloning vehicle. Annu Rev Genet 15:295.

Fuerst TR, Earl PL, Moss B (1987): Use of a hybrid vaccinia virus-T7 RNA polymerase system for expression of target genes. Mol Cell Biol 7:2538.

Gold L, Pribnow D, Schneider T, Shinedling S, Singer BS, Stormo G (1981): Translational initiation in procaryotes. Annu Rev Microbiol 35:365.

Gruss P, Lai C-J, Dhar R, Khoury G (1979): Splicing as a requirement for biogenesis of functional 16S mRNA of simian virus 40. Proc Natl Acad Sci USA 76:4317.

Hall CV, Jacob PE, Ringold GM, Lee F (1983): Expression and regulation of *Escherichia coli* lacZ gene fusions in mammalian cells. J Mol Appl Genet 2:101.

Karin M, Cathala G, Nguyen-Huu MC (1983): Expression and regulation of a human metallothionein gene carried on an autonomously replicating shuttle vector. Proc Natl Acad Sci USA 80:4040.

Kaufman RJ, Murtha P, Davies MV (1987): Translational efficiency of polycistronic mRNAs and their utilization to express heterologous genes in mammalian cells. EMBO J 6:187.

Kaufman RJ, Murtha P, Ingolia DE, Yeung C-Y, Kellems RE (1986): Selection and amplification of heterologous genes encoding adenosine deaminase in mammalian cells. Proc Natl Acad Sci USA 83:3136.

Kaufman RJ, Sharp PA (1982): Amplification and expression of sequences cotransfected with a modular dihydrofolate reductase complementary DNA gene. J Mol Biol 159:601.

Kikuchi Y, Yoda K, Yamasaki M, Tamura G (1981): The nucleotide sequence of the promoter and the amino-terminal region of alkaline phosphatase structural gene (phoA) of *Escherichia coli*. Nucleic Acids Res 9:5671.

Law M-F, Byrne JC, Howley PM (1983): A stable bovine papillomavirus hybrid plasmid that expresses a dominant selective trait. Mol Cell Biol 3:2110.

Lindenmaier W, Hauser H, Greiser I, de Wilke, Schutz G (1982): Gene shuttling: Moving of cloned DNA into and out of eucaryotic cells. Nucleic Acids Res 10:1243.

Luckow VA, Summers MD (1988): Trends in the development of baculovirus expression vectors. BioTechnology 6:47.

Lupton S, Levine AJ (1985): Mapping genetic elements of Epstein-Barr virus that facilitate extrachromosomal persistence of Epstein-Barr virus-derived plasmids in human cells. Mol Cell Biol 5:2533.

Maniatis T, Goodbourn S, Fischer JA (1987): Regulation of inducible and tissue-specific gene expression. Science 236:1237.

Marquis DM, Smolec JM, Katz DH (1986): Use of a portable ribosome-binding site for maximizing expression of a eucaryotic gene in *Escherichia coli*. Gene 42:175.

Mulligan RC, Berg P (1980): Expression of a bacterial gene in mammalian cells. Science 209:1422.

Nevins JR (1983): The pathway of eucaryotic mRNA formation. Annu Rev Biochem 52:441.

Padgett RA, Grabowski PJ, Konarska MM, Seiler S, Sharp PA (1986): Splicing of messenger RNA precursors. Annu Rev Biochem 55:1119.

Pavirani A, Skern T, Le Meur M, Lutz Y, Lathe R, Crystal RG, Fuchs J-P, Gerlinger P, Courtney M (1989): Recombinant proteins of therapeutic interest expressed by lymphoid cell lines derived from transgenic mice. BioTechnology 7:1049.

Sambrook J, Fritsch EF, Maniatis T (1989): Molecular Cloning. Cold Spring Harbor, NY: Cold Spring Harbor Laboratory.

Schimke RT (1984): Gene amplification in cultured animal cells. Cell 37:705.

Shatzman A, Ho Y-S, Rosenberg M (1983): Use of a phage λ regulatory signals to obtain efficient expression of genes in *Escherichia coli*. In Inouye M (ed): Experimental Manipulation of Gene Expression. New York: Academic Press, p 1.

Shatzman AR, Rosenberg M (1987): Expression, identification, and characterization of recombinant gene products in *Escherichia coli*. Methods Enzymol 152:661.

Talmadge K, Kaufman J, Gilbert W (1980): Bacteria mature preproinsulin to proinsulin. Proc Natl Acad Sci USA 77:3988.

DISCUSSION

DR. HERR: Our experience with endogenous β-galactosidase and the potential problems using β-gal-fusion proteins is restricted to one injection in each of two rabbits. We monitored the animals over a period of 8 weeks, and, although there was some weight loss, there were no visible signs of pathology.

DR. CHIN: β-Galactosidase immunologic activity has been found in a number of cells, in particular in the pituitary. I would be interested in hearing if other investigators have observed such reactions.

DR. O'RAND: We have experience in making a number of antibodies against fusion proteins. In fact, we purified the β-galactosidase from testes because we were concerned that antibodies to that part of the fusion protein might cause problems. As far as we have observed, the mammalian β-galactosidase is totally different from that of *E. coli* in terms of chemical and enzymatic properties, and there is no immunological cross-reactivity between them. These enzymes appear to be very different, and the bacterial form should not be a problem as part of a fusion protein immunogen.

DR. DUNBAR: We agree. We have used zona pellucida antigen–β-gal-fusion protein in rabbits, and, although we did not make antibodies to the rabbit zona proteins, we saw no side effects from the use of fusion protein in these long-term immunizations.

29

cDNA Cloning and Its Application to Cell Surface Proteins

R.G. Sutcliffe, A.M. Hundal, D.A. Nickson, S. Zeinali, M. McBride, and S.-L. Wang

The surface proteins of sperm and trophoblast represent potential targets for the immunological control of fertility, and considerable effort is being expended to find surface proteins of suitable tissue specificity for vaccine development. Molecular cloning provides a powerful way to investigate the structure and function of such proteins and to express them for large-scale antigen production. This chapter provides an overview of complementary DNA (cDNA) cloning strategies for the analysis of new membrane proteins. It also discusses a way in which techniques of molecular genetics may enable new membrane proteins to be discovered directly through the manipulation of cDNA, without the initial raising of monoclonal antibodies.

Since the availability of reliable methods for the synthesis and cloning of cDNA, an ever-increasing number of cDNAs have been identified as encoding defined proteins. There are several factors that have contributed to this rapid progress. The first is the creation of libraries large enough to represent most nearly the full diversity of mRNA species within the cell type or tissue. A given cell type may contain 1 pg of mRNA or some 500,000 molecules, representing 10,000–40,000 different mRNA species of which 25% are at very low abundance [see Williams, 1981]. To be 99% certain of cloning at least one representative of each messenger species, 2×10^5 recombinants are required [Maniatis et al., 1982]. These recombinants are generated by a series of steps, starting with the synthesis of cDNA, its

Gamete Interaction: Prospects for Immunocontraception, pages 435–458
© 1990 Wiley-Liss, Inc.

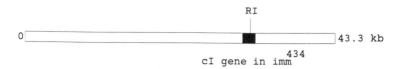

Fig. 1. λgt10, showing the EcoRI (RI) cloning site in the cI gene.

ligation into a vector, and the transformation of bacterial cells. Only when the library DNA is in bacterial cells as a set of independent and replication-competent transformants can the effective size of the library be estimated. The major advantage of using λ-derived cloning vectors (λgt10, λgt11, λZAP), is that the vector (plus insert DNA) can be packaged into phage heads in vitro with an efficiency of 10^{-1}. Packaged phage heads can transform *Escherichia coli* with an efficiency of close to unity. This is a very much higher frequency than can be achieved for plasmids, where with the best transformation efficiencies (10^8/μg) only 0.1% of the ligated vector ends up as transformants. In earlier days [see Maniatis et al., 1982], when bacterial transformation frequencies were commonly two orders of magnitude lower, plasmid cloning systems could not be applied with confidence to the search for rare cDNAs. More recently, the convenience of plasmid vectors has been combined with the packaging efficiency of λ vectors in commercially available kits (Stratagene LAMBDA ZAP and pBluescript).

The second requirement is to identify specific clones within the library that encode the required polypeptide. These requirements have most frequently been met, to date, by using derivatives of bacteriophage λ as vector and by screening with nucleic acid probes (notably in λgt10) or with specific antibodies to detect expressed protein epitopes (notably in λgt11). In both cases, phage plaques provide a better screening system, with a lower background, than do bacterial colonies.

λGT10: SCREENING BY NUCLEIC ACID HYBRIDIZATION

λgt10 (Fig. 1) is an insertion vector that will accept inserts up to 7 kb in length. The cloning site is an EcoRI site in the *cI* repressor gene. The vector's biological properties are that it grows as a lysogen, yielding turbid plaques on wild-type *E. coli* or strains such as L87. Lysogeny is directed primarily by the *cI* gene, in which mutations (including insertions of cDNA) disrupt the function of the repressor, leading to lytic growth and to the accumulation of large amounts of phage DNA. After restriction with EcoRI, λgt10 should be phosphatased before ligation of cDNA to reduce the yield of parental phage. It is possible to distinguish parental from recombinant phage by plating out the library on *E. coli hfl⁻* strains, where the lysogenic state is so favored that parental *cI⁺* phages do not form plaques. Even so, it is necessary to check that lytic plaques have genuine cDNA inserts rather than RI linkers, small fragments of other DNA, or *lacZ* deletions. λgt10 libraries are screened by nucleic acid hybridization, using labeled probes. Duplicate filters are screened for each set of plaques to allow the exclusion of spurious signals, and several rounds of plaque-purification are necessary to isolate a pure clone. There are several different types of probes. First, there are cross-hybridizing cDNA or genomic subclones that have previously been obtained to related members of a gene family or to similar proteins in other species. Examples abound of this type of probe, but particularly relevant ones include the isolation of HLA-C clones from the human trophoblastic choriocarcinoma cell lines BeWo and JEG-3 [Ellis et al., 1989; Rinke de Wit et al., 1990; Ward et al., manuscript in preparation, 1990].

The second class of hybridization probe is obtained by deduction from the partial sequence of a polypeptide, as was first achieved for β_2-microglobulin [Suggs et al., 1981]. Although it is relatively easy to obtain unblocked amino-terminal sequence, the codons corresponding to this protein sequence are located at the 5' end of the sense strand of cDNA, which may not have been cloned in an oligo(dT)-primed library. This complication may be avoided by screening a large random-primed library in which first strand synthesis of cDNA is not solely primed from the 3' end of the message. However, improvements in gas-phase sequencing of peptides recovered from two-dimensional acrylamide gels now make it easier to get multiple internal peptide sequences from single proteins cleaved either by cyanogen bromide (at methionine residues) or by V8 or other proteases [Kennedy et al., 1988]. Obviously, the longer the nucleic acid probe, the greater will be its specificity; however, because of the degeneracy of the genetic code, not all protein sequences will yield equally useful and lengthy oligonucleotide probes. With probes of 20 bases or more, a few mismatched bases can occur without disrupting the duplex, and, with probes of over 50 bases, mismatches of 20% can be tolerated without significant loss of specificity [Duby, 1987]. Tolerance of mismatches allows the selection at degenerate sites of codons of maximum likelihood based on codon utilization frequencies, dinucleotide frequencies and other considerations [Lathe, 1985]. Degeneracy in shorter sequences (<20–23 bases) is a more serious difficulty, because the thermal stability of the DNA duplex is low. The most obvious approach is to incorporate all alternative bases at all degenerate sites. However, it is difficult to be sure that the alternative bases will be incorporated at equal frequencies into the oligonucleotide [see Huynh-Dinh et al., 1988]. Furthermore, as the level of degeneracy rises, 1) the specific activity of the truly complementary oligonucleotide falls and 2) hybridization may occur between some species of oligonucleotide and irrelevant cDNA clones. The latter complication can be avoided if there is sufficient protein sequence to design two consecutive oligonucleotide probes to screen duplicate filters of the library [Wallace and Miyada, 1987]. Although there are formulae relating to the melting temperature of hybrid to the GC content of DNA [Lathe, 1985], the optimum stringency conditions for hybridization and subsequent washing have to be determined empirically. This is especially so with a very degenerate population of oligonucleotides that have a wide range of GC contents, though such difficulties of optimization have been avoided by the use of tetramethylammonium chloride, which abolishes the preferential melting of AT versus GC base pairs [Hanks, 1987; Wood et al., 1985].

To minimize these difficulties, bases and base analogs have been tested for their ability to form stable duplex structures with more than one of the natural bases in DNA. Deoxyinosine, 2-amino-2'-deoxyadenosine, and phenyl derivatives have been used to prepare unique complements to degenerate bases [Huynh-Dinh et al., 1985; Takahashi et al., 1985]. The stability of mismatches involving these analogs is not high, but at least for inosine the mismatch does not disrupt complementary base pairing on either side. Deoxyguanosine (dG) mismatches in a relatively stable manner with thymidine and thus can be used to complement C/T ambiguities [Millican et al., 1984]. 5-Fluorodeoxyuridine (FdU) matches relatively stably with deoxyadenosine and deoxyguanosine. This has led to a proposal that dG and FdU act as "spacer" purines and pyrimidines, respectively, at sites of ambiguity, with both being used at sites of fourfold ambiguity [Habener et al., 1988].

AMPLIFICATION OF CODING SEQUENCES BY POLYMERASE CHAIN REACTION

Polymerase chain reaction (PCR) is a method whereby microgram quantities of a short sequence of DNA (commonly up to a few kilobases) can be amplified from an initial template of nanogram quantities of high complexity DNA [see White et al., 1989]. This permits genetic analysis on single diploid cells and single sperm [Li et al.,

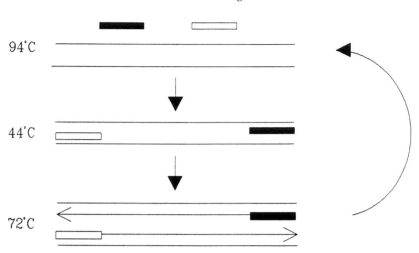

Fig. 2. The polymerase chain reaction (PCR). At 94°C the template DNA exists as single strands (shown as two lines) and the primers (shown as black and white boxes) do not hybridize to the DNA. At the optimal temperature for the primer sequences involved (shown here as 44°C) the primers anneal to complementary sites on the DNA. The optimal temperature for Taq polymerase is 72°C and the enzyme extends the primers from their 3′ ends to form new complementary DNA strands (arrowed lines). When the extension is complete, the PCR begins a new cycle of DNA melting, primer annealing, and primer extension. The quantity of DNA synthesized increases twofold each cycle; thus the reaction requires a vast excess of primers over template for the first cycle.

1988]. The system requires the presence of two primer sites on the same piece of template DNA. After the DNA has been rendered single stranded by heating to 94°C, the temperature is reduced so that the primers can anneal to the template DNA. If the primers anneal close enough together at sites on complementary strands of DNA and with their 3′ ends facing inward (Fig. 2), then DNA synthesis can extend those 3′ ends past the opposite primer site, thereby creating a new template for a further round of PCR. The result is the amplification of a short piece of DNA whose ends are precisely defined by the primers employed. DNA synthesis is catalyzed by Taq polymerase, which is sufficiently thermostable to withstand 40 cycles of temperature of up to 94°C and hence yield microgram quantities of amplified DNA. The inclusion of restriction sites at the 5′ ends of the PCR primers allows amplified DNA to be cloned into vectors for sequencing and other work.

PCR has been used in several ways to assist in cDNA cloning, both to create new clones ab initio (see below) and to extend the cloning of rare cDNAs to the full length of their corresponding transcripts

[O'Hara et al., 1989; Frohman et al., 1988]. Using the genetic code, PCR primers can be designed from protein sequence. As discussed above, the degeneracy of the code can lead to a large number of possible oligonucleotides. Degenerate oligonucleotides have been successfully used to clone protein coding sequences from cDNA libraries or from genomic DNA and, in the case of the 54 kd subunit of signal recognition particle, from a single sequence of 30 amino acids [Bernstein et al., 1989]. Some base pair mismatching between primer and template may be tolerated [Gould et al., 1989], provided there is a stable duplex at the 3' end of the primer so that DNA synthesis can occur. However, there are complications.

First, in highly degenerate mixtures of oligonucleotides, the concentration of each species of primer can be as little as less than 1/4,000 of the total primer. Thus it is possible for the supply of the appropriate primer to run out during a PCR reaction and so prevent the appearance of product as a major band on a gel. To overcome this problem, some investigators have reduced the annealing temperature of the first few rounds of PCR; others have incorporated the base deoxyinosine at positions of fourfold degeneracy in the primer [Knoth et al., 1988].

A second complication of PCR relates to the formation of primer–dimers [see Pauli et al., 1989]. Short lengths of homology between the 3' ends of primers can lead to the synthesis of extended primers. This can be seen when ^{32}P-labelled PCR products are resolved on a sequencing gel. The products are small and are not template dependent (Fig. 3). Primer–dimers are a particular hazard when short-range amplifications are attempted, especially when using highly degenerate primers. Although the formation of dimers may not be favored by the temperature of the PCR, a few rare dimers are all that is required to take over the PCR reaction.

DIRECTIONAL cDNA CLONING

Directional cDNA cloning is necessary for the efficient formation of subtraction libraries (see below) and should increase the efficiency of formation of other libraries. In conventional cloning into bacteriophage λ, double-stranded cDNA is ligated to EcoRI linkers and cloned in either orientation into the vector. In directional cloning, the cDNA is oriented by placing different restriction sites at either end. Several approaches have been devised, but assessment of their relative efficiencies has yet to emerge [see Kaiser, 1990a]. Uni-ZAP XR is a kit available from Stratagene that, like several other methods, employs a hybrid primer for the synthesis of the first strand of

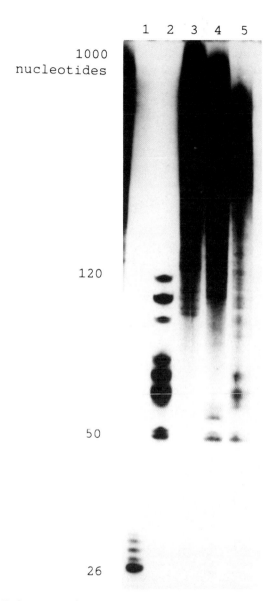

Fig. 3. Polymerase chain reaction (PCR) products labeled with α-^{32}P-labeled
nucleotide triphosphates, resolved on a 12.5% polyacrylamide sequencing gel
and detected by autoradiography. PCR was carried out on a placental cDNA
library in pCDM8, using in each case a single primer of degeneracy 2^{12}. Primer
A (shown as end-labeled DNA in track **1**) was used to generate the PCR products
seen in tracks **2** and **5**. Primer B was used for tracks **3** and **4**. Template DNA
(human genomic) was only present in the PCR reactions of tracks **3**, 4, and 5.
Note that, in the absence of template (track 2), primer A generates primer–dimer
products 50 nt and larger (50–120 nt). These products are also made when
template is present in the reaction (track 5), but not when the different primer
(B) is used (tracks 3 and 4).

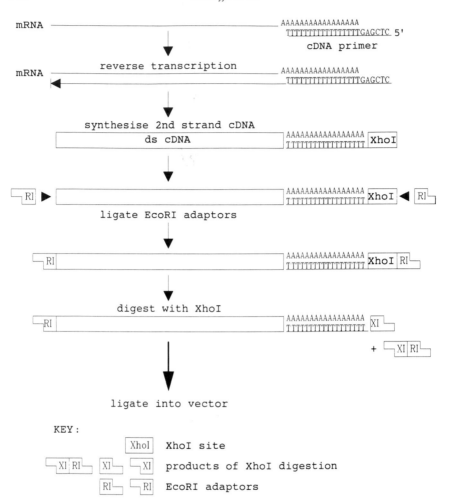

Fig. 4. Directional cloning of a cDNA molecule. See text for explanation. Details of the protection of the cDNA against XhoI digestion are not shown (see Stratagene manufacturer literature for Uni-ZAP XR).

cDNA. At the primer's 3' end is the oligo (dT) tract to prime reverse transcriptase; 5' to this is the sequence of an XhoI restriction site (Fig. 4). After the second strand of cDNA has been synthesized and the duplex cDNA has been flush ended, an EcoRI linker is ligated to both ends of the molecule. Cleavage with EcoRI and XhoI cuts the linker and the primer, yielding a cDNA with directionally oriented "sticky" ends for insertion into a vector with an oriented cloning site. In outline, this methodology is similar to standard bidirectional cloning methods and requires the protection of restriction enzyme sites within the cDNA sequence to be cloned.

THE DETECTION OF DIFFERENTIALLY EXPRESSED cDNAs BY SUBTRACTED PROBES AND SUBTRACTION LIBRARIES

The detection of differentially expressed gene products, such as those that are tissue specific, hormonally or virally induced, or heat-shock associated, is of great interest in both fundamental and applied research. *Plus and minus screening* has been employed to detect differentially expressed gene products whose mRNAs have an abundance of more than about 0.1% of the total cellular mRNA. In this technique, mRNA is made from the tissue of interest, and a cDNA library is prepared. mRNA is also made from a control tissue in which the genes to be cloned are either not expressed or expressed at a much lower level. Duplicate filters of the library are screened with labeled first-strand cDNA from mRNA of the tissue of interest and of the control tissue. Clones that hybridize to one cDNA probe but not the other are likely to be differentially expressed [Williams and Lloyd, 1979; Rowekamp and Firtel, 1980].

Subtractive methods are necessary to detect genes whose mRNAs have an abundance of less than 0.1% of the total cellular mRNA [Sargent, 1987]. The principle of the method is as follows. Consider two expressed nucleic acid sequences: S is tissue specific to spermatocytes and U is unspecific and is present in other tissues, including testis. If first-strand cDNA is made to testis mRNA and purified, an excess of mRNA from another tissue (e.g., fibroblasts) can be added under hybridization conditions. Because the single-stranded cDNA molecules are reverse transcripts, the U-type cDNAs will form hybrids with U-type mRNA from fibroblasts. These heteroduplexes are then separated by hydroxylapatite chromatography from the small proportion of single-stranded cDNA that remains [Davis, 1986; Sargent, 1987]. The latter is enriched in S-type sequences and is available either as a subtracted probe or to be cloned into a phage vector to yield a subtracted library. The subtracted probe can be used at high specific activity to screen a conventional phage or plasmid library, and the clones thus isolated can be checked for tissue specificity through Northern blots [Timberlake, 1980]. Subtracted libraries are technically difficult to make, because only a very small quantity of unsubtracted cDNA is available and it will be difficult to obtain a representative library. The addition of homopolymer tails to the 3' ends of the first-strand cDNA (see next section) may provide a means of amplifying the subtracted cDNA by PCR and hence cloning it more efficiently into phage.

A potentially more economical approach is to create a large conventional (U + S) library first and then subtract U-type sequences from it. This approach was used in the experiments on scrapie virus–modulated RNAs by Duguid et al. [1988]. Here, unoriented cDNA from scrapie-induced and -uninduced cells were made in pCDM8 (see below). Single strands were run off the library from the M13 origin, using a helper phage system, and the single strands from the uninduced library were labeled with biotin. Because the orientation of the M13 origin was the same in both libraries, the single vector strands would not hybridize together. However, the cDNA inserts were in either orientation in the two libraries. Thus uninduced cDNA sequences could form duplexes with the complementary strands from either library. To subtract the duplexes containing uninduced-type sequences, the DNA was passed over an avidin chromatography column that removed the biotinylated strands. By exposing the scrapie cDNA strands to an excess of biotinylated cDNA, the strands from the scrapie-induced preparation were successively depleted of uninduced sequences. The residual cDNA was made double stranded and transformed into *E. coli*. The transformants were then screened by colony hybridization with radiolabeled cDNA from induced and uninduced mRNA. Colonies that showed marked hybridization with the induced probe were selected and analyzed.

This type of subtraction library work could be developed in several ways. If the induced and uninduced cDNAs had been cloned in *opposite* directions into the vector to create the two libraries, there would have been no hybridization between single-stranded DNAs from within each library. This would have increased the efficiency of the subtraction. Second, the use of unselected cDNA as a probe for colony hybridization limits the sensitivity of the technique. Removal of U-type sequences from the probe will reduce the specific activity of the U component, making it more possible to pick up weaker signals from clones hybridizing with less abundant S-type cDNAs in the probe. Thus the use of a subtracted probe would improve this screening step, as would the transfer of the subtracted library into a λ phage vector, which can be screened with nucleic acid probes most efficiently.

LIBRARIES FROM SMALL NUMBERS OF CELLS

Conventional cDNA cloning is relatively routine, at least at the level of forming a representative library, if there are 10^7 or more cells available to provide the 200–1000 ng of mRNA required to create a library. However, there are circumstances in which tissue is in limited supply, for example, in work on early embryos or on nonproliferative cells explanted or dissected from complex tissues. In the last 2 years workers have begun to devise ways of scaling down the number of cells and mRNA required to create a representative library. It may be possible to scale down the isolation of poly(A)$^+$ RNA to an input of RNA from 10^3 cells [Tam et al., 1989]. Alternatively, and more attractively, Belyavsky et al. [1989] and Lu and Werner [1988] report that total cellular RNA is a satisfactory source for the synthesis of oligo(dT)-primed cDNA. Because small amounts of mRNA template can only yield small amounts of cDNA, PCR is the essential next step if sufficient cDNA is to be made to clone into a vector. Belyavsky et al. [1989] have used homopolymer tailing to add poly(dG) to the 3' end of the first-strand cDNA. Poly(dC) can then be used as a primer for second-strand synthesis at the start of a PCR reaction cycle. When duplex cDNA has been made, it can be amplified up to submicrogram amounts by suitable primers (Fig. 5). Such primers contain poly(dC) and poly(dT), respectively, as well as specific 5' *anchor sequences* on each primer to improve the fidelity of the PCR reaction and to provide a means of directional cloning.

The ability to make libraries from small numbers of cells will be important in reproductive biology, especially when the study of early embryonic or trophoblast cell populations is concerned. However, the methodology is now just emerging, and the reader is referred to a review by Kaiser [1990b] for detailed discussion.

λGT11

The significance of phage λ has already been discussed in that its highly efficient DNA packaging system enables the creation of large and representative cDNA libraries. In this section, we review the use of λgt11 as an expression vector and later compare it with a mammalian expression system.

λgt11 [Young and Davis, 1983] (Fig. 6) can accept cDNA sequences of up to about 7 kb in length into a unique EcoRI site 53 bases before the stop codon of the *lacZ* gene, which encodes β-galactosidase. Any adjacent open reading frame in a cDNA insert can be expressed as a fusion polypeptide with the β-galactosidase protein. Cloning is not directional, and the frequency with which a cDNA will be expressed in the correct frame and orientation will therefore be 1/6. Stratagene's recent Uni-ZAP XR system provides directional cloning into lacZ in a λ-based system. Like λgt10, λgt11 must be phosphatased before

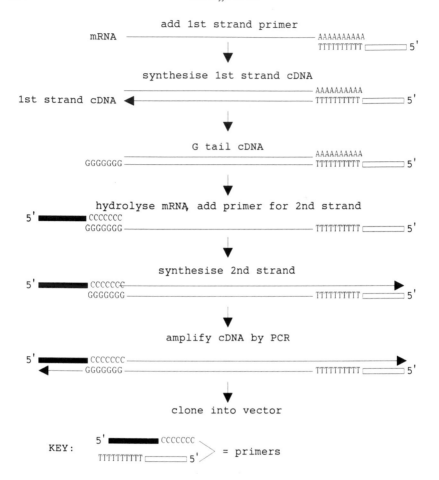

Fig. 5. Synthesis of cDNA molecules with primer sequences at either end. The primer sequences allow small quantities of cDNA to be amplified by polymerase chain reaction (PCR). Based on work by Belyavsky et al. [1989].

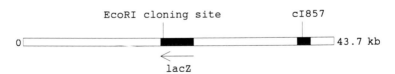

Fig. 6. λgt11, showing the EcoRI cloning site close to the end of the coding sequence for lacZ and the temperature-sensitive cI857 allele.

ligation of cDNA to reduce the yield of parental phage. Unlike λgt10, there is no system for suppressing parental phage. Thus it is important to have a low frequency of parental (nonrecombinant) phage;

otherwise very large screens are necessary to prevent rare recombinants being obscured by the overgrowth of parental phage. λgt11 has the *cI857* repressor allele, which encodes a temperature-sensitive cI repressor. At 42°C the repressor is inactivated and the phage will enter lytic growth.

To screen a λgt11 library, phage can be adsorbed to protease-deficient *lon⁻* Y1090 *E. coli*, plated, and incubated at 42°C for 3.5 hr to induce lysogens. The plates are then covered with dry nitrocellulose filters impregnated with the lac inducer isopropylthiogalactoside (IPTG). The plates are left at 37°C for 3–4 hr before antibody screening. The IPTG inducer relieves *lac* repression. Some workers find that lysogen induction or even IPTG induction is unnecessary, and some incubate their filters overnight.

Several protocols exist for antibody staining of nitrocellulose filters [see Mierendorf et al., 1987]. The prime requirements are for a low background and high sensitivity. Because an incomplete length of polypeptide is being expressed as a fusion protein in *E. coli*, it is wise to screen for as many epitopes on the protein as possible. Monoclonals that react with antigen in Western blots are more likely to combine with stable epitopes. Mixtures of monoclonal antibodies are preferable to single ones. Polyclonal antibodies are probably most useful, especially if there is a source of purified antigen to act as an adsorption control. It will often be necessary to adsorb antisera with *E. coli* cells, and prefiltration through 0.2 μm filters can also reduce background staining, possibly because of the removal of serum lipoproteins. A wide variety of commercial antibody detection systems are available, using ^{125}I-labeled protein A or protein G, biotin–avidin–horseradish peroxidase, or alkaline phosphatase.

SELECTION OF CLONES THROUGH TRANSIENT EXPRESSION IN MAMMALIAN CELLS

The use of mammalian cells for the expression and screening of cDNA clones is an attractive alternative to λ cloning. The polypeptide can be expressed in its native conformation with the appropriate pattern of post-translational modification. Such a system is the pCDM vector system of Seed and colleagues, which has been conspicuously successful in the cloning of a series of membrane proteins, most of which were defined by single or by a few monoclonal antibodies [Seed and Aruffo, 1987; Aruffo and Seed, 1987; Simmons and Seed, 1988]. pCDM8 (Fig. 7) is a shuttle vector with an SV40 origin (SV40 ori; Fig. 7), which allows the plasmid to replicate episomally in COS cells. COS cells contain a chromosomal copy of the

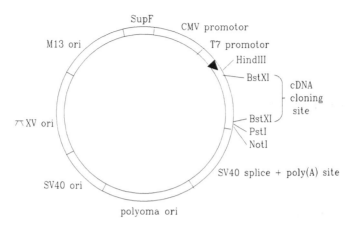

Fig. 7. pCDM8, a eukaryotic expression vector [Seed and Aruffo, 1987].

gene for the SV40 T antigen, which drives plasmid replication. Transient expression of cDNA sequences is initiated by the CMV promoter and enhancer 5′ to the cDNA cloning site, enabling transient expression of cDNA sequences. In contrast to the λgt11 system, no fusion protein is formed, and the cDNA should therefore contain the entire coding sequence of the polypeptide. The cDNA is therefore size selected before the library is made, because small cDNA inserts are unlikely to contain a complete coding sequence. A useful detail in the design of the BstXI cloning site increases the efficiency of ligation of cDNA into the vector. BstXI sites are interrupted palindromes, of sequence 5′CCAN5/NTGG3′. The middle six bases are in inverted orientation in the two sites, yielding identical and noncomplementary sticky ends after cleavage. These will not religate without an insert sequence, obviating the need to phosphatase the vector. The cDNA is then ligated into the vector via BstXI adaptors. A commercial version of pCDM8, pCDNA I, is now available from Invitrogen. Some of the original pCDM8 restriction sites have been removed, enabling the creation of a polylinker cloning site which includes two BstXI sites. Also included is an SP6 promoter for expressing antisense RNA in vitro.

The cDNA library in pCDM8 is transferred into *E. coli* MC1061/P3 and grown up under antibiotic selection. To maintain sequence representation, it is important to use a high efficiency transformation method. Seed and Aruffo [1987] made transformation-competent *E. coli* by a variation of the $CaCl_2$ procedure. In our hands this has an efficiency of 5×10^6 to 5×10^7/μg DNA. More recently we have found bacterial electroporation (Biorad Gene Pulser) to be more convenient, yielding efficiencies of $1-8 \times 10^7/\mu g$ DNA.

After amplification in *E. coli*, the library is expressed in COS cells so that clones can be expressed and immunoselected. For the immunoselection procedure, transfected COS cells are mixed with the specific antibody of interest and kept on ice in the presence of NaN_3. The cells are then pelleted through Ficoll to remove unbound antibody and then placed on bacteriological dishes coated with a second antibody. Cells coated with primary antibody attach to the dish through the second antibody bridge, and the unbound cells are discarded. This procedure is known as *panning*. The attached cells are then lysed to yield their plasmids, which are then purified and amplified by retransformation into MC1061/P3 cells.

To obtain specific clones, three cycles of expression, immunoselection, and amplification are usually required. In the first cycle the COS cells can be transformed with the library in the form of purified DNA, using DEAE dextran and DMSO shock. This transforms COS cells at a high frequency (10–40%) and allows a library to be panned from about 5×10^6 cells. However, with this approach the cells receive a mixture of plasmids, so that cells that are then panned with a specific antibody will contain a large number of different "passenger" clones as well as the cDNA encoding the required epitope. Further cycles of DEAE dextran transformation and panning will not reduce the complexity of these clones beyond 10^2 to 10^3 (A. Arrufo, personal communication). Transformation by spheroplast fusion has a lower efficiency (1–5%), and transformants are most likely to result from the fusion of a single *E. coli* cell with a single COS cell. This method is therefore used in the second and third rounds of selection. The technique requires practice.

The advantage of the COS cell system is that antigens or receptors can be expressed in their native state as full-length polypeptides on the surface of mammalian cells. Thus monoclonal or polyclonal antibodies, or other ligands, can be used to select cells expressing the clones. However, there are some limitations. It is difficult to clone full-length cDNA for long polypeptides, and it will not usually be possible to clone a protein whose antigenicity requires the presence of two different polypeptide chains unless one of the chains is normally expressed in COS cells. Next, the antibody or ligand must be able to bind the antigen or receptor when it is in the membrane. Antibodies to hidden determinants will be ineffective. It is therefore wise to show that the ligand will pan cells that naturally express the protein to be cloned. Furthermore, the selective antibody must not cross-react with COS cells or with mock transfected COS cells. If

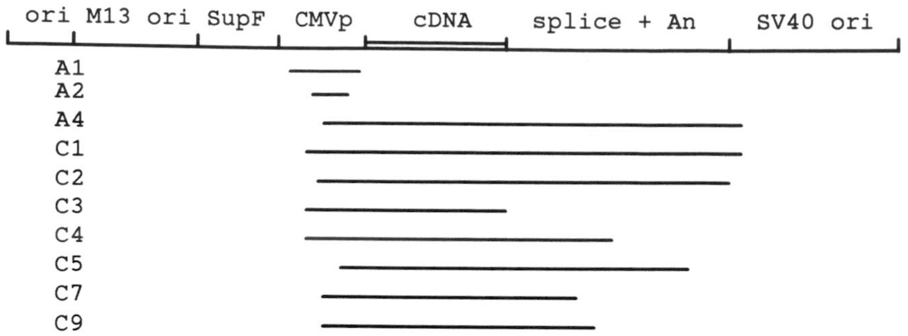

```
ori M13 ori SupF  CMVp      cDNA     splice + An    SV40 ori
└──┴─────┴───┴───┴────┴══════════┴──────────────┴──────────┘
      A1                ───────
      A2               ──
      A4                   ──────────────────────────────────
      C1            ──────────────────────────────────────
      C2            ──────────────────────────────────────────
      C3            ────────────────────
      C4            ──────────────────────────────
      C5               ───────────────────────────
      C7           ────────────────
      C9           ─────────────────────────
```

Fig. 8.   Deletion maps of 10 independent cDNA clones isolated as small plasmids from COS cells. In each case a deletion has occurred in the cytomegalovirus promoter region (CMVp).

there is cross-reaction, particularly if it involves a mouse monoclonal antibody, it may be possible to express pCDM8 in mouse WOP cells, using the plasmid's polyoma origin. Polyoma virus is very closely related in structure to SV40 but replicates in mouse cells. WOP cells are analogous to COS cells, because they have a chromosomal copy of polyoma virus big T antigen and can therefore drive the polyoma origin of replication in pCDM8.

A final word of caution relates to observations of our own that extensive deletions of the pCDM8 library can sometimes occur in COS-7 cells (Fig. 8). This can be extremely damaging, occurring at a rate that prevents the isolation of a clone. Analysis of deletants that have been recovered by back-transformation into *E. coli* MC1061/P3 cells show deletions in the nonreplicative parts of the plasmid. These can be observed even when the transfected DNA has been prepared from single colonies of pCDM8 or of CD2 in pCDM8. Deletions occur in DNA whether it has been transfected by DEAE dextran or by spheroplast fusion. It is necessary to incubate *E. coli* overnight in chloramphenicol or spectinomycin to prepare effective spheroplasts. Although this step arrests protein synthesis and chromosome replication, it does not generate deletants in spheroplasts before PEG fusion.

When deleted plasmids occur in a particular cycle of selection, they are found to occur at an increased frequency after the next round of selection. We suspect that this is due to an increased replication rate of the smaller plasmids. We are currently determining the effect on deletion rate of the type of COS cell lines we use and on the density and replication rate of the cells during and after transfection.

TRANSIENT EXPRESSION OF HYBRID MEMBRANE PROTEINS IN COS CELLS

λgt11, λZAP [Short et al., 1988], pCDM8, and similar expression systems require a specific antibody or other ligand to be available to identify and select the appropriate clones. The advantage of the present pCDM8 system is that it expresses eukaryotic membrane proteins in a native state, in which they are most likely to react with monoclonal antibodies. However, the rate at which new membrane proteins are cloned still depends on the rate at which monoclonal antibodies are raised and analyzed. Large numbers of monoclonal antibodies have not been raised against the surface proteins of many tissues. It is very unlikely that early embryonic and extra embryonic tissue will be available in sufficient quantities to allow a saturation analysis of surface proteins through the raising of monoclonal antibodies. One way round this problem is to raise monoclonals against tissue that *is* available, such as placenta, and the WHO Task Force on Vaccines for Fertility Regulation has initiated a program in this area. Because far less tissue is required to make a full cDNA library than to raise a panel of monoclonal antibodies, we have started to explore the possibility that cDNA sequences encoding membrane protein anchoring domains could be directly selected in a fusion protein expression system based on pCDM8.

Integral membrane proteins can be divided into four classes on the basis of their topology (Fig. 9). Class I proteins (e.g., HLA, Ig, and EGF receptor) have a cleaved leader sequence, which generally contains a string of 8–12 uncharged and very hydrophobic amino acids [von Heijne, 1985]; these may interact with the methionine bristle structure on the surface of the 54 kd protein of the signal recognition particle [Bernstein et al., 1989].

Transmembrane sequences (Tm sequences) are of approximately 21 amino acids long and can form into an α-helix that will span the nonpolar part of the membrane. The basic residues arginine and lysine are usually to be found adjacent to their cytoplasmic ends [von Heijne, 1985, 1986; von Heijne and Gavel, 1988]. There are no general sequence motifs within Tm regions. The amino acid sequence seems to be random and subject to the single requirement of a very high overall hydrophobicity. This hydrophobicity is extreme and has been shown to be greater than that found in most prokaryotic and eukaryotic proteins that are not associated with plasma membranes [von Heijne, 1981, 1986; Eisenberg et al., 1984].

It is established that transmembrane sequences can anchor unrelated membrane proteins or foreign proteins in the plasma mem-

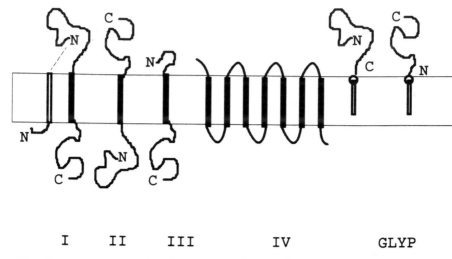

I   II   III   IV   GLYP

Fig. 9.   Diagram showing the different classes of membrane proteins. The horizontal shaded area represents the cell membrane; the black vertical rectangles
represent transmembrane regions of proteins. Classes I, II, III, and IV are integral membrane proteins. GLYP represents those membrane proteins that are
anchored by glypiation tails (see text). For class I integral membrane proteins,
the N-terminal leader sequence (left open box) is shown cleaved (dotted line)
from the N terminus of the mature protein. The number of transmembrane
sequences of class IV proteins need not be seven, and the orientation of their N
and C termini need not be as shown.

brane [Zerial et al., 1987; Yost et al., 1983]. We are therefore developing the approach shown in Figure 10. A vector based on pCDM8
contains the cDNA for an antigenic polypeptide that is *secreted* from
COS cells. The cDNA has several cloning sites immediately 5′ to the
translational termination codon. Placental cDNA sequences will be
cloned into these sites, and COS cells will be panned for the expression of the antigenic polypeptide on the cell surface. cDNA inserts
that stop the transfer of the expressed protein into the endoplasmic
reticulum could encode classic Tm polypeptides or sites for the attachment of glypiated tails [Ferguson and Williams, 1988; Zuber et
al., 1989]. Figure 10 shows the anchoring domain located at the carboxy terminus of the protein; insertions at the amino terminus can
also be designed to mimic the structure of class II integral membrane
proteins (Fig. 9).
    As an initial step in the design of the cloning system, we took the
full-length clones for the human T-cell erythrocyte receptor, CD2
[Seed and Aruffo, 1987]. This is a 332 amino acid class I integral
membrane protein that is a member of the immunoglobulin super-

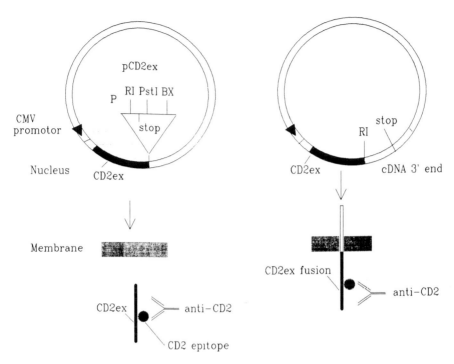

Fig. 10. Cloning vector for transmembrane sequences. On the **left** the CD2 external domain is encoded by the plasmid pCD2ex and is secreted form the COS cell. On the **right**, the CD2 external domain is fused to transmembrane and cytoplasmic domains from another protein, encoded by the cDNA insert ("cDNA 3' end"). The CD2ex fusion is located in the membrane, and the COS cell is panned with anti-CD2.

family. It is believed to consist of two external domains, the car-boxyterminal one being stabilized by an intrachain disulfide bond [see Williams, 1987]. By comparison with the β-pleated sheets of immunoglobulin, the disulfide bridge in the CD2 domain II occurs between the cysteines at positions $+127$ and $+167$. The Tm sequence of CD2 is located between amino acid residues 191 and 216.

When cloned into pCDM8, the cDNA strongly expressed CD2 antigen on the surface of COS cells, as detected by immunofluorescence (Fig. 11a), and cells expressing the clone can be panned with monoclonal anti-CD2. When CD2 was truncated by deletion of codons 183–332 (CD2-Tm), CD2 expression on the membrane was abolished (Fig. 11b) and transfected cells could not be panned. The truncated CD2 sequence (codons -19 to $+182$) was joined in frame through an EcoRI linker to the final 92 codons of the HLA B7 allele (CD2 + B7Tm). This included the last 44 codons of the B7 α3 external

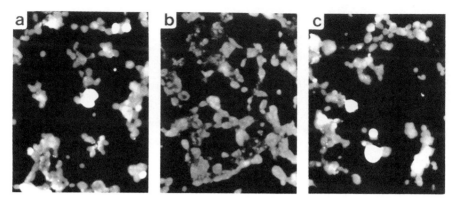

Fig. 11.   Indirect immunofluorescent staining of COS cells containing CD2 constructs. **a:** full-length CD2. **b:** CD2-Tm, the truncated CD2 without a transmembrane or cytoplasmic domains. **c:** CD2 + B7Tm, the CD2 + HLAB7 fusion construct; see text.

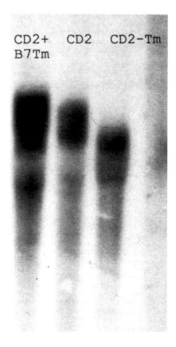

Fig. 12.   Northern blot of total RNA from COS cells transfected with CD2, the truncated form of CD2 (CD2-Tm) and the CD2 + B7 fusion construct (CD2 + B7Tm). The blot was probed with cDNA for CD2. Untransfected COS cells gave no signal with CD2 probes.

domain, including a cysteine at position +259 that forms an intra-chain disulfide bond in the B7 α3-domain. This fusion construct expressed CD2 on the cell membrane (Fig. 11c), and COS cells transfected with the construct could be as efficiently panned with anti-CD2 as those transfected with the original CD2 clone. This indicates that the CD2 epitope was not disrupted in the fusion protein. Northern blot analysis showed that all three constructs expressed approximately the same amount of mRNA in COS cells (Fig. 12). We deduce that the external domain of CD2 can be effective as an immunoselectable domain for the cloning of Tm sequences. We are presently using it for that purpose with the aim of screening cloned Tm sequences for tissue specificity using subtracted hybridization probes.

ACKNOWLEDGMENTS

This work was supported by a grant from the WHO Special Programme of Research, Development and Research Training in Human Reproduction. A.M.H. was supported by an MRC research studentship. S.L.W. is supported by a visiting fellowship from the British Council. We are grateful to Dr. Kim Kaiser for discussion and access to preprints.

REFERENCES

Aruffo A, Seed B (1987): Molecular cloning of a CD28 cDNA by a high efficiency COS cell expression system. Proc Natl Acad Sci USA 84:8573–8577.

Belyavsky A, Vinogradova T, Rajewsky K (1989): PCR-based cDNA library construction: General cDNA libraries at the level of a few cells. Nucleic Acids Res 17:2919–2932.

Bernstein HD, Portiz MA, Strub K, Hoben SJ, Brenner S, Walter P (1989): Model for signal sequence recognition from amino-acid sequence of 54K subunit of signal recognition particle. Nature 340:482–486.

Davis MM (1986): Subtractive hybridisation and the T cell receptor genes. In Weir DM (ed): Handbook of Experimental Immunology, Cellular Immunology Vol 2, 4th ed. Oxford: Blackwell, pp 7601–7613.

Duby A (1987): Synthetic oligonucleotides as probes. In Ansubel FM, Brent R, Kingston RE, Moore DD, Seidman JG, Smith JA, Struhl K (eds): Current Protocols in Molecular Biology. New York: Wiley-Interscience, pp 641–645.

Duguid JR, Rohwer RG, Seed B (1988): Isolation of cDNAs of scrapie-modulated RNAs by subtractive hybridisation of a cDNA library. Proc Natl Acad Sci USA 85:5738–5742.

Eisenberg D, Schwartz E, Komarony M, Wall R (1984): Analysis of membrane and surface protein sequences with the hydrophobic moment plot. J Mol Biol 179:125–142.

Ellis SA, Strachan T, Palmer MS, McMichael AJ (1989): Complete nucleotide sequence of a unique HLA class I C locus product expressed on the human choriocarcinoma cell line BeWo. J Immunol 142:3281–3286.

Ferguson MAJ, Williams AF (1988): Cell-surface anchoring of proteins via glycosyl-phosphidylinositol structures. Annu Rev Biochem 57:285–320.

Frohman MA, Dush MK, Martin GR (1988): Rapid production of full-length cDNAs from rare transcripts: Amplification using a single gene-specific oligonucleotide primer. Proc Natl Acad Sci USA 85:8998–9002.

Gould SJ, Subramani S, Scheffer IE (1989): Use of the DNA polymerase chain reaction for homology probing. Proc Natl Acad Sci USA 86:1934–1938.

Habener JF, Vo CD, Le DB, Gryan GP, Ercolani L (1988): 5-Fluorodeoxyuridine as an alternative to the synthesis of mixed hybridisation probes for the detection of specific gene sequences. Proc Nat Acad Sci USA 85:1735–1739.

Hanks SK (1987): Homology probing: Identification of cDNA clones encoding members of the protein-serine kinase family. Proc Natl Acad Sci USA 84:388–392.

Huynh-Dinh T, Duchange N, Zakin MM, Lemarchand A, Igolen J (1988): Modified oligonucleotides as alternatives to the synthesis of mixed probes for the screening of cDNA libraries. Proc Natl Acad Sci USA 82:7510–7514.

Kaiser K (1990a): New directions in cDNA cloning: 1. Directional cloning. Technique 2:1–17.

Kaiser K (1990b): New directions in cDNA cloning: 2. Towards a library from a single cell. Technique 2:51–64.

Kennedy TG, Wager-Smith K, Barzilai A, Kandel ER, Sweatt JD (1988): Sequencing proteins from acrylamide gels. Nature 336:499–500.

Knoth K, Roberds S, Poteet C, Tamkun M (1988): Highly degenerate, inosine-containing primers specifically amplify rare cDNA using the polymerase chain reaction. Nucleic Acids Res 16:10932.

Lathe R (1985): Synthetic oligonucleotide probes deduced from amino acid sequence data. The theoretical and practical considerations. J Mol Biol 183:1–12.

Li H, Gyllenstten UB, Cui X, Saiki RK, Erlich HA, Arnheim N (1988): Amplification and analysis of DNA sequences in single human sperm and diploid cells. Nature 335:414–417.

Lu X, Werner D (1988): Construction and quality of cDNA libraries prepared from cytoplasmic RNA not enriched in poly(A)RNA. Gene 71:157–164.

Maniatis T, Fritsch EF, Sambrook J (1982): Molecular Cloning: A Laboratory Manual. Cold Spring Harbor, NY: Cold Spring Harbor Laboratory.

Millican TA, Mock GA, Chauncey MA, Patel TP, Eaton MAW, Gienning J, Cutbuch SD, Neidle S, Mann J (1984): Synthesis and biophysical studies of short oligodeoxynucleotides with novel modifications. Nucleic Acids Res. 12:7435–7453.

Mierendorf RC, Percy C, Young RA (1987): Gene isolation by screening λgt11 libraries with antibodies. Methods Enzymol 152:458–468.

O'Hara O, Dorit RL, Gilbert W (1989): One-sided polymerase chain reaction: The amplification of cDNA. Proc Natl Acad Sci USA 86:5673–5677.

Pauli U, Beutler B, Peterhans E (1989): Porcine tumor necrosis factor alpha: Cloning with the polymerase chain reaction and determination of the nucleotide sequence. Gene 81:185–191.

Rinke de Wit TF, Vloemans S, van den Elsen PJ, Ward J, Sutcliffe RG, Glazebrook J, Haworth A, Stern PL (1990): Novel class I genes are expressed by tumour cell lines representing embryonic and extramembryonic tissues. J Immunogenet (in press).

Rowekamp W, Firtel RA (1980): Isolation of developmentally regulated genes in *Dictyostelium* Dev Biol 79:409–419.

Sargent T (1987): Isolation of differentially expressed genes. In Berger SL, Kimmel AR (eds): Methods Enzymol 152:423–432.

Seed B, Aruffo A (1987): Molecular cloning of the CD2 antigen, the T-cell erythrocyte receptor, by a rapid immunoselection procedure. Proc Natl Acad Sci USA 84:3365–3369.

Short JM, Fernandez JM, Sorge JA, Huse W (1988): λZAP: An expression vector with in vivo excision properties. Nucleic Acids Res 16:7583–7599.

Simmons D, Seed B (1988): The Fc receptor of natural killer cells is a phosospholipid-linked membrane protein. Nature 333:568–570.

Suggs SV, Wallace RB, Hirose T, Kawashima EH, Itakura K (1981): Use of synthetic oligonucleotides as hybridisation probes: Isolation of cloned cDNA sequences for human β_2-microglobulin. Proc Natl Acad Sci USA 78:6613.

Takahashi Y, Kato K, Hayashizaki Y, Wakabayashi T, Ohtsuka E, Matsuki S, Ikehara M, Matsubara K (1985). Molecular cloning of the human cholecystokinin gene by use of a synthetic probe containing deoxyinosine. Proc Natl Acad Sci USA 82:1931–1935.

Tam AW, Smith MM, Fry KE, Larrick JW (1989). Construction of cDNA libraries from small numbers of cells using sequence independent primers. Nucleic Acids Res 17:1269.

Timberlake WE (1980): Developmental gene regulation in *Aspergillus nidulans*. Dev Biol 78:497–509.

von Heijne G (1981): Membrane proteins: The amino acid composition of membrane-penetrating segments. Eur J Biochem 120:215–218.

von Heijne G (1985): Structural and thermodynamic aspects of the transfer of proteins into and across membranes. Curr Top Membr Transport 24:151–179.

von Heijne G (1986): The distribution of positively changed residues in bacterial inner membrane proteins correlates with the trans-membrane topology. EMBO J 5:3021–3027.

von Heijne G, Gavel Y (1988): Topogenic signals in integral membrane proteins. Eur J Biochem 174:671–678.

Wallace RB, Miyada CG (1987): Oligonucleotide probes for the screening of recombinant DNA libraries. Methods Enzymol 152:423–432.

Williams AF (1987): A year in the life of the immunoglobulin superfamily. Immunol Today 8:298–303.

Williams JG (1981): The preparation and screening of a cDNA clone bank. In Williamson AR (ed): Genetic Engineering. New York: Academic Press, pp 2–22.

Williams JG, Lloyd MM (1979): Changes in the abundance of polyadenylated RNA during slime mold development measured using cloned molecular hybridisation probes. J Mol Biol 129:19.

White TJ, Arnheim N, Erlich HA (1989): The polymerase chain reaction. Trends Genet 5:185–189.

Wood WI, Cutschier J, Lasky LA, Lawn RM (1985): Base composition-independent hybridisation in tetramethylammonium chloride: A method for oligonucleotide screening of highly complex gene libraries. Proc Natl Acad Sci USA 82:1585–1588.

Yost CS, Hedgpeth J, Lingappa VR (1983): A stop transfer sequence confers predictable transmembrane orientation to a previously secreted protein in a cell-free system. Cell 34:759–766.

Young RA, Davis RW (1983): Efficient isolation of genes by using antibody probes. Proc Natl Acad Sci USA 80:1194–1198.

Zerial M, Huylebroeck D, Garoff H (1987): Foreign transmembrane peptides replacing the internal signal sequence of transferrin receptor allow its translocation and membrane binding. Cell 48:147–155.

Zuber MX, Strittmatter SM, Fishman MC (1989): A membrane-targeting signal in the amino terminus of the neuronal protein GAP-43. Nature 341:345–348.

DISCUSSION

DR. MITCHISON: When you insert cDNA into your CD2 expression vector, why do you have to nibble off the 5' end of the coding sequence corresponding to the amino terminus of the polypeptide? Is it that you can't get these molecules into that cloning site?

DR. SUTCLIFFE: 5' untranslated regions may contain stop codons, and we should also delete leader sequences. Hence the nibbling step. I like the idea of nibbling a large amount or a small amount and seeing what will generate the largest number of recombinants.

DR. MITCHISON: You said that you used a nibble of HLA molecule and that you succeeded. But do you know that you couldn't have done it without nibbling?

DR. SUTCLIFFE: No. We don't know that, although we had to remove the leader sequence or there could have been problems.

DR. MITCHISON: What is the possibility of combining that with subtraction in order to do as much as possible at the DNA level before you have to do a panning experiment?

DR. SUTCLIFFE: Certainly, I think that we must go in with subtractive techniques.

30

Antisperm Assays

Warren R. Jones

Many different methods have been used to detect antisperm antibodies. There has been less interest in the possible role and assessment of cell-mediated immunity to sperm in infertility. Over the years major concerns about the immunological validity, interpretation, and standardization of antisperm antibody tests have arisen. This has been attended by compounding confusion regarding the clinical significance of some of the laboratory assays. The situation has been clarified somewhat in recent years by critical collaborative studies of reproducibility, validation, and correlation of standard sperm antibody tests (see Chapter 23, this volume). The advent of new and more meaningful assays such as the immunobead test (IBT) and an understanding of the importance of the sites, modes of action, and immunoglobulin (Ig) class of sperm antibodies have contributed to a new degree of scientific order. Selected collaborative and critical reviews of antisperm tests provide a detailed overview and historical perspective on this difficult area [Jones, 1976; Boettcher et al., 1977; Beer and Neaves, 1978; Jones, 1980; Bronson et al., 1984; Haas, 1987; Jones, 1987]. This chapter discusses the nature and clinical utility of sperm antibody assays; in vitro tests of sperm–ovum interaction are considered in other chapters.

THE SIGNIFICANCE OF SPERM IMMUNITY

Several key "rules of thumb" have evolved in relation to the relative importance and clinical significance of antisperm tests:

1   Sperm antibodies are of more clinical significance than is cell-mediated immunity (CMI) to sperm.

2   Local genital tract antibodies are more important than systemic antibodies except when antibodies transudate into the

Gamete Interaction: Prospects for Immunocontraception, pages 459–470
© 1990 Wiley-Liss, Inc.

fallopian tube or reach there in follicular fluid and interfere
with fertilization or with embryonic development.

3   Sperm immunity is more clinically significant in the male
than in the female. Here, again, the presence of antibodies
bound to sperm or in seminal plasma is more significant
than their detection in serum.

4   Men with sperm autoimmunity may be more likely to have
female partners who also demonstrate immunity to sperm.

5   Sperm immunity is unrelated to clinically significant systemic immunological or general medical disease.

EFFECTOR MECHANISMS IN SPERM IMMUNITY

Autoimmune (in the male) and isoimmune (in the female) reactions to sperm may influence fertility in the following ways:

1   Disruption of spermatogenesis
2   Disordered sperm transport in the male genital tract
3   Autoagglutination of ejaculated sperm
4   Cytotoxic (immobilizing) action on sperm in the female
genital tract
5   Antibody-enhanced phagocytosis of sperm in the female
tract
6   Prevention of cervical mucous penetration because of agglutination or to more subtle mechanisms such as the
"shaking" phenomenon
7   Interference with sperm capacitation
8   Inactivation of sperm enzymes, thereby inhibiting cumulus dispersal or zona penetration
9   Inhibition of the acrosome reaction
10   Blockage of sperm–ovum interaction
11   Postfertilization disruption of the peri-implantation embryo, since sperm antigens may be incorporated into the
zygote

METHODS FOR SPERM ANTIBODY DETECTION

Immune reactions to sperm are mostly tissue specific rather than
individual specific, although there is some evidence for allogeneic
variation in sperm antigens. Therefore, sperm antibody titers may be
higher when autologous sperm (for autoantibodies in the male) or
husband's sperm (for isoantibodies in the female) and used compared with donor sperm [Mather et al., 1983]. For practical purposes,

however, donor sperm provide a suitable and satisfactory antigen substrate for all sperm antibody tests. Although not optimal, it is possible to use cryopreserved and subsequently thawed sperm for antibody assays, since the relevant antigens are conserved during this process [Haas et al., 1984; Phillip et al., 1984].

Sperm Antibody Tests

A catalog of tests that have been used for the assessment of sperm antibodies is listed together with supporting references.

1. Tray agglutination test (TAT)—Agglutination of sperm observed in microtiter trays
   Fribert [1974]
   Rose et al. [1976]
   Boettcher et al. [1977]

2. Tube-slide agglutination test (TSAT)—Agglutination of sperm observed on a microscope slide after transfer from a test tube
   Franklin and Dukes [1964]
   Rose et al. [1976]
   Boettcher et al. [1977]

3. Gelatin agglutination test (GAT)—Agglutination of sperm in gelatin medium in a test tube
   Kibrick et al. [1952]
   Rose et al. [1976]
   Boettcher et al. [1977]

4. Sperm immobilization test (SIT)—Complement-dependent immobilization of sperm observed on microtiter trays
   Isojima et al. [1986]
   Husted and Hjort [1975]
   Rose et al. [1976]
   Boettcher et al. [1977]
   Chen and Jones [1981]

5. Sperm cytotoxicity test—Standard dye exclusion test on microscope slide
   Husted and Hjort [1975]
   Mathur et al. [1980]
   Jager et al. [1984b]

6. Immunofluorescence antibody tests—Antibody localization usually using indirect label on fixed sperm
   Hjort and Hansen [1971]
   Hansen and Hjort [1971]

Rose et al. [1976]
Haas and Cunningham [1984]

7   Mixed antiglobulin reaction (MAR)—Assay for sperm-bound antibodies using Ig-coated erythrocytes or latex particles and anti-Ig antibodies
Jager et al. [1978]
Hendry et al. [1982]
W.H.O. [1987]
Hinting et al. [1988]

8   Radiolabeled antiglobulin test (RAT)—Same principle as MAR with radiolabeled marker rather than cells or particles
Haas et al. [1980]

9   Immunobead test (IBT)—Assay for sperm-bound antibodies using anti-Ig–coated immunobeads
Bronson et al. [1981]
Bronson et al. [1985]
Clarke [1984, 1987]
Clarke et al. [1985]

10   Passive hemagglutination—The agglutination of sensitized erythrocytes by sperm antibodies in test sera
Mathur et al. [1979]

11   Enzyme-linked immunosorbent assay (ELISA)—Detection of sperm antibodies that recognize a solid-phase antigen substrate of whole sperm or sperm extracts using enzyme-conjugated second antibodies directed against immunoglobulins
Wolf et al. [1982]
Zanchetta et al. [1982]
Alexander and Bearwood [1984]
Ing et al. [1985]
Mettler et al. [1986]

12   Sperm–cervical mucous contact test (SCMC-T)—Detection of sperm "shaking" because of cross-linkage of cervical mucous micelles with motile sperm by antisperm antiboides present either on the sperm surface or in the mucus
Kremer and Jager [1976, 1980]

Testing Cervical Mucus

Cervical mucus is most easily and appropriately collected at midcycle; the volume of mucus available for testing may be increased by preovulatory estrogen therapy. Theoretically, for the specific purpose of sperm antibody assessment, the timing of collection is irrelevant, because there tends to be an inverse relationship between the amount of cervical mucus produced and its immunoglobulin concentration. While unprocessed mucus is used for sperm penetration and SCMC tests, for the purposes of direct sperm antibody assessment one of several techniques must be employed to liquify the mucus and render the immunoglobulins accessible to testing [Chen and Jones, 1981; Jager et al., 1984a; Clarke et al., 1984]. In brief, the principles involved in these several techniques are as follows:

1   Ultracentrifugation to produce a supernatant; this tends to exclude a large portion of the antibodies
2   Extraction with a physiological buffer followed by centrifugation to produce an antibody-containing supernatant
3   Liquefaction with bromelin, a proteolytic enzyme (while, theoretically, it might be thought advisable to avoid the use of such an agent, bromelin treatment does not appear to distort the results of immunoglobulin or specific antibody measurement)
4   Physical liquefaction by either repeated passage through a 21 guage needle or by mechanical shaking with glass beads

Methods (3) and (4) have proved satisfactory and are recommended for routine use. Both "neat" cervical mucus and extracted fractions from liquefaction procedures can be stored, if necessary, at −20°C until required for testing.

Tests of Cell-Mediated Immunity

The assessment of systemic (and local) CMI to spermatozoal and testicular antigens has been complicated by technical and interpretational difficulties. Notwithstanding these problems, there is evidence from in vitro studies of sperm antigen–induced lymphocyte responses that CMI may participate in the autoimmune reaction to genital tract disruption in the male [El-Alfi and Bassili, 1970; Mancini and Andrada, 1971; Nagarkatti and Rao, 1976; Dorsman et al., 1978]. Lymphocytic infiltration has also been described in 5% of routine testicular biopsy specimens from men with oligo- and azoospermia.

In the female, any role for CMI to sperm in the genesis of immunological infertility has been overshadowed by the more obvious and measurable effects of sperm antibodies. The insemination of sperm into the female genital tract, either experimentally or by coitus, induces a physiological leukocytic response in the cervix and uterus [Pandya and Cohen, 1985]. There is little evidence, however, that this phenomenon, which can be readily identified in cervical aspirates, has any immunological role beyond the removal of redundant or dead sperm and bacteria. More specific evidence for a cellular attack on sperm is based on the observation that peritoneal macrophages exhibit enhanced phagocytosis and lysis of sperm that are coated with antibodies [London et al., 1985]. This finding suggests that an additional (but logistically undiagnosable) role for sperm immunity may involve a cellular response in the upper genital tract.

Studies of lymphokine production as an index of effector CMI to sperm in infertile women have yielded conflicting results. Mettler and Shirwani [1975] and Tait et al. [1976] found no difference in responses from infertile and fertile women using, respectively, assays for leukocyte inhibitory factor and macrophage migration-inhibitory factor. On the other hand, McShane et al. [1985] reported evidence of cellular immunity to sperm using the leukocyte inhibitory factor assay in infertile women who had no evidence of sperm antibodies. The final answer on the role of CMI to sperm awaits improvements in techniques, particularly the use of purified soluble sperm antigens in tests of both the recognition and effector arms of the CMI response.

Choice of Sperm Antibody Methods

The author has previously expressed a degree of circumspection and healthy scepticism about, respectively, the selection of sperm antibody tests for common use and the interpretation of their results [Jones, 1980]. Methodological advances and a more critical appraisal of the basis and limitations of tests of sperm immunity [Haas, 1987] have modified this former view. The deployment of these tests as an aid to the clinical management of infertility will obviously depend on their local availability. Ideally, the assessment of sperm immunity should form part of the comprehensive investigation of all infertile couples. If selection is necessary, however, it is logical to test patients in the following categories:

1   "Unexplained" infertility
2   Abnormal postcoital test
3   Failed vasectomy reversal
4   Abnormal semen profile
        a. oligozoospermia

b. low sperm motility

c. sperm autoagglutination

5   History of male genital tract infection, mumps orchitis, or testicular trauma

In selecting appropriate and valid tests for sperm antibodies, the following caveats should be kept in mind:

1   In general, bioassays (e.g., TAT, SCMC-T) and antibody-binding assays using live sperm (e.g., IBT) are more clinically relevant and correlate better among themselves than do radio- and enzyme-binding assays using dead sperm substrates or solubilized sperm fractions.

2   Antibodies in the IgA class are probably the main mediators of infertility caused by sperm immunity.

3   Agglutination tests (TAT, TSAT, GAT) may yield false positive results because of nonantibody agglutinating factors. They also detect antibodies in both IgG and IgM classes; the latter do not gain access to the male or female genital tracts except indirectly via peritoneal or follicular fluid.

4   The SIT also suffers the disadvantage of detecting both IgG (two of the four subclasses) and IgM antibodies. Care must be taken in controlling assays for nonspecific toxicity in both guinea pig and human complement. Because complement-dependent sperm immobilization requires the presence of Fc fragments of two IgG antibodies to be present in close proximity on the sperm surface, the SIT is less sensitive than agglutination tests.

5   Immunofluorescence antibody tests using methanol (or other) fixation of sperm recognize subsurface antigens that are of no relevance to the biological activity of sperm antibodies in vivo.

6   The IBT is more robust than the MAR test (using either erythrocytes or latex particles) and is more easily adapted to test IgA antibodies.

7   Sperm antibody levels in body fluids, particularly in serum, may fluctuate from time to time, and repeated testing may be necessary to identify a pathogenic pattern. This may be due, in part, to the incorporation of sperm antibodies into circulating immune complexes with the disappearance of free antibodies from the serum.

8   The assays described above test only for the presence of antibodies on sperm and their effects on viability and trans-

port. The effects of sperm antibodies on sperm–ovum interaction and on the peri-implantation embryo require separate
assessment (e.g., zona-free hamster test, hemizona assay,
human IVF; see Chapter 31, this volume).

In summary, a suggested scheme for the investigation of sperm
antibodies in clinical practice is as follows:

1   On female serum, TAT, SIT (+ indirect IBT)
2   On male serum, TAT, SIT (+ indirect IBT)
3   On cervical mucus, SCMC-T (+ indirect IBT)
4   On semen, TAT, SCMC-T, direct IBT (+ indirect IBT if in-
    sufficient sperm present for direct)

REFERENCES

Alexander HJ, Bearwood D (1984): An immunosorption assay for antibodies to spermatozoa in comparison with agglutination and immobilization tests. Fertil Steril 41:270–
276.

Beer AE, Neaves WB (1978): Antigenic status of semen from the viewpoint of the female
and male. Fertil Steril 29:3–21.

Boettcher B, Hjort T, Rumke P, Shulman S, Vyazov O (1977): Auto- and iso-antibodies to
antigens of the human reproductive system. Acta Pathol Microbiol Scand (Sect C Suppl)
258:1–69.

Bronson R, Cooper G, Hjort T, Ing WR, Wang SX, Mathur S, Williamson HO, Rust PF,
Fudenberg HH, Mettler L, Czuppon AB, Sudo N (1985): Anti-sperm antibodies, detected
by agglutination, immobilization, microcytotoxicity and immunobead-binding assays. J
Reprod Immunol 8:279–299.

Bronson R, Cooper G, Rosenfeld D (1981): Membrane-bound sperm-specific antibodies:
Their role in infertility. In Vogel H, Jagiello G (eds): "Bioregulators in Reproduction." New
York: Academic Press, pp 521–527.

Bronson R, Cooper G, Rosenfeld D (1984): Sperm antibodies: Their role in infertility. Fertil
Steril 42:171–183.

Chen CYH, Jones WR (1981): Application of a sperm micro-immobilisation test to cervical
mucus in the investigation of immunologic infertility. Fertil Steril 35:542–545.

Clarke GN (1984): Detection of anti-spermatozoal antibodies of IgG, IgA and IgM immunoglobulin classes in cervical mucus. Am J Reprod Immunol 6:195–197.

Clarke GN (1987): An improved immunobead test procedure for detecting sperm antibodies in serum. Am J Reprod Immunol Microbiol 13:1–3.

Clarke GN, Elliott PJ, Smaila C (1985): Detection of sperm antibodies in semen using the immunobead test: A survey of 813 consecutive patients. Am J Reprod Immunol Microbiol 7:118–123.

Clarke GN, Stojanoff A, Cauchi MM, McBain JC, Spiers AL, Johnston WIH (1984): Detection of anti-spermatozoal antibodies of IgA class in cervical mucus. Am J Reprod Immunol 5:61–65.

Dorsman BG, Tumboh-Oeri AG, Roberts TK (1978): Detection of cell-mediated immunity to spermatozoa in mice and man by leukocyte adherence-inhibition test. J Reprod Fertil 53:277–283.

El-Alfi OS, Bassili F (1970): Immunological aspermatogenesis in man. I. Blastoid transformation of lymphocytes in response to seminal antigen in cases of non-obstructive azoospermia. J Reprod Fertil 21:23–28.

Franklin RR, Dukes CD (1964): Anti-spermatozoal antibody and unexplained infertility. Am J Obstet Gynecol 89:69.

Friberg J (1974): A simple and sensitive micromethod for demonstration of sperm agglutinating activity in serum from infertile men and women. Acta Obstet Gynecol Scand Suppl 36:21–29.

Haas GG (1987): How should sperm antibody tests be used clinically? Am J Reprod Immunol Microbiol 15:106–111.

Haas GG, Cines DB, Schreiber AD (1980): Immunologic infertility: Identification of patients with antisperm antibody. N Engl J Med 303:722–727.

Haas GG, Cunningham ME (1984): Identification of antibody laden sperm by cytofluorometry. Fertil Steril 42:606–613.

Haas GG, Cunningham ME, Culp L (1984): The effect of freezing on sperm-associated immunoglobulin G (IgG). Fertil Steril 42:761–764.

Hansen KB, Hjort T (1971): Immunofluorescent studies on human spermatozoa. II. Characterisation of spematozoal antigens and their occurrence in the male partners of infertile couples. Clin Exp Immunol 9:21–31.

Hendry WF, Stredonska J, Lake RA (1982): Mixed erythrocyte-spermatozoa antiglobulin reaction (MAR test) for IgA antisperm antibodies in subfertile males. Fertil Steril 37:108–112.

Hinting A, Vermuelen L, Comhaire F (1988): The indirect mixed antiglobulin reaction test using a commercially available kit for the detection of antisperm antibodies in serum. Fertil Steril 49:1039–1044.

Hjort T, Hansen KB (1971): Immunofluorescent studies on human spermatozoa. I. The Detection of different spermatozoal antibodies and their occurrence in normal and infertile women. Clin Exp Immunol. 8:9–23.

Husted S, Hjort T (1975): Microtechniques for simultaneous determination of immobilising and cytotoxic sperm antibodies. Clin Exp Immunol 22:256–264.

Ing RMY, Wang S-X, Brennecke AM, Jones WR (1985): An improved indirect enzyme-linked immunosorbent assay for the detection of anti-sperm antibodies. Am J Reprod Immunol 8:15–19.

Isojima S, Li TS, Ashitaka Y (1968): Immunologic analysis of sperm immobilising factor found in sera of women with unexplained infertility. Am J Obstet Gynecol 101: 677–683.

Jager S, Kremer J, de Wilde-Janssen IW (1984a): Are sperm immobilizing antibodies in cervical mucus an explanation for a poor post-coital test? Am J Reprod Immunol 5: 56–60.

Jager S, Kremer J, von Slochteren-Draaisma T (1978): A simple method for screening for anti-sperm antibodies in the human male: Detection of spermatozoal surface IgG with the direct mixed antiglobulin reaction carried out on fresh untreated human semen. Int J Fertil 23:12–21.

Jager S, Kuiken J, Kremer J (1984b): Comparison of two supravital stains in examination of human semen and in tests for cytotoxic antibodies to human spermatozoa. Fertil Steril 41:294–297.

Jones WR (1976): Immunological aspects of infertility. In Scott JS, Jones WR (eds): Immunology of Human Reproduction. London: Academic Press, pp 375–414.

Jones WR (1980): Immunologic infertility—Fact or fiction? Fertil Steril 33:577–586.

Jones WR (1987): Immunological factors in infertility. In Pepperell R, Hudson B, Wood C (eds): The Infertile Couple. Melbourne: Churchill Livingstone, pp 158–180.

Kibrick S, Belding DL, Merrill B (1952): Methods for the detection of antibodies against mammalian spermatozoa. I. A modified macroscopic agglutination test. Fertil Steril 3: 419–429.

Kremer J, Jager S (1976): The sperm–cervical mucus contact test: A preliminary report. Fertil Steril 27:335–340.

Kremer J, Jager S (1980): Characteristics of anti-spermatozoal antibodies responsible for the shaking phenomenon with special regard to immunoglobulin class and antigen-reactive sites. Int J Androl 3:143–152.

London SN, Haney AF, Weinberg JB (1985): Macrophages and infertility: Enhancement of human macrophage-mediated killing by anti-sperm antibodies. Fertil Steril 43:274–278.

Mancini RE, Andrada JN (1971): Immunological factors in human male and female infertility. In Samter M (ed): Immunological Diseases. Boston: Little Brown, pp 1240–1252.

Mathur S, Williamson HO, Derrick FC, Madyastha PR, Melchers JT, Holtz GL, Baker ER, Smith CL, Fudenberg HH (1980): A new microassay for spermocytotoxic antibody: Comparison with passive haemagglutination assay of antisperm antibodies in couples with unexplained infertility. J Immunol 126:905–909.

Mathur S, Williamson HO, Genco PV, Koopmann WR, Rust PF, Fudenberg HH (1983): Sperm immunity in infertile couples: Antibody titres are higher against the husband's sperm than to sperm from controls. Am J Reprod Immunol 3:18–22.

Mathur S, Williamson HO, Landgrebe SG, Smith CL, Fudenberg HH (1979): Application of passive haemagglutination for evaluation of anti-sperm antibodies and a modified Coombs' test for detecting male autoimmunity to sperm antigens. J Immunol Methods 30:381–393.

McShane PM, Schiff I, Trentham DE (1985): Cellular immunity to sperm in infertile women. J Am Med Assoc 253:3555–3558.

Mettler L, Czuppon AB, Alexander M, D'Almeida MD, Haas GG, Hjort T, Jensen JM, Ing RMY, Jones WR, Wang S-X, Witkin SS, Bongiovanni AM (1986): Antibodies to spermatozoa and seminal plasma detected by various enzyme-linked immunosorbent (ELISA) assays. J Reprod Immunol 8:302–312.

Mettler L, Shirwani D (1975): Macrophage migration inhibitory factor in female infertility. Am J Obstet Gynecol 121:117–120.

Nagarkatti RS, Rao SS (1976): Cell-mediated immunity to homologous spermatozoa following vasectomy in the human male. Clin Exp Immunol 26:239–342.

Pandya IJ, Cohen J (1985): The leukocytic reaction of the human uterine cervix to spermatozoa. Fertil Steril 43:417–421.

Phillip M, Kleinman D, Potashnik G, Insler V (1984): Antigenicity of sperm cells after freezing and thawing. Fertil Steril 41:615–619.

Rose NR, Hjort T, Rumke P, Harper MJK, Vyazov O (1976): Techniques for the detection of iso- and auto-antibodies to human spermatozoa. Clin Exp Immunol 23:175–199.

Tait BD, Barrie JU, Johnston I, Morris PJ (1976): Cellular immunity to lymphocyte antigens in huan infertility. Fertil Steril 27:389–396.

Wolf DP, Rowlands DT, Haas GG (1982): Antibodies to sperm-associated antigens detected by solid phase assay. Biol Reprod 26:140–146.

World Health Organisation (1987): WHO Laboratory Manual for the Examination of Human Semen and Semen–Cervical Mucus Interaction. Cambridge: Cambridge University Press.

Zanchetta R, Busolo F, Matrogiacomo L (1982): The enzyme-linked immunosorbent assay for the detection of anti-spermatozoal antibodies. Fertil Steril 38:730–734.

DISCUSSION

DR. ISOJIMA: I think that in the immunobead test and the MAR test, we are accepting antibody binding. The immobilization antibody reaction or maybe the hemizona test will reveal a more biological reaction. At first screening, the immunobead test may appear adequate. But if the results are not completely related to the infertility, perhaps we need a more biological test.

DR. JONES: I agree that you need to use a combination of tests.

DR. HJORT: I note that other people use the MAR test over alternative tests and the tray agglutination test over the other agglutination tests. I am sorry that you relegated the gelatin agglutination to a historical perspective, as it is really the most reliable in my laboratory. I've run more gelatin than tray agglutination tests.

DR. JONES: Thanks. I would have been very disappointed if you had not said that.

DR. HJORT: The problem is that if you try to put tests into such categories, often, when one uses them, they are criticized.

DR. JONES: I feel that the tray agglutination test probably achieves the same thing as the gel agglutination test, so why have the pain of setting up the gel agglutination test?

31

Antifertilization Assays

Sergio Oehninger, Nancy J. Alexander,
Daniel R. Franken, Charles C. Coddington,
Lani J. Burkman, Thinus F. Kruger,
Anibal A. Acosta, and Gary D. Hodgen

The hemizona assay (HZA) has been introduced as a new diagnostic test for the binding of human spermatozoa to human zonae pellucidae to predict fertilization potential [Burkman et al., 1988]. In the HZA the two matched zona hemispheres, created by microbisection, provide three main advantages: 1) the two halves (hemizonae) are functionally equal surfaces, allowing a controlled comparison of binding and reproducible measurements of sperm binding from a single oocyte; 2) the limited number of available human oocytes is amplified, because an internally controlled test can be performed in a single oocyte; and 3) because the oocyte is split microsurgically, even fresh oocytes cannot lead to inadvertent fertilization and pre-embryo formation [Hodgen et al., 1988].

It is accepted that before a spermatozoon can penetrate the zona pellucida, there is a specific need for firm attachment between them. When spermatozoa and zona are mixed in vitro, some of the spermatozoa adhere rapidly and irreversibly to the zona by a process called *sperm attachment*. Subsequently, an irreversible adhesion occurs between the two gametes; this phase is called *binding*. Both specific and nonspecific binding in mammals is attributed to the presence of complementary binding sites or receptors on the surface of the gametes. Typically these factors manifest a high degree of species specificity [Ahuja, 1985]. The HZA is thus a unique test, an internally controlled, homologous bioassay that evaluates tight binding of human spermatozoa to the zonae pellucidae of human oocytes in vitro. Because the binding of gametes is a critical initial step in fertilization and embryo development, the HZA has multiple poten-

Gamete Interaction: Prospects for Immunocontraception, pages 471–486
© 1990 Wiley-Liss, Inc.

tial uses in reproductive medicine. Although initially developed as a test to investigate male infertility and predict fertilization potential, this bioassay has potential application in contraceptive technology. As has often been the case, the difference in projecting new findings in reproductive medicine toward infertility or contraceptive technology is merely the plane of our interest [Hodgen, 1989].

In this chapter, we summarize the information gained thus far from application of the HZA in three main areas: prediction of human spermatozoa fertilization potential, physiological studies, and possible applications for contraception. Detailed descriptions of oocyte collection, handling, and micromanipulation, as well as semen processing and sperm suspension preparations for the HZA, have been described elsewhere [Burkman et al., 1988; Franken et al., 1989a,b].

HZA AS A PREDICTOR OF HUMAN SPERMATOZOA FERTILIZATION POTENTIAL

Overstreet and Hembree [1976] were the first to use nonliving, unfertilized human oocytes to assess the zona-penetrating capacity of human spermatozoa. However, in their studies, sperm binding to the zona pellucida was not used as the assay end point. They described the storage of human oocytes in a dimethylsulfoxide (DMSO) solution at ultralow temperatures, with the oocytes subsequently thawed and used in the sperm penetration assay. In 1979, Yanagimachi and colleagues showed that highly concentrated (hyperosmolar) salt solutions provided effective storage of hamster and human oocytes while preserving the biological properties of the zonae. Thus it became apparent that salt storage represents a simple, inexpensive means of accumulating and transporting human zonae pellucidae.

In previous studies [Burkman et al., 1988], we examined the feasibility and kinetics of sperm binding to the human zona pellucida, showing maximum binding after 4 to 5 hr of coincubation. Spermatozoa from fertile men showed equivalent binding to DMSO (2.0 M solution)–frozen/stored and salt (MgCl$_2$, 1.5 M solution)–stored human zonae with a similar shape of the binding curve for zonae stored by either method over a period of 6 to 30 days [Franken et al., 1989a] (Figs. 1, 2).

In a blinded study we initially investigated the relationship between sperm binding to the hemizona and in vitro fertilization (IVF) success in 36 patients [Burkman et al., 1988; Franken et al., 1989b]. Nonliving human oocytes, recovered from surgically removed ovaries and salt stored, were used in these experiments. For the HZA,

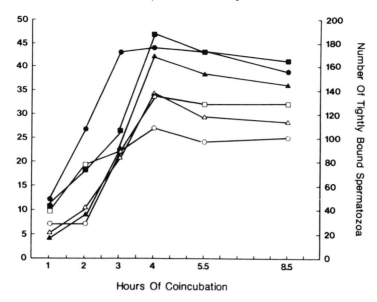

Fig. 1. The number of spermatozoa from fertile men that bound to hemizonae from oocytes stored in DMSO or salt solution for 6 days. Each curve represents the mean binding for two matching hemizonae. For experiment 1, a separate y-axis scale is shown on the right. △, ▲ Experiment 1, fertile male A. ○, ●, Experiment 2, fertile male B. □, ■, Experiment 3, fertile male B. Open symbols are salt-stored oocytes; closed symbols are DMSO-stored oocytes. [Reproduced from Franken et al., 1989a, with permission of the publisher.]

one hemizona was exposed to a droplet of abnormal spermatozoa (standardized to 100 μl of 500,000 motile sperm per ml), while the matching hemizona was exposed to a control droplet of normal spermatozoa. After 4 hr, the number of tightly bound spermatozoa was counted. Binding to the zona was significantly higher in patients with IVF success (mean of 36.1 ± 7 SE tightly bound sperm) than in the IVF failure group (10.4 ± 4; $P < 0.05$). Fewer sperm from the failure group had normal morphology, as evaluated by the strict criteria used in our laboratory [Kruger et al., 1988] (Table 1). Tight binding was significantly correlated with the percentage of motile sperm, normal morphology, and seminal sperm concentration. These initial results enhanced our confidence that the HZA is a potential diagnostic test for identification of patients at high risk for failure of fertilization in IVF.

This line of investigation was extended in subsequent experiments. A new prospective, blinded study was designed for two purposes: to assess the relationship between tight binding in the HZA and IVF outcome and to determine the sensitivity and specificity of

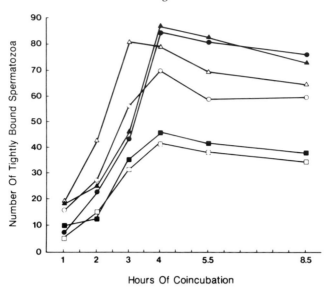

Fig. 2.   The number of spermatozoa from fertile men that bound to hemizonae from oocytes stored in DMSO or salt solution for 30 days. Each curve represents the mean binding for two matching hemizonae. △, ▲ Experiment 7, fertile male A. ○, ●, Experiment 8, fertile male A. □, ■, Experiment 9, fertile male B. Open symbols are salt-stored oocytes; closed symbols are DMSO-stored oocytes. [Reproduced from Franken et al., 1989a, with permission of the publisher.]

TABLE 1. Number of Sperm That Bound Tightly to Hemizonae During the Hemizona Assay (HZA) for Patients in the Successful IVF Group Versus Patients in the IVF Failure Group and the Corresponding Group Semen Parameters (Mean ± SE)[a]

	Group	
Parameter	Fertilization (N = 27)	Failure (N = 9)
HZA: No. tightly bound sperm	36.1 ± 6.8	10.4 ± 3.6*
Percent normal morphology	12.7 ± 1.5	3.2 ± 0.9*
Sperm concentration (× 10^6/ml)	74.2 ± 10.0	54.8 ± 7.8
Percent motility	45.2 ± 4.0	33.3 ± 6.2

[a]Reproduced from Franken et al. [1989b], with permission of the publisher.
*Mean is significantly less than the value for the fertilization group ($P < 0.05$).

the HZA. For optimal results, two strict criteria were established: 1) only proven fertile donors with normal semen parameters were used as internal controls in each test and 2) only IVF patients with at least

TABLE 2. Sperm Parameters and Hemizona Assay (HZA) Results According to IVF Outcome[a]

	Group 1 (Fertilization rate of preovulatory oocytes, ≥65%; N = 22)	P	Group 2 (Fertilization rate of preovulatory oocytes, <65%; N = 6)
Part A			
Patients' IVF samples			
Concentration	116.0 ± 16.6	0.1 > P > 0.05	49.0 ± 14.5
Percent motility	71.3 ± 3.3	<0.01	31.5 ± 6.3
Percent normal morphology	9.7 ± 1.3	0.1 > P > 0.05	4.3 ± 2.1
Patients' HZA samples			
Concentration	93.3 ± 13.9	0.2 > P > 0.1	51.0 ± 12.3
Percent motility	54.2 ± 3.4	<0.02	33.1 ± 1.4
HZA binding	62.1 ± 10.9	<0.02	7.3 ± 1.4
HZA index	120.4 ± 18.3	<0.02	29.5 ± 7.5
Part B			
Controls' HZA samples			
Concentration	150.5 ± 13.3	>0.5	142.8 ± 16.6
Percent motility	64.6 ± 1.7	>0.5	66.8 ± 3.5
HZA binding	59.5 ± 11.2	>0.5	40.6 ± 11.9*

[a]Reproduced from Oehninger et al. [1989a], with permission of the publisher.
*$P<0.02$ (controls' versus patients' HZA binding within group 2, paired t test).

two mature preovulatory oocytes at retrieval were included in the study [Oehninger et al., 1989a].

Twenty-eight infertile men participating in the Norfolk IVF program were allocated to the study group. Similar to our previous study, patients with poor fertilization rates in IVF had significantly lower binding than patients with successful fertilization (7.3 ± 1.4 tightly bound sperm vs. 62.1 ± 10.9, respectively; $P < 0.02$) (Table 2). Based on current standards, the HZA predicted fertilization accurately in 26 of 28 cases, with a sensitivity of 95%, specificity of 83%, and a positive predictive value of 95% (Table 3). In addition, sperm concentration, percentages of motility and morphology, mean number of sperm bound in the HZA, and the HZA index (number of sperm bound for an abnormal sample/normal sample × 100) differed significantly when infertile patients with normal semen values were compared with male factor patients (Table 4).

Thus the HZA discriminated by identifying patients at risk for poor or failed fertilization. However, more experiments are needed

TABLE 3. Ability of the Hemizona Assay (HZA) to
Predict IVF Outcome[a]

HZA index	Poor fertilization	Good fertilization	Total
≤36	5	1	6
>36	1	21	22
Total	6	22	28

[a]Reproduced from Oehninger et al. [1989a], with permission of the publisher.

TABLE 4. Hemizona Assay (HZA) Results According to Sperm
Quality in Patients With Normal Semen and in Male
Factor Patients[a]

	Normal sperm parameters[b] (N = 17)	Male factor patients (N = 11)
Concentration	126.0 ± 18.2	64.2 ± 17.6*
Percent motility	75.5 ± 2.5	42.9 ± 6.5[†]
Percent normal morphology	12.1 ± 1.2	3.1 ± 0.9[†]
HZA binding	72.2 ± 17.6	16.7 ± 5.0[‡]
HZA index	124.5 ± 23.2	59.2 ± 13.0[‡]

[a]Reproduced from Oehninger et al. [1989a], with permission of the publisher.
[b]Sperm concentration, >20 million/ml; motility, >50%; and normal morphology, ≥14%.
*$P < 0.05$.
[†]$P < 0.001$.
[‡]$P < 0.005$.

to establish the threshold HZA index value and the intra-assay variation. In addition, to maximize application of the HZA and its power of discrimination, it may be necessary to establish a minimal number of tightly bound sperm (probably a minimum of 20 to 30, according to our current information) for the fertile sample to the control hemizona, thus assuring an acceptable oocyte-binding capacity and a valid HZA [Franken et al., 1990; Hodgen et al., 1988].

No assay, especially a bioassay, can be absolute in its predictive value. In the HZA, false-positive results can occur, because other physiologic steps follow the binding of sperm to the zona and are necessary for fertilization and development. False-negative results could also be the consequence of interegg variation in binding ability or interassay variation. Establishment of a minimal binding threshold for the control specimen may overcome false results.

These clinical studies show that, in the HZA, male factor patients and those with poor fertilization rates in IVF have lower binding ability than selected fertile controls. The HZA is therefore a valuable tool for evaluating dysfunctional sperm–zona binding, with good predictive value for IVF results.

PHYSIOLOGICAL STUDIES

Variability in Sperm Binding Capacity of Zonae Pellucidae

Franken et al. [1990] evaluated the number of sperm bound to different zonae pellucidae during the HZA. For 15 immature (germinal vesicle) oocytes collected from surgically removed ovaries, they reported a large variability between unmatched hemizonae. For HZA performed with normal semen from fertile donors, they found wide confidence intervals and a large coefficient of variation (approximately 30%) for that group of oocytes. Although the interassay variability in the HZA seemed high, because of interegg variability, they obtained statistically reliable data by using matched hemizonae. As mentioned above, a minimal binding threshold should be determined to give validity to the assay. Furthermore, despite the fact that all the oocytes used in the study were immature (prophase I), there was variability in binding, even excluding eggs of poor quality (very low binding). Perhaps judging oocyte maturity by nuclear status alone is not a satisfactory indicator of zona pellucida maturity. More data are needed to determine how human oocytes in the same apparent maturational nuclear stage possess different sperm-binding capacities in the HZA.

Variation in the Zona Pellucida–Binding Potential of Spermatozoa From Fertile Men Measured Over a 3 Month Period

Franken et al. [1990] also investigated tight zona binding of sperm from fertile men using three samples collected at 1 month intervals over a period of 3 months from each individual. The results of these experiments showed that after the determination of the lower 95% confidence interval, all fertile men bound >40 sperm after 4 hr of coincubation (immature oocytes). This finding suggests that the spermatozoa from these men did not lose binding ability during the 3 month interval. Thus it appears that, if the sperm from a fertile male bind well initially, adverse changes will not be noted over 3 months, provided that he remains healthy. This reassures his qualification as a control in the HZA.

Comparison of Tight Sperm Binding to the Zona Pellucida in the HZA With Fresh and Cryopreserved Semen

In artificial insemination by donor (AID) programs, pregnancy rates seem to be lower with the use of cryopreserved–thawed semen than with fresh samples. The nature of injury to spermatozoa caused by the freezing process has not been defined, although functional and morphological abnormalities have been well documented. Coddington et al. [1989b] showed in a preliminary report that in three of five fertile men tested in the HZA, tight sperm binding was 30% to 50% lower with the use of frozen semen than with fresh semen from the same male. Although decreased binding was observed, the binding kinetics were equivalent for fresh and frozen semen, with peak binding at 3 to 4 hr of coincubation. The decrease in binding of frozen–thawed sperm may thus be a contributory factor to its decreased effectiveness during AID.

Recent unpublished results have corroborated these findings in the cynomolgus monkey. The number of spermatozoa tightly bound in the HZA was significantly lower for cryopreserved–thawed semen than for fresh samples, using standards similar to the human studies. Similar results were obtained with immature (prophase I) and preovulatory (metaphase II) monkey oocytes. The number of sperm bound to the zonae was markedly enhanced when the number of motile frozen–thawed spermatozoa was increased in the coincubation suspension with the hemizonae. This observation has also been found in our IVF program, as recently reported by Morshedi et al. [1989].

Relationship Between Sperm Acrosomal Status and Binding to the Zona Pellucida

The HZA has been successful in evaluating the acrosomal status of tightly bound sperm to the human zona pelludica using the T-6 monoclonal technique (Humagen, Charlottesville, VA) and fluorescent staining [Fulgham et al., 1989]. The rate of acrosome reaction was assessed at different intervals (0 to 4 hr) after swim-up separation and following 15 to 45 min of coincubation with the hemizonae. For each interval and at each coincubation time, the percentage of acrosome-reacted sperm bound to the zonae was measured by the T-6 antibody. This preliminary study suggests that the acrosome reaction can occur within 15 min of coincubation under HZA conditions, regardless of the time interval preceding coincubations. Based on this evidence, a hypothesis is that the acrosome reaction occurs asynchronously in human spermatozoa.

These findings are similar to those obtained with transmission electron microscopy (TEM), as described by Oosthuizen and colleagues [1990]. These authors investigated the morphological features of spermatozoa bound to the hemizonae after 4 hr of coincubation in the HZA, following processing for TEM. The results illustrated acrosome-reacted and partially acrosome-reacted sperm firmly bound to the zonae or beginning entry. In addition, both acrosome-intact and partially reacted spermatozoa were observed within the inner zone, clearly leaving a digestive pathway or tunnel through the zona substance. These TEM observations stress the earlier reports dealing with the retention of the zona's biological characteristics when stored in highly concentrated salt solutions. Apart from retaining their sperm-binding properties, the zona glycoproteins also seem to maintain their ability to allow spermatozoa to penetrate the zona substance at least partially.

A new series of experiments [Burkman et al., 1989] simultaneously studied acrosome reaction, zona binding, and hyperactivated sperm motility. Here, with proven fertile specimens, the highest rate of acrosome reactions was initiated about the time that hemizona binding peaked. The peak rate of the acrosome reaction occurred just after the maximal incidence of hyperactivated motility. These three events, on a per sperm basis, may be closely linked temporarily.

Effects of Sperm Autoantibodies on Binding to the Zona Pellucida

The HZA was used to compare the effect of several IgG mouse antihuman sperm monoclonal antibodies on sperm–zona interactions. When spermatozoa were coincubated with the antibody for 1 hr, different monoclonal antibodies affected binding dissimilarly. For example, MA-7 (1:500 dilution) and MA-10 (1:100 and 1:50) showed no effect on binding. MA-14 (1:100) showed a 40% inhibition of binding, whereas at a 1:50 dilution the inhibition reached 45% [Coddington et al., 1989a]. Thus exposure to antisperm antibodies appears to play a role in zona binding, suggesting that both in vitro and in vivo effects can be expected in the homologous human system.

Validation of the HZA in the Monkey and Influence of Oocyte Maturational Stages

As mentioned above, the HZA has been successfully used in the cynomolgus monkey, according to standards reported for human studies. The monkey model allows researchers the freedom to pur-

TABLE 5. Hemizona Assay (HZA; Tight Sperm Binding) in the
Cynomolgus Monkey: Results According to Stage of
Oocyte Maturation[a]

	Prophase I (N = 8 oocytes, 16 hemizonae)	Metaphase I (N = 6 oocytes, 12 hemizonae)	Metaphase II (N = 7 oocytes, 14 hemizonae)
No. of sperm bound/ matched hemizonae	25–15	37–20	25–37
	16–14	17–23	50–64
	20–15	57–64	75–60
	52–13	57–76	102–115
	13–21	49–63	80–97
	11–18	38–27	83–75
	10–5		43–58
	43–48		
Mean ± SE	21.1 ± 3.4	44.0 ± 5.4*	68.9 ± 5.8[†]
Mean value of the difference between the two halves	10.1 ± 3.9	12.3 ± 2.0	14.2 ± 0.8[‡]

[a]Reproduced from Oehninger et al. [1989b], with permission of the publisher.
*$P < 0.01$ compared with prophase I and metaphase II oocytes.
[†]$P < 0.001$ compared with prophase I oocytes.
[‡]No significant differences among the groups.

sue aggressive protocols without the ethical contraints that could limit similar clinical studies in humans, i.e., experimental studies on preovulatory oocytes from women undergoing IVF.

In a recent investigation, Oehninger and colleagues [1989b] evaluated the binding pattern of cynomolgus monkey spermatozoa to the zonae pellucidae of immature (prophase I) and mature (metaphase I and II) monkey oocytes. Semen was obtained from anesthetized animals by electroejaculation. Oocytes were obtained by laparascopic retrieval following stimulation with human menopausal gonadotropin (Serono Laboratories, Randolph, MA). Metaphase II oocytes showed significantly more tight binding than did prophase I oocytes, while metaphase I oocytes showed intermediate binding ability (Table 5). It can therefore be postulated that oocyte meiotic competence seems to be accompanied by an increase in zona-binding potential. Mature, preovulatory oocytes may have a greater ability to bind sperm because of special rearrangements of zona glycoproteins during the late stages of maturation, dependent on either intrinsic oocyte factors or influences derived from cumulus-granulosa cells. In ongoing experiments we are testing the effects of luteinizing hormone in in vitro and HZA studies.

POTENTIAL USES OF THE HZA IN CONTRACEPTION

Being a functional bioassay that evaluates sperm–oocyte interaction (tight binding in vitro)—the requisite first step in fertilization and development—the HZA has a potential role in contraception technology. For example, contraceptive vaccines that depend on blocking the antigens essential to sperm and oocyte functions inherent in sperm binding require some means for prediction of clinical success. Such biological end points would help to monitor effective antibody titer attainment and maintenance during and after the immunization regimen. HZA could add a measure of ethical assurance before exposure of treated subjects to the risk of an unwanted pregnancy [Hodgen et al., 1988].

Similarly, the use of gonadotropin-releasing hormone agonists (GnRHa), usually in combination with androgen replacement therapy to attain fertility control in men via suppression of spermatogenesis, is fraught with concern that persistent oligospermia or episodic "escape phenomena" might leave some subjects at risk for unwanted fertility. Even though there is evidence to suggest that these "residual" sperm may be qualitatively abnormal, their fertilizing potential may be high. Achievement and maintenance of absolute azoospermia in all men receiving GnRHa or other hormonal protocol seems an elusive and perhaps impractical goal. Thus a biological test that can reliably show the fertilizing potential of sperm may be scientifically and ethically informative during early clinical trials [Hodgen et al., 1988]. Ongoing experiments are assessing the potential use of the HZA in predicting contraceptive efficacy in these circumstances.

Compelling evidence has demonstrated that sperm surface carbohydrate-binding proteins mediate gamete recognition by binding with high affinity and specificity to complex glycoconjugates of the zona pellucida [Macek and Shur, 1988]. For example, L-fucose and/or fucoidin (a polymer of L-fucose) inhibits gamete attachment in many animal species [Ahuja, 1985; Macek and Shur, 1988]. We therefore used the HZA as an internally controlled bioassay to evaluate the effects of fucoidin and other complex polysaccharide moieties on the tight binding of human spermatozoa to the zonae pellucidae of salt-stored human oocytes. These experiments showed that preincubation of sperm with fucoidin (for 15 to 60 min at a concentration of 1 mg/ml) significantly inhibited binding by >85% compared with

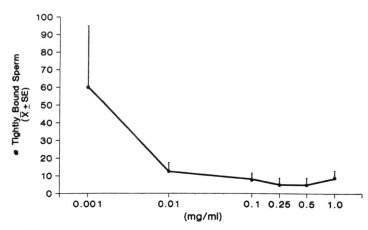

Fig. 3.   Effects of different fucoidin concentrations on the number of sperm with tight binding in the hemizona assay (1 hr preincubation). Note that abscissa is in logarithmic scale. [Reproduced from Oehninger, et al., 1990, with permission of the publisher.]

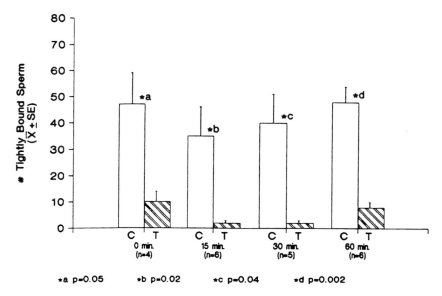

Fig. 4.   Effect of different fucoidin preincubation periods (1.0 mg per ml) on hemizona assay results. C, control; T, test; n, number of oocytes per experiment. [Reproduced from Oehninger et al., 1990, with permission of the publisher.]

sugar-free controls (Fig. 3). Similarly, lesser fucoidin concentrations (0.5, 0.25, and 0.01 mg/ml) were markedly inhibitory (Fig. 4). Heparin sulfate at a concentration of 1.0 mg/ml was also a potent binding inhibitor [Oehninger et al., 1990].

Thus for the first time we have presented evidence that fucoidin and heparin sulfate are potent inhibitors of tight binding under HZA conditions. Potential barrier contraceptive methods, based on adding complex saccharides to spermicidal formulations, seem plausible if these carbohydrate moieties are effective and well tolerated in vivo.

SUMMARY

The HZA is a unique, internally controlled, reproducible homologous bioassay that has a high predictive value for human IVF. It has become a valuable experimental tool for physiological and cellular analysis of the early events requisite for human fertilization. Thus its potential usefulness in predicting contraceptive efficacy and reversibility deserves immediate exploration.

REFERENCES

Ahuja KK (1985): Carbohydrate determinants involved in mammalian fertilization. Am J Anat 179:207–223.

Burkman LJ, Coddington CC, Franken DR, Kruger TF, Rosenwaks Z, Hodgen GD (1988): The hemizona assay (HZA): Development of a diagnostic test for the binding of human spermatozoa to the human zona pellucida to predict fertilization potential. Fertil Steril 49:688–697.

Burkman LJ, Johnson D, Fulgham D, Alexander NJ, Hodgen GD (1989): Temporal relationships between zona binding, hyperactivated motion, and acrosome reactions in sperm from fertile men. Abstract: Serono Symposium on Gamete Physiology. Newport Beach, California, November 6–10, 1989.

Coddington CC, Alexander NJ, Fulgham D, Johnson D, Hodgen GD (1989a): Mouse and human sperm antibodies may modulate sperm binding to the zona pellucida as shown by the hemizona assay (HZA). Abstract: VIth World Congress in In Vitro Fertilization and Alternate Assisted Reproduction. Jerusalem, April 2–7, 1989, p 54.

Coddington CC, Oosthuizen W, Franken D, Burkman L, Hodgen GD (1989b): Comparison of tight sperm binding to the zona pellucida in the hemizona assay utilizing fresh versus frozen sperm from the same male. Abstract: 14th Annual Meeting of the American Society of Andrology. New Orleans, April 13–16, 1989, p 16.

Franken DR, Burkman LJ, Oehninger S, Coddington CC, Veeck LL, Kruger TF, Rosenwaks Z, Hodgen GD (1989a): Hemizona assay using salt-stored human oocytes: Evaluation of zona pellucida capacity for binding human spermatozoa. Gamete Res 22:15–26.

Franken DR, Coddington CC, Burkman SL, Oosthuizen WT, Kruger TF, Hodgen GD (1990): Defining the valid hemizona assay: accounting for binding variability within zonae pellucidae and within semen samples from fertile males. Fertil Steril (submitted).

Franken DR, Oehninger S, Burkman LJ, Coddington CC, Kruger TF, Rosenwaks Z, Acosta AA, Hodgen GD (1989b): The hemizona assay (HZA): A predictor of human sperm fertilizing potential in in vitro fertilization treatment. J In Vitro Fert Embryo Transfer 6:44–50.

Franken DR, Oosthuizen WT, Cooper S, Kruger TF, Burkman LJ, Coddington CC, Hodgen GD (1990): Electron microscopic evidence on the acrosomal status of bound sperm and their penetration into human hemizonae pellucida after storage in a buffered salt solution. Andrologia (in press).

Fulgham DL, Johnson D, Coddington CC, Herr J, Alexander NJ, Hodgen GD (1989): Human sperm acrosome reaction rate in zona pellucida: A time course study. 45th Annual Meeting of the American Fertility Society. San Francisco, November 11–16, 1989.

Hodgen GD, Burkman LJ, Coddington CC, Franken DR, Oehninger S, Kruger TF, Rosenwaks Z (1988): The hemizona assay (HZA): Finding sperm that have the "right stuff." J In Vitro Fert Embryo Transf 5:311–313.

Kruger TF, Acosta AA, Simmons KF, Swanson RJ, Matta JF, Oehninger S (1988): Predictive value of abnormal sperm morphology in in vitro fertilization. Fertil Steril 49:112–117.

Macek MB, Shur BD (1988): Protein–carbohydrate complementarity in mammalian gamete recognition. Gamete Res 20:93–109.

Morshedi M, Oehninger S, Acosta A, Veeck L, Bocca S, Swanson RJ (1989): Cryopreserved semen for in vitro fertilization: Comparison of results using semen from fertile donors and infertile patients. Abstract: 14th Annual Meeting of the American Society of Andrology. New Orleans, April 13–16, 1989, p 74.

Oehninger S, Acosta AA, Hodgen GD (1990): Antagonistic and agonistic properties of saccharide moities in the hemizona assay. Fertil Steril 53:143–149.

Oehninger S, Coddington CC, Scott R, Franken DR, Burkman LJ, Acosta AA, Hodgen GD (1989a): Hemizona assay: Assessment of sperm dysfunction and prediction of in vitro fertilization outcome. Fertil Steril 51:665–670.

Oehninger S, Scott RT, Coddington CC, Franken DR, Acosta AA, Hodgen GD (1989b): Validation of the hemizona assay in a monkey model: Influence of oocyte maturational stages. Fertil Steril 51:881–881.

Overstreet JW, Hembree WC (1976): Penetration of zona pellucida of nonliving human oocytes by human spermatozoa in vitro. Fertil Steril 27:815–831.

Yanagimachi R, Lopata A, Odom CB, Bronson RA, Mahi CA, Nicolson GL (1979): Retention of biologic characteristics of zona pellucida in highly concentrated salt solution: The use of salt-stored eggs for assessing the fertilizing capacity of spermatozoa. Fertil Steril 31:562–574.

DISCUSSION

DR. MORALES: How do you ensure that the sperm is tightly bound? Do you do any method to separate the loosely bound from the tightly bound? And with such a long coincubation, aren't you afraid to lose some sperm that penetrate the hemizona and swim away?

DR. ALEXANDER: To assess tight binding, the zonae pellucidae are washed thoroughly before the sperm are counted. Thus all those sperm that are loosely bound should wash off during this process. It is true that you see some low amount of binding to the inner surface of the zona. And it is also possible that some spermatozoa could have swum through. That is why a time-course study was conducted and 4 hr was determined to be the most appropriate amount of time to assess binding.

DR. ISOJIMA: In what you said about the hemizona test, you indicated that a serum positive for agglutination and immobilization decreases the binding of spermatozoa, but fertility could still result. I agree, but I think that this finding means that the antibody may bind with spermatozoa, but not necessarily to a key point on the spermatozoa.

DR. ALEXANDER: We have not yet found an antibody that totally covers the sperm-binding sites that interface with the surface of the zona. Perhaps this is because of the way that the test is set up and that all of the binding sites cannot interact with antibody. Antibodies are important as a cause of infertility, although some people may have antibodies to sperm that are unrelated to fertility. The Norfolk group and the South African group have demonstrated that anti-sperm antibody effects can be bypassed by in vitro fertilization. After fertilization occurs, the pregnancy rate is the same as that found in normal couples.

DR. ISOJIMA: There are pregnancies in women with antibodies as measured by immunobead and mixed agglutination reaction tests. Biological testing is very important. People may misunderstand that if the immunobead test is positive, this is not very correlative with infertility. So I insist that a biological test and a hemizona test are important to check fertility.

DR. ALEXANDER: Thank you.

DR. GUPTA: Do you have any data on preincubation of zona with antizona antibodies and whether that would stop induction of the sperm acrosome reaction? If it was found to be positive, an important functional assay could be to test for antizona antibodies.

DR. ALEXANDER: That is a good idea. We did not do that.

DR. AHUJA: With certain monoclonals that were raised against specified saccharides, the binding to the outer surface of mouse and hamster zona was found to be uniform. About 20–30% of the zonae show very big binding forces with antibodies. I noticed that in using the hemizona assay, you used zona sliced into two halves. Do you see the binding to be uniform? Or, did you observe dispersed batches or cases in which there was no binding at all?

DR. ALEXANDER: That is why there were so many assessment at the beginning of the development of this assay. We wanted to be sure that the binding on both halves of the zona was similar. So many of the zona were cut and then incubated with normal sperm, i.e., control sperm on both sides, and the number on both sides counted in order to determine whether there was uniformity in the numbers bound on both sides. If there was a region on the zona that did not allow much binding, then we would expect that our assay some times would not be effective. We did not find that to be the case.

DR. GOLDBERG: I know that you did a study of the effect of sperm concentration on zona binding, but I am concerned about the high concentration of sperm that are used in the in vitro assay. If you are really interested in effective antibody, what about the effect of sperm concentration under those conditions or any of those other factors that you might add to perturb the binding by extraneous agents?

DR. ALEXANDER: You are correct that a more physiological circumstance would involve many fewer sperm. But any time researchers develop an in vitro test, they try to telescope the assay into a reasonable time frame. Based on our temporal and concentration studies, this seemed the most appropriate approach. I think that it is of particular interest that the use of fucoidin could so rapidly and effectively reduce sperm binding. But I agree it is not the same as you would find in the human body.

DR. DACHEUX: Why did the frozen sperm bind less than normal ones?

DR. ALEXANDER: I don't know. Some of those sperm may actually be injured, and, therefore, there may have been leakage from their acrosome so, as a result, they may not be in the same physiological condition to initiate zona binding.

DR. DACHEUX: Is motility of sperm important?

DR. ALEXANDER: In each case, we used 500,000 motile sperm. And it was not just a question of motility, it was a question of other physiologic changes, as well.

32

Primate Models for Research in Reproduction

M.A. Isahakia and C.S. Bambra

When compared with other laboratory animals, nonhuman primates are more difficult to maintain in captivity. Many are seasonal breeders and do not adapt well to captive conditions. Females of most primates are characterized by long ovarian cycles, pregnancies, and generation intervals. This makes establishment of self-sustaining captive colonies both a long-term and an expensive undertaking. Use of primates as experimental animals should therefore only be considered when other laboratory animals are unsuitable.

Development of new methods of fertility regulation involves many important facets such as efficacy, safety, and mechanism of action. Such studies need to be done in nonhuman primates. An example would be the development of a sperm-based vaccine. For an antisperm vaccine to be effective in women, antibodies must be able to gain access to the reproductive tract lumen in sufficient quantities to neutralize the large numbers of spermatozoa deposited in the vagina. The cervix in humans is a major barrier to sperm ascending the reproductive tract.

Great apes are closest to man in many anatomical and physiological aspects of reproduction. However, because all of them are protected, endangered species in the wild, they are not practical models for research for most studies. The baboon may be a suitable substitute. Detailed accounts of its implantation and fetal development are available [Hendrickx, 1971]. It is a proven model for applied aspects of endocrinology, teratology, and testing of steroidal contraceptive agents. The baboon is a continuous breeder and is a convenient size if large numbers of recurrent blood samples are required or complex experimental surgery is to be conducted. It has a straight cervix,

Gamete Interaction: Prospects for Immunocontraception, pages 487–500

which makes it an acceptable animal for the development of IUDs or vaginal rings. It breeds well in captivity and has a perineal skin that indicates the stage of menstrual cycle with relative precision. The use of the baboon as a model for studies in development of immunocontraceptive methods in both males and females will now be considered.

IMMUNOCONTRACEPTION

Male Immunocontraception

Studies with male gamete antigens. Recent advances in immunology and molecular biology have enhanced research efforts toward identifying sperm-specific antigens that can be used in fertility regulation. Several such antigens have been identified and described by various investigators in the last 5 years [Isahakia and Alexander, 1984; Saling et al., 1985; Naz et al., 1984]. Rodents have been mostly used as models to document development of gamete antigens in the male and to assess the effect of antibodies on fertilization. However, marked differences occur between rodent species and even between strains of the same species. It has been shown that the pattern of spermatogenesis in the baboon is intermediate between rats and man [Chowdhury and Steinberger, 1976].

Several antigens have been characterized in the baboon sperm using monoclonal antibodies [Isahakia, 1988, 1989]. Some of these antigens also cross-react with human sperm. With one such antibody (BSA-4), development of the acrosomal region of the sperm during spermatogenesis and spermiogenesis was traced. This particular antibody also cross-reacts with rat and mouse. In the baboon this antibody recognizes a 43 kd determinant that is first expressed in postmeiotic round spermatids. Several stages of acrosome development were recognized by the avidin–biotin immunoperoxidase method, namely, cap, acrosome, and maturational stages of spermiogenesis (Fig. 1). Better understanding of the spermiogenesis process and expression of gene products on mature sperm is necessary for development of novel methods of fertility regulation. Because many of the monoclonal antibodies produced against baboon sperm cross-react with human sperm, it is possible to carry out such studies in this appropriate animal model. Moreover, many of the antigens recognized by these antibodies have a testicular origin. Recently, a monoclonal antibody reacting with the midpiece region of both human and baboon sperm has been raised in our laboratory. This antibody (SCA-1) was found to react with Sertoli cells in both human and baboon testes (Fig. 2).

Sertoli cells play both structural and sustentacular roles in promoting mammalian spermatogenesis. Besides having hormonal interactions, these epithelial cells are known to secrete a variety of substances and indeed transfer vital macromolecules into germ cells through an exocytotic–endocytotic mechanism. It has also been shown that transfer of Sertoli cell hyaloplasm into spermatid cytoplasm takes place in the latter half of spermiogenesis. This complex process is presumed to serve as a mechanism for transferring macromolecules to the spermatid during the crucial period of flagella formation and nuclear transformation. With this novel exocytotic–endocytotic process and with recent developments in immunology and genetic engineering, it may be possible to target monoclonal antibodies to the appropriate antigen determinants and thereby effectively "neutralize" sperm function. Using the baboon as a model, we hope to understand better these and other related mechanisms that might yield new contraceptive methods.

Studies on vaccine development. Primates have also been used in immunization studies undertaken to evaluate the potential of both sperm and male hormone antigens as contraceptive agents. However, very few studies have been done with sperm antigens. Female baboons have been immunized with lactic dehydrogenase isoenzyme (LDH-C$_4$) [Goldberg et al., 1981]. These animals subsequently developed antibodies against native LDH-C$_4$, and matings resulted in a 70% decrease in the fertility rates of the female baboon. No immunopathological side effects were apparent with the use of this vaccine. This experiment confirms feasibility and appropriateness of using the baboon as a model for testing candidate sperm vaccines.

Hormonal methods for male contraception are also being studied in primates. Luteinizing hormone-releasing hormone (LHRH) and follicle-stimulating hormone (FSH) have been studied extensively. It has been shown that oligozoospermia induced by active immunization with FSH in bonnet monkeys results in infertility in all immunized animals, and no long-term side effects were apparent in these animals [Moudgal et al., 1988].

Female Immunocontraception

Studies with chorionic gonadotrophin. A number of hormones have been proposed as immunogens over the last few years, and from these human chorionic gonadotropin (hCG) appears to be the most promising [Stevens, 1986; Talwar and Singh, 1988]. This hormone and its β-subunit have been evaluated as possible vaccine candidates in immunization studies carried out in both humans and

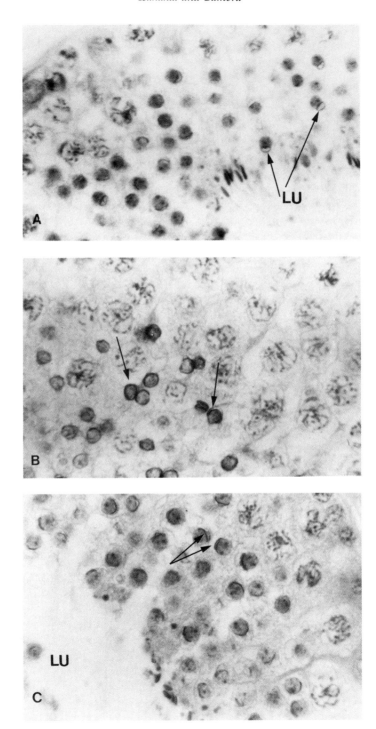

primates. Three candidate preparations have been used in human phase I clinical trials. Antibodies generated in these studies have been shown to have an antifertility effect. This effect may be mediated through ablation of the luteotrophic signal of CG [Talwar and Singh, 1988] or other events occurring at the fetal level [Hearn, 1980]. The mechanisms of action of anti-CG at the embryonic level are not known. Such studies cannot be done in women for ethical reasons, and a suitable animal model must be identified. Previous studies on the development of the CG vaccine have been done largely in the baboon [Stevens, 1980; Talwar, 1980].

Studies done at the Institute of Primate Research (IPR) have examined the effects of antibodies to CG at the embryonic level. A procedure has been developed for preparing and culturing baboon trophoblast cells derived from placentae obtained at 33 days of gestation (Fig. 3). These cultured cells have been characterized and found to be mostly cytotrophoblast (Fig. 4) and can be maintained in vitro for up to 6 days [Bambra, 1989]. Preliminary studies designed to evaluate effects of CG antibodies on these cultured trophoblast cells have been done [Bambra and Tarara, 1989]. It has been shown that this baboon trophoblast culture system can be used to study aspects of the mechanism of action of CG antibodies in pregnancy termination in a homologous situation.

Studies with trophoblast antigens. The trophoblast, which forms a continuous interface of the maternofetal junction, has always been of particular interest to biologists. An area of recent activity is the search for trophoblast-specific antigens [Johnson et al., 1981; Loke and Day, 1984; Hsi and Yeh, 1986]. Identification and characterization of these antigens has many practical applications such as in development of birth control vaccines [Anderson et al., 1987]. Trophoblast-specific antigens can be identified with monoclonal antibodies. Monoclonal antibodies recognizing specific antigens on human syncytiotrophoblast [Sunderland et al., 1984; Johnson et al., 1981; Brown et al., 1983] and cytotrophoblast [Loke and Day, 1984; Butterworth et al., 1985] have been produced.

Development of a trophoblast birth control vaccine is dependent

Fig. 1. **A:** Antibody BSA4 reacts with the developing acrosome in the baboon testis (arrows). Lu, lumen. ×400. **B:** Antibody BSA-4 reacts with a more advanced stage of the developing acrosome (arrows). ×400. **C:** Antibody BSA-4 reacts with the acrosome that has spread laterally, forming a distinct crescent. Both inner and outer acrosomal membranes are stained (arrows). ×400.

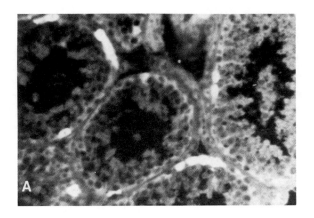

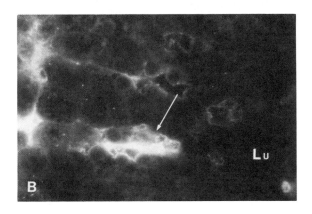

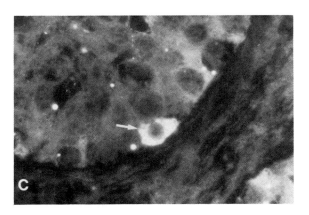

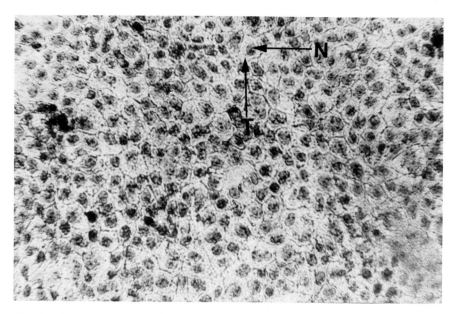

Fig. 3.   A photomicrograph of a monolayer derived from day 33 baboon placenta, showing closely packed oval mononuclear cells with no obvious intercellular spaces. T, trophoblast cell; N, nucleus. ×280.

on the identification of one or more antigens that are expressed on the very early trophoblast and whose recognition by immunological means will prevent or disrupt pregnancy. Such developmental studies cannot be done in humans for ethical reasons. Even though baboon cross-reactivity with several human trophoblast monoclonal antibodies has been claimed [Anderson et al., 1987] it is very weak or only apparent on frozen sections. Precise cross-reactivity with baboon tissues is not known. An alternative approach is the generation of nonhuman primate trophoblast monoclonal antibodies and testing their reactivity with human trophoblast. This would be an important step toward development of a trophoblast vaccine, because extensive efficacy and safety studies could then be done.

Monoclonal antibodies that are specific to baboon cytotrophoblast or syncytiotrophoblast have been produced at IPR. Staining charac-

Fig. 2.   **A:** Antibody SCA-1 reacts with Sertoli cells in baboon testicular sections. ×400. **B:** The intercellular spaces between the developing spermatid cells occupied by Sertoli cell cytoplasmic projections are distinctly stained by antibody SCA-1 (arrow). Lu, lumen. ×800. **C:** Antibody SCA-1 cross-reacts with human Sertoli cells (arrow). ×600.

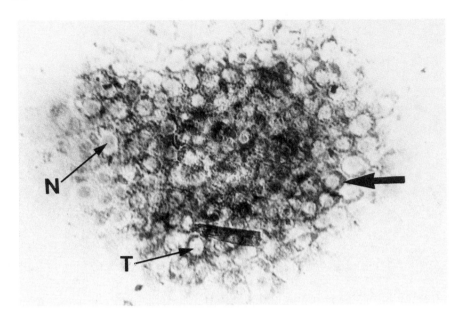

Fig. 4. A monolayer reacted with cytotrophoblast-specific monoclonal antibody (BM-2), showing cytoplasmic localization of the reaction product (arrow). T, trophoblast cell; N, nucleus. ×440.

teristics of some of these antibodies have recently been described [Bambra and Isahakia, 1989]. One of these antibodies (BM-3) recognizes antigens that are restricted to the apical syncytial membrane in baboon placenta (Fig. 5). This antibody has been found to cross-react with first-trimester human placenta but with different staining characteristics. Preimplantation baboon embryos can be recovered using a nonsurgical procedure [Pope et al., 1980]. This procedure has been developed at IPR, and recovered embryos can be maintained in vitro for up to 14 days. During this period blastocysts attach to culture dishes (Fig. 6) and give rise to extensive trophoblast outgrowths (Fig. 6). The baboon placental monoclonal antibodies are currently being screened against this early "pregnancy" trophoblast material.

Studies with zona pellucida antigens. The zona pellucida (ZP) is an extracellular matrix that surrounds the ovum. It plays a key role in the process of sperm–egg interaction in mammals. A variety of mammalian species have been immunized with ZP glycoproteins. In these studies the antibodies produced were found to inhibit fertilization by preventing the binding of the spermatozoa to the surface of ZP [Aiken, 1988; Skinner et al., 1984]. Such studies have led to the belief than an effective immunologic contraceptive method may be developed with ZP antigens.

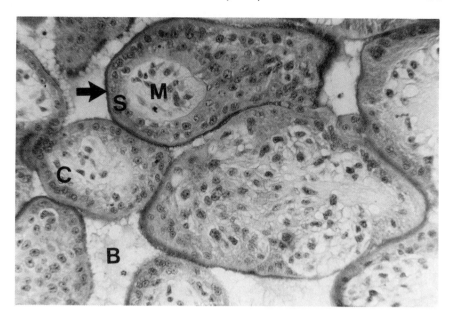

Fig. 5. Antibody BM-3 reacts with the apical surface of syncytiotrophoblast (arrow) on sections of baboon chorionic villous. B, maternal blood spaces; S, cytotrophoblast; M, mesenchyma. ×280.

Use of monoclonal and polyclonal antibodies has shown that the antigenicity and immunogenicity of mammalian ZP is complex [Drell and Dunbar, 1984; Marresh and Dunbar, 1987; Timmons et al., 1987]. Multiple antigens are associated with ZP, and both shared and unique antigenic determinants are associated with the ZP of different mammalian species. Even carbohydrate moieties of the ZP can affect immunogenicity and antigenicity of ZP [Sacco et al., 1986].

Even though an antifertility effect has been observed in ZP-immunized animals of various species, the adverse effect on the ovarian follicles has been of major concern [Skinner et al., 1984]. It is believed that these problems can be overcome by using ZP proteins produced by recombinant deoxyribonucleic acid (DNA) technology or by synthetically produced peptides. These types of peptides will be devoid of carbohydrate structures. It has been shown that immunization of baboons with denatured and deglycosylated ZP does result in production of antibodies that recognize antigenic determinants on ZP [Dunbar et al., 1989]. However, these antibodies did interfere with the normal ovarian function of the immunized baboons. Currently, IPR is evaluating synthetic ZP peptides in terms of their immunogenicity and effects on ovaries in baboons in collaboration with Dr. B. Dunbar.

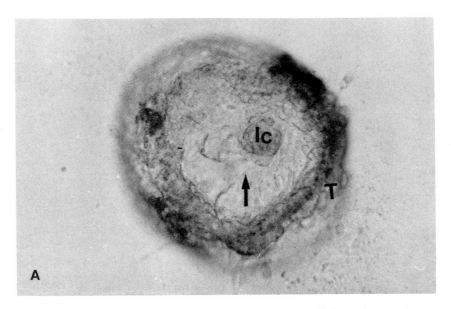

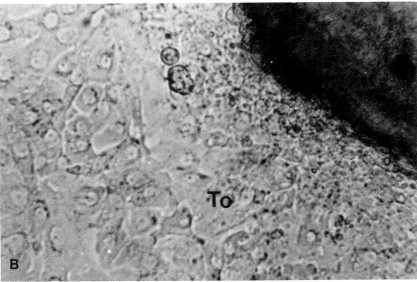

Fig. 6. **A:** Hatched blastocyst recovered by nonsurgical uterine flushing implanting (arrow) on the culture dish. Ic, inner cell mass; T, trophoblast outgrowth. ×440. **B:** Attached embryo showing extensive trophoblast outgrowth (To) after 14 days in culture. ×280.

FUTURE DEVELOPMENTS

The anatomical similarities between human and primates coupled with the phsyiologically similar responses to endocrine stimuli make nonhuman primates suitable models for the evaluation and development of novel methods of contraception. Cellular and humoral immunological parameters in the baboons have been found to be very similar to those of humans [Mendelow et al., 1980]. In this regard baboons provide the most suitable model in terms of the information available on placentation, embryogenesis, pregnancy development, and immunology in this animal.

Production of monoclonal antibodies against gamete antigens has been in progress for some time, whereas isolation and mass production of specific gamete antigens by recombinant DNA technology has been recently initiated. These purified materials promise to make available an acceptable gamete-based vaccine for human use. The efficacy and safety of these vaccines will need to be evaluated in primates prior to human use. In this respect it will be essential to understand not only the local immune response mechanisms to antigens but also systemic immune responses in the animal model. Few such studies have been done in primates. Preliminary studies done at IPR suggest that immunized baboons develop very low systemic antibody levels, with 30% animals not showing any response at all. Primate models will continue to be needed for some time to come for in vivo studies on various aspects of contraceptive development.

ACKNOWLEDGMENTS

We acknowledge financial support from the World Health Organization Special Programme for Research, Development, and Research Training in Human Reproduction and from the Rockefeller Foundation.

REFERENCES

Aiken J (1988): Contraceptive potential of antibodies to the zona pellucida. J Reprod Fertil 83:325–331.

Anderson DJ, Johnson PM, Alexander NJ, Jones WR, Griffin PD (1987): Monoclonal antibodies to human trophoblast and sperm antigens: Report of two WHO-sponsored workshops, June 30, 1986, Toronto, Canada. J Reprod Immunol 10:231–257.

Bambra CS (1989): Characterization of dispersed baboon placental cells grown in vitro using monoclonal antibodies. J Reprod Immunol 16:217–224.

Bambra CS, Isahakia M (1989): Monoclonal antibodies to baboon syncytio- and cyto-trophoblast. J Reprod Immunol 16:207–216.

Bambra CS, Tarara R (1989): Effects of baboon chorionic gonadotrophin antibodies on placental derived baboon trophoblast cells in vitro. J Reprod Immunol 16:225–238.

Brown PJ, Molony CM, Johnson PM (1983): Immunohistochemical identification of human trophoblast membrane antigens using monoclonal antibodies. J Reprod Immunol 5:351–361.

Butterworth BH, Khong TY, Loke YW, Robertson WB (1985): Human cytotrophoblast populations studied by monoclonal antibodies using single and double biotin–avidin–peroxidase immunochemistry. J Histochem Cytochem 33:977–983.

Chowdhury AK, Steinberger E (1976): A study of germ cell morphology and duration of spermatogenic cyle in the baboon *(Papio anubis)*. Anat Rec 185:115–170.

Drell DW, Dunbar BS (1984): Monoclonal antibodies to rabbit and pig zona pellucida distinguish species specific and shared antigenic determinants. Biol Reprod 30:435–444.

Dunbar BS, Lo C, Powell J, Stevens VC (1989): Use of a synthetic peptide adjuvant for the immunization of baboons with denatured and deglycosylated pig zona pellucida glyco-proteins. Fertil Steril 52:311–318.

Goldberg E, Wheat TE, Powell JE, Stevens VC (1981): Reduction of fertility in female baboons immunized with lactate dehydrogenase C_4. Fertil Steril 35:214–217.

Hearn JP (1980): The immunology of chorionic gonadotrophin. In Hearn JP (ed): Immunological Aspects of Reproduction and Fertility Control. Lancaster: MTP Press, pp 229–244.

Hendrickx AG (1971): Embryology of the Baboon. Chicago: University of Chicago Press.

Hsi BL, Yeh CG (1986): Monoclonal antibody GB 25 recognizes human villous trophoblast. Am J Reprod Immunol Microbiol 12:1–3.

Isahakia M (1988): Characterization of baboon testicular antigen using monoclonal antis-perm antibodies. Biol Reprod 39:889–899.

Isahakia M (1989): Monoclonal antibody localization of sperm surface antigens secreted by the epididymis of the baboon *(Papio cynocephalus)*. J Reprod Fertil 86:51–58.

Isahakia M, Alexander NJ (1984): Interspecies cross-reactivity of monoclonal antibodies directed against human sperm antigens. Biol Reprod 30:1015–1026.

Johnson PM, Cheng HM, Moloy CM, Stern CMM, Slade BM (1981): Human trophoblast-specific surface antigens identified using monoclonal antibodies. Am J Reprod Immunol 1:246–254.

Loke YW, Day S (1984): Monoclonal antibody to human cytotrophoblast. Am J Reprod Immunol 5:106–108.

Marresh GA, Dunbar BS (1987): Antigenic comparison of five species of mammalian zonae pellucidae. J Exp Zool 244:299–306.

Mendelow B, Grobicki D, Hunt M, Marcus F, Metz J (1980): Normal celluar and humoral immunologic parameters in the baboon *(Papio ursinus)* compared to human standards. Lab Anim Sci 30:1018–1021.

Moudgal NR, Murthy GS, Ravindranath N, Rao AG, Prasad MRN (1988): Development of a contraceptive vaccine for use by the human male: Results of a feasibility study carried out in adult male bonnet monkeys *(Macaca radiata)*. In Talwar GP (ed): Contraception Research for Today and the Nineties. New York: Springer Verlag, pp 253–258.

Naz RK, Alexander NJ, Isahakia M, Hamilton D (1984): Monoclonal antibody against human germ cell membrane glycoprotein that inhibits fertilization. Science 225:342–344.

Pope CE, Pope VZ, Beck LR (1980): Nonsurgical recovery of uterine embryos in the baboon. Biol Reprod 23:657–662.

Sacco AG, Yurewicz EC, Subramanian MG (1986): Carbohydrate influences the immunogenic and antigenic characteristics of the 2P3 macromolecule (Mr 55,000) of the pig zona pellucida. J Reprod Fertil 76:575–584.

Saling PM, Irons G, Waibel R (1985): Mouse sperm antigens that participate in fertilization. I. Inhibition of sperm fusion with egg plasma membrane using monclonal antibodies. Biol Reprod 33:515–526.

Skinner SM, Mills T, Kirchick HJ, Dunbar BS (1984): Immunization with zona pellucida proteins results in abnormal ovarian follicular differentiation and inhibition of gonadotropin-induced steroid secretion. Endocrinology 115:2418–2423.

Stevens VC (1980): The current status of anti-pregnancy vaccines based on synthetic fractions of HCG. In Hearn JP (ed): Immunological Aspects of Reproduction and Fertility Control. Lancaster: MTP Press, pp 203–216.

Stevens VC (1986): Current status of antifertility vaccines using gonadotropin immunogens. Immunol Today 7:369–374.

Sunderland CA, Redman CWG, Stirrat GM (1984): Monoclonal antibodies to human syncytiotrophoblast. Immunology 43:541–546.

Talwar GP (1980): Vaccines based on the beta-subunit of HCG. In Hearn JP (ed): Immunological Aspects of Reproduction and Fertility Control. Lancaster: MTP Press, pp 217–228.

Talwar GP, Singh O (1988): Birth control vaccines inducing antibodies against chorionic gonadotrophin. In Talwar GP (ed): Contraception Research for Today and the Nineties. New York: Springer-Verlag, pp 183–197.

Timmons TM, Maresh GA, Bundman DS, Dunbar BS (1987): Use of specific monoclonal and polyclonal antibodies to define distinct antigens of porcine zona pellucida. Biol Reprod 36:1,275–1,284.

DISCUSSION

DR. SWERDLOFF: I was curious about the patchy nature of the staining of the testes in the passively immunized animals. Since we know that germ cells mature in a stage-specific fashion, I wonder if you had observed whether the Sertoli cells that expressed antigens had associations with certain germ cells of a specific stage. Perhaps that would give us some insight into factors that might be responsible for the orderly maturation of spermatogenesis.

DR. ISAHAKIA: Yes. This particular antibody that recognizes Sertoli cell products was just recently raised, and the data presented are from studies that we have just done. Specifically, we need to do more studies to define the problems this antigen might have in terms of Sertoli cell interaction with some of the germinal cells.

DR. PRIMAKOFF: Clinical data have shown that human sperm with antibody on their surface become immobilized in cervical mucus. Is that true in any of the primate species that you have tested?

DR. ISAHAKIA: Our study was conducted mainly on male baboons. Obviously we would like to go to females and switch the model because of SIV concerns, but the assumption is that the mechanisms would essentially be the same. I think the cervix and cervical mucus is an area that needs additional study in terms of its role as a major barrier to primate sperm. We know that unlike in rodents, in which sperm are deposited directly into the uterus, sperm in humans and primates are deposited into the vagina. Clearly, the cervix is a major barrier. This is something that we need to remember in terms of the antifertility effects of the vaccines we might study in some of the rodent models.

DR. ANDERSON: Is there a good in vitro fertilization model for the baboon? And, can you examine the sperm–egg reactions in vitro? Also, do human sperm bind to zona from baboons?

DR. ISAHAKIA: We haven't done any of those studies. In fact, a major drawback in terms of selecting some of these antigens for possible contraceptive value has been the lack of reliable in vitro assays, particularly concerning whether these antibodies have a functional effect. While the antigens cross-react with human sperm, the human sperm hamster egg penetration assay has obviously been the choice assay to use. In terms of the baboon in vitro assay, very few studies have been done in primates.

DR. ANDRADA: Can you detect antigens in younger monkeys?

DR. ISAHAKIA: No. We don't detect any of these antigens in immature testes. That is something that we have looked for, but thus far none of the antigens that we have identified with these antibodies are expressed in immature testes.

33

Strategy of Vaccine Development

David Griffin

Traditionally, vaccines have been designed and developed to elicit a protective immune response against microorganisms causing disease. They exhibit, therefore, the following general properties and characteristics:

1   They provide protection against debilitating and often life-threatening infectious diseases.
2   They are often the only means available for protecting against, or controlling the effects of, these diseases.
3   They are designed to generate long-term (ideally lifetime) protective immunity, often aided by natural boosting throughout the lifetime of the individual as a result of intermittent, subclinical exposure to the natural antigen.
4   They are based on and directed against immunologically "foreign" or "nonself"-antigens.

In contrast, the properties and characteristics of antifertility vaccines differ markedly from antidisease vaccines in that

1   The vaccines will be used by healthy, fertile individuals to protect against an unwanted pregnancy.
2   Several alternative methods of family planning are already available.
3   The vaccine-induced immunity will be of a predictable and comparatively short duration and, to avoid permanent infertility, will not be naturally boosted by exposure to the target antigens.

Gamete Interaction: Prospects for Immunocontraception, pages 501–522
© 1990 Wiley-Liss, Inc.

4   The vaccines will be directed against isologous antigens.

However, in spite of the substantial differences in the requirements and intended uses of these two types of vaccines, the overall
strategies for their development are essentially the same and can be
broadly divided into the following major steps:

1   The identjfication of target events
2   The selection of target molecules
3   The engineering of prototype vaccines
4   The preclinical testing of vaccines
5   The clinical testing of vaccines

With regard to the development of fertility-regulating vaccines,
these five steps can be defined, more precisely, as follows:

1   The identification of events in the process of reproduction
      that are accessible to immunological intervention
2   The identification and selection of molecules necessary for,
      and essential to, the reproductive process whose elimina-
      tion or neutralization by immunological means will result in
      a safe, effective, and acceptable antifertility effect
3   The development of vaccines using natural or synthetic im-
      munogens derived from these molecules
4   The preclinical evaluation of vaccine safety and efficacy in
      relevant animal models
5   The clinical testing of vaccine safety and efficacy

A detailed review of this area has been carried out recently in a
WHO Symposium on the Assessment of the Safety and Efficacy of
Antifertility Vaccines [Ada and Griffin, 1990]. This chapter will not
attempt to repeat that review but will, instead, present an overview
of the five main steps involved in the development of antifertility
vaccines, the issues that are presented by this work, and the points
that need to be considered when planning studies in this area.

EVENTS IN THE PROCESS OF REPRODUCTION THAT ARE ACCESSIBLE TO IMMUNOLOGICAL INHIBITION

Mammalian reproduction is a complex sequence of events that
can, for convenience, be divided into three stages: the production of
the male and female gametes; the interaction of the gametes leading
to fertilization; and the process of implantation of the developing

embryo. All of these events can be inhibited immunologically by eliciting an immune response directed against virtually any of the functionally and structurally important molecules that are involved in, or produced during, these three stages. These molecules include the hypothalamic gonadotropin-releasing hormone (GnRH), the pituitary gonadotropins follicle-stimulating hormone (FSH) and luteinizing hormone (LH), the gonadal steroids (testosterone, estrogen, and progesterone), and tissue-specific products and components of the mature gametes and the early conceptus.

In a large number of studies carried out over the past two decades, it was clearly demonstrated that passive and/or active immunization with many of these molecules, in either their natural or modified forms, can produce varying types and degrees of antifertility effects through neutralization of the biological actions of hormones, through inhibition of enzyme activities, and through a variety of cytolytic and cytotoxic actions. However, when some of these molecules are used in prototype vaccines, they produce immediate endocrine and other metabolic disturbances and/or have the potential for eliciting immunopathology.

It is necessary, therefore, to establish a number of criteria for the identification of those molecules that represent suitable candidates for development into vaccines for clinical use.

CRITERIA FOR THE SELECTION OF CANDIDATE MOLECULES FOR VACCINE DEVELOPMENT

Relevance

A necessary prerequisite for an antifertility immunogen is that it should be based on a molecule involved in, and essential for, the process of reproduction so that immunological neutralization or removal of the target antigen will result in an antifertility effect.

Specificity

It is important that the molecules selected for vaccine development exhibit tissue specificity, that is, they are secreted by or expressed on the intended target tissue only. This will avoid cross-reactions of the vaccine-elicited immune response with nontarget tissues that could lead to unacceptable metabolic disturbances and immunopathological changes.

In addition, the target antigen should, ideally, have an identical or closely related form and function in an animal model in which extensive immunization studies can be carried out. This will permit relevant and meaningful preclinical safety and efficacy studies to be conducted with the vaccine prior to clinical trials.

Accessibility

For an antifertility immune response to be effective, the target antigen must be accessible to antibodies and sensitized lymphocytes in the circulation and/or in the lumen of the genital tract of the vaccine recipient. This requires that the target is either secreted by, or expressed on, the outer surface of the target cells.

Location

If the immune attack is concentrated in the lumen of either the male or female genital tracts, adverse reactions are likely to be minimized. However, the potential for producing immediate and delayed-type hypersensitivity reactions and other inflammatory responses in these locations must be considered. In contrast, an immune attack against molecules that appear in the vaccine recipient's circulation and/or find their way into other tissues and body fluids must not result in adverse reactions in any of these locations.

Quantity

The relative proportions of antigen to antibody, as well as the frequency and duration of appearance of the target molecules, are important factors from the point of view of the potential safety and efficacy of an antifertility vaccine. In terms of safety, the immediate and long-term consequences of the formation and deposition of insoluble immune complexes in vascular and other sites where they might provoke pathology need to be considered. In terms of efficacy, the level of immunity elicited by the vaccine must be sufficient to neutralize or remove all of the target antigen.

Transience

Ideally, antifertility vaccines should be directed against molecules that are present only transiently and/or in low concentrations. This would have the following advantages: The risk of chronic formation of immune complexes and possible subsequent immune complex disease will be minimized; the immune effect will only be called into play when antigen is present; and the immune response is unlikely to be overwhelmed by an excess of antigen.

Synthesizable

An important consideration when selecting molecules for development into antifertility vaccines is the ability to prepare them in sufficient quantities for large-scale vaccine production. As it is unlikely that starting materials will be obtained from natural sources, the ability to prepare these immunogens by classic chemical synthesis procedures or by the more modern biosynthetic approaches is a necessary practical requirement.

CANDIDATES FOR ANTIFERTILITY VACCINE DEVELOPMENT

The criteria referred to in the previous section have been established to minimize unacceptable side effects, to maximize efficacy, and to facilitate the production of antifertility vaccines. From these criteria it appears that the ideal target for such a vaccine would be a molecule that

1 When eliminated or neutralized by immunological means, will result in a safe, effective, and acceptable means of fertility regulation
2 Is specific to the intended target
3 Is present in a site where a controlled immune response will not lead to immunopathology
4 Is present transiently and/or at low levels compared with the anticipated immune response
5 Will not elicit other undesirable immune responses, such as IgE production and subsequent allergic reactions
6 Is, or can be, chemically characterized and easily produced

The many molecules involved in the different stages of reproduction do not represent equally attractive candidates for antifertility vaccine development and can be broadly classified into the following two categories by the extent to which they satisfy the above criteria.

More Attractive Candidates

Immunization against molecules expressed on, or produced by, the mature gametes and the trophectoderm of the preimplantation conceptus does not appear to lead to metabolic disturbances or local or systemic immunopathological side effects and, provided an adequate level of immunity is generated, also results in a high level of efficacy. Many of these molecules, for example, sperm antigens in the female, have the additional advantage of being immunologically "foreign."

Less Attractive Candidates

Immunization against the pituitary gonadotrophins FSH and LH produces a pronounced antifertility effect in males and females with no evidence of secondary endocrine or other metabolic disturbances. However, the long-term (lifetime) consequences of persistent immunity to these constantly present normal body constituents has yet to be determined, and the theoretical potential for inducing immunopathology in the pituitary and/or FSH and LH target tissues remains a concern.

Immunization against GnRH has an indirect antifertility effect but is associated with major endocrine disturbances and associated anatomical and behavioral changes. Although these can be overcome, in the male, by the frequent administration of exogenous testosterone, the need for this concomitant treatment and the theoretical potential for immunopathology in the hypothamus and/or pituitary makes this approach less attractive for a contraceptive vaccine. An anti-GnRH vaccine may prove suitable, however, in the treatment of benign prostatic hyperplasia and prostatic tumors.

Experiments of Nature

A substantial amount of evidence has been collected concerning the possible role of naturally occurring antisperm immunity in men and women with otherwise unexplained infertility. The majority of these individuals are healthy and exhibit no physiological disturbances or overt side effects, apart from their infertility. These experiments of nature suggest that an antisperm vaccine might be a clinically acceptable approach to fertility regulation and provide some encouragement for further studies in this area.

PRECLINICAL STAGES OF VACCINE DEVELOPMENT

Design of Prototype Antifertility Vaccines

As with any new prophylactic or therapeutic preparation, the development of antifertility vaccines proceeds through a series of steps involving the selection and testing of various prototype formulations before a safe, effective, and clinically acceptable product can be identified. This process is particularly complex in the case of vaccines, because, unlike most pharmaceuticals, they often contain several components with different biological functions, such as the B-cell immunogen, T-cell stimulating carrier, and one or more immunostimulants.

Composition of Antifertility Vaccines

With the possible exception of antisperm vaccines to be used by women, antifertility vaccines will be based on "self" or "self-like" molecules to which the vaccine recipient is immunologically tolerant and that are likely to be only weakly immunogenic. These molecules need to modified, therefore, either by chemical alteration, by conjugation to macromolecular carriers, or by synthesis as analogs of the parent molecule, in order to increase their immunogenicity.

In addition, potent immunostimulants may need to be included in the vaccine formulation to elicit an immune response of the desired magnitude. Furthermore, the vaccine formulation must have the appropriate physicochemical properties to persist at the site of administration long enough to elicit an immune response of the desired duration.

Type of Immune Response

Depending on the intended target of the vaccine, and its known or suspected mechanism of action, either a predominantly antibody-mediated or predominantly cell-mediated immune response may be required. For example, antibodies alone may be sufficient to inhibit gamete interactions by immobilizing sperm and/or by coating the surface of the zona pellucida. Similarly, removal of human chorionic gonadotropin (hCG) from the maternal circulation may be accomplished by antibodies alone, whereas an effective cytotoxic attack on the trophectoderm may require both antibodies and sensitized lymphocytes. An important part of vaccine development, therefore, involves monitoring the qualitative nature of the immune response, in relation to its efficacy and safety, to ensure that the vaccine produces appropriate responses.

Site of Immune Response

The optimal site of the immune response generated by antifertility vaccines will depend on the location of the intended target. In the case of antigamete vaccines, adequate levels of antibodies and sensitized lymphocytes will be needed in the lumen of the female genital tract in order to inhibit fertilization, blastocyst hatching, and/or implantation. This may require formulating and delivering the vaccine in ways that will favor the production of local secretory immunity, as sufficient quantities of antibodies and sensitized lymphocytes may not reach the lumen of the genital tract by transport from the circulation. By contrast, an immune response restricted to the circulation of the vaccine recipient may be sufficient for other targets, such as hCG, although there is some evidence that the antifertility effect of anti-hCG vaccines may involve a direct antibody-mediated effect on the trophectoderm.

Duration of Immune Response

Unlike antidisease vaccines, antifertility vaccines are not intended to provide lifetime immunity but rather to produce an effective immune response of predictable and comparatively short duration. For example, an antifertility vaccine with a duration of effect of 12–24 months may be a useful and attractive addition to the existing family planning armamentarium. However, vaccines with a shorter duration of effect may prove attractive alternatives to injectable contraceptive steroids, and vaccines with a longer duration of effect may be attractive alternatives to surgical sterilization for those individuals seeking a long-term or irreversible method, provided such vaccines are free of major side effects.

Magnitude of Immune Response

The magnitude of the immune response must be sufficient to neutralize or remove all of the target antigen at an acceptable point in the reproductive process. This may be easier to achieve with a vaccine directed against the female gamete, such as an antizona pellucida vaccine, where the target is a discrete entity of known size and quantity, and with an anti-hCG vaccine, where the range of hCG produced by the preimplantation blastocyst is known. It may be more difficult to achieve, however, with an antisperm vaccine, where the concentration of target antigen can vary greatly depending on the frequency of intercourse.

SELECTION OF ANIMAL MODELS

The ease with which appropriate animal models can be identified and selected for the preclinical testing of vaccine efficacy and safety depends, to a large extent, on the nature of the intended target molecule. In some cases, such as certain sperm antigens, the molecule can be widely conserved—in terms of structure, location, and function—across many animal species, and any one of these may be suitable as an animal model. In other cases, however, such as the chorionic gonadotropins, the molecule is restricted to the higher primate species, necessitating extensive use of these animal models in the preclinical phases of vaccine development. The criteria by which animal models in which to carry out the necessary preclinical safety and efficacy evaluations of antifertility vaccines are identified and selected, as well as some of the problems presented in this area, are summarized below.

Relevance to the Human

Relevance is probably the most important and difficult question to be addressed when identifying animal models for the preclinical safety and efficacy evaluations of antifertility vaccines intended for human use. Many factors need to be taken into consideration, depending on the particular vaccine to be studied, the objectives of the study to be conducted, and the parameters to be measured. These factors include the similarities of the animal models to the human in terms of their reproductive biology, immunological responsiveness (both quantitative and qualitative), as well as the antifertility mechanism and immunopathological reactions, and their sequelae, associated with the use of the vaccine. Other important factors to be taken into consideration include what is known about the various animal models in terms of their reproductive performance; the incidence of naturally occurring pathology and fetal abnormalities in the species; their susceptibility to disease; and known reactions to experimentation involving the administration of drugs or the injection of vaccines [Berry and Barlow, 1976].

Availability in Sufficient Numbers

Another important consideration is the availability of the animals in sufficient numbers to carry out the proposed studies in a way that will permit the generation of statistically valid data. This is not a problem if mice, rats, and rabbits are considered appropriate animal for these studies, but major supply difficulties can be encountered if more exotic species, such as the higher primates, are required.

Feasibility of Studies Required

For antifertility vaccines based on and directed against primate-specific antigens, the use of appropriate infrahuman primates is an important part of their preclinical development and evaluation. However, major logistical, financial, and legal limitations can be encountered in the use of primates in experiments requiring invasive procedures and autopsies. The following questions must be considered, therefore, when planning the nature and range of studies to be conducted:

1   Can the vaccine be administered by the proposed route and at the required frequency and dose?
2   Can body fluids and tissues be taken in the quantities required for the laboratory examinations to be carried out during the in-life phase of the studies?
3   Can the animals be autopsied during and at the end of the study for postmortem examinations and analysis?

The last question takes on particular significance with regard to the protected status of some of the higher primate species, particularly the apes.

PRELIMINARY TESTING OF VACCINE SAFETY AND EFFICACY IN ANIMALS

Immunogenicity of the Prototype Vaccine

The development and selection of a prototype antifertility vaccine for eventual preclinical and clinical evaluation involves a large number of studies to compare different ratios of the vaccine constitutents, different doses of the vaccine, different routes of administration, and different methods of formulation in order to generate the desired type of immunity as well as to optimize the magnitude and duration of the immune response. These studies usually involve some evaluations of species differences in immunoresponsiveness to the vaccine, compared with expected human responses, to ensure the development of a preparation relevant for clinical use.

Specificity of the Elicited Antibodies

The specificity of the antibodies elicited by the vaccine will depend primarily on the nature of the immunogen used but can also be influenced by the animal species in which the antibodies are raised.

Although there will be both quantitative and qualitative differences in the immune responses of animals and humans to the same vaccine formulation, if a prototype antifertility vaccine elicits antibodies in animals that cross-react with nontarget tissues, this would argue against further development of that particular vaccine formulation.

On the other hand, the production of target-specific antibodies in one or more animal models does not mean that the same vaccine formulation will generate an immune response with the same specificity in humans. A careful examination of the sera obtained from volunteers taking part in clinical trials of prototype vaccines is needed, therefore, to determine if any potentially hazardous cross-reacting antibodies are produced and, if so, to identify the tissues and molecules with which they cross-react.

Evidence of Actual or Potential Antifertility Efficacy In Vitro and/or In Vivo

Preliminary information on the potential efficacy of antifertility vaccines can sometimes be obtained in studies carried out in vitro, for example, the ability of antisera raised by antigamete vaccines to inhibit sperm–ovum interactions and/or blastocyst hatching in vitro and the ability of antibodies raised to an antitrophectoderm vaccine to lyse trophoblast cells in culture. However, the significance of results obtained under these unnatural conditions compared with the situation that prevails in vivo must be constantly questioned.

More relevant information is gained in in vivo studies carried out in relevant animal models. As indicated earlier, the animal models in which the efficacy of a prototype antifertility vaccine is to be assessed must take into account the type of vaccine being evaluated, the species specificity of the antigen on which it is based, and its expected/intended mechanism of action. For example, rodents may be suitable models in which to carry out a preliminary evaluation of a vaccine based on a sperm antigen that is conserved across species but would be inappropriate for a vaccine based on a primate-specific antigen such as chorionic gonadotrophin.

PRECLINICAL STUDIES OF VACCINE SAFETY

In view of their novelty, the amount of previous relevant experience with fertility-regulating vaccines is limited, and, consequently, the regulatory requirements for the preclinical toxicological testing of such vaccines are not clearly defined. The studies proposed by the World Health Organization [WHO, 1967, 1975] and by national regulatory authorities [Department of Community Services and Health, 1987] for the preclinical reproductive toxicity and teratogenicity testing of new drugs are designed to identify drug-associated adverse effects at three susceptible stages of reproduction: gametogenesis, fetal organogenesis, and peri- and postnatal development [Berry and Barlow, 1976]. In principle, the same studies could be carried out with antifertility vaccines, although some studies, such as those on the effect on gametogeneis in the male, would not be relevant for vaccines directed against oocyte, placental, and other female-specific antigens, and vice versa. In the absence of established national and international guidelines on appropriate preclinical safety studies to be carried out with prototype antifertility vaccines, the following information is based on studies conducted and/or proposed by the WHO Task Force on Vaccines for Fertility Regulation in connection with its anti-hCG vaccine development program.

Toxicology and Immunosafety

The pre-phase I anti-hCG vaccine toxicology and immunosafety studies carried out by the Task Force [Stevens and Jones, 1983] were based largely on those used for assessment of new drugs, irrespective of composition, mode of action, and intended use. These studies involved conventional assessments of acute, subacute, and chronic toxicities of the complete vaccine formulation, as well as various combinations of its constituents, and were carried out at several dose levels in mice, rats, rabbits, and baboons. In addition, a hyperimmunization study was carried out in baboons as part of the immunosafety evaluation of the vaccine. Because of the nature of the preparation, these studies included assessment of chemical toxicity, similar to those carried out for new drugs, and specific tests for immunotoxicity of the vaccine.

Chemical toxicity. The purpose of chemical toxicity studies is to determine if the complete vaccine formulation and its individual components will be free of undesirable or unacceptable toxic side effects at the dose proposed for clinical use. The studies include assessments of acute and subacute toxicity in mice and rats and intramuscular tolerance studies in rabbits. Typically, acute toxicity studies are restricted to body weight measurements and daily observations for detection of gross and overt changes in general health status, whereas subacute toxicity studies include in-life hematological, biochemical, and urine analyses and postmortem macroscopic and histological examinations of the injection site and of other body tissues. Although multiples of the intended human dose are administered in these studies, demonstration of finite toxicity by determining the LD_{50} dose is usually not feasible or relevant for vaccines.

Immunotoxicity. The purpose of immunotoxicity studies is to determine if the immune response elicited by the vaccine produces any adverse and undesirable side effects. Such events could include:

1. The formation of immune complexes, which in certain forms and under certain circumstances may produce pathology in susceptible sites such as the renal glomerulus and choroid plexus
2. Disturbances in the complex systems involved in homeostasis as a result of the removal or neutralization of the target antigen
3. Unexpected and unpredicted cross-reactive immunity to other, nontarget tissues because of the hitherto unknown presence of the target molecule in tissues other than those of the intended target, or to molecular mimicry

Teratology

Before conducting clinical trials in fertile volunteers, it is essential that studies are carried out to determine if fetal anomalies occur in immunized animals that become pregnant in the presence of ineffective levels of immunity. As for the toxicity studies mentioned earlier, these studies can also be divided into two types.

Chemical teratology. Chemical teratology might be manifested through one or both of the following two mechanisms. 1) The components of a fertility-regulating vaccine—in combination or in isolation, as parent compounds or breakdown/metabolic products—may have a direct or indirect effect on the gametes, in both males or females, that results in subsequent lethal or sublethal defects in the fetus. 2) Fetal exposure to these same compounds may occur as the result of immunization during the early stages of an undetected pregnancy or as the result of pregnancy occurring below the efficacy threshold during the waxing and waning phases of the immune response.

Immunoteratology. The maternal immune response elicited to a fertility-regulating vaccine might have a teratological effect on the developing fetus, either indirectly as a result of subtle alterations in the maternal physiology on which the fetus is dependent or directly as a result of antibodies passing across the placenta and being deposited in, or reacting with, fetal tissues. The nonovert consequences of such events may not be detectable until the offspring reach sexual maturity, in which case their fertility and the normality of their off-spring might also need to be assessed.

Carcinogenicity and Mutagenicity

The nature and extent of carcinogenicity and mutagenicity studies that should be carried out with antifertility vaccines and the stages of clinical testing at which such animal studies should be carried out are less easy to define [WHO, 1969, 1971]. In view of the small quantities of vaccine to be administered, the infrequency of their administration, and their intended comparatively short duration of effect, it may not be relevant to conduct conventional carcinogenicity and mutagenicity studies with these preparations.

CLINICAL STAGES OF VACCINE DEVELOPMENT

Clinical Trials of Vaccine Safety, Efficacy, and Acceptability

The various stages of clinical testing of a novel antifertility vaccine are similar to those used in the evaluation of a new contraceptive drug. However, because the immune response elicited by a vaccine is an active process, controlled to a large extent by the genetics of the recipient, the time course of the trial and the parameters to be assessed will be different from those evaluated in a pharmacodynamic/pharmacokinetic study of a pharmaceutical preparation. For all clinical trials, care needs to be taken to determine relevant and essential inclusion and exclusion criteria for the trial volunteers and to ensure that recruitment is based on fully informed consent.

Phase I

The primary objective of a phase I clinical trial of a new antifertility vaccine is to determine the safety of the preparation in humans. Therefore, volunteers taking part in phase I trials need to be regularly monitored for evidence of adverse signs or symptoms during physical examinations and for evidence of abnormal findings in laboratory tests of immunological, endocrinological, and other systems.

Phase I studies are carried out in volunteers of reproductive age who are not at risk of becoming pregnant either because they have been previously sterilized or because they are using a reliable method of contraception (such as an intrauterine device) that will not interact or interfere with the action of the vaccine. However, an indication of potential efficacy can also be obtained in a phase I trial by assessing the immune response elicited by the vaccine and relating this to the level of immunity calculated to confer efficacy in fertile individuals. Phase I studies are usually carried out as dose-finding exercises, involving the allocation of subjects to different dose groups, with the first group to be immunized receiving the lowest dose of vaccine.

In view of the exploratory nature of a phase I clinical trial of a novel antifertility vaccine, the number of subjects recruited to a phase I clinical trial should be kept to the minimum needed to obtain statistically reliable data in order not to expose any more subjects than necessary to an unknown risk. The overall length of a phase I trial is determined largely by the duration of the immunity elicited by the vaccine together with an initial period for the screening of potential trial subjects and for follow-up during the time of waning immunity. A period of 1–3 years is usually sufficient for this purpose.

Phase II

The principal purpose of a phase II clinical trial of an antifertility vaccine is to determine the efficacy (i.e., prevention of pregnancy) of a selected dose of vaccine in healthy, fertile volunteers. In addition, the effects of giving at least one booster injection of the vaccine, as well as further studies of safety and the relationship between the subjects' genetic constitution and immune response, may also be assessed.

The efficacy of the vaccine is determined by comparing the pregnancy rates in the trial subjects and in a group of noncontraceptors in the study population. The minimum number of cycles of theoretical protection against pregnancy provided by the vaccine can be deduced from the antibody titer data obtained in the phase I trial, and, from this figure, the number of subjects required for the phase II study can be readily calculated.

The protocol needs to include a record of sexual activity to determine, retrospectively, the number of menstrual cycles in which intercourse took place during the fertile phase of the cycle. In addition, the timing of discontinuation and resumption of alternative contraception needs to be carefully defined to avoid exposure to the risk of pregnancy during the waxing and waning phases of the immune response. Again, the overall length of a phase II trial is determined by the duration of the immunity elicited by the vaccine and the time required for screening of potential trial subjects and for post-treatment follow-up. A period of 2–3 years is usually sufficient for this purpose.

Phase III

The primary objectives of a phase III clinical trial of an antifertility vaccine are to determine its efficacy and safety in the general population and in varied service settings. In addition, some indication of the acceptibility of the vaccines will also be gained. A phase III trial also offers the opportunity to assess the vaccine in a situation when it is given on a repeated basis, i.e., when booster immunizations are provided after initial immunity has waned.

Depending on the duration of effective immunity elicited by the vaccine, determined from phase II trials, phase III studies may require in excess of 2,000 subjects. Ideally, these trials should be randomized, controlled comparisons between the vaccine and an established family planning method, such as an intrauterine device. The studies should be designed with sufficient statistical power to demonstrate a clinically important difference between treatment groups, with regard to both efficacy and side effects.

Population differences may affect the results of large clinical trials in terms of both efficacy and side effects, and this needs to be taken into account in the design and subsequent analysis of the study. These considerations are particularly important for vaccines, where the immune response may be modified by genetic variations and by the influence of intercurrent endemic illnesses. Because of the large number of subjects to be recruited and the time required for analysis of the trial data, phase III clinical trials can require between 4 and 6 years for completion.

TIME AND COST ESTIMATES FOR ANTIFERTILITY VACCINE DEVELOPMENT

The figures often quoted by the pharmaceutical industry for the time and costs required to bring a new drug from initial compound elucidation to final product are minima of 15 years and US $80 million, respectively. Much of this time and cost is taken up by preclinical toxicity studies and clinical trials.

Because of their novelty and experimental status, there are no corresponding industry-derived figures for the time and costs required for the development of antifertility vaccines. However, in view of their intended long duration of action, their dependence on an active and ongoing response by the recipient, and the comparative lack of previous experience with these vaccines, it can be reasonably argued that at least the same amounts of time and money will be needed to bring these novel preparations to the product registration stage as are required for new pharmaceuticals.

The rapidly developing field of "vaccinology" is constantly adding to our knowledge of the immune system and ways in which prototype vaccines can be engineered to elicit responses of the desired type, magnitude, and duration. It is likely that this information will lead to significant savings in both the time and costs required to produce vaccines for preclinical animal studies and, eventually, clinical trials. It is unlikely, however, that the time or costs involved in the clinical phases of the development and assessment of antifertility vaccines can be significantly reduced.

PRACTICAL ASPECTS OF VACCINE PRODUCTION AND USE

Antifertility vaccines need to satisfy a number of requirements relevant to their production, distribution, formulation, administration, and cost if they are to be considered viable additions to the options available to both the users and providers of family planning services and thereby achieve wide and continued use.

Production

All components of the vaccine must be capable of large-scale production under conditions satisfying national regulatory requirements for manufacture and quality assurance. Ideally, the method of preparation should avoid the use of toxic chemicals and biological reagents that, as residual contaminants, may represent potential hazards.

Distribution and Storage

The vaccine and, particularly, the immunogen component of the vaccine should be stable under a wide range of environmental conditions in order that it can be shipped and stored for long periods without deterioration. The stability of the vaccine should be confirmed at regular intervals by chemical analysis, by testing its immunogenic potency, and by assessing the target specificity of the immune response it elicits.

Formulation and Dosage Form

For the foreseeable future, vaccine immunogens are likely to be nonglycosylated peptides prepared by solid-phase synthesis or nonglycosylated or glycosylated peptides prepared by biosynthetic procedures. This will permit the immunogen to be packed as a lyophilized preparation, greatly enhancing its stability and perhaps permitting formulation of the vaccine immediately before administration using a nonreusable, multichamber syringe containing the separated vaccine components.

The dosage form should be easily prepared and should elicit a predictable and prolonged immune response of the intended magnitude and duration. This may involve the use of vaccine vehicles and delivery systems consisting of emulsions with predetermined stability and/or microcapsules and microspheres made from biodegradable/biocompatible polymers.

Administration

The first generation of antifertility vaccines to be used on a large scale are likely to be administered as viscous emulsions by intramuscular injection. A sufficiently high viscosity will be required to ensure the persistence of the vaccine at the injection site needed for a prolonged immune response, but this must not be so high that it requires the use of an unacceptably large needle for administration.

Because the majority of antifertility vaccines will exert their primary effect in the lumen of the male or female genital tract, local rather than systemic immunity might be more effective and more acceptable. This may lead to the development of vaccines that can be administered orally and that will predominantly, or selectively, elicit secretory immune responses in these locations.

Cost

The overall cost of the vaccine, including production, packing, shipping, storage, and administration, should be competitive with other methods of family planning used over equivalent periods of time. The ability to dispense with a cold-chain, to provide preloaded syringes, and, eventually, to provide orally active preparations should all prove important factors in reducing the overall cost of these vaccines.

Monitoring of Level of Immunity

One of the major advantages of antifertility vaccines is their long duration of effect and the continuation of their contraceptive action without intervention by the recipient. Although the duration of effect might be predictable within certain limits, individual variations in immune responsiveness are to be expected. This necessitates the development of simple, rapid, inexpensive, and reliable kits with which vaccine recipients can monitor their level of immunity and determine whether they are still protected by the vaccine.

RESEARCH NEEDS RELEVANT TO THE DEVELOPMENT OF ANTIFERTILITY VACCINES

In spite of the major advances that have been made over the last decade or so, we are still a long way from understanding all of the complex interactions that are responsible for the production and maintenance of effective immunity and that are central to vaccine development. A large number of studies can be readily envisaged under the general heading of "vaccinology" that would provide valuable information in this regard. These include studies on:

Vaccine composition and formulation
  Immunogen design
    Linear peptides
    Conformational peptides
    Mimotopes
    Expression products
  Carriers
    Defined chemicals
    Fusion proteins
    T-cell peptides
  Adjuvants
    Immunogen specific
    Immunogen nonspecific
  Vehicles and delivery systems
    Emulsions
    Microcapsules
Vaccine characteristics
  Rate of release in vivo
    Constant release
    Intermittent release
    Programmed release
  Vaccine dose
    Dose–response effects
  Effects of varying composition
  Frequency of administration
  Number of injections per administration
  Route of administration

    Oral
    Transdermal
    Intradermal
    Subdermal
    Intramuscular
    Intraperitoneal
  Site of administration
    Local versus systemic immunization
    Local versus systemic responses
  Selective production of secretory immunity in the lumen of the
    female genital tract
Control of the immune response
  Role of immunogenetics
    Magnitude of response
    Duration of response
  Role of different classes of immunoglobulins
  Relative benefits of IgG versus IgA
    Systemically
    Locally
    For all targets
    For selected targets
  Boosters
  Use of immunostimulants and interleukins
  Inhibition and reversibility of immunity
  Animal models
    Necessity of in vivo systems
    Development of in vitro systems

It is obvious that a systematic assessment of these and other issues requires a major investment in both time and money, but this may be necessary if safe, effective, and acceptable antifertility vaccines are to be developed and made available.

REFERENCES

Ada GL, Griffin PD (1990): The Assessment of the Safety and Efficacy of Vaccines to Regulate Fertility. Proceedings of a World Health Organization Symposium, June 12–16, 1989, Geneva (in press).

Berry CL, Barlow S (1976): Some remaining problems in the reproductive toxicity testing of drugs. Br Med Bull 32:34–38.

Department of Community Services and Health (1987): Guidelines for Preparation and Presentation of Applications for Investigational Drugs and Drug Products Under the Clinical Trials Exemption Scheme. Canberra: Australian Government Publishing Service.

Stevens VC, Jones WR (1983): Preclinical safety studies on a hCG vaccine. In Isojima S, Billington WD (eds): Reproductive Immunology. Amsterdam: Elsevier, p 233.

World Health Organization (1967): Principles for the Testing of Drugs for Teratogenicity. Technical Report Series, No. 364. Geneva: WHO.

World Health Organization (1969): Principles for the Testing and Evaluation of Drugs for Carcinogenicity. Technical Report Series, No. 426. Geneva: WHO.

World Health Organization (1971): Evaluation and Testing of Drugs for Mutagenicity. Technical Report Series, No. 482. Geneva: WHO.

World Health Organization (1975): Guidelines for Evaluation of Drugs for Use in Man. Technical Report Series, No. 563. Geneva: WHO.

DISCUSSION

DR. HANDELSMANN: One of my concerns as a requirement for contraceptive methodology is reversibility. One issue that always concerns me when thinking about vaccines is the inability, or lack of priority, accorded to switching off the immune system. I would certainly consider that to be a higher priority in designing and advocating immunocontraceptive methods. Could you comment on that?

MR. GRIFFIN: The question concerns reversal on demand—simply terminating the effect of the vaccine. That would be dealt with in the same way that you would, for instance, deal with an injectable steroid. You would inform recipients that they would have to accept that the vaccine would be active for the stated duration of time, whether 1 year, or 2 years, or however long. And you would also inform them that it is irreversible during that period. I think that it is not unreasonable to consider, at this stage, the feasibility of eventually providing a vaccine of 1 or 2 years duration.

DR. MITCHISON: The first question is "Why do you need a vaccine?" And does it have to be reversible? Perhaps there are certain circumstances in which permanent contraception is what is wanted.

MR. GRIFFIN: In answer to your first question, there is an increasing amount of dissatisfaction in many countries with currently available contraceptive methods. And, there are a number of theoretical advantages to a vaccine over the available methods, namely, the lack of conventional pharmacological activity, the long duration of effect, the ready acceptance of the vaccination principle, and the comparative costs once these are produced on a large scale. Thus there is ample justification for developing a contraceptive vaccine. The question of reversibility is always going to arise, and, as I mentioned, it may be acceptable to have a permanent vaccine for a certain segment of the "contracepting" population, for instance, women who are reaching the end of their reproductive life who would normally have sought surgical sterilization. In many developing countries, tubal ligation remains an in-patient procedure. An alternative method of sterilization that is nonpharmacological and nonsurgical would have some advantages. But, initially, we are aiming for something that is reversible within a predicted period of time.

MR. SPIELER: One in eight couples around the world practice sterilization as a method of birth control. And there are numerous organizations that are interested in looking at nonsurgical methods of sterilization. So, for a segment of the population who do not want to have any more children, a vaccine may be a very nice and acceptable form of nonsurgical sterilization.

DR. SWERDLOFF: Concerning the issue of efficacy and reversibility, is there a great deal of heterogeneity between people, in terms of the persistence of the immune response? Do some have a very long, protracted effect and some have a duration of action and reversibility that is much shorter?

MR. GRIFFIN: There is much evidence indicating a wide variation in the responsiveness, both in magnitude and duration, to the same vaccine in an outbred population. The advantage of synthetic vaccines, however, and the new delivery systems is that we can predict the persistence of the immunogen much more accurately with these preparations. That helps us to predict the duration of the immunity that is generated by them.

DR. SWERDLOFF: It seems that the degree of predictability in duration of effect is going to be an important consideration in the utilization of these techniques.

MR. GRIFFIN: I agree. I think we merely have to wait for the clinical trials to determine the range of effects in terms of duration and magnitude.

34

Immunoactivator Properties of RWJ 21757, a Substituted Guanosine With Adjuvant Activity

D.W. Anderson and R.J. Capetola

The immune system is divided into two separate but interacting responses: T-cell (cell-mediated) and B-cell (humoral) immunity. This conceptual and experimental separation of immunities can be used to describe three major classes of primary immune deficiency diseases: isolated T deficiency, isolated B deficiency, or combined T and B deficiencies with accompanying functional defects in cellular, humoral, or both types of immunity. There are a variety of clinical symptomatologies associated with these disease states, but the one central problem is a decrease in antibody production, causing susceptibility to a variety of microbial pathogens. While these genetic and congenital primary disorders are rare, there is a class of secondary immunodeficiency disease states common to a significant number of individuals. Included in this class of immunodeficiencies are patients with acquired immunodeficiency syndrome (AIDS), patients undergoing immunosuppressive therapy (antimetabolite, corticosteroid, radiation) for cancer or transplantation, victims of burns or massive trauma, leukemia and lymphoma patients, cancer patients, patients with chronic infections, and a number of persons with metabolic disorders (e.g., diabetes mellitus, nephrotic syndrome, hepatic disease, uremia, protein-losing enteropathies). In addition, there is also an age-associated senescence of the immune response. All of these disorders, while greatly varied in nature, share one thing in common—immune deficiency. This is often expressed

Gamete Interaction: Prospects for Immunocontraception, pages 523–548
© 1990 Wiley-Liss, Inc.

clinically by an increased susceptibility to infections, autoimmune disease, neoplasia, and vascular disease. Perhaps most important is the increase in disease and death resulting from infectious processes caused by lack of antibody production [Buckley, 1987; Green and Faist, 1988]. Therefore, a therapeutic entity that could restore or enhance the production of antibody should prove invaluable in helping these individuals fight life-threatening infections. Improved immune function would reduce the incidence of infections and neoplastic diseases and provide an improved sense of well-being and quality of life for these individuals. Concomitantly health care expenditures would decrease.

Depending on the extent and nature of the immune dysfunction, the principal modes of therapy for immunodeficiency disorders, whether inherited or acquired, include protective isolation; use of antibiotics for eradication or prevention of bacterial, parasitic, fungal, and a few viral infections; antibody replacement; and bone marrow transplantation. While all of these have demonstrated a degree of efficacy, each is beset with problems. Therefore, there is a medical need for pharmacologic agents functioning as immunopotentiators to restore defective immune responses.

Agents that enhance or potentiate the immune response are termed *adjuvants*. For many years there has been an attempt to develop these immunopotentiators to enhance the efficacy of vaccines, to modulate the host's natural defenses against microorganisms and cancer, and to restore impaired immune functions. A wide variety of materials have been demonstrated to have adjuvant activity. Some of the sources include bacteria, plants (Table 1), natural substances such as vitamins and antibiotics (Table 2) and the immune system itself (Table 3). Recently, a number of synthetic compounds have provided for a new class of immunopotentiators (Table 4).

As varied as are the types of agents with adjuvant activity, so too are the potential mechanisms by which these agents augment the immune response. Table 5 lists the means by which a number of adjuvants act as immunopotentiators. There are many sites of adjuvant action within the immune response that adjuvants operate. A number of recent reviews have been published that discuss the preclinical and clinical profiles of many adjuvants being developed for vaccines or immunotherapy [Altman and Dixon, 1989; St. Georgiev, 1988; Klausner, 1988; Ruzzala-Mallon et al., 1988; Warren and Chedid, 1988]. The purpose of this chapter is to focus on the immunopharmacology and adjuvant activity of C8-substituted guanosine ribonucleosides, with special emphasis on 7-allyl-8-oxoguanosine (RWJ 21757).

TABLE 1. Adjuvants: Bacterial, Fungal, or Plant Origin

Bacteria
  Bacillus Calmette-Guérin (BCG)
  Corynebacterium parvum (Propionobacter)
  Bordetella pertussis
Bacterial origin: Derived or synthesized
  BCG extracts
  MDP/murabutide
  LPS (detoxified)
  Lipid A analogs
  Biostim (RU 41740; *Klebsiella*)
  OK 432 (picibanil)
  Ribomunyl (ribosomes from various species)
  Ovamid (trahalose dimycolate; *C. parvum*)
  Forphenicinol (actinomyces)
Fungal or plant origin: Derived or synthesized
  Bestatin *(Streptomyces)*
  Glucan *(Saccharomyces)*
  Krestin *(Coriolus)*
  Aristolochic acid *(Aristolochia)*
  FK 156 analogs (gludapcin; *Streptomyces*)
  Swainsonine

TABLE 2. Adjuvants: Biological Substances

Vitamines and naturally occurring substances
  Vitamin A and Derivatives
  Vitamin E
  Lysolecithins
  Lipoidalamines
  Lynestrenol (progesterone-like agent)
Antibiotics
  Amphotericin B
  Nystatin
  Pyrrolomycin B
  Cefactor
  Cefodizime

ACTIVATION OF B LYMPHOCYTES BY C8-SUBSTITUTED GUANOSINE DERIVATIVES

Activation of B lymphocytes to become antibody-producing cells involves both proliferation and differentiation events and appears to be initiated when antigen and information-bearing molecules (lym-

TABLE 3. Adjuvants From the Immune System

Biological polypeptides
   Interferons
   Lymphokines/interleukins (e.g., IL-1, IL-2)
   Thymic factors
   Tuftsin
Oligo- and polynucleotides
   Poly A:U and Poly I:C
   tRNA
   dsRNA
   Transfer factor

TABLE 4. Adjuvants: Synthetic Heterocycles

Sulfur-containing compounds
   Levamisole
   Cimetidine
   Tilomisole (Imidazothiazole)
   Fanetizole Mesylate
   CL 259,763
Purine- and pyrimidine-like compounds
   Inosiplex (isoprinosine)
   Hydroerythranol (NPT-15392)
   Pyrimidinones
   C8-substituted guanosines (RWJ 21757)
Miscellaneous heterocycles
   Azimexon
   Therafectin
   CL 246,738
   Azarole
   Tilorone
   Traxanox
   Oxamisole
Nonheterocycles
   Imuthiol
   Thiabendazole
   Pimelautide
   Lobenzarit

phokines or interleukins) interact with specific receptors located in the plasma membrane [Jelinek and Lipsky, 1987]. These interactions are thought to perturb receptors, causing new associations between membrane proteins that ultimately lead to the transduction of intra-

TABLE 5. Various Materials With Adjuvant Activity and Possible Sites/Mechanisms of Action[a]

Materials	Functions
Protein carriers: Protein containing appropriate T-cell epitopes	Mobilization of T-cell help
Inert carriers: Alum, bentonite, latex, acrylic particles	Aggregation of soluble antigens, induction of T-cell help, focus for congregation of lymphoid cells in different areas of lymphoid organs
Hydrophobic antigen: Addition of lipid tail to proteins, adding MDP to antigen in oil	Localization of Ag in T-dependent areas, generation of effector T cells (DTH), formation of amphipathic structures?
Depot formers: Water–oil and oil–water emulsions, some polysaccharides	Delayed release of antigen, leading to prolonged immune response; recruitment of memory cells?
Surface-active materials: Saponin, lysolecithin, retinal, Quil A, some liposomes, pluronic polymer formulations (e.g., SAF-1)	Facilitate cell–cell interaction, aggregate antigen in specific way (e.g., immunostimulating complexes, ISCOMs)
Macrophage (APC) stimulators: MDP and derivatives, LPS, various factors, from microorganisms	Synthesis of factors: IL-1, IL-6, IFNs, CSFs, complement components
Polyclonal activators of T cells: PPD, poly A:U, poly I:C, heterocycles	Provide additional T-cell help (lymphokines), secondary activation of macrophages
B-cell activators (membrane): Antigen-polymerizing factors, B-cell mitogens, e.g., LPS	Modulate Ig receptors on B cells

(continued)

TABLE 5. Various Materials With Adjuvant Activity and Possible
Sites/Mechanisms of Action (Continued)

Materials	Functions
B-cell activators (intracellular?): Substituted guanosines	Activation of B-cell proliferation and differentiation via intracellular pathway(s), bypass surface membrane events
Alternate pathway complement activators: Inulin, zymosan, endotoxin, levamisole, *Corynebacterium parvum*	Focus of antigen on and stimulation of leukocytes with C3 receptors, e.g., macrophages, B cells, follicular dendritic cells

[a]Adapted from Paul WE, 1989.

TABLE 6. Evidence That C8-Substituted Guanine
Ribonucleosides Act at an Intracellular Site

Observation	Consistent with intracellular activation	Consistent with plasma membrane activation
Carrier-mediated transport	+	−
8MGuo Sepharose conjugate fails to activate	+	−
Poly 8Br guanylic acid fails to activate	+	−
Membrane rigidification fails to impede activation	+	−
Cross-linking surface IgM with whole antibody fails to impede activation	+	−

cellular biochemical signals across the membrane. While it is now considered that B-cell signal transduction is mediated by phospho-inositide degradation and calcium mobilization [Bijsterbosch et al., 1985], at the time this research was initiated one of the internal messengers of B-cell activation was thought to be cyclic guanosine-3′-5′-monophosphate (cGMP).

Experimental studies conducted by Goodman and Weigle [1981a] centered on investigating the role of substituted guanosine compounds in the activation of B lymphocytes and the increased production of antigen-specific antibody induced by these agents. In early studies examining the effects of guanosine analogs on the proliferation of B lymphocytes (mitogenic assay), dibutyryl cGMP was shown to be ineffective but 8-bromo-cGMP consistently induced a three- to fivefold stimulation of B-cell proliferation [Goodman and Weigle, 1981a]. These data suggested that the nature of the substituent on the cyclic nucleotide was more important than the cyclic phosphodiester moiety of the compound. Subsequent experiments confirmed this hypothesis by demonstrating that 8-bromoguanosine (8-BrGuo) was 1.5–2 orders of magnitude more potent as a B-lymphocyte stimulant than was 8-bromo-cGMP [Goodman and Weigle, 1981b]. Mechanistic studies suggested that these C8-substituted guanosines had to be transported across the cell membrane to be active, implying that they were acting as intracellular activators of proliferation [Lafer et al., 1981]. Furthermore, these compounds do not act as substrates for guanylate cyclase, and they do not stimulate the activity of this enzyme [Goodman and Weigle, 1982]. Therefore, the C8-substituted guanosines apparently act as intracellular signals independent of guanylate cyclase activity (Table 6).

Following identification of 8-mercaptoguanosine (8-MGuo) as a lead compound, additional studies were performed to describe further the immunobiological profile of this compound and thus the activity of the C8-substituted guanosines in general. Studies designed to examine the cellular specificity of the immunoactivation properties were conducted comparing the activity of 8-Mercaptoguanosine (8-MGuo) on cell cultures that were either B-cell or T-cell enriched. Using the uptake of radiolabeled thymidine as an indication of DNA synthesis, 8-MGuo was capable of stimulating B-cell proliferation but had no effect on either thymocyte or splenic T-cell proliferation [Goodman and Weigle, 1983]. Additional studies using spleen cells from congenitally athymic (nu/nu) mice, which lack T lymphocytes, confirmed that B lymphocytes proliferate in response to substituted guanosines [Goodman and Weigle, 1983a]. Taken together, these results established that cells of the B-lymphocyte lineage are the major target of the proliferative properties of C8-derivatized nucleosides and suggest that the activation of these cells results from a direct interaction between the nucleoside and the target cells (Tables 7, 8). For a comprehensive review of the immunological activities, see the review by Goodman [1984].

With this background information, the R.W. Johnson Pharmaceutical Research Institute and the Scripps Clinic initiated a joint program of analoging and testing, focusing on the parent guanosine structures with the goal of discovering more potent candidates that could be used for clinical evaluation. The potential benefits of an agent with potent immunoactivating or T-cell replacement properties

TABLE 7. Characterizations of C8-Derivatized Guanosine
Responsive and Unresponsive Lymphocytes

8MGuo responsive	8MGuo unresponsive
nu/nu Spleen cells	Thymocytes
Splenic B cells (Thy 1.2−)	Splenic T cells (NW passed)
FcR$^+$ cells	FcR$^-$ cells
μ^+ cells	μ^- cells
δ^+ cells	Most δ^- cells
Ia$^+$ cells	Most Ia$^-$ cells
CR$^+$ cells	Most CR$^-$ cells
Lyb 3/5/7$^+$ cells	Most Lyb 3/5/7$^-$ cells

TABLE 8. Effects of C8-Derivatized Ribonucleosides on
Humoral Immunity

Polyclonal activation of B cells to secrete immunoglobulin
Antigen-specific enhancement of
Primary in vitro response to T-dependent antigens
Secondary in vitro IgM and IgG responses to T-dependent
antigen; no enhanced IgE synthesis
Primary in vitro response to T-dependent antigens (TI-2, TI-1)
Primary in vivo response to T-dependent antigens
T-cell-like inductive signal for B cells presented with T-dependent
Antigens
Occurs independently of T cells and T-cell-derived lymphokines
Is enhanced synergistically by T cells and T-cell-derived lymphokines

rest in the possibility of restoring a significant degree of immune function to individuals with compromised immunity. This report describes the pharmacological profile of RWJ 21757 (7-allyl-8-oxoguanosine; Fig. 1), a newly synthesized analog of the C8-substituted guanosines. Although the immunoactivator property of RWJ 21757 is qualitatively the same as the other C8-substituted guanosines, RWJ 21757 has greater potency and activity and a favorable toxicology profile warranting further testing as a clinical candidate.

IN VITRO IMMUNOENHANCING EFFECTS OF RWJ 21757

Mitogenic Properties

RWJ 21757 has the ability to induce lymphocyte proliferation in murine spleen cell cultures of various strains of mice. Murine spleen cells cultured 1 day with increasing concentrations of the nucleoside were pulsed 24 hr with ^{3}H-TdR as a measure of cell proliferation. As

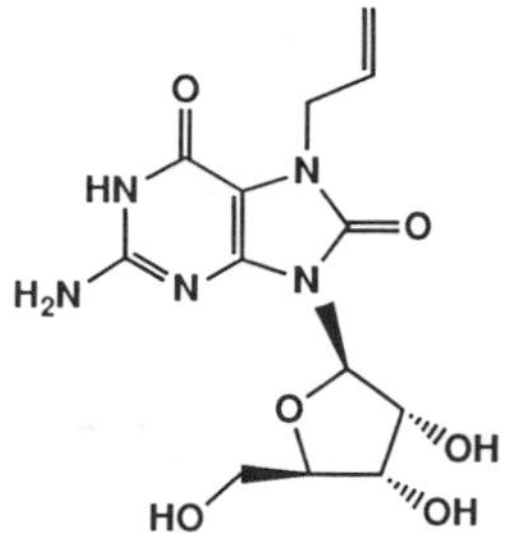

RWJ 21757

7-ALLYL-8-OXOGUANOSINE

Fig. 1. Structure of the immunoactivator RWJ 21757 (7-allyl-8-oxoguanosine.

can be seen in Figure 2, RWJ 21757 induced lymphocyte proliferation in a dose-dependent fashion and was approximately three times more potent than another substituted guanosine, RWJ 21765 (7-methyl-8-oxoguanosine).

Effects of RWJ 21757 on Antibody-Producing Cells

The Jerne plaque assay was used to evaluate the number of splenic B cells making antibody to sheep red blood cells (SRBC) following in vitro immunization. Figure 3 demonstrates that RWJ 21757 has a significant augmenting effect on the number of antibody-producing cells or plaque-forming cells (PFC) against the nominal antigen when added to the incubation system. At 30 μM, the compound induced the maximum increase in specific antibody-producing cells (PFC's) that was more than 100-fold greater than control cultures without RWJ 21757. This indicates that the compound not only induces lymphocyte proliferation but has an adjuvant effect as expressed by the increase in antigen-specific antibody-producing cells. Four other guanosines were devoid of activity, indicating that the immunoenhancing effect is not a general effect of all guanosine compounds.

Kinetics of In Vitro Adjuvanticity

The kinetics of the adjuvanticity of RWJ 21757 in normal mouse spleen cell cultures is shown in Figure 4. When addition of either 10 or 30 μM RWJ 21757 to SRBC-stimulated spleen cells was delayed, antibody production was increased even if the compound was added 1 or 2 days after addition of antigen at the initiation of culture. If 3

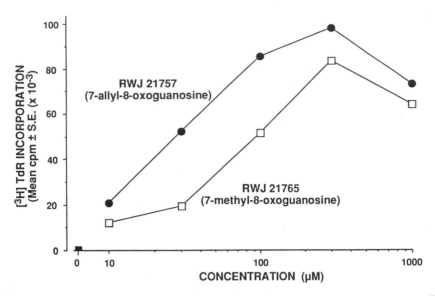

Fig. 2.   Stimulation of murine spleen cells by RWJ 21765 and RWJ 21757: 5×10^5 viable CBA/CaJ spleen cells were cultured with incremental concentrations of nucleoside as indicated. Cultures were harvested 2 days later following a 24 hr pulse of ^{3}H-TdR during the final day. Each point represents arithmetic means of five replicate cultures $\pm$ SE. Spleen cells without drug gave 6,075 $\pm$ 201 cpm.

days passed between antigen stimulation and compound addition, little adjuvant effect was observed with RWJ 21757. These data demonstrate the in vitro antibody-augmenting effect of RWJ 21757 when given within 2 days of antigen. This suggests that this compound acts at an intermediate stage of B-cell activation/differentiation for antibody synthesis and that only certain populations of B cells at such a stage will be responsive. This may explain the antigen dependency of augmentation of antibody production observed with RWJ 21757.

B-Cell-Stimulatory Effects

The effects of RWJ 21757 on the number of cells producing immunoglobulin in cell cultures of purified B cells from normal mice is shown in Table 9. These data demonstrate that RWJ 21757 stimulates immunoglobulin secretion by B cells in a dose-dependent fashion, with greater than 50 times the number of immunoglobulin-producing cells at 100 μM compared with control cultures without RWJ 21757. These data also demonstrate that the stimulatory activity

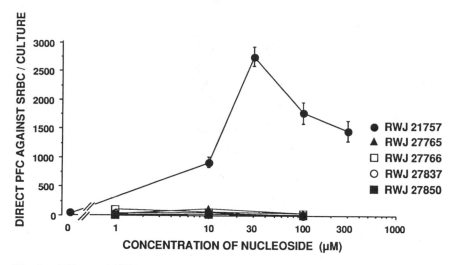

Fig. 3.   Effects of RWJ 21757 on antibody-producing cells in vitro: 5 × 10^6 viable CBA/CaJ spleen cells were cultured with 2 × 10^6 sheep red blood cells (SRBC): Various doses of RWJ 21757 were added at the initiation of culture. Direct plaque-forming cell (PFC) responses to SRBC were determined 4 days after incubation at 37°C. Results are expressed as the arithmetic means of triplicate cultures ± SE. The control response to SRBCs alone was 20 PFCs.

of RWJ 21757 can operate on pure B-cell cultures without the influence of T-helper cells or T-cell-derived lymphokines. The ability of 100 μM (33 μg/ml) RWJ 21757 to induce immunoglobulin synthesis is more potent on a weight basis than is the B-cell stimulator lipopolysaccharide (LPS).

T-Cell-Replacing Activity

Figure 5 illustrates that in B-cell cultures, without the influence of T cells and specific antigen, RWJ 21757 induces a small increase in antibody production (i.e., without SRBC). However, when antigen is supplied (i.e., with SRBC), there is a pronounced dose-dependent enhancement of the production of antigen-specific antibody, despite the continued absence of T-helper cells. At 100 μM, RWJ 21757 induced an 30-fold increase in PFCs compared with controls without the compound.

Two conclusions can be drawn from these last two experiments. First, RWJ 21757 has the ability to stimulate purified B cells by providing an alternate, T-cell-like, signal. This has been demonstrated by others evaluating C8-substituted guanosines [Feldbush and Ballas, 1982; Dosch et al., 1988]. Second, while there is a small degree of

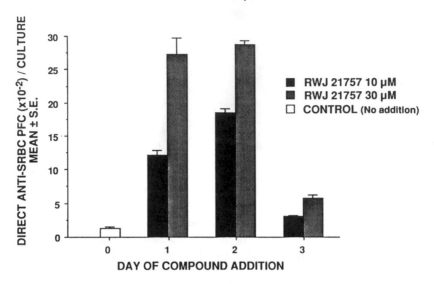

Fig. 4. Kinetics of RWJ 21757 addition to sheep red blood cell (SRBC)-stimulated spleen cells: 5×10^6 viable CBA/CaJ spleen cells were cultured with 2×10^6 SRBC, and 30 μM RWJ 21757 (10 μg/ml) was added to cultures 1, 2, or 3 days later. Direct plaque-forming cell (PFC) responses to SRBC were determined 4 days after culture initiation. Results are expressed as the arithmetic means of triplicate cultures $\pm$ SE.

TABLE 9. Induction of Immunoglobulin Secretion By RWJ 21757 in B Cells From Normal Mice[a]

Concentration of RWJ 21757	Direct anti-SRBC PFC per culture	E/C[b]
None	8 ± 1	1.00
3 μM	62 ± 1	7.75
10 μM	143 ± 37	17.88
30 μM	223 ± 12	27.88
100 μM	472 ± 17	59.00
LPS Control (100 μg/ml)	1,150 ± 212	70.60

[a]5×10^6 viable CBA/CaJ B cells were cultured in the presence of incremental concentrations of RWJ 21757 in a volume of 1 ml of 5% fetal bovine serum containing medium. Direct plaque forming cells (PFC) to sheep red blood cells (SRBC) were evaluated after 4 days of culture. Results are presented as the arithmetic mean of triplicate cultures $\pm$ SE.
[b]E/C = experimental to control ratio of activity.

antigen-independent activation, the maximum augmentation of antibody production occurs when specific antigen is present during activation, the difference between the two response curves (Fig. 5) representing the antigen-dependent enhancement.

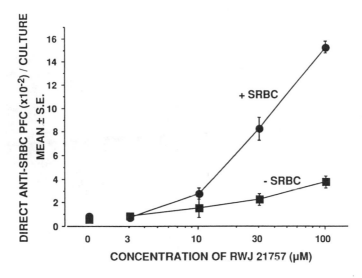

Fig. 5. T-cell-replacing activity of RWJ 21757 supports antigen-specific antibody responses in B-cell cultures: 5 × 10⁶ viable CBA/CaJ B lymphocytes were cultured in the presence or absence of 2 × 10⁶ sheep red blood cells (SRBC) together with incremental concentrations of RWJ 21757. The inability of purified B cells to respond to antigen in the absence of nucleoside is seen by comparing the two points at lower left with no added nucleoside. Direct plaque-forming cell (PFC) responses to SRBC were determined after 4 days of culture. Results are expressed as the arithmetic means of triplicate cultures ± SE.

Immunorestorative Properties

Cyclosporin A (CsA) is a drug that experimentally and clinically suppresses immune responses by inactivating helper T cells (Columbani and Hess, 1987). It is known to suppress lymphokine production by helper T cells, which play a role in immune regulation and antibody synthesis [Hess et al., 1986; Thomson et al., 1983]. The addition of CsA to spleen cell cultures immunized with antigen in vitro suppresses the level of antigen-specific antibody-producing cells [Goodman and Weigle, 1983]. The effects of RWJ 21757 on antibody response in the presence of CsA were examined. The B-cell-stimulatory activity of RWJ 21757 (10 μM) was evident in the murine spleen cell Jerne plaque assay system in the presence of CsA at concentrations up to 100 ng/ml (Fig. 6). In the absence of RWJ 21757, the PFC response to antigen was inhibited in a dose-dependent fashion until, at 100 ng/ml CsA, it fell below background levels [Goodman and Weigle, 1983b]. These data again demonstrate the ability of RWJ 21757 to act directly on B cells and further suggest that this compound may replace lymphokine helper activity provided by T

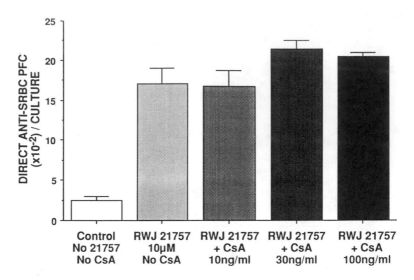

Fig. 6. Ability of RWJ 21757 to overcome the immunosuppressive effects of cyclosporin A: 5×10^6 viable CBA/CaJ spleen cells were cultured with 2×10^6 sheep red blood cells (SRBC) and 10 μM RWJ 21757 in the presence or absence of incremental concentrations of cyclosporin A (CsA) to inhibit production of lymphokines and monokines. Direct plaque-forming cell (PFC) responses to SRBC were determined 4 days later. Results are expressed as the arithmetic means of triplicate cultures ± SE. Control response in the absence of CsA was 220 ± 59 PFC, whereas the response at the highest dose of CsA (100 ng/ml) is typically suppressed 100%.

cells. In addition, RWJ 21757 demonstrated the ability to overcome the drug-induced immunosuppression, which may have clinical relevance.

The CBA/N strain of mice manifests an X-linked immunodeficiency that results in a profound inability to respond to most antigens. Low serum IgM and IgG_3 levels, abnormal B-cell maturation, and an increased susceptibility to certain parasitic and bacterial pathogens are also hallmarks of these animals [Scher, 1982; Duran and Metcalf, 1987]. The effects of RWJ 21757 on the antibody response to SRBC for CBA/N spleen cells was compared with the response of spleen cells from normal mice of the same genetic background (CBA/CaJ). As shown in Figure 7, cells from the immunodeficient mice do not make antibody under normal circumstances (12 PFC without antigen and 8 PFC with antigen vs. 265 PFC with antigen in cells from normal mice). Treatment with RWJ 21757 (3–30 μM) stimulated the production of antibody PFC in a dose-dependent fashion equal to that of normal mice (CBA/CaJ) at the 30 μM dose.

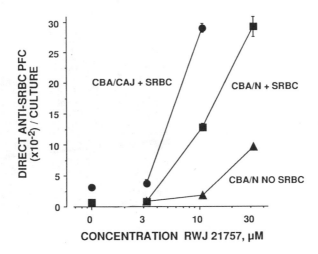

Fig. 7. Reconstitution of the primary humoral immune response to sheep red blood cells (SRBC) by RWJ 21757 in X-linked immunodeficient (CBA/N) mice in vitro: 5×10^6 viable CBA/N or CBA/CaJ spleen cells were cultured together with or without 2×10^6 SRBC and incremental concentrations of RWJ 21757 in 1 ml of medium containing 5% FCS. Direct plaque-forming cell (PFC) responses to SRBC were determined after 4 days of culture. Results are expressed as the arithmetic means of triplicate cultures ± SE.

IN VIVO IMMUNOENHANCING ACTIVITY OF RWJ 21757

Effects of Different Vehicles on Adjuvanticity

The in vivo activity of RWJ 21757 was studied in a variety of vehicles to determine whether solubilization or depot formation could convey greater adjuvant effects. As shown in Figure 8, the greatest activity of RWJ 21757 was seen when the compound was administered subcutaneously (s.c.) in sesame oil or in incomplete Freund's adjuvant (IFA) rather than in an aqueous solution in carboxymethylcellulose (CMC). While there was only a small increase in the number of PFCs induced by RWJ 21757 in CMC over the sesame oil control (2,500 ± 240 PFC), there was a sixfold to ninefold increase in PFCs induced by the compound in oil-based vehicles. These data suggest that a depot form of the compound has greater adjuvant activity than a more readily absorbed form and that slow absorption of the compound is a more desirable method of administration. The use of oil-based vehicles will also most likely enhance the delivery of the compound to the lymphatics (Friend and Pangburn, 1987). Early metabolism studies in dogs show a fivefold increase in the level of radiolabeled compound in the draining lymph nodes compared with plasma levels when administered intramuscularly in sesame oil.

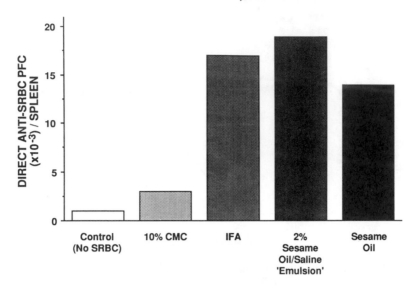

Fig. 8. In vivo adjuvanticity of RWJ 21757: Presentation in an array of vehicles. Groups of five CBA/CaJ mice were injected with 2×10^6 sheep red blood cells (SRBC) i.p. followed by no nucleoside or 1 mg/kg of RWJ 21757 s.c. in a volume of 0.2 ml of the following vehicles: 10 mg/ml carboxymethylcellulose (CMC) in saline; incomplete Freund's adjuvant (IFA) emulsified with saline; 2% sesame oil in saline; 100% sesame oil. Seven days following immunization, a plaque assay was carried out on spleens from these mice. Data represent average plaque-forming cells (PFC) for five mice per group.

Effects of RWJ 21757 on the Primary IgG Serum Antibody Response to Sheep Red Blood Cells

The response exhibited by the mice immunized intraperitoneally (i.p.) with a 10% (approximately 3×10^8 SRBC) suspension of SRBC is considered an optimal response, because previous studies have shown that doses of 1.0% SRBC (approximately 3×10^7 cells) or higher elicit an antibody response similar in magnitude. RWJ 21757, administered s.c., produced a dose-related enhancement of the IgG anti-SRBC antibody response approaching a near optimal level in animals injected, i.p. with a suboptimal dose of 0.03% SRBC (approximately 1×10^6 SRBC; Fig. 9); at doses of 3–20 mg/mouse, total antigen-specific immunoglobulins (IgG and IgM) are consistantly enhanced four- to sixfold over vehicle control (data not shown). These results support the data obtained in the PFC assay, which demonstrate that RWJ 21757 induced an increased number of antigen-specific antibody-producing cells. The data obtained from these experiments indicate that this recruitment of PFC by RWJ 21757 translates

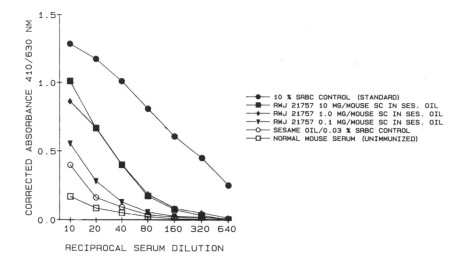

Fig. 9. Dose-related enhancement of RWJ 21757 on the antibody response to a suboptimal challenge of sheep red blood cells (SRBC) in mice. Animals were immunized i.p. with SRBC, treated with drug or vehicle s.c. 3 hr later, and bled by cardiac puncture at 14 days. Serum antibody titers were determined by ELISA. Each point represents the average of duplicate determinations on dilutions of pooled serum samples of 10 mice per dose level.

into an increased titer of antigen-specific serum antibody and therefore a higher level of immunity.

Induction of Memory for Antibody Synthesis

The results shown in Figure 10 demonstrate that a 20 mg/mouse dose of RWJ 21757 given on day 0 (the day of primary immunization) was effective at increasing the serum IgG anti-SRBC antibody compared with control mice treated with sesame oil. However, the effects of RWJ 21757 are much more pronounced after the secondary boost of SRBC (without additional compound) given on day 18. The data clearly demonstrate that both the 20 and 2.0 mg doses of RWJ 21757 given on day 0 produced an effect on the immune response to SRBC other than just an increase in antibody titer alone. The 2.0 mg dose of RWJ 21757 had no effect on the primary antibody response to SRBC (day 18). However, when antigen was presented again, the animals treated with 2.0 mg as well as with 20 mg RWJ 21757 exhibited a classic secondary antibody response—that is, a rapid rise in antibody titer 2–4 days after a booster injection of antigen. The control mice did not exhibit a secondary response, and the low dose (0.2 mg) of RWJ 21757 also did not produce a response. These data sug-

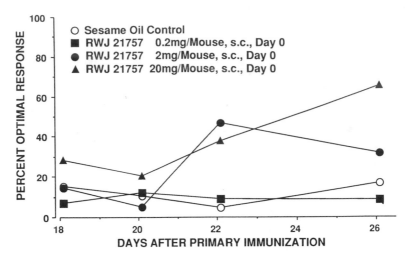

Fig. 10.   In vivo induction of immunological memory in mice with RWJ 21757.
Groups of 20 C57BL/6J mice were immunized i.p. with 0.2 ml of a 0.03% suspension of sheep red blood cells (SRBC) and treated with RWJ 21757, suspended
in sesame oil, s.c., immediately thereafter. Five mice per group were bled on day
18 and the remainder boosted with 0.03% SRBC as in the primary immunization.
Five mice in each group were bled on days shown and their serum IgG anti-
SRBC antibody level determined by ELISA. An additional group of 10 mice were
immunized on day 0 with 0.2 ml of a 3% suspension of SRBC and bled on day
18. These mice served as optimal responders. Data represent averages of duplicate determinations on pooled serum samples of five mice per time point.

gest that RWJ 21757 may exert its effects by inducing a clonal expansion of antigen-specific memory B cells during the primary antigen
challenge. Upon a secondary challenge, these antigen-primed cells
responded rapidly by differentiating into antibody-secreting plasma
cells, which can contribute to the increase in serum antigen-specific
antibody. Therefore, RWJ 21757 not only has the ability to enhance a
primary immune response but also appears to increase the number
or responsiveness of memory B cells expressed as a heightened secondary response to suboptimal primary antigenic challenge.

Adjuvant Effect on Guinea Pig Antibody Response to Synthetic Peptide Vaccine

The potential use of RWJ 21757 as an adjuvant for vaccines, that is,
to bolster the antibody response to a vaccination and also to decrease
the amount of vaccine needed to elicit a response, was investigated
in guinea pigs immunized with a peptide from the foot and mouth
disease virus (FMDV). RWJ 21757 with IFA caused a 10-fold increase

TABLE 10. Adjuvanticity of RWJ 21757 for FMDVp 141–160 in the Guinea Pig[a]

Immunogen	Adjuvant	ELISA titer
FMDVp (141–160) TT	IFA	1,280
FMDVp (141–160) TT	IFA/10 mg RWJ 21757	12,800

[a]Groups of guinea pigs (N = 3) were injected s.c. with 100 μg foot and mouth disease virus peptide (FMDVp) amino acids 141–160 coupled to tetanus toxoid (TT) and given as an emulsion in incomplete Freund's adjuvant (IFA) alone or with 10 mg RWJ 21757. Animals were bled 4 weeks later and anti-FMDVp ELISA titers evaluated.

in antibody titer compared with IFA alone, as determined by an antigen-specific enzyme-linked immunosorbent assay (Table 10). Therefore, the adjuvant effect of the potent IFA can be enhanced further by RWJ 21757 to achieve significantly higher titers.

Antibody Synthesis in Mongrel Dogs

RWJ 21757 was tested for its ability to enhance the antibody response to human serum albumin (HSA) in mongrel dogs as a large animal model of immunization. The dose of antigen used was suboptimal—that is, a dose of antigen that elicits a weak but measuable antibody response as determined from previous research. This allowed for drug-induced augmentation of the antibody response toward an optimal level. The results (Fig. 11) of the study indicate that a single 100 mg intramuscular injection of RWJ 21757 in sesame oil administered immediately after immunization enhanced the IgG anti-HSA antibody response compared with controls as measured by an enzyme-linked immunosorbent assay. The enhancement was seen as early as 7 days after immunization and persisted for the duration of the study (49 days). Figure 12 shows the titration curves of sera from the day 35 bleeds and indicates that the response of RWJ 21757-injected animals was enhanced toward the optimal level seen in control dogs immunized with HSA emulsified in complete Freund's adjuvant (CFA). These data demonstrate that RWJ 21757 is capable of enhancing the antibody response to a suboptimal dose of a specific antigen in normal dogs similar to the potent CFA. This suggests that RWJ 21757 may be capable of enhancing the antibody response to poor immunogens or vaccines that only elicit a weak antibody response in normal individuals and, by doing so, afford greater immunological protection.

UNDESIRABLE SIDE EFFECTS OF ADJUVANTS

While many materials can act as adjuvants and enhance an immune response, untoward or toxic effects have precluded the clinical

542   *Anderson and Capetola*

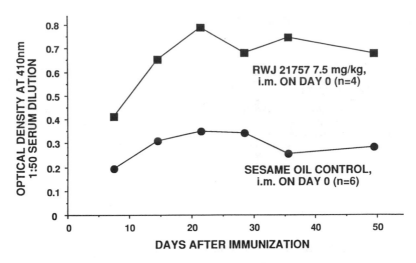

Fig. 11.   Effect of RWJ 21757 on the antibody response to human serum albumin (HSA) in mongrel dogs. Adult mongrel dogs were immunized i.v. with 1.0 mg HSA in saline and treated with sesame oil (1.0 ml) or RWJ 21757 (100 mg in sesame oil) immediately thereafter. Dogs were bled periodically to determine IgG anti-HSA antibody titers by ELISA. Data points represent means of duplicate values for each dog.

use of many of these potential immunoactivators. Table 11 lists the major concerns related to side effects. A review of the toxicology of RWJ 21757 is beyond the scope of this chapter. However, a brief summary of the key points is given.

Pyrogenicity

RWJ 21757 did not demonstrate fever-inducing activity when administered intravenously in an oil-in-water emulsion (Intralipid A®). As a control, an endogenous pyrogen, interleukin-1 (IL-1; 36.3 ng) and the inducer of endogenous pyrogens LPS (1 mg) were administered. The characteristic biphasic febrile response was seen (Fig. 13).

Induction of Autoimmune Responses

The possibility of inducing autoimmune responses is a major concern when using adjuvants clinically. The unlikely possibility that RWJ 21757 would have this problem is based on the following: 1) lack of enhanced pathology in the adjuvant rat model of arthritis by RWJ 21757 at high levels (100 mg/kg), 2) lack of immune complexes or other immune abnormalities in rats or dogs receiving multiple

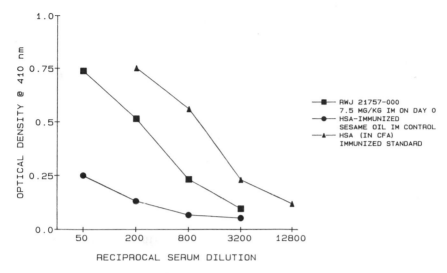

Fig. 12.   Serum titration of the dog anti-human serum albumin (HSA) antibody response. RWJ 21757 produced a shift of the antibody titer toward an optimal level as seen with HSA in complete Freund's adjuvant (CFA)-immunized standard. Data represent means of duplicate values for each dog.

TABLE 11. Undesirable Side Effects of Adjuvants

Pyrogenicity
Induction of autoimmune responses
  Arthritis
  Vasculitis
Induction of allergies (IgE synthesis)
Inflammatory, granulomatous, necrotizing, or other unacceptable
  reactions at injection sites

courses of RWJ 21757 (10, 20, and 40 mg/kg) and evaluated at various times during and after drug treatment, and 3) lack of the ability of substituted guanosine adjuvants to exacerbate the autoimmune condition (i.e., anti-single-stranded DNA, rheumatoid factor, immune complexes) in NZB × NZW F_1 males, B × SB females, and MRL +/+ males and females (1 mg/mouse every other week for 1 year) relative to controls (vehicle only).

Local Inflammatory Reactions

RWJ 21757 in sesame oil does not cause significant inflammation at the site of injection that might preclude its clinical use. This was determined by histologic assessment in animal studies.

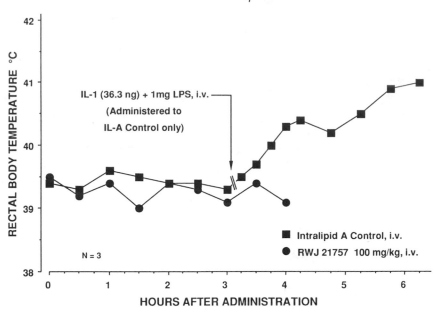

Fig. 13.   Rabbit pryogen test for RWJ 21757 (100 mg/kg) in Intralipid A®. Body temperatures were monitored rectally using a sensortek thermistor and recorded every 30 min. Neither vehicle nor RWJ 21757 administered i.v. (6 ml total volume given over 6 min) were pyrogenic. A positive response induced by a mixture of interleukin-1 (IL-1) and lipopolysaccharide (LPS) gave a temperature rise of greater than 2°C.

SUMMARY

Table 12 summarizes the immunopharmacology of RWJ 21757. Because of its unique immunoactivator properties and its favorable toxicology, we feel that this compound has the potential to be an adjuvant for vaccines and to be an immunotherapeutic agent in a variety of clinical settings, including those listed in Table 13.

ACKNOWLEDGMENTS

We are glad to acknowledge the following collaborators: M. Goodman (Scripps), W. Weigle (Scripps), J. Bittle (Scripps), D. Argentieri (R.W. Johnson Pharmaceutical Research Institute), C. Bishop (R.W. Johnson Pharmaceutical Research Institute), and D. Ritchie (R.W. Johnson Pharmaceutical Research Institute).

TABLE 12. RWJ 21757

Immunopharmacologic activity

Adjuvant-like activity enhances antibody production in response to specific foreign antigens in normal *and* immunodeficiency states (genetic and drug induced)

Selective stimulation of B-cell growth and differentiation via lymphokine-like signals

Mimics the intracellular consequence of receptor triggering or amplifies the signals generated following B-cell activation

Bypasses need for T-cell derived lymphokines/interleukins, thereby enhancing antibody response in the absence of T cells

Active in vivo (mg/kg levels) in mice, guinea pigs, dogs, monkeys and enhances antibody production by human lymphocytes in vitro (mM levels)

Devoid of any significant polypharmacology at 10–20 times anticipated clinical dose of 5–10 mg/kg

TABLE 13. Clinical Utility of RWJ 21757

Immunoprophylactic therapy: Useful as adjuvant for vaccines to increase quantity and quality of antibody response, thus affording greater protection

    Vaccines (cancer antigens; recombinant peptides for viruses, bacteria, or parasites)

    Immunotherapy for allergy patients

Immune augmenting: Potential use as immunotherapeutic in immunodeficiency states caused by deficiency of T-cell numbers, T-cell function, B-cell hypofunction, or combination of the above

Primary immunodeficiency diseases. SCID, CVH

Secondary immunodeficiencies

    Leukemia/lymphomas

    Metabolic disorders (e.g., diabetes mellitus, uremia, nephrotic syndrome)

    Viral infections: AIDS

    Immunosuppressive therapy: Cancer, transplantations (antimetabolites, corticosteroids, radiation)

    Surgical and trauma patients (e.g., burns)

    Aging

LAK cell therapy for cancer patients (IL-2 "sparing")

REFERENCES

Altman A, Dixon F J (1989): Immunomodifiers in vaccines. Adv Vet Sci Comp Med 33:301–343.

Bijsterbosch M K, Meade C J, Turner G A, Klaus G G (1985): B lymphocyte receptors and polyphosphoinositide degradation. Cell. 41(3):999–1006.

Buckley R H (1987): Immunodeficiency diseases. JAMA 258(20):2841–2850.

Columbani P M, Hess A D (1987): (Commentary) T-lymphocyte inhibition by cyclosporine-potential mechanisms of action. Biochem Pharmacol 36:3789–3793.

Dosch H, Osundwa V, Lam P (1988): Activation of human B lymphocytes by 8 substituted guanosine derivatives. Immunol Lett 17(2):125–131.

Duran L W, Metcalf E S (1987): Antibody-defective, genetically susceptible CBA/N mice have an altered *salmonella typhimurium*-specific B cell repertoire. J Exp Med 165(1):29–46.

Feldbush T L, Ballas Z K (1985): Lymphokine-like activity of 8-mercaptoguanosine: Induction of T and B cell differentiation. J Immunol 134(5):3204–3211.

Friend D R, Pangburn S (1987): Site-specific drug delivery. Medicinal Res Rev 7(1):53–106.

Goodman M G (1984): Inductive and differentative signals delivered by C8-substituted guanine ribonucleosides. Immunol Today 5:319–324.

Goodman, M.G and Weigle, W.O. (1981a): Activation of lymphocytes by brominated neucleoside and cyclic nucleotide analogus implications for the "second messenger" function of cyclic GMP. Proc Natl Acad Sci USA 78(12):7604–7608.

Goodman M G, Weigle W O (1981b): Induction of immunoglobulin secretion by a simple nucleoside derivative. J Immunol 128:2399–2404.

Goodman M G, Weigle W O (1982): Bromination of guanosine and cyclic GMP confers resistance to metabolic processing by B cells. J Immunol 129(6):2715–2717.

Goodman M G, Weigle W O (1983a): Activation of lymphocytes by a thiol-derivatized nucleoside: Characterization of cellular parameters and responsive subpopulations. J Immunol 130(2):551–557.

Goodman M G, Weigle W O (1983b): T-cell replacing activity of C-8 derivatized guanine ribonucleosides. J Immunol 130(5):2042–2045.

Goodman M G, Weigle W O (1984): Intracellular lymphocyte activation and carrier-mediated transport of C8-substituted guanine ribonucleosides. Proc Natl Acad Sci USA 81(3): 862–866.

Green D R, Faist E (1988): Trauma in the immune response. Immunol Today 9:253–255.

Hess A D, Colombani P M, Esa A H (1986): Cyclosporine and the immune response: Basic aspects. CRC Crit Rev Immunol 6(2):123–149.

Jelinek D F, Lipsky P E (1987): Regulation of human B lymphocyte activation, proliferation and differentiation. Adv Immunol 40:1–59.

Klausner A (1988): A real shot in the arm for recumbent vaccines. Biotechnology 6:773–782.

Lafer E M, Moller A S, Nordheim A, Stollar B D, Rich A (1981): Antibodies specific for left-handed Z-DNA. Proc Natl Acad Sci USA 78(6):3546–3550.

Paul WE (1989): Fundamental Immunology. New York: Raven Press, p 1008.

Ruszala-Mallon V, Lin Y-I, Durr F E, Wang B S (1988): Low molecular weight immunopotentiators. Int J Immunopharmacol 10:497–510.

Scher I (1982): The CBA/N mouse strain: An experimental model illustrating the influence of the X-chromosome on immunity. Adv Immunol 33:1–71.

St. Georgiev V (1988): New synthetic immunomodulating agents. Trends Pharmacol Sci 9:446–451.

Thomson A W, Moon D K, Geczy C L, Nelson D S (1983): Cyclosporin A inhibits lymphokine production but not the responses of macrophages to lymphokines. Immunology 48:291–299.

Warren H S, Chedid L A (1988): Future prospects for vaccine adjuvants. CRC Crit Rev Immunol 8(2):83–101.

DISCUSSION

Dr. THAU: How far are these two new adjuvants that you presented from practical application?

Dr. CAPETOLA: One of them is going into clinical trials in February of 1990.

Dr. STEVENS: Regarding the two amino groups, are they primary or secondary amines, and does conjugation at this point destroy their immunoreactivity? Could you provide the antigen simultaneously with your compounds in the first injection, or was it necessary to have presensitized activated B cells in order to stimulate a good immune response?

DR. CAPETOLA: In answer to your second question, the adjuvant compound can be administered at the same time as the antigen or up until 3 days after the antigen is injected. Perhaps this means that actively dividing clones, or clonal expansion, is not necessary for the adjuvant effect of these compounds. Concerning your first question, I think the only substitutions on the two amino groups have been changes to render them electronegative, and not large or bulky groups.

DR. STEVENS: Will these compounds stimulate resting B cells in vitro?

DR. CAPETOLA: I don't think that that has been looked at specifically.

DR. DONCEL: Do you have any information about side effects of the use of these adjuvants?

DR. CAPETOLA: Yes. After 1 year of a toxicology profile with complete histopathology, there is no evidence of any systemic toxicology. There is some local irritation at the injection site in some of the dogs. The concern that we have with a compound like this is the induction of autoimmune responses. A 12 month study was carried out with a previous analog in MRL and NZB mice, with no apparent increase in mortality, morbidity, or anti-DNA titers, etc. The current compound is being evaluated in a similar study that has been underway for only 9 months, so we don't know the answer yet. If it induces autoimmune responses, then we would not be very interested in it.

DR. MITCHISON: Have you compared it with the "gold standard," complete Freund's adjuvant?

DR. CAPETOLA: I don't think that any adjuvant compound that I know of can consistently bring an antibody titer to the level attained with complete Freund's adjuvant. Of course, the goal is to find a compound that produces comparable results, works by a different mechanism, and does not have the attendant side effects of complete Freund's adjuvant. But to answer your question, it does not produce titers as high as those elicited by complete Freund's adjuvant.

DR. MITCHISON: Are you releasing this compound for experimental studies?

DR. CAPETOLA: We are about to begin so, very soon.

DR. BIALY: Have you tested this compound and others for antiviral activity?

DR. CAPETOLA: The compound itself has very weak reverse transcriptase inhibitory activity. I am not sure that it would have a meaningful application, though, because the IC_{50} was on the order of 100 μM, compared with AZT, which is on the order of 0.1 μM.

35

Studies of Various Delivery Systems for a Human Chorionic Gonadotropin Vaccine

V.C. Stevens, John E. Powell, Michael Rickey, Arthur C. Lee, and D.H. Lewis

The question of which medium is optimal for administering vaccine components to humans to date has not been clearly answered. Separate from antigen and adjuvant requirements for triggering high and sustained antibody levels, the characteristics of vehicles containing these components can influence the responses obtained. The classic dogma among immunologists is that a compound or bacterial particle must be present for activating antigen-presenting cells, and a depot effect of a thick emulsion or precipitate is needed for the prolonged release of antigen into the lymphatic system. These interpretations may be correct, but few data were heretofore available to document these phenomena, particularly the need for sustained antigen delivery. Several vehicles for antigen delivery have been tested as a part of the development of a vaccine against the reproductive hormone human chorionic gonadotropin (hCG) by the WHO Special Programme of Research, Development, and Research Training in Human Reproduction. Following the identification of a candidate immunogen and adjuvant compound, experiments were initiated to identify a suitable medium for delivering these components to vaccine recipients.

Gamete Interaction: Prospects for Immunocontraception, pages 549–563
© 1990 Wiley-Liss, Inc.

IMMUNOGEN AND ADJUVANT COMPOUND

The immunogen used in these studies was a synthetic peptide representing the carboxyl terminal 37 amino acids of the β-subunit of hCG covalently coupled to diphtheria toxoid (DT) in a peptide:carrier ratio of 24–28 peptides per 100 kd of DT. The adjuvant compound employed was a synthetic analog of a surface component of mycobacteria (MDP-N-acetyl-nor-muramyl-L-alanyl-D-isoglutamine). Detailed descriptions of these components are described elsewhere, [Stevens et al., 1986a,b].

CONTROLLED RELEASE OF IMMUNOGEN AND ADJUVANT COMPOUND

To gain some insight regarding the timing of optimal delivery of antigen and adjuvant to the lymphatic drainage, experiments were conducted in rabbits whereby the components were delivered intramuscularly either together or separately by injection or via an osmotic pump. These experiments were designed to ascertain 1) whether sustained antibody levels could best be obtained by bursts of antigen delivery or by continuous release, 2) whether the adjuvant compound was needed throughout the period of antibody production or only periodically, and 3) whether antibody levels could be maintained in the absence of antigen. It was recognized that high antibody levels would not be induced following delivery of these highly soluble components in saline because of rapid clearance, but it was believed that relative responses would provide useful data. The following four groups of rabbits were studied: group 1, immunogen and adjuvant released constantly via a miniosmotic pump (Alzet) in saline for 28 days (The rate of release was 0.07 mg/day for the immunogen and 0.035 mg/day for the adjuvant); group 2, immunogen delivered constantly for 35 days (0.07 mg/day) and adjuvant (0.5 mg) injected in saline on days 0, 14, and 28; group 3, immunogen (0.5 mg) injected in saline on days 0, 14, and 28 and adjuvant delivered constantly for 35 days (0.35 mg/day); group 4, both immunogen and adjuvant (0.5 mg each) injected in saline on days 0, 7, 14, and 21.

The mean antibody levels elicited in each of these groups (N = 4) are shown in Figures 1–4, respectively. As anticipated, no group produced high antibody levels as compared with immunizations in Freund's complete adjuvant (FCA). However, these data indicate that the highest antibody levels were attained in groups 1 and 2 in which the immunogen was delivered continuously whether the ad-

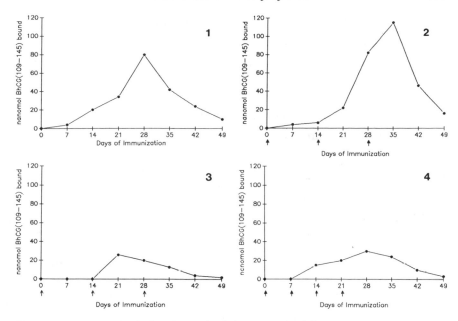

Fig. 1. Mean antibody levels to the hCG peptide following continuous intramuscular delivery of the peptide–carrier conjugate and synthetic adjuvant via an osmotic pump.

Fig. 2. Mean antibody levels to the hCG peptide following continuous delivery of the peptide–carrier conjugate and the separate injection of the synthetic adjuvant.

Fig. 3. Mean antibody levels to the hCG peptide following intramuscular injections of the peptide–carrier conjugate and the continuous delivery of the synthetic adjuvant.

Fig. 4. Mean antibody levels to the hCG peptide following intramuscular injection of both peptide–carrier conjugate and the synthetic adjuvant.

juvant was delivered concomitantly with the immunogen or injected separately. In the two groups (3 and 4) in which the immunogen was injected, antibody levels were lower. Constant infusion of the adjuvant did not promote noticeably different responses from those occurring when it was injected together with the immunogen. In both groups 1 and 2, antibody levels fell promptly when the osmotic pumps were removed.

These and other experiments suggested that 1) antigen availability is necessary to sustain antibody levels, 2) constant release (at the rates studied) of immunogen was immunogenic and not tolerogenic, and 3) the adjuvant compound did not need to be continuously present and probably was not essential beyond the first few days after the primary immunization. While it was recognized that these studies were preliminary, they did provide a general guide to the design of other studies for developing vaccine delivery systems.

WATER–OIL EMULSIONS

One of the first means explored to deliver vaccine components was to mimic FCA using materials that would be acceptable for human use. Squalene was a suitable substitute for mineral oil as it is biodegradable, and the MDP analog selected for the adjuvant compound was found to be an aequate replacement for intact mycobacteria. Mannide monooleate (MM) was selected as the most effective emulsifier for establishing an emulsion of squalene and water. A series of experiments, conducted over several years, established the optimal formulation for administering the experimental vaccine to women. A summary of the findings is reported below.

Some of the factors effecting emulsion stability were found to be

1   Oil:water ratio
2   Concentration of protein (immunogen)
3   Physical–chemical properties of immunogen
4   Concentration of emulsifier
5   Shear forces applied

Certain of these factors were fixed and others were varied to determine the most suitable combination to deliver the specific components in the hCG vaccine. In early studies with rabbits, mice, and baboons as recipients, a formulation was selected employing a squalene:MM ratio of 4:1 and emulsifing this "oil phase" with an equal volume of physiological saline. The concentration of the immunogen and adjuvant compound in the emulsion was 1.0–2.0 mg/ml prepared by forcing water and oil back and forth through a three-way stopcock attached to two glass syringes. Shear force (number of strokes) was applied as needed to establish a thick water-in-oil emulsion that showed no separation of phases after 24 hr. Animals were injected intramuscularly usually at 3 week intervals three times. An example of a typical response is shown in Figure 5. This formulation served to evaluate numerous study parameters such as evaluations of carriers, adjuvants, and immunosafety of the vaccine.

Despite the routine use of this method of emulsion preparation in our laboratory for several years with "in-house" reagents, its use by others with a different immunogen source, different equipment, and

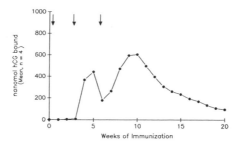

Fig. 5. Mean antibody levels reactive with hCG following immunization of rabbits with conjugate and adjuvant contained in a squalene–water emulsion prepared using two glass syringes connected by a three-way stopcock. The water:oil ratio was 50:50, and the immunogen concentration was 1.0 mg/ml. Arrows indicate the time of injections.

certified "pure" reagents, yielded variable results. During a phase 1 clinical trial of the vaccine, establishing emulsions was a problem in several instances, and complete phase separation was sometimes observed [Jones et al., 1988]. Subsequent to these studies an effort was made to define a method of establishing stable emulsions that could be prepared at a central facility some months before use and shipped, without significant change in properties, to the site of clinical trials. This task was accomplished by adding aluminum monostearate to the oil phase and by reducing the immunogen concentration. Both water-in-oil and oil-in-water emulsions of high stability (6–12 months) were prepared by use of a machine (Microfluidizer Model 110S, Microfluidics Corporation) for applying controlled high shear forces. Examples of immune responses to these formulations are shown in Figures 6 and 7. It was apparent that while both types of emulsions were highly stable, the oil in-water emulsion did not delay the release of antigen significantly following each injection and antibody levels were not sustained over an extended period. Conversely, the water-in-oil emulsion delayed responses well after the last injection but elicited relatively low antibody levels immediately after the primary immunization. Because of this latter finding and because aluminum monosterate precipitated from the oil phase upon storage, this approach to providing vaccine emulsions for clinical studies was abandoned.

Efforts returned to defining an emulsion formulation that could be prepared at the site of clinical studies but could be expected to remain stable for an extended period and elicit the desired immune response. It was found that the concentration of immunogen that could be contained in a water-in-oil emulsion depended on the concentration of emulsifier at a fixed water:oil ratio. Under conditions

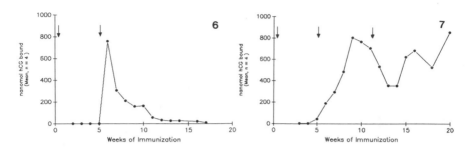

Fig. 6. Mean antibody levels reactive with hCG in rabbits immunized with conjugate and adjuvant in a oil-in-water squalene–water emulsion prepared in a mechanical emulsifier. The water:oil ratio was 70:30. Arrows indicate the time of injections.

Fig. 7. Mean antibody levels reactive with hCG after immunization with the hCG peptide conjugate in an emulsion of squalene–water containing aluminum monostearate as a stabilizer. The mechanical device (Microfluidizer) was used to prepare the emulsion of 1 part water and 1 part squalene containing 4% monostearate. Arrows indicate the time of injections.

practical for individual "on-site" emulsion preparation, an appropriate volume for vaccine injection to deliver the desired immunogen dose was established with a squalene:MM ratio of 4:1. Fixing this variable, the immunogen concentration and shear forces applied, various water:oil ratios were tested. Shown in Figures 8, 9, and 10 are responses in rabbits to the vaccine in emulsion with water:oil ratios of 45:55, 50:50, 60:40, respectively. The viscosity of the emulsion increased with an increase in emulsion water content. All emulsions were stable for at least 1 week, although those used for immunizations were administered to animals within 1 hr after preparation. No major difference in antibody levels was seen, but higher water:oil ratios delayed immune responses.

Another variable found to be important in emulsion stability and immune responses was the amount of shear force applied during preparation. With a fixed squalene:MM ratio, water:oil ratio, protein concentration, and volume of emulsion, several emulsions were prepared with various sizes of orifices through which components were forced during emulsification. The double-syringe method was used, but plungers of the two syringes were pushed by a mechanical device rather than by hand. The number of strokes (once back and once forth) was standardized to 25 per emulsion. Orifice sizes tested were equivalent to a circular orifice of 25, 22, and 18 gauge and no restriction between syringes. The stability of the emulsions, as measured by phase separation, microscopic evaluation of water droplet size distribution, viscosity, and creaming (oil leakage from emulsion),

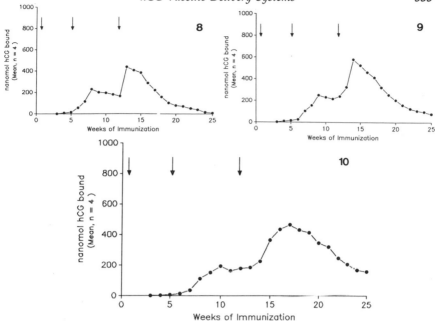

Fig. 8. Mean antibody levels reactive with hCG following immunization of rabbits with immunogen and adjuvant in a squalene–water emulsion using a water:oil ratio of 45:55. Arrows indicate the time of injections.

Fig. 9. Mean antibody levels reactive with hCG following immunization of rabbits with immunogen and adjuvant in a squalene–water emulsion using a water:oil ratio of 50:50. Arrows indicate the time of injections.

Fig. 10. Mean antibody levels reactive with hCG following a squalene–water emulsion using a water:oil ratio of 60:40. Arrows indicate the time of injections.

varied inversely with orifice size. Emulsions prepared with the smallest orifice were stable up to 6 weeks at room temperature. Those made with no restriction between syringes showed complete phase separation within 12 hr. Emulsion viscosity was directly related to stability.

The immune responses to these formulations are shown in Figures 11–14. It is readily apparent that the rate of antigen release at the injection site is related to emulsion stability and viscosity. However, it was somewhat surprising that the most stable emulsions elicited neither the highest antibody levels nor the most sustained responses. While the most unstable emulsions initiated a prompt booster response at the second injection, levels dropped rapidly thereafter, suggesting rapid clearance of immunogen. Conversely, the most stable ones failed to elicit "spikes" of antibody following

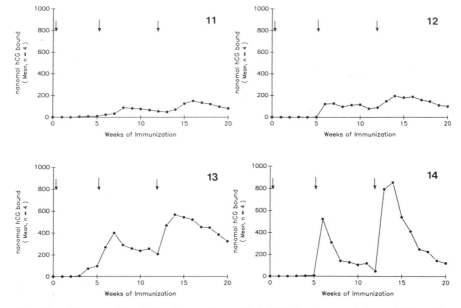

Fig. 11.   Mean antibody levels reactive with hCG after immunizing rabbits with immunogen in squalene–water emulsion by forcing components through a circular orifice equivalent to 25 gauge. Arrows indicate the time of injections.

Fig. 12.   Mean antibody levels reactive with hCG after immunizing rabbits with immunogen in squalene–water emulsion by forcing components through a circular orifice equivalent to 22 gauge. Arrows indicate the time of injections.

Fig. 13.   Mean antibody levels reactive with hCG after immunizing rabbits with immunogen in squalene–water emulsion by forcing components through a circular orifice equivalent to 18 gauge. Arrows indicate the time of injections.

Fig. 14.   Mean antibody levels reactive with hCG after immunizing rabbits with the immunogen in an unstable squalene–water emulsion prepared by passing the oil and water phases back and forth between two syringes with no restriction between them. Arrows indicate the time of injections.

booster injections, suggesting an inadequate immunogen release rate. Optimal responses (based on the injection intervals used) were obtained from emulsions prepared using an 18 gauge orifice.

These studies reflect the need to establish ideal conditions for preparing emulsions on an individual immunogen basis. Different conditions for establishing stable emulsions for BSA or DT are required from those described herein for the hCG immunogen. Likewise, should a different injection interval be needed, the characteristics of the emulsion used would need to be changed. As emulsions,

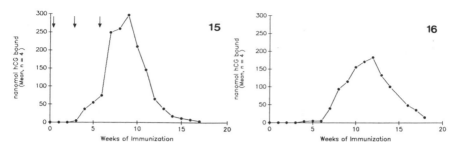

Fig. 15.   Mean antibody levels reactive with hCG from rabbits immunized with the immunogen and adjuvant encapsulated into liposomes. Liposomes suspended in saline were injected intramuscularly at 0, 3, and 6 weeks. Arrows indicate the time of injections.

Fig. 16.   Mean antibody levels reactive with hCG following immunization of rabbits with immunogen and adjuvant entrapped in liposomes. A single injection of liposomes suspended in saline was made at 0 time.

by definition, are unstable mixtures of two immiscible liquids, the degree of stability can be varied. In the examples described here, a compromise in stability and immunogen release is needed to produce the desired immune response. It may be possible to optimize responses by preparing different emulsion stabilities for the primary and subsequent immunization injections.

LIPOSOMES AND ISCOM SYSTEMS

A limited number of experiments were conducted using the hCG immunogen and adjuvant compound incorporated into liposomes and immunostimulating complexes (ISCOMs). Collaboration was established with G. Gregoriadis (London) for testing liposomes. This investigator incapsulated vaccine components into eight separate liposome formulations. Details of the procedures are provided elsewhere [Gregoriadis et al., 1987]. Some preparations were injected intramuscularly into rabbits three times in saline, whereas others were administered only once via the same route and vehicle. Examples of the best responses obtained from the two sets of experiments are shown in Figures 15 and 16. While multiple injections elicited responses comparable to a water–oil emulsion delivery system, the single injection formulation provided nearly the same pattern with a delayed response. These data demonstrate the utility of liposomes for successful immunogen delivery, but the duration of elevated antibody levels from one immunization was limited to 3–4 months.

A system for absorbing immunogens in a matrix of micelles

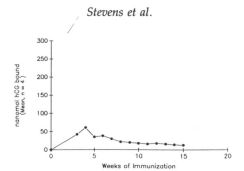

Fig. 17. Mean antibody levels reactive with hCG from immunizations of rabbits with the immunogen entrapped in Quil A ISCOMs. A single injection of the particles suspended in saline was made.

(ISCOMs) of an organic substance Quil A was developed by B. Morien (Uppsala) [Morien et al., 1984]. This scientist collaborated with the authors in testing this system for delivering the hCG vaccine components. As the properties of immunogens bound by these particles require a very hydrophobic molecule, the hCG peptide was coupled to an influenza virus envelope protein before incorporation into ISCOMs. These insoluble particles were administered to rabbits in a similar manner as described above for liposomes. The data obtained are shown in Figure 17. Like liposome entrapped vaccine, significant responses at very low doses on immunogen were obtained but the response was of short duration.

An explanation of the results of these studies is not readily apparent. It can be speculated that, while significant triggering of the immune response was induced by both liposomes and ISCOMs, release of the hCG immunogen was complete within a few weeks. As this immunogen is very hydrophilic, its presence outside the delivery system is followed by a rapid clearance. Thus, while the process of immune response initiation was quite effective, sustained slow release of vaccine antigen by these systems is not accomplished with the particular immunogen tested.

BIODEGRADABLE MICROSPHERE SYSTEMS

Although the systems described above provided means to deliver the vaccine components during vaccine development and preliminary clinical testing, none were found effective for providing a sustained level of antibodies for an extended period from a single injection. As multiple (three or more) injections were required to sustain theoretically effective levels of antibodies for several months, the use of these systems would not be practical for routine vaccine application in a large population of recipients. For this reason, studies were conducted to ascertain whether incorporation of the vaccine immunogen and adjuvant compound into biodegradable polymers of lactic acid and glycolic acid (and copolymers of these) would provide a delivery system capable of maintaining a sustained level of immunity for a sufficient period of time that would make vaccine application practical.

The successful use of these polymers for the controlled release of pharmaceuticals has been known for many years [Beck et al., 1979; Lewis and Tice, 1983]. Their nontoxic properties and tolerability in clinical trials has been well established. To date, no vaccine formulation has been put into use employing these materials, and there are no guidelines for instant preparation of vaccine materials. Furthermore, as with the other delivery systems described, the composition of an effective system depends on the characteristics of the component(s) to be incorporated, and a formulation for suitable release of one molecule will not likely be appropriate for another. Thus microspheres of lactide–glycolide acid polymers for the controlled release of the hCG vaccine had to be developed on a "custom" basis.

The biodegradation rates of these polymers are known. Polylactide materials degrade slower than copolymers of lactide and glycolide, with the fastest rate of decay occurring when a copolymer comprising 50% of each monomer is used. The molecular weight of the polymer also effects the rate of polymer breakdown, and they are generally inversely related to each other. Other factors that effect release of molecules entrapped in microspheres are the size of the spheres and the density (load) of the compound in the spheres. As the size of microspheres is increased, the duration of release of entrapped material is also increased. As the load of entrapped substance is increased, the rate of release is faster. Thus there are several variables that can be manipulated to provide release characteristics suitable for a particular need.

Using these parameters, numerous microsphere–hCG vaccine preparations were developed and tested. Dry microspheres were suspended in appropriate vehicles to maintain a uniform suspension and to attract lymphoid cells to the site of injection. Antibody levels were monitored weekly usually beginning 2 weeks after the single injection intramuscularly into rabbits. Early experiments demonstrated that significant levels of antibodies were elicited from a single injection but fell to very low levels by 15–20 weeks after immunization (Fig. 18). Further studies to evaluate spheres with longer degradation times were conducted. While antibody levels were present for a longer time after immunization (Fig. 19), the levels were slower to rise and were generally lower than when using the more rapidly

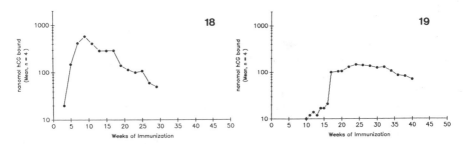

Fig. 18.   Mean antibody levels (on log scale) reactive with hCG after a single injection of the immunogen and adjuvant entrapped in polylactide microspheres.

Fig. 19.   Mean antibody levels (on log scale) reactive with hCG after a single injection of the immunogen and adjuvant entrapped in polylactide–glycolide copolymer formulation.

degrading polymers. This led us to prepare mixtures of fast, intermediate, and slowly degrading microspheres for vaccine delivery. Some examples of the profiles of antibody levels using this approach are shown in Figures 20–22. Some of the latter formulations were able to deliver immunogen over an extended period sufficient to maintain antibody production for more than 1 year following a single injection. We believe that should similar profiles be obtained from immunizations of women, a delivery system for practical application of the vaccine would be available.

DISCUSSION

The studies reported here shed some light on the requirements of a vaccine delivery system to provide elevated and sustained antibody levels. However, they also point out the complexity of designing an optimal system for a particular vaccine preparation. Clearly, the chemical and immunological characteristics of various immunogens will dictate which system and which conditions are most suitable for a particular vaccine. For example, many examples are available in which excellent immune responses were obtained when vaccine components were injected adsorbed to aluminum hydroxide precipitates [Bomford, 1980]. Experiments using our hCG immunogen delivered by adsorption to alum were ineffectual, as were emulsions using various vegetable oils. Most bacterial or viral vaccines use no special vehicle at all and are administered in water suspensions. Thus we wish to point out that the procedures tested here might

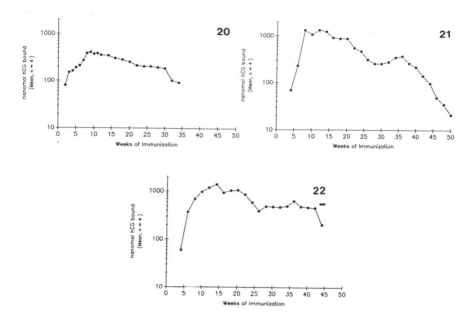

Fig. 20. Mean antibody levels (on log scale) reactive with hCG after a single injection of the immunogen and adjuvant entrapped in a blend of polylactide and lactide–glycolide copolymer microspheres.

Fig. 21. Mean antibody levels (on log scale) reactive with hCG after a single injection of the immunogen and adjuvant entrapped in a blend of polylactide and lactide–glycolide copolymer microspheres.

Fig. 22. Mean antibody levels (on log scale) reactive with hCG after a single injection of the immunogen and adjuvant entrapped in a blend of polylactide and lactide–glycolide copolymer microspheres.

have suggested use for other immunogens only if they are highly hydrophilic molecules with similar molecular weights.

We have tried to separate "adjuvant" activity (i.e., the vaccine component principally involved in macrophage activation) from the vehicle or medium controlling the rate of immunogen release at the injection site. In reality, it is likely that these are dependent variables in the immune response. It can be recalled that the simultaneous delivery of immunogen and adjuvant via the osmotic pump did not elicit high levels of antibodies despite the fact that both adjuvant (MDP) and the hCG immunogen were delivered to an intramuscular site in adequate quantities for a protracted period. When the same components were delivered via an oil–water emulsion, the oil component clearly played a role in attracting and/or activating macrophages. Such actions are known to occur also from injections of alum and nonionic block polymers [Hunter and Bennett, 1986]. Furthermore, booster injections several months after the last immunization will elevate antibody levels using immunogen alone with some antigens, but with others elevated levels can be obtained only if both antigen and adjuvant are injected (V. Stevens, unpublished observations). Also, the rate of proteolytic degradation of protein antigens will vary, which affects their availability to the immune system. Despite the limitations on conclusions that can be drawn from data collected here, the approaches taken may provide useful information for designing delivery systems for other vaccines.

ACKNOWLEDGMENTS

The investigations reported here received financial support from the WHO Special Programme of Research, Development, and Research Training in Human Reproduction.

REFERENCES

Beck LR, Cowsar DR, Lewis DH, Gibson JW, Flowers CE (1979): New long-acting injectable microcapsule contraceptive system. Am J Obstet Gynecol 135:419–426.

Bomford R (1980): Effect on the antibody response to bovine serum albumin and sheep red blood cells of Freund's incomplete and complete adjuvants, alhydrogel, *Corynebacterium parvum, Bordetella pertussis,* muramyl dipeptide and saponin. Clin Exp Immunol 39:426–434.

Gregoriadis G, Davis D, Davies A (1987): Liposomes as immunological adjuvants: Antigen incorporation studies. Vaccine 5:145–151.

Hunter RL, Bennett B (1986): The adjuvant activity of nonionic block polymer surfactants. Scand J Immunol 23:287–300.

Jones WR, Bradley J, Judd SJ, Denholm EH, Ing RMY, Mueller UW, Powell JE, Griffin PD, Stevens VC (1988): Phase I clinical trial of a World Health Organization birth control vaccine. Lancet 1:1295–1298.

Lewis DH, Tice TR (1983): Polymeric considerations in the design of microencapsulated contraceptive steroids. In Zatuchni GI (ed): Long Acting Contraceptive Delivery Systems. Philadelphia: Harper & Row, pp 77–95.

Morien B, Sundquist B, Hoglund S, Dalsgaard D, Osterhaus A (1984): ISCOM, a novel structure of antigenic presentation of membrane proteins from enveloped viruses. Nature 308:457–459.

Stevens VC, Cinader B, Powell JE, Lee AC, Koh SW (1986a): Preparation and formulation of a hCG antifertility vaccine: Selection of a peptide immunogen. Am J Reprod Immunol 1:306–314.

Stevens VC, Cinader B, Powell JE, Lee AC, Koh SW (1986b): Preparation and formulation of a hCG antifertility vaccine: Selection of adjuvant and vehicle. Am J Reprod Immunol 1:315–321.

DISCUSSION

DR. GABELNICK: On a number of occasions, you have indicated that microcapsules as well the vehicles are important. Is that still the case?

DR. STEVENS: Yes. When you inject these in saline, they are completely inert. There is no cellular infiltration around the site at all. So you must conclude that there is something in the vehicle in addition to the microcapsules that will attract lymphoid cells to the site.

DR. GABELNICK: Can you disclose what this magic ingredient is?

DR. STEVENS: It is not mine. It belongs to the Stolle Corporation, but I don't believe there is a patent on it. I think they are still experimenting with what will be the most effective and safe vehicles. But some of these particular vehicles have not had toxicology studies done and, thus, may not be safe for human applications.

DR. BIALY: We have worked with progestin esters. When we incorporated some of them in a saline type of suspension, we could get 1 year of biological activity. Every time I have discussed the issue of very long-acting compounds, I have been told that you do not want something that you inject and that can be active for as long as 1 year. What has been the thinking of your group about the maximum duration of a nonretrievable type of an injection system from the body?

DR. STEVENS: That is a very good question. One of our problems with emulsions is that we can't get a long enough duration of response from a single injection. So, we have to administer them every 2 or 3 months. Obviously, we can make them last for shorter periods, almost as short as we wish. You can make them last for 6 weeks, but the advantage of the method would then be lost. The question was raised earlier this morning about the reversibility of the immune response. I think it would have to be made very clear to the user of any of these products, whether it be sperm, zona, hCG, or any other vaccine, that there is some risk involved with this particular kind of contraceptive method, and that there is not yet a way that we can stop the immune response. Obviously, depending on the vaccine, we can override the immune response sometimes and allow fertility to be regained. But, one has to live with a certain duration of immunity if this method of birth control is to be used.

36

Immunosafety Aspects of Fertility Control Vaccines

G.L. Ada

Vaccines have been developed over the last two centuries to protect against infectious disease. For vaccines, there were two main criteria: safety and efficacy. As control was gained over endemic and epidemic infectious diseases in industrialized countries, the question of safety became paramount and efficacy, though obviously important, took a somewhat lower profile. Some vaccines either previously or currently in use that were licensed for use many years ago might have difficulty in passing the licensing authorities in some countries today. In contrast, the situation is reversed for vaccines for veterinary and particularly livestock use, when efficacy becomes the dominant factor.

SPECIAL EXPECTATIONS AND REQUIREMENTS OF FERTILITY CONTROL VACCINES

In discussing fertility control vaccines for human use, several differences compared with traditional vaccines are immediately apparent.

1   In both cases, the vaccine would usually be administered to normal healthy people, but with the difference that the fertility control vaccine is to prevent a normal physiological process, not an otherwise potentially deadly disease. This is not to deny that there is a certain morbidity and mortality rate resulting from pregnancy, depending on many factors, and that this rate may be very high in some developing countries (sometimes 100-fold) compared with that in developed countries.

Gamete Interaction: Prospects for Immunocontraception, pages 565–578

2   Vaccines to control infectious disease ideally achieve long-lived immune responses, i.e., the aim is irreversibility. For most family planning purposes, fertility control vaccines should be reversible after a predetermined period of time, generally considered to be 1–2 years after vaccination. There may be situations in which a longer lasting contraceptive effect would be suitable. One concern is how uniformly reversible will the vaccine be? Will there be great variation in the length of response, and how will this be monitoried?

3   In contrast to vaccines that are based on all or part of a foreign agent to control infectious diseases, fertility control vaccines will be based on a self or self-like antigen. Theoretically, the risk of inducing autoimmunity or initiating a nonphysiological response is higher than with a vaccine against an infectious agent. This risk may be enhanced if a powerful adjuvant is incorporated into the formulation. This aspect in particular will be discussed later.

4   Depending on the success of this approach, the vaccine may be administered rather more often (e.g., at frequent intervals during much of the childbearing life span of a fertile, healthy woman) than is the case with existing vaccines with conceivably a greater risk of increased side effects.

5   The benefits of a contraceptive vaccine need to be weighed against the advantages and disadvantages of other forms of contraception, including those for which there is now a vast amount of experience in some countries.

All these considerations point to one major requirement: Fertility control vaccines for human use must pass very stringent safety tests. Their development, therefore, will be both expensive and very time-consuming. If successful, they may become one of the most important mechanisms for allowing personal control over fertility. The goal is worth the effort.

IMMUNOLOGICAL RESPONSES EXPECTED OF A VACCINE

Our knowledge of the important immune responses to all of the successful medical vaccines that control an infection is rudimentary. Other than measurement of antibody and sometimes using a functional test such as neutralization of infectivity, no systematic effort seems to have been made to assay other parameters. Our understanding of the essential requirements of a vaccine comes from studies of model systems, particularly the response to an acute infectious agent. It is thought that such a system mimics to a reasonable extent the use of many live attenuated viral vaccines that have in general been highly effective. The important attributes of a vaccine to prevent or control an infection have been summarized as follows [Ada, 1990]:

1   Activate the immune system, particularly the antigen-presenting cells, so that the appropriate cytokines are produced and secreted.

2   Generate a large pool of both T and B memory cells. This is because a vaccine administered sometime before exposure to the wild-type agent exploits the adaptive component of the immune response. If the vaccine is administered where the infectious disease is endemic, nonadaptive responses may also contribute.

3   Possess or, in the case of an infectious agent, induce favorable kinetics of antigen accumulation and persistence in such a form and in the appropriate location to recruit the B memory cells to form antibody-secreting cells, thus providing a protective level of antibody. The most likely site for localization of antigen to have this function is the follicular dendritic cells in the follicles or germinal centers in lymphoid tissues.

4   Contain sufficient B-cell and T-cell (including T-helper and cytotoxic T) epitopes to overcome the genetic polymorphism in the major histocompatibility complex (MHC) antigens in outbred populations. This will ensure that the great majority of people will recognize and respond to at least some of the epitopes.

On the other hand, there are some consequences we would wish vaccination not to have. Apart from autoimmunity, which is discussed later, this includes the avoidance of polyclonal activation of T and/or B cells. This activation occurs during the immune response to some infections such as malaria and, in general, is undesirable, as the specific component is swamped by an excess of nonspecific responses. The requirements of a vaccine to control human fertility will differ in some ways from the above.

DEVELOPMENTAL OPTIONS FOR FERTILITY CONTROL VACCINES

Most vaccines, either current or under trial, are composed of either a component of the entire infectious agent or the whole agent, which, in most cases, can be grown or produced in vitro in sufficient amount. The "raw" material to produce vaccines on the large scale envisaged to control fertility is unlikely to be so readily available and thus alternative approaches are mandatory. These are of two general types:

1   The synthesis of peptides corresponding to B-cell epitopes and possibly T-cell epitopes. It is more likely that T-cell epitopes will be provided by conjugating the B-cell epitopes to a protein carrier, most likely of viral or bacterial origin.

2   Use of recombinant DNA coding for the antigens concerned to transfect appropriate cells that will then express the product. Because of the need for reversibility, it is unlikely that an engineered live vector, viral or bacterial, will be considered in the near future.

To achieve the different ideal properties of a vaccine described above, it is most likely that such preparations will need to be administered with an adjuvant, which achieves two purposes. One is to activate the antigen-presenting cells so that the antigen is presented with the production of appropriate lymphokines. A second is to allow for persistence of antigen; the use of controlled-release devices may be highly successful in achieving this [V.C. Stevens, personal communication].

THE PROSPECT OF AUTOIMMUNITY AND AUTOIMMUNE DISEASE

Vaccines to control fertility may involve immunization against a normal host antigen, e.g., zona pellucida vaccines. A major concern is the generation of autoimmunity, which may lead to a disease situation. This section will address the following questions:

1   What is the nature of autoimmunity?
2   What are the steps between autoimmunity and autoimmune disease initiation?
3   Can the risk of autoimmune disease be reasonably assessed?

4   If autoimmune disease occurs, can it be alleviated in any way?

The Nature of Autoimmunity

There are two completely conflicting ideas about autoimmunity. The first stems from the clonal selection theory of Burnet [1957], which states that clones of cells specific for self-antigens are "forbidden," i.e., they are eliminated so that only responses to foreign antigens are mounted. Autoimmune disease represented a failure to eliminate forbidden specificities. The second concept [Coutinho, 1989; Rossi et al., 1989] considers that autoimmunity is part of an idiotypic/anti-idiotypic network organization and should be considered as a normal physiological situation.

While the general concept of clonal selection as the basis of the immune system has been amply verified, Burnet was only partly correct in his concept of "forbidden clones," as became obvious shortly after the enunciation of the theory. Examination of human populations showed that a high proportion of otherwise healthy people contained autoantibodies to a variety of self-antigens. The following observations are relevant [Rose et al., 1990]:

1   Autoantibodies to many self-antigens are commonly found. There seems to be some exceptions; autoantibodies to MHC antigens have not been convincingly demonstrated.
2   T cells with high affinity to self-epitopes are eliminated in the thymus. T cells with lower affinity receptors escape, are present in the periphery, and may be activated under certain conditions.
3   Molecular mimicry, i.e., some homology between amino acid sequences of self-antigens and "foreign" antigens, occurs at a relatively high frequency [Lernmark et al., 1988].
4   Autoimmune disease may be T-cell mediated or antibody mediated; it may be initiated by antibody but, particularly in the case of intracellular antigens, is more likely to be T-cell initiated.

Is there any evidence to favor the network organization theory? First, it has been shown that the prevalence of clones of B cells with a particular self-reactivity is as high as is the case with clones to many foreign specificites. Second, the sera of patients who have recovered from autoimmune disease are found to contain anti-idiotypes to the specific autoantibody. Functionally more impressive is the demonstration that administration of very large quantities of pooled normal serum, containing polyspecific immunoglobulins, to patients with one of several different autoimmune diseases resulted in clinical improvement and/or a decrease in circulating antibody titer [Rossi et al., 1989]. There is also evidence for anti-idiotypic or clonotypic T cells that may help in controlling autoimmune reactivity [Cohen, 1986]. Perhaps we should now accept the point of view that many, if not the majority, of autoimmune reactions are physiologically normal and thus their occurrence should not be of great concern.

Autoimmunity Following Vaccine Administration

Some vaccines, particularly those administered as part of the World Health Organization's Expanded Programme of Immunization (bacillus Calmette-Guérin [BCG], measles, polio, pertussis, diphtheria, and tetanus toxoids) have now been administered to billions of recipients. Is there any evidence of autoimmunity or autoimmune disease occurring following administration of such vaccines?

It seems reasonable to state that if a significant level of autoimmune disease had occurred subsequent to the administration of any of these vaccines, it would have been detected and the use of the vaccine at least questioned. This has not occurred. The development of autoimmunity following vaccination seems not to have been closely examined, but there are sufficient indications to suggest that this is probably widespread. In one study [Srinivasappa et al., 1986], up to 3.5% of monoclonal antibodies prepared against 11 viruses were found to react with normal tissue. Database searches [Oldstone et al., 1986] have also demonstrated considerable homology between viral and tissue proteins. Furthermore, rabbits immunized with a decamer from a hepatitis B antigen that showed 60% homology with the encephalitogenic site of rabbit myelin basic protein developed both humoral and cell-mediated immune responses to the native myelin protein, and several developed pathological lesions [Fujinami and Oldstone, 1985]. There are of course even greater opportunities in the case of bacteria. Some have been documented in great detail, e.g., *Mycobacterium tuberculosis*–induced arthritis [van Eden et al., 1988] and streptococcal cell wall–induced arthritis [Cromartie et al., 1977; Beachey et al., 1988]. In both models, bacterium-specific T lymphocytes were shown to play a crucial role [van der Broek et al., 1989].

If these reactions occur after vaccination, why do they not lead to autoimmune disease? A definitive answer cannot be given at present, but there are two interesting possibilities. One [Rose, 1988, as cited in Lernmark et al., 1988] is that the host will respond poorly to a molecule sharing self-sequences because of the existence of a tolerant state. Thus the group B meningococcus polysaccharide, a polymer of N-acetylneuraminic acid, is poorly immunogenic and stimulates at best short-lived IgM responses of low affinity. It is generally thought that the reason for this is the fact that this molecule occurs very widely in normal tissue proteins. Possibly, use of a potent stimulus (e.g., an adjuvant) could overcome the tolerance, and in fact one person has been found [Kabat et al., 1986] with a benign monoclonal gammopathy (23 mg/ml of IgM anti-poly-a(2-8) of N-acetylneuraminic acid).

The other possibility stems from the recent finding [van Eden et al., 1988; van der Broek et al., 1989] that pretreatment of animals with the mycobacterial 65kd heat shock protein *prevents* the induction of *M. tuberculosis*–induced arthritis. It seems that prior treatment with the heat shock protein may induce the formation of suppressor T cells. As heat shock proteins are highly conserved in nature, a possible scenario is that immunization with BCG may induce preferentially a suppressor T-cell response so that autoimmune disease rarely, if ever, occurs. This is clearly a very interesting finding, and further studies should reveal more detail about the nature and specificity of the suppressive effect.

Autoimmune Disease Initiation

The induction of autoimmunity depends in the first place on the location of the self-antigen. Generally, the host will be tolerant, but some antigens, such as sperm- and eye lens-associated proteins, may be sufficiently sequestered from the immune system that tolerance has not developed.

Circulating antigens and those present at cell surfaces are obvious targets for antibody-mediated reactions. Immunity to antigens circulating at low concentrations, e.g., thyroglobulin, is generally more readily achieved than, say, to albumin, which occurs at high concentrations, but the reverse rarely holds. Autoantibodies to nonidiotypic regions of immunoglobulins are found under special conditions, e.g., rheumatoid factors. Autoantibodies to cell surface components, such as cellular receptors, may directly initiate cellular disturbances or cause damage by inducing, with complement, cell lysis. In some situations, the presence of relatively high-affinity IgG antiself antibodies is an indication of a disease situation and should not necessarily imply that autoantibody initiated the disease process.

Antigen–antibody complexes contribute to the pathogenesis of many diseases. Their continuing presence in the bloodstream indicates inefficient removal and/or continuing release of antigen into the system with continuing antibody production. The complexes are removed either by the scavenging cells of the reticuloendothelial system (RES) or by filtration through the glomerular membrane. The former is more likely to be dominant if the lesion occurs locally, as in the Arthus reaction. When immune complexes are deposited in the glomerula loops, binding of complement can induce glomerular nephritis and proteinuria. However, considering the frequency of occurrence of autoantibodies, the relative rarity of autoimmune lesions is striking.

There is increasing evidence that the target antigens in many autoimmune diseases are intracellular [e.g., Mackay and Gershwin, 1989; Demaine, 1989] and do not exist as intact antigen either outside or at the cell surface. As neither antibodies nor immune cells can normally penetrate cells, recognition must occur at the cell surface, and this is now generally acknowledged to be a peptide derived from the protein, expressed at the cell surface associated with MHC molecules and recognized by T cells. The recognition may be by class I MHC-restricted T cells that are cytotoxic, thus lysing the cell and releasing antigens that may then initiate an antibody response. Such cells have been shown to occur in some autoimmune reactive tissues. The alternative is recognition by class II MHC-restricted cells that have helper activity; once activated, these cells can initiate a humoral response that may result in the generation of high-affinity IgG antibody. Various mechanisms have been proposed whereby this activation of the T cell may be promoted [Blanden et al., 1987; Ada and Rose, 1988]. It is also possible that the activated T-helper cell, through liberation of factors, might initiate damage to the target cell.

Assessment of the Risk of Autoimmune Disease

On the assumption that all the necessary immunological tests to detect immunological and other abnormalities have been carried out on subjects prior to their enrollment in a clinical trial, a sequence of tests have been published as an algorithm for the stepwise characterization of any autoimmune reaction [Rose et al., 1990]. Except perhaps in the very early stages of disease, a cell-mediated immune response is accompanied by the presence of specific antibody so that the initial screen is the examination of a wide variety of tissue sections with antibody from immunized hosts and using either immunofluorescence or immunoperoxidase. If negative, the risk of autoimmune disease is considered to be negligible. If the autoreaction has occurred after immunization, it should be straightforward to see whether T-cell activation has occurred by seeing whether the self-antigenic component that was used in the immunization schedule will induce proliferation of peripheral blood T lymphocytes from the immunized host. This is not an option if the self-antigen is unknown.

Provided that staining artifacts, e.g., nonspecific binding and binding via Fc receptors, are eliminated, a positive reaction with labeled antibody will indicate not only the organ and cell type involved but also the localization of the antigen—plasma membrane associated or intracellular—which can be further refined by electron microscopy if desired. The specificity of the binding, i.e., the antibody responsible for the reaction can be absorbed out with the antigen (hapten) used for immunization, should be adequately checked.

If plasma membrane associated and if the cell type can be isolated, tests can be carried out to determine the nature of the reactive antigen, such as a known cellular receptor or otherwise. If intracellular, an extensive program of cell fractionation procedures could be undertaken, but the need to do this would be influenced by the strength of the observed reaction, the frequency of the reaction using different antisera, and the nature of the reactive cell. For example, if the cell is known to produce an important hormone(s) of the endocrine system and the antigen in the immunization schedule is hormone derived, the antibody specificity with regard to this and related hormones should be checked.

It may also be possible in some cases to carry out functional assays. For example, hormone levels in vivo or possibly in vitro using tissue slices might be measured to ascertain whether an autoimmune reaction had interfered with the production of the hormone. This scheme for analysis will first be followed in the animal model used in the preclinical studies and will involve studying the animals for sufficient time to establish whether there is any indication of autoimmune disease.

Can Autoimmune Disease Be Alleviated?

Any vaccine to control human fertility that was shown to induce autoimmune disease during clinical testing or even at the postregistration stage would be considered unsafe for general use. As with many vaccines, however, such reactions might be seen at very low frequencies, when tens or hundreds of thousands of people had received the vaccine. This would mean a careful assessment of the

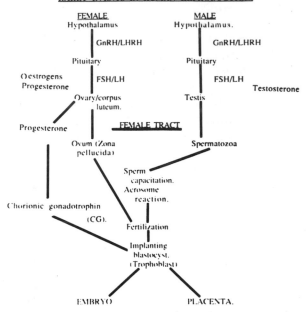

Fig. 1.   Early events in human reproduction. GnRH, LHRH; gonadotropin and luteinizing hormone-releasing hormone, respectively; FSH, follicle stimulating hormone; LH, luteinizing hormone; CG, chorionic gonadotropin.

risk/benefit ratio of the particular vaccine. It would be helpful if there was a means of alleviating the effects of an autoimmune disease in these rare cases. Recent work mentioned above has indicated possible approaches to such therapy, particularly if T-cell activation is clearly the initiating mechanism.

The Nature of Immunological Hazards in the Use of Fertility Control Vaccines

Leading antigen candidates for fertility control vaccines are of two classes: hormones of the endocrine system and cell-associated antigens [Ada and Griffin, 1990]. Figure 1 illustrates the events leading to fertilization of the ovum and the development of the trophoblast. The hormone that best fulfills the requirements of a target for vaccination is the human chorionic gonadotropin (hCG) hormone, and three major research groups in this area (WHO, The Population Council, and the National Institute of Immunology, New Delhi) have focused their studies on this hormone [Rose et al., 1990]. The candidate vaccines contain either the complete B chain of hCG or the C-terminal 37 amino acid sequence (which is unique to hCG among hormones). The mode of action of these vaccines is generally considered to be antibody mediated, but it has not been excluded that cell-mediated immunity may also play some role. If in fact antibody per se is shown to be completely contraceptive, it could be argued that the "haptenic" group in any vaccine that contained a carrier from other sources (e.g., diphtheria or tetanus toxoids) might contain only B-cell epitopes and thus minimize the risk of inducing autoimmunity by T-cell activation.

Antibody from some volunteers immunized with the vaccine candidate consisting of the 37 amino acid component of hCG conjugated to diphtheria toxoid [Jones et al., 1988] has reacted with some human tissues, particularly a cytoplasmic component in somatostatin-secreting pancreatic cells. Absorption with the hCG peptide, but not with somatostatin, removed this reactivity. This reaction was not associated with abnormalities in blood glucose levels, and there is no homology between the peptide and somatostatin.

There is a variety of nonhormonal potential targets for vaccine development. These include sperm antigens, antigens of the zona pellucida, and antigens of the trophoblast, all of which have been discussed in other chapters. Again, most attention is given to the development of humoral immunity to these candidate antigens, but the possibility of a vaccine based on cellular immunity is also receiving attention [Anderson and Hill, 1988a]. CMI responses are known to occur in both the male and female reproductive tracts [Anderson and Hill, 1988b], and certain lymphokines have been shown to interfere with sperm function [Hill et al., 1987b], trophoblast immunogenicity and viability [Head et al., 1987], and with embryo development [Hill et al., 1987a]. Although there has been some success in predicting T-cell epitopes [Berzofsky, 1985] that might then form part of a vaccine, it is debatable whether a continuing cell-mediated immune response to an antigen, say, on sperm in the male reproductive tract would be desirable. Again, there would be a need to look for molecular mimicry, this time in T-cell epitopes, about which very little is currently known. In view of the fact that peptides recognized by class I or II MHC antigens are relatively small and that sequence rather than conformation is critical, there would seem to be considerable opportunities for cross-reactivity.

CONCLUSION

Vaccines to control human fertility in theory run a higher risk of inducing antiself reactions compared with vaccines to control infectious diseases, and this risk may be greater still if powerful adjuvants are used and the vaccine is administered frequently. Safety, particularly the avoidance of autoimmune disease, is a dominant factor in their acceptability. Despite conflicting concepts about whether autoimmunity is a normal or abnormal manifestation, both autoantibodies and self-reactive T cells occur in otherwise normal individuals. There is a growing concensus that the main mechanism for induction of autoimmune disease is activation of T cells, which are normally anergic, controlled by suppressor mechanisms, or of low affinity. One way to minimize the chances of activation of antiself T cells is to use a "foreign" carrier protein as the main or only source of T-cell epitopes in the vaccine. A vaccine that induced autoimmune disease during clinical trials would be unacceptable. Should cases occur in very low frequency, however, it is encouraging that recent work in model systems shows promise of being able to prevent or minimize the pathological manifestation of at least some autoimmune reactions.

REFERENCES

Ada GL (1990): Strategies for exploiting the immune system in the design of vaccines. Mol Immunol (in press).

Ada GL, Griffin PD (1990): The process of reproduction in humans: Antigens for vaccine development. In Griffin PD, Ada GL (eds): Symposium on the Assessment of Safety and Efficacy of Vaccines To Control Human Fertility. Cambridge: Cambridge University Press.

Ada GL, Rose NR (1988): The initiation and early development of autoimmune diseases. Clin Immunol Immunopathol 41:3–9.

Anderson DJ, Hill JA (1988a): Should cell-mediated immunity be considered in the implementation of anti-fertility vaccines? In Talwar GP (ed): Contraception Research for Today and the Nineties. Berlin: Springer-Verlag, pp 285–292.

Anderson DJ, Hill JA (1988b): Cell-mediated immunity in infertility. Am J Reprod Immunol Microbiol. 17:22–30.

Beachey EH, Bronze M, Dale JB, Kraus W, Poirier T, Sargent S (1988): Protective and autoimmune epitopes of streptococcal M proteins. Vaccine 6:192–196.

Berzofsky JA (1985): Intrinsic and extrinsic factors in protein antigenic structure. Science 229:932–940.

Blanden RV, Hodgkin PD, Hill A, Sinikas VG, Mullbacher A (1987): Quantitative considerations of T-cell activation and self tolerance. Immunol Rev 98:75–93.

Burnet FM (1957): A modification of Jerne's theory of antibody production using the concept of clonal selection. Aust J Sci 20:67–70.

Cohen IR (1986): Regulation of autoimmune disease: Physiological and therapeutic. Immunol Rev 94:5–31.

Coutinho A (1989): Beyond clonal selection and network. Immunol Rev 110:63–88.

Cromartie WJ, Craddock JG, Schwab JH, Anderle SK, Yang C (1977): Arthritis in rats after systemic injection of streptococcal cells or cell walls. J Exp Med 146:1585–1596.

Demaine AG (1989): The molecular biology of autoimmune disease. Immunol Today 10: 357–361.

Fujinami RS, Oldstone MBA (1985): Amino acid homology between the encephalitogenic site of myelin basic protein and virus: Mechanism for autoimmunity. Science 230:1043–1045.

Head JR, Drake BL, Zuchermann FA (1987): Major histocompatibility antigens on trophoblast and their regulation: Implication in the materno-foetal relationship. Am J Reprod Immunol 15:12–18.

Hill JA, Hacmovici F, Anderson DJ (1987a): Products of activated lymphocytes and macrophages inhibit mouse embryo development in vitro. J Immunol 139:2250–2254.

Hill JA, Hacmovici F, Politch JA, Anderson JA (1987b): Effects of soluble products of activated lymphocytes and macrophages (lymphokines and monokines) on human sperm motion parameters. Fertil Steril 47:460–465.

Jones WR, Bradley J, Judd SJ, Denholm EH, Ing RMY, Mueller UW, Powell J, Griffin PD, Stevens VC (1988): Phase 1 clinical trials of a World Health Organization birth control vaccine. Lancet 1:1295–1298.

Kabat EA, Nickerson KG, Liao J, Grossbard L, Osserman EF, Glickman E, Chess L, Robbins JB, Schneerson R, Yang YA (1986): A human monoclonal macroglobulin with specificity for a (2–8) linked poly-N-acetylneuraminic acid, the capsular polysaccharide of group B meningococci and *Eschericia coli* K1 which crossreacts with polynucleotides and with denatured DNA. J Exp Med 164:642–654.

Lernmark A, Dryberg T, Terenius L, Hokfelt B (eds) (1988): Molecular Mimicry in Health and Disease. Exerpta Medica: Amsterdam.

Mackay IR, Gershwin ME (1989): Molecular basis of mitochondrial autoreactivity in primary biliary cirrhosis. Immunol Today 10:315–318.

Oldstone MBA, Schwimmbeck P, Dyrberg T, Fujinami R (1986): Mimicry by virus of host molecules: Implications for autoimmune disease. Prog Immunol 6:787–798.

Rose NR, Wick G, Berger P, Ada GL (1990): Immunological hazards associated with human immunization with self or self-like antigens. In Griffin PD, Ada GL (eds): Symposium on the Assessment of the Safety and Efficacy of Vaccines To Regulate Fertility. Cambridge: Cambridge University Press (in press).

Rossi F, Dietrich G, Kazatchkine MD (1989): Anti-idiotypes against autoantibodies in normal immunoglobulins: Evidence for network regulation of human autoimmune responses. Immunol Rev 110:135–150.

578   *Ada*

Srinivasappa J, Saeguse J, Prabhakar BS, Gentry MK, Buchmeir MJ, Wicktor TJ, Koprowski H, Oldstone MB, Notkins AL (1986): Molecular mimicry: Frequency of reactivity of monoclonal antiviral antibodies with normal tissues. J Virol 57:397–401.

van Eden W, Thole JER, van der Zee R, Noordzij A, van Embden JDA, Henson EJ, Cohen IR (1988): Cloning of the mycobacterium epitope recognized by T lymphocytes in adjuvant arthritis. Nature 331:171–173.

van der Broek MF, Hogervorst EJM, van Bruggen MCJ, van Eden W, van der Zee R, van den Berg WB (1989): Protection against Streptococcal cell wall–induced arthritis by pretreatment with the 65-kD mycobacterial heat shock protein. J Exp Med 170:449–466.

37

Experiences of the Anti-hCG Vaccine of Relevance to Development of Other Birth Control Vaccines

G.P. Talwar, O. Singh, R. Pal, and K. Arunan

The human chorionic gonadotropin (hCG) vaccine, the first potential vaccine to be developed for birth control, faces various problems peculiar to being first. Vaccines hitherto were made against pathogens. The idea of mobilizing the immune system to intercept a process within the body was conceptually new and evoked the following type of questions: Is it feasible? Will it lead to autoimmune reactions? Will it be reversible? What are its side effects?

The answers to most, albeit not all, of these questions are available from the studies carried out by three major groups engaged in research on the hCG vaccines over the last 15 years. These will be discussed briefly in this chapter. We also propose to mention some of the birth control vaccine requirements for efficacy and applicability to a genetically diverse population. The latter have evolved primarily from results of three successive clinical trials conducted with our vaccine(s) and the strategies adopted to meet the problems. The prototype vaccine that we proposed initially was the β-subunit of hCG linked in defined molar proportions to tetanus toxoid (TT) as carrier (βhCG-TT) [Talwar et al., 1976; see also articles in the February 1976 issue of *Contraception*]. Conjugation of βhCG to this carrier was conceived with two objectives in mind: to overcome immunological tolerance of women to hCG and simultaneously to confer immunoprophylactic benefit against tetanus, a major cause of mortality among women in developing countries at the time of delivery.

Gamete Interaction: Prospects for Immunocontraception, pages 579–593
© 1990 Wiley-Liss, Inc.

Probing phase I clinical trials with this vaccine conducted in six centers located in five countries revealed that the vaccine design fulfilled the basic requirements of inducing anti-hCG and antitetanus antibodies in women, that the response was reversible, and that no side effects of any significance occurred [Kumar et al., 1976; Hingorani and Kumar, 1979; Nash et al., 1980; Shahani et al., 1982]. However, the shortcoming of this prototype vaccine was the large variability of response in recipients, and those with low titers were not protected from becoming pregnant. This led to the search and inclusion of an adjuvant to the vaccine that was hitherto adsorbed on alum. The intrinsic immunogenicity of βhCG was improved by associating it with the α-subunit of ovine luteinizing hormone (LH). The heterospecies dimer generated conformational antibodies of higher bioefficacy [Talwar et al., 1988].

Another phase I clinical trial was conducted in 101 women with the "improved" formulations. These formulations were more immunogenic; *all* women, without exception, responded by making high antibody titers [Singh et al., 1989]. They had high avidity and enhanced bioefficacy. These trials also brought out a new feature. Repeated immunization of some women with TT-linked vaccine induced hypersensitivity and immunosuppression. This response was overcome by employing the vaccine conjugated to two different carriers, TT and diphtheria toxoid (DT) used in an alternate sequence [Gaur et al., 1990]. The progression of this vaccine from laboratory experimental stages to clinical use has brought out issues relevant to other promising candidate antigens for birth control vaccines.

FEASIBILITY

The answer to whether a contraceptive vaccine is feasible is not yet available. Only after phase II clinical efficacy studies in women will the workability of efficacy of an hCG vaccine for control of fertility be clear. Nonhuman primates immunized with βhCG linked to a carrier such as TT [Talwar et al., 1980] or βhCG given with Freund's complete adjuvant (FCA) [Hearn, 1976] rendered these animals infertile. However, these primates are not identical to humans. The duration and pattern of chorionic gonadotropin (CG) secretion in these species is different. In molecular terms, hCG differs from the primate CG. Immunologically, antibodies against βhCG have only 1 to 10% cross-reactivity with the baboon or monkey CG. The cross-reaction with the human carboxy terminal peptide (CTP) is even lower, if not completely absent [Chen and Hodgen, 1976]. These considerations are important in determining the suitability of the experimental

TABLE 1. Efficacy Testing of hCG Vaccines in a Subhuman Primate Model (*Macaca radiata*)[a]

Monkey No.	Immunogen	Ka for hCG (nM^{-1})	Bioneutralization capacity (IU/liter)		Fertility status
			hCG	mCG	
100	αoLH-βhCG-TT	0.7	1,120	450	Inf
		21.6	760	0	P
110	βhCG-TT + βoLH-TT	4.2	600	320	Inf
		30.3	960	0	P
161	βhCG-TT + βoLH-TT	0.4	430	240	Inf
		7.1	250	0	P
164	βhCG-TT + βoLH-TT	0.3	450	320	Inf
		9.0	605	0	P
177	βhCG-TT + βoLH-TT	0.3	440	250	Inf
		2.6	200	0	P
178	βhCG-TT + βoLH-TT	0.1	280	270	Inf
		2.3	180	0	P
180	βhCG-TT + βoLH-TT	0.1	580	1,080	Inf
		0.5	700	0	P
162	LDH-C_4–βhCG-TT	0.3	800	680	Inf
		17.6	690	0	P
163	LDH-C_4–βhCG-TT	0.8	800	800	Inf
		4.2	900	5	P
173	LDH-C_4–βhCG-TT	0.5	630	640	Inf
		4.7	740	0	P

[a]Various formulations of βhCG vaccines inducing antibodies against hCG prevented bonnet monkeys from getting pregnant only when the antibodies had bioneutralization capacity against monkey CG. This property was not directly related to hCG bioneutralization capacity. Inf, infertile; P, pregnant. [Data are from Rao et al., 1988.]

model for testing a candidate vaccine. For example, bonnet monkeys immunized with anti-hCG vaccines demonstrated infertility unrelated to anti-hCG titers, the measurement of vaccine response. Instead, the block of fertility was related to the extent that the antibodies inactivated the bioactivity of the monkey CG (Table 1). Thus the usual parameter employed, i.e., titers of antibodies against the human CG, was an inappropriate and erroneous criterion with which to evaluate the efficacy of a vaccine formulation in a nonhuman experimental model. It is further apparent that the higher the affinity of antibodies to hCG, the lower the cross-reactivity with primate CG and the less suitable the heterologous experimental animal model.

AUTOIMMUNE REACTIONS

An immunological approach, especially against a self-protein or an internally located process, demands careful screening for type and range of cross-reactions. Usually immune response is both humoral and cell mediated (CMI). The former is easier to monitor, but methods have to be devised to assess the safety of the latter, a likely response to immunization with many gamete antigens. In the case of hCG, immune response is predominantly humoral, CMI being restricted to the carrier (TT or DT). Termination of pregnancy can be affected by passive administration of anti-hCG antibodies [Hearn, 1976; Stevens, 1976; Tandon et al., 1981]. Sera should be evaluated for reactions with other hormones and tissues. Vaccines employing the entire β-subunit of hCG induce antibodies cross-reactive with human LH, but these are devoid of cross-reactivity with human follicle stimulating hormone (FSH) and thyroid-stimulating hormone (TSH) [Singh et al., 1989]. The degree of cross-reaction with LH does not, however, impede ovulation [Thau et al., 1979; Nash et al., 1980; Talwar et al., 1990]. Similar observations have been made in ongoing phase I clinical studies with βhCG-TT vaccine in Helsinki (Dr T. Luukkainen), Santiago (Dr. H. Croxatto), and Santa Domingo (Dr. F. Alvarez). It is possible that the cross-reactive antibodies are of low affinity [Shastri et al., 1978] or that the human LH surge, encountered once a month, has surplus of the hormone vis-à-vis the amount needed to induce ovulation. Whatever be the mechanism, this type of cross-reaction does not seem to cause any unacceptable side effects. Menstruation is maintained by and large with no bleeding irregularities [Kharat et al., 1990]. The antibodies do not manifest adverse tissue reactivities, and DNA, rheumatoid factor, thyroid, adrenal, pituitary, nuclear, and islet cells reactivities are not observed (S. Sehgal, unpublished data). At times unexpected cross-reactions occur, even when devising a strategy that obviates anticipated cross-reaction with a hormone. For example, the vaccine based on the CTP of βhCG engenders antibodies free of cross-reaction with human LH [Jones et al., 1988]; however, the antibodies cross-react with pancreatic cells and pituitary [Rose et al., 1988]. The cross-reaction is due to the CTP, as it is absorbable with the peptide. Long-term effects of such cross-reactions, if any, are not known.

Studies on the long-term effects of immunization can only be conducted in vivo. For the βhCG-TT vaccine, toxicology studies were conducted in rhesus monkeys [Nath et al., 1976; Gupta et al., 1978].

No deposits of immune complexes were found in kidney and choroid plexus. Pituitaries and other tissues were normal. A long-term (5 to 7 year) study was conducted in rhesus monkeys hyperimmunized with ovine β-LH (β-oLH) employing FCA [Thau et al., 1987; Thau, 1988]. These studies demonstrated a lack of immunopathological consequences after immunization with LH cross-reactive immunogens. In view of the fact that immunological tolerance to a self-protein, hCG, is overcome by linkage with a carrier, a natural question was whether the manipulation would in any way compromise the T-cell nonreactivity to other self-molecules. That this does not happen is clear from numerous toxicology studies conducted in India [Nath et al., 1976; Gupta et al., 1978], by the Population Council in New York [Thau et al., 1987; Thau, 1988], and by the WHO Task Force on Vaccines for Fertility Regulation [Stevens and Jones, 1983].

Another issue of concern was the possible booster effect of hCG produced as a result of conception. If this were to occur, an immune response would develop progressively, resulting in permanent fertility block. To evaluate this possibility, women immunized with βhCG-TT were challenged with single or multiple doses of hCG [Ramakrishnan et al., 1976; Talwar et al., 1976]. Administration of hCG resulted in a decrease in antibody titers, indicating the hCG recognition by antibodies. The immune complexes were biologically inactive. Antibody titers returned to about the same levels as prevailed at the time of challenge within 23–25 days (Fig. 1). The antitetanus antibody titers did not change during the treatment. These studies show that hCG per se does not boost the immune response. Furthermore, the titers increase within 1 month so as to withstand the possible challenge of hCG in the subsequent cycle. Of course antibodies of adequate titers to meet the challenge are necessary.

Similar clearance studies have been done in recent phase I clinical trials. Women's antibody titers of 60 to 3,500 ng/ml hCG-binding capacity could combine with hCG given in the form of four to six daily injections of increasing amounts of the hormone (500, 1,000, 1,500, 3,000, 6,000 and 10,000 IU of hCG). No evidence of boosting of anti-hCG titers was noticed (unpublished data).

Similar studies are strongly recommended for sperm antigens. In contrast to hCG, many sperm proteins are intrinsically "foreign" to the immune system, and coitus may cause boosting of immunity. Long-lasting, if not permanent, infertility caused by immunological factors has been described in the clinical literature [Isojima, 1969; Hjort and Hansen, 1971].

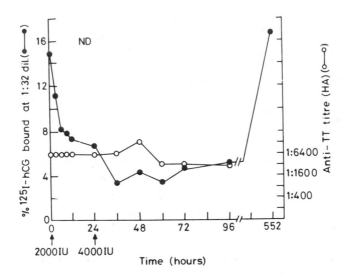

Fig. 1.   Effect of hCG administration on a human subject (N.D.) immunized
with βhCG-TT. hCG was given in two doubling doses of 2,000 and 4,000 IU,
which resulted in temporary decline of anti-hCG titer but not that of anti-TT.
Anti-hCG titer returned to pre-hCG challenge levels within 23 days. [Repro-
duced from Ramakrishnan et al., 1976.]

REVERSIBILITY

Immunization of rodents, nonhuman primates, and women with
βhCG-carrier vaccines has been observed to be reversible in all cases.
Antibody titers decline with time. Animals regain fertility, and the
progeny born are normal in every respect [Talwar et al., 1980]. This
may not be the case with gamete antigens; antisperm antibodies in
some vasectomized men are long lasting, and a percentage of vasectomized men do not regain fertility [for review, see Talwar, 1980]. In
addition, immunization of rabbits with porcine zona pellucida plus
FCA causes atresia of follicles and permanent sterility [Skinner et al.,
1984]. A moderate degree of immunization achieved with purified
zona antigens, however, may not cause irreversible impairment of
fertility [Aitken et al., 1984; Bamezai et al., 1986; Upadhyay et al.,
1989].

SAFETY

At the time that the hCG vaccine evolved, no safety guidelines
formally existed for testing safety. Some recommendations were
made by the WHO Steering Committee on Immunological Methods
for Fertility Regulation [1978]. The Indian Council of Medical Re-

search also established guidelines for birth control vaccines in 1985. In mid-1989, WHO convened another meeting of experts to review further and to establish safety guidelines in light of the latest knowledge. These should soon appear in print and will be useful as various birth control vaccines are developed. In contrast to other drugs, the active principle in the vaccines is not what is injected but what is produced by the body in response.

EFFICACY

Along with safety, a primary requirement of a vaccine is its efficacy, which must be evaluated in suitable models. The experimental model and parameters to be monitored vary depending on the mode by which efficacy is exercised. Knowledge in many cases may be partial; for example, it is believed that the main functions of hCG are to sustain the corpus luteum (CL) and to maintain progesterone production to prepare the endometrium for implantation of the embryo. If these are the sole functions of hCG, the ability of antibodies to inactivate the steroidogenic function of hCG can be tested in a variety of in vivo and in vitro systems not restricted to the species. hCG acts on the CL and Leydig cells of rodents and other easily available species. This may, however, not be the only site of action. Marmoset embryos exposed to anti-hCG antibodies failed to implant [Hearn et al., 1988].

NATURE AND QUANTUM OF IMMUNE RESPONSE

Having antibodies against the putative target molecule as measured by radioimmunoassay in no way guarantees the efficacy of immunization. For example, women became pregnant at anti-hCG titers of less than 10 ng/ml [Shahani et al., 1982]. Thus antibody levels above a threshold are required. The threshold for a given antigen may only be determinable by actual phase II efficacy studies. Furthermore, antibodies have to be of the right class and present at the right site. For gamete antigens, immunity in local genital tract may be necessary. Affinity or avidity of antibodies for the antigen has to be higher than the affinity of the antigen to its receptor. The association constant of hCG for the ovarian receptors is of the order of 10^{10} M^{-1} [Dufau et al., 1973]. Thus antibodies must have an equivalent or higher association constant for hCG to prevent it from binding to CL receptors. It was because of low affinity that Matsuura et al. [1979] observed that antibodies against the 30 amino acid CTP of βhCG, even though active in vitro, were devoid of efficacy in vivo.

ADJUVANTS

To obtain adequate antibody (or CMI) response, it is usually necessary to employ immunopotentiating agents. At present, alum is the only universally accepted adjuvant for human vaccines. Sodium phthalyl derivative of lipopolysaccharide from gram-negative bacteria (SPLPS) is an excellent nonpyrogenic adjuvant. It must be given with the first injection only. As an additive to alum, it improves antibody titers against luteinizing hormone-releasing hormone (LHRH) and hCG [Singh et al., 1982]. Several derivatives of muramyl dipeptide (MDP) have also been prepared that lack the pyrogenicity and other side effects of MDP. They, however, must be used, in most cases, as water-in-oil emulsions, in contrast to alum or SPLPS, which are usable in aqueous phase.

BIOEFFECTIVE EPITOPES

Antibodies to hCG of even high titer are not necessarily bioeffective. Louvet et al. [1974] reported the inability of high-titer antibodies (as determined by RIA), generated by the 23 amino acid CTP of βhCG, to inactivate hCG bioactivity. Similarly, antibodies against β-TSH did not inactivate TSH [Beall et al., 1973]. These observations point to the importance of the epitopes against which antibodies are directed to achieve efficacy. Every antibody reactive with sperm may not necessarily impair its fertilizing capability.

HOW TO ENSURE NEAR 100% RESPONSE

The effective agent in a birth control vaccine is the immune response generated and not the vaccine administered. Individuals respond in a variable manner to a given antigen. The genetic basis for differences in immunological responsiveness are becoming increasingly clear. A given epitope has to be read in context with products of immune response genes or MHC class II antigens. Hyporesponders to a given antigen are to be expected. This is especially likely to occur when the antigen has a single or limited number of determinants. Even for a larger protein, such as TT (with a molecular weight of 150 kd), used as a carrier, about 40% of immunized monkeys are hyporesponders even though *all* of them do make antibodies because of the multiplicity of determinants on the molecule. βhCG being a self-molecule, it requires coupling to a carrier to be

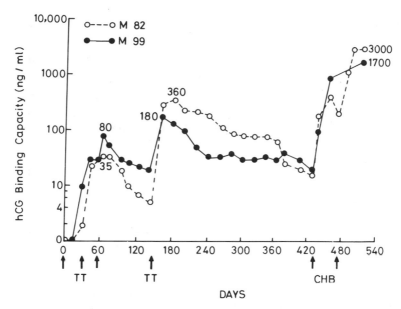

Fig. 2. Effect of immunization with gonadotropin conjugated to cholera toxin chain B (CHB) in two bonnet monkeys producing low anti-hCG titers with TT conjugate. [Reproduced from Talwar et al., 1987.]

rendered immunogenic. TT was initially used as the carrier for several reasons [Talwar et al., 1976]: It was available as a pure protein; it is approved for human use; a large body of past experience exists with this vaccine; it induces useful prophylaxis against a disease that contributes to maternal mortality at the time of delivery in the developing countries; and repeated injections are practiced as and when injury occurs without any apparent contraindication. βhCG vaccines linked to TT as carrier generated high antibody titers to hCG in about 60% of monkeys. In the rest, it was of a low order. Repeated booster injections with the vaccine presented on the same carrier did not appreciably increase the anti-hCG titers in these monkeys. We contended that the low responsiveness may be due to the genetic inability of these monkeys to respond to TT, because the carrier TT was responsible for T-helper activity. To verify the validity of this hypothesis and to devise a method to get high anti-hCG response in the hyporesponder monkeys, we presented βhCG to these monkeys on an alternate carrier, cholera toxin chain B (CHB). This resulted in induction of a high anti-hCG response (Fig. 2). Thus diversification of carriers may be one way of getting an adequate antibody response in all recipients.

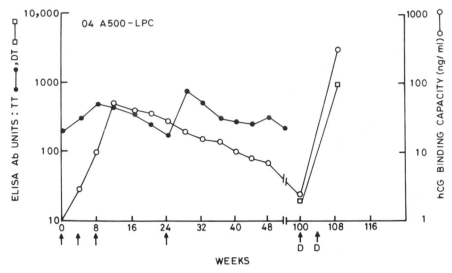

Fig. 3. Effect of booster injection with alternate carrier diphtheria toxoid (D) in a subject (LPC) showing no enhancement of anti-hCG titers following a booster with gonadotropin (500 μg) conjugated to TT. [Reproduced from Gaur et al., 1990.]

CARRIER-INDUCED IMMUNOSUPPRESSION

A large molecule such as TT has several determinants, some activating helper T cells against discrete genetic backgrounds, others inducing suppression. Carrier-induced suppression was initially observed in mice by Herzenberg et al. [1983]. We noted a similar phenomenon in women during phase I clinical trials with βhCG-TT and related vaccines. A few women failed to show enhancement of anti-hCG titers at the time of the booster injection. These women were immunized with TT prior to their enrollment in the anti-hCG vaccine trial. It is possible that repeated administration of a TT-linked vaccine at short intervals may have resulted in building up of suppression. Why it happened only in these women and not in others is unclear. There were other women in the trial whose preimmunization blood samples revealed prevalence of fairly high antitetanus antibodies. A study of the major histocompatibility complex (MHC) is under way, but conclusive results will not be possible on small numbers of subjects. Of interest is the generation of high anti-hCG titers in these subjects when βhCG (or related peptides) was presented on an alternate carrier, such as DT (Fig. 3) [Gaur et al., 1990].

MULTIVALENT VACCINES

Given the importance of class II MHC products in the generation of an effective immune response, it will be beneficial to employ antigens with several determinants. Another useful strategy will be to employ multiple vaccines. Not only will they enhance the chances of universal responsiveness, but their efficacy will be higher in view of multiple sites for interception of fertility. We are investigating such vaccines employing βhCG linked to purified zona proteins and sperm antigens.

CONCLUSIONS

For an antifertility vaccine to become workable in humans, several considerations have become evident from the experience with anti-hCG vaccines. It is important to assess satisfactorily the efficacy of immunization with putative vaccine candidates for control of fertility in suitable experimental models. It will be useful to delineate the nature of immune response implicit in efficacy, namely, humoral, cell mediated, or both. Passive immunization experiments can help define the role of antibodies. The avidity of antibodies for effective response may be a consideration for some vaccines. The site at which immune response needs to be generated for efficacy may be important for gamete antigens, such as local immunity in the genital tract. The immune response has to be adequate in magnitude, above a threshold to ensure efficacy. This has been demonstrated time and again for various antigens. Vaccine design should aim to present "bioeffective" epitopes. Various studies point to the presence in macromolecules of determinants that generate irrelevant antibodies and others that induce bioeffective antibodies. Delineation of these epitopes would be useful. It is further recommended that *multiple* determinants of this type, rather than a single one, be included, so as to overcome immunogenetic restrictions for response to a given determinant. Self-molecules and short peptides would require linkage to immunogenic carriers. Here again diversity of the carriers would ensure wider range of responsiveness and avoidance of hypersensitivity to a given carrier administered repeatedly.

ACKNOWLEDGMENTS

The work on the hCG vaccine was supported by grants from the Science and Technology Mission Project of the Department of Biotechnology, Government of India, the International Development

Research Centre (IDRC) of Canada, and the Rockefeller Foundation and benefited from cooperative interaction with the International Committee for Contraception Research of the Population Council, New York.

REFERENCES

Aitken RK, Richardson DW, Hulme M (1984): Immunological interference with the properties of the zona pellucida. In Creighton DB (ed): "Immunological Aspects of Reproduction in Mammals." London: Butterworth, pp 305–325.

Bamezai AK, Suman K, Das C, Talwar GP (1986): Effect of immunization against porcine zona pellucida (PZP) on steroid hormone profile and fertility in primates. J Reprod Immunol (Suppl):85.

Beall GN, Chopra IJ, Solomon DJ, Pierce JC, Cornell JS (1973): Neutralizing and non-neutralizing antibodies to bovine thyroid stimulating hormone and its subunits. J Clin Invest 52:2979–2985.

Chen HC, Hodgen GD (1976): Primate chorionic gonadotropins: Antigenic similarities to the unique carboxy terminal peptide of hCGβ subunit. J Clin Endocrinol Metab 43:1414–1417.

Dufau ML, Charreau EH, Catt KJ (1973): Characteristics of a soluble gonadotropin receptor from the rat testis. J Biol Chem 248:6973–6982.

Gaur A, Arunan K, Singh O, Talwar GP (1990): Bypass by an alternate carrier of acquired unresponsiveness to hCG upon repeated immunization with tetanus conjugated vaccine. Int Immunol 2:151–155.

Gupta PD, Nath I, Talwar GP (1978): Immunofluorescence and electron microscopic studies on kidney, choroid plexus and pituitary in rhesus monkeys immunized with the anti-hCG vaccine Pr-β-hCG-TT. Contraception 18:91–104.

Hearn JP (1976): Immunization against pregnancy. Proc R Soc Lond [Biol] 195:149–160.

Hearn JP, Gidley-Baird AA, Hodges JK, Summers PM, Wibley GE (1988): Embryonic signals during the preimplantation period in primates. J Reprod Fertil 36(Suppl):49–58.

Herzenberg LA, Tokuhisa T, Hayakawa K (1983): Epitope specific regulation. Annu Rev Immunol 19:609–623.

Hingorani V, Kumar S (1979): Anti-hCG immunization—Phase I clinical trials. In Talwar GP (ed): "Recent Advances in Reproduction and Regulation of Fertility." Amsterdam: Elsevier, pp 467–472.

Hjort T, Hansen KB (1971): Immunofluorescent studies on human spermatozoa. 1. The detection of different spermatozoal antibodies and their occurrence in normal and infertile women. Clin Exp Immunol 8:9–23.

Isojima S (1969): Relationship between antibodies to spermatozoa and sterility in females. In Edwards RG (ed): "Immunology and Reproduction." London: IPPF, pp 267–277.

Jones WR, Bradley J, Judd SJ, Denholm EH, Ing RMY, Mueller UW, Powell J, Griffin

PD, Stevens VC (1988): Phase I clinical trials of a World Health Organization birth control vaccine. Lancet 1:1295–1298.

Kharat I, Nair NS, Dhall K, Sawhney H, Krishna U, Shahani SM, Banerjee A, Roy S, Kumar S, Hingorani V, Om Singh, Talwar GP (1990): Analysis of menstrual records of women immunized with anti-hCG vaccines inducing antibodies partially cross-reactive with hLH. Contraception 41:293–299.

Kumar S, Sharma NC, Bajaj JS, Talwar GP, Hingorani V (1976): Clinical profile toxicology studies on four women immunized with Pr-β-hCG-TT. Contraception 13:252–267.

Louvet JP, Ross GT, Birken S, Canfield RE (1974): Absence of neutralizing effect of antisera to the unique structural region of human chorionic gonadotropin. J Clin Endocrinol Metab 39:1155–1158.

Matsuura S, Ohashi M, Chen HC, Hodgen GD (1979): A human chorionic gonadotropin specific antiserum against synthetic peptide analogues to the carboxy terminal peptide of its β-subunit. Endocrinology 104:396–401.

Nash H, Talwar GP, Segal S, Luukkainen T, Johannsson EDB, Vasquez J, Coutinho E, Sundaram K (1980): Observations on the antigenicity and clinical effects of a candidate anti-pregnancy vaccine: β-Subunit of human chorionic gonadotropin linked to tetanus toxoid. Fertil Steril 34:328–335.

Nath I, Gupta PD, Bhuyan UN, Talwar GP (1976): Autopsy report on rhesus monkeys immunized with Pr-β-hCG-TT vaccine. Contraception 13:213–224.

Ramakrishnan S, Dubey SK, Das C, Salahuddin M, Talwar GP, Kumar S, Hingorani V (1976): Influence of hCG and tetanus toxoid injections on the antibody titres in a subject immunized with Pr-β-hCG-TT. Contraception 13:245–251.

Rao LV, Singh O, Talwar GP (1988): Immunological cross-reactivity of antibodies with species chorionic gonadotropin is a critical requirement for efficacy testing of human chorionic gonadotropin vaccines in sub-human primates. J Reprod Immunol 13:53–63.

Rose NR, Burek CL, Smith JP (1988): Safety evaluation of hCG vaccine in primates: Autoantibody production. In Talwar GP (ed): Contraception Research for Today and the Nineties. New York: Springer-Verlag, pp 231–239.

Shahani SM, Kulkarni PP, Patel KL, Salahuddin M, Das C, Talwar GP (1982): Clinical and immunological responses with Pr-β-hCG-TT vaccine. Contraception 25:421–434.

Shastri N, Dubey SK, Vijay Raghvan S, Salahuddin M, Talwar GP (1978): Differential affinity of anti-Pr-β-hCG-TT antibodies for hCG and hLH. Contraception 18:23–34.

Singh O, Rao LV, Gaur A, Sharma NC, Alam A, Talwar GP (1989): Antibody response and characteristics of antibodies in women immunized with three contraceptive vaccines inducing antibodies against human chorionic gonadotropin. Fertil Steril 52:739–744.

Singh O, Shastri N, Narang BS, Talwar GP (1982): Immuno-prophylaxis: Search for an adjuvant acceptable in humans. In Cellular and Humoral Mechanism in Immune Response. New Delhi: Department of Atomic Energy, pp 114–118.

Skinner SM, Mills T, Kirchick HJ, Dunbar BS (1984): Immunization with zona pellucida proteins results in abnormal ovarian follicular differentiation and inhibition of gonadotropin induced steroid secretion. Endocrinology 115:2418–2432.

Stevens VC (1976): Perspectives of development of a fertility control vaccine from hormonal antigens of the trophoblast. In Development of Vaccines for Fertility Regulation. Copenhagen: Scriptor, pp 93–110.

Stevens VC, Jones WR (1983): Pre-clinical studies on an HCG vaccine. In Isojima S, Billington WD (eds): Reproductive Immunology. Amsterdam: Elsevier, pp 233–237.

Talwar GP (1980): Immunology of Contraception. London: Edward Arnold Publishers.

Talwar GP, Das C, Tandon A, Sharma MG, Salahuddin M, Dubey KS (1980): Immunization against hCG: Efficacy and teratological studies in baboons. In Anand Kumar TC (ed): Non-Human Primate Models for Study of Human Reproduction. Basel: Karger, pp 190–201.

Talwar GP, Hingorani V, Kumar S, Roy S, Banerjee A, Shahani SM, Krishna U, Dhall K, Sawhney H, Sharma NC, Singh O, Gaur A, Rao LV, Arunan K (1990): Phase I clinical trials with three formulations of anti-human chorionic gonadotropin vaccine. Contraception 41:301–316.

Talwar GP, Sharma NC, Dubey SK, Salahuddin M, Das C, Ramakrishnan S, Kumar S, Hingorani V (1976): Isoimmunization against human chorionic gonadotropin with conjugates of processed β-subunit of the hormone and tetanus toxoid. Proc Natl Acad Sci USA 73:218–222.

Talwar GP, Singh O, Rao LV (1988): An improved immunogen for anti-human chorionic gonadotropin vaccine eliciting antibodies reactive with a conformation native to the hormone without crossreaction with human follicle stimulating hormone and human thyroid stimulating hormone. J Reprod Immunol 14:203–212.

Talwar GP, Singh O, Singh V (1987): Birth control vaccines. In Diczfalusy E, Bygdeman (eds): Fertility Regulation Today and Tomorrow. New York: Raven Press, pp 43–54.

Tandon A, Das C, Jailkhani BL, Talwar GP (1981): Efficacy of antibodies generated by Pr-β-hCG-TT to terminate pregnancy in baboons: Its reversibility and rescue by medroxyprogesterone acetate. Contraception 24:83–95.

Thau RB (1988): Active immunization of rhesus monkeys against the β-subunit of ovine luteinizing hormone: Evaluation of safety and effectiveness of antigonadotropin vaccine. In Talwar GP (ed): Contraception Research for Today and the Nineties. New York: Springer-Verlag, pp 217–230.

Thau RB, Sundaram K, Thornton YS, Seidman LS (1979): Effects of immunization with the β-subunit of ovine luteinizing hormone on corpus luteum function in the rhesus monkeys. Fertil Steril 31:200–204.

Thau RB, Wilson CB, Sundaram K, Phillips D, Donelly T, Halmi NS, Bardin CW (1987): Long-term immunization against the β-subunit of ovine luteinizing hormone (oLHβ) has no adverse effect on pituitary functions in rhesus monkeys. Am J Reprod Immunol Microbiol 15:92–98.

Upadhyay SN, Thillaikoothan P, Bamezai A, Jayaraman S, Talwar GP (1989): Role of adjuvants in inhibiting influence of immunization with porcine zona pellucida antigen (ZP-3) on ovarian folliculogenesis in bonnet monkeys: A morphological study. Biol Reprod 41:665–673.

WHO Task Force on Immunological Methods for Fertility Regulation (1978): Evaluating the safety and efficacy of placental antigen vaccines for fertility regulation. Clin Exp Immunol 33:360–375.

DISCUSSION

DR. BIALY: How do you check that when you use the αoLH, some viral particles may not be present?

DR. TALWAR: Extensive purification procedures exclude the carry over of viral particles. In the long run, it will be taken care of by the fact that peptides will be made by the DNA recombinant approach.

MR. SPIELER: Concerning the slide on antibody titers using your C terminal preparation, you got an antibody titer, but does that antibody have any bioactivity? You showed that it was of low avidity.

DR. TALWAR: Adjuvants, such as alum, give very low titers with C-terminal peptide. But if you use complete Freund's adjuvant, you can get high RIA titers against the 45 C-terminal peptide (CTP). They are bioeffective in vitro, but not in vivo, probably because of low avidity.

DR. SUTCLIFFE: Could you tell us a little more about the hCG and the anchor sequence in vaccinia.

DR. TALWAR: The βhCG anchor construct was made by my colleagues, Srinivasan and Chakravarty. It is the gene for the 49 amino acid peptide of vasicularstomatitis virus glycoprotein that is tagged to the βhCG gene. This construct gives a very good immune response in comparison to the βhCG gene alone expressed by the vaccinia promoter. The latter is not as immunogenic.

DR. SUTCLIFFE: I would like to ask about the concept of the anchor to enhance immunogenicity.

DR. TALWAR: Most likely, the peptide expressed along with the transmembrane anchor is put on the membrane of the infected cell, and that sensitizes lymphocytes. This is the only way we can explain the higher immunogenicity of this construct and not of the construct where βhCG is expressed alone. The peptide in that case is released and thrown into circulation.

MR. GRIFFIN: What is the probability of introducing a lifetime immunity with that particular vaccinia-based vaccine system? Also, what is the risk of transmission from one individual to another?

DR. TALWAR: In the case of vaccinia rabies vaccine made and evaluated by our group, it has been possible to study the transmission of the virus to other co-caged animals. Thus far, a transmission has not been observed. I don't think that lifelong immunity is caused by vaccinia-delivered vaccines. In these studies, we note that a booster is necessary after a certain period of time to sustain the antibody titers.

38

Lessons From an Antihuman Chorionic Gonadotropin Contraceptive Vaccine Trial

Warren R. Jones

This chapter describes and discusses the issues and problems arising during the preparation for and conduct of a phase I clinical trial of a contraceptive vaccine directed against the pregnancy hormone human chorionic gonadotropin (hCG).

DEVELOPMENT OF AN hCG VACCINE

The World Health Organization (WHO), through its Special Programme of Research, Development, and Research Training in Human Reproduction, has been involved since 1974 in the development of an anti-hCG vaccine for fertility regulation [Stevens et al., 1982; Jones, 1982; Ada et al., 1985; Griffin, 1986, 1988]. The precise mechanism(s) by which such a vaccine might exert antifertility effects are unknown. The most likely major mechanism is the stimulation of antibodies that neutralize the luteotrophic effect of hCG. This would result in regression of the corpus luteum and disruption of implantation. Another possible action is by a direct immune attack on the hCG-producing cells of the peri-implantation blastocyst.

Whatever the mode of action, data on actively immunized marmosets [Hearn, 1976] and baboons [Stevens, 1976] indicate that an hCG vaccine is capable of blocking fertility at an early stage of pregnancy, with no discernible alterations in the menstrual cycle. This method, therefore, should be a highly acceptable birth control strategy.

Gamete Interaction: Prospects for Immunocontraception, pages 595–605
© 1990 Wiley-Liss, Inc.

THE ANTIGEN

hCG is a glycoprotein with a molecular weight of approximately 38 kd and a carbohydrate content of 30%. The hCG molecule consists of two dissimilar noncovalently linked subunits designated α and β. These subunits have been dissociated and purified and their primary structures established. The α-subunit, consisting of 89 to 92 amino acids, is quite similar in structure to that of pituitary glycoprotein hormones except for its content of β-galactose and sialic acid. There are, however, chemical differences between the β-subunit of hCG (β-hCG) and those of the pituitary hormones. Notwithstanding this, β-hCG and the β-chain of human luteinizing hormone (β-hLH) have 94 (85%) of the first 110 amino acids in common. However β-hLH has only 115 residues, whereas β-hCG has 145. Except for one position between residues 111 and 115, the 35 amino acid sequence of the carboxyl terminal (CT) end of β-hCG is not represented in β-hLH. These extra residues confer potentially unique antigenic properties on hCG and provide the basis for immunogen capable of provoking antibodies with specificity for hCG.

THE VACCINE

The vaccine strategy adopted by the WHO Task Force on Fertility Regulating Vaccines involved the use, as antigen, of a synthetic oligopeptide corresponding to the amino acid sequence 109–145 of the CT region of β-hCG. It was thereby aimed to achieve specificity and to avoid the possibility of cross-reactive autoimmunity involving β-hLH. To optimize immunogenicity, this antigen was synthesized and conjugated to diphtheria toxoid to form a hapten–carrier complex. The remaining components of the vaccine were a water-soluble synthetic muramyl dipeptide (MDP) analog as adjuvant and a saline–oil emulsion vehicle with an oil phase consisting of 4 parts squalene to 1 part mannide monooleate (Arlacel-A) as an emulsifying agent.

PRETRIAL ASSESSMENT

This prototype vaccine proved efficacious in baboons and was subjected to detailed toxicological and immunosafety testing [Stevens and Jones, 1983]. Preclinical assessment involved acute toxicology in the mouse and rat, subacute toxicology in the rat, and rabbit muscle irritancy studies. Immunosafety studies were conducted in baboons receiving three intramuscular injections of 0.5 ml vaccine volume at 28 day intervals. Clinical, hematological, biochemical, and urinary parameters were assessed together with in vivo testing for hypersensitivity, tissue autoantibodies, immune complexes, and hormone antibody cross-reactivity. Histopathology was assessed extensively following sacrifice 90 days after the last injection. Additional studies involved a separate group of baboons hyperimmunized with the vaccine or its individual components by six injections at fortnightly intervals.

THE PHASE I CLINICAL TRIAL

A Phase I clinical trial of the safety and immunogenicity of this vaccine was approved by the U.S. Food and Drug Administration in 1984 and subsequently by the Australian Department of Health in 1985. The trial was conducted during 1986 and 1987, and details of its design and results were published subsequently [Jones et al., 1988]. In brief, 30 premenopausal female subjects who had been surgically sterilized previously were assigned to five dosage groups of six subjects each and received the vaccine by intramuscular injection on two occasions 6 weeks apart. In each group four subjects received the full vaccine and two received the adjuvant and vehicle alone in a similar injection volume. The highest vaccine dose comprised 1.0 mg peptide–carrier conjugate in 0.5 ml vehicle. Immunogenicity and safety parameters were intensively monitored over a 6 month follow-up period, with further follow-up assessment as indicated.

LESSONS FROM THE TRIAL

In terms of concept, intended mode of action, and therapeutic rationale, vaccines directed against the physiological process of conception pose complex and novel problems in vaccine development. Additional complexities (and expense) include the special requirements for preclinical testing and the sophisticated and extensive safety monitoring in phase I and, to a lesser extent phase II trials, to accomodate any potential untoward interactions between the immune, reproductive, and endocrine systems and to monitor for cross-reactive autoimmunity. Further potential problems are added to the conduct of clinical trials of contraceptive vaccines by the ethical and legal issues they raise and by the novelty of the concepts they pose to drug regulatory agencies and to the community at large.

Ethical Aspects

Unlike strictly therapeutic drugs, a contraceptive method is intended for general use by individuals for prolonged periods of their reproductive life rather than for the treatment of specific disease. This imparts an added dimension of ethical responsibility to the conduct of clinical trials of contraceptives, an imperative that assumes an even sharper focus when vaccination against reproduction is contrasted with vaccination against infectious diseases. Moreover, more frequent, repeated immunization may be necessary to maintain contraceptive levels of immunity than disease-protecting immunization.

The ethical principles guiding the conduct of biomedical research involving human subjects are laid down in The Declaration of Helsinki of the World Medical Association as revised by the 29th World Medical Assembly in Tokyo in 1975 and in the *Proposed International Guidelines for Biomedical Research Involving Human Subjects*, published by the Council for International Organizations of Medical Science in Geneva in 1982. These guidelines state that a clinical trial, and its protocol, should be reviewed by an independent ethics committee. In practice, therefore, an antifertility vaccine clinical study will require ethical approval at several levels, for example, an international agency, if such is involved as sole or joint sponsor of the trial; a national body; and an institutional ethics committee.

Legal Aspects

There are two areas of biomedical research in which it is particularly difficult and expensive to obtain liability insurance protection, namely, for the development of contraceptives and of vaccines. When the two areas are combined in an antifertility vaccine, the problem is greatly compounded. Therefore, investigators will be wise to clarify the nature and extent of their legal indemnity and of potential subject compensation, particularly in relation to early phase trials. For example, most professional indemnity and insurance organizations will not accept liability for non-negligent trial-related mishaps. There may also be limitations on the extent to which trial sponsors will accept liability. For example, the WHO claims "global immunity" to claims for subject compensation in its research programs. Thus investigators should seek confirmation, in writing, of the extent of legal responsibility for trial mishaps that will be accepted by each of the involved parties, which may include international agencies, phamaceutical companies, government agencies, implementing institutions, and organizations providing liability insurance.

Drug Regulatory Aspects

Until relatively recently, national drug regulatory authorities have had no specific criteria for dealing with the normal aspects of anti-fertility vaccines. Experience in gaining drug regulatory approval for the CT peptide βhCG vaccine gave promise that an ongoing process of consultation with trial investigators and relevant experts will facilitate the processing of future trial applications. Central to this process will be the sharing of information on protocol format and trial problems between investigators, consultation between national regulatory agencies on assessment guidelines and strategies, and an advisory role for involved international agencies such as the WHO.

Community Reactions

Ethical and social concerns about the mode of action and potential for abuse of some contraceptive vaccines may lead to adverse community reactions to the conduct of trials. These reactions may be particularly fierce in minority religious or "right to life" groups who seek to impose their views on the community as a whole. The anti-hCG vaccine, apparently intercepting pregnancy before the process of implantation is completed, is regarded in selective religious and secular opinions as an abortifacient. Trial staff and subjects may be subject to at least indirect community abuse, and more serious attempts may be made at a government level to disrupt trials even though they have been fully sanctioned by the scientific, legal, and regulatory processes of the country involved. For example, in Australia, at the time of the phase I trial, a federal senator acting on behalf of a "right to life" organization adopted the following strategies: 1) a public campaign accusing the investigators of "experimenting with human embryos," 2) an attempt to block Australian government contributions to the WHO, and 3) an application under the federal Freedom of Information Act for disclosure of the Investigational New Drug (IND) application documents for the trial. This latter intrusion proved particularly burdensome and involved WHO, the pharmaceutical sponsors and affiliates, the institution, and the investigators in considerable time and cost (Aus$25,000) in responding to the application (which itself cost Aus$128). The outcome of this exercise was the release of a mutilated document that contained less information than was already in the public domain through reports, publications, and media releases.

Subject Recruitment

The recruitment of subjects for a phase I clinical trial of an anti-fertility vaccine is logistically difficult and time consuming. Detailed explanation is required for the trial staff and volunteers covering the aims of the trial, the criteria for inclusion, and the commitment necessary for successful completion. Potential subjects may be identified by approaches to selected community groups, for example, family planning clinics and women's organizations. It is also helpful to encourage sympathetic media coverage as a means of soliciting subjects.

As a result of these strategies, recruitment for the phase I trial in Australia resulted in 181 telephone enquiries from female volunteers, of which 89 were potentially suitable for inclusion. Of these, 57 were interested in participating and underwent the screening process. At this point 13 were excluded for the following reasons: carrier protein (DT) skin test positive (N = 2), HLA-B27 positive (2), subclinical autoimmune thryoiditis (1), acute autoimmune thrombocytopenia (1), decision to seek sterilization reversal (2), premenstrual tension/menstrual problems (2), husband opposed to trial (1), work commitments (1), and sudden death of husband (1). This left a final group of 44 to provide for 30 subjects plus reserves. Volunteers were motivated to participate by personal concern about currently available contraceptives ("I want a better method for my daughters") and by a desire to help women in third world countries.

Informed Consent

Volunteers for a clinical trial must be fully informed of the nature, risks, and benefits of the study. Specific features of contraceptive vaccine trials require particular emphasis, and the informed consent requirements vary with the trial phase. For example, in a phase I trial the participants receive no therapeutic benefit from the agent administered, and in both phase I and II trials, subjects must understand that reversibility cannot be assured.

Relevant issues regarding informed consent to participate in antifertility vaccine trials are as follows:

1   The experimental nature of the vaccine; the goals of the study; the nature of the antigen used and its role in reproduction; the likely mechanism of action; and the results of

previous preclinical and clinical studies of the vaccine, including adverse reactions

2   Theoretical risks, including adverse reactions not seen in previous studies; irreversibility of antifertility effect; failure of antifertility effect resulting in unplanned pregnancy (phase II–IV)

3   Options for dealing with unplanned pregnancy should it occur, including termination, if legal, and carrying the pregnancy to term with possible risk of an adverse outcome (phase II–IV)

4   Alternative methods of contraception available (for later phase trials); likely advantages of this form of contraception; real and theoretical benefits from participation in the study

5   Reimbursement for lost earnings and other legitimate expenses; Compensation available for subjects who experience adverse reactions, perhaps including the source of compensation and the spectrum of coverage (e.g., medical treatment, lost income, pain and suffering)

6   Study design, including eligibility criteria; number of participants and centers; duration; number of vaccine doses and route of administration; number and nature of visits; nature of invasive procedures (e.g., blood drawing, HIV testing, physical examinations, injections)

7   The need to be recontacted in the course of follow-up studies

8   The nature of any research related to, but not directly involved in, the aims of the trial (the subject must be given the option of participating in the main study but not in ancillary studies; Also, if it becomes apparent subsequent to the commencement of the trial, that the subject's participation may lead to other research goals, particularly if they have commercial implications, then separate and additional informed consent must be sought)

9   Confidentiality of subject records and safeguards against subject identification in publications

10   The name and telephone numbers of two persons (one independent of the trial staff) who may be contacted for further information or for reporting adverse reactions

After ensuring that all the relevant information has been provided and understood, the investigator will ask the subject to sign a consent form in the presence of a witness who also endorses the form.

Logistical Problems

The complexity and special requirements of a phase I clinical trial of a contraceptive vaccine may be associated with practical problems, some of which can be anticipated but others that may be unexpected. Examples from the Australian trial are as follows:

1   Three subjects had to be withdrawn before receiving their second injection. One had severe marital problems, one had a recurrence of a parasitic intestinal disorder, and one had converted to carrier (DT) skin test positive following the first injection.

2   The intensity of monitoring was somewhat daunting to subjects on occasions. Some traveled long distances for their assessments (one covered 1,200 km over the period of the trial). Multiple investigations on the one day caused some stress, for example, when a fasting blood sample was taken, followed by a skin test, ECG, and ophthalmoscopy; the latter resulting in blurred vision and a delay in departure from the hospital. An attempt was made to restrict blood sampling to a maximum of 30 ml. The average volume of blood required during the course of the trial was 750 ml.

3   There were difficulties in appropriating scarce in-patient beds for subjects requiring acute phase monitoring for 48 hr following injections.

4   An inquiry was received from the local blood transfusion service concerning the suitability of one of the vaccine recipients for blood donation. Since preclinical data suggested that passively induced abortion could be a remote consequence of transfused anti-hCG antibodies, trial subjects were advised against donating blood until their antibody levels had subsided.

5   A shipment of vaccine components was mislaid en route from New York to Adelaide, creating temporary difficulties in the progressive entry of subjects into the trial.

Quality Control

Stringent quality control requirements had to be met in the phase I trial of the complex CT peptide βhCG vaccine with its multiple components. The components were reconstituted and manually emulsified on the day of administration. Despite all attempts to standardize this procedure, it became clear that emulsion stability was suboptimal in some preparations, particularly in the highest dosage group. This problem, once recognized, required the replacement of 10 subjects in the original trial group and a review of the emulisification procedure. It also foreshadowed the need for a technical modification to ensure consistent vaccine emulsion stability for any future human trials using this vaccine formulation.

It is clear, therefore, that quality assurance may pose special problems in clinical trials particularly if complex vaccine delivery systems are utilized for injectable preparations. Careful clinical surveillance is necessary to identify local reactions and evidence of variable release rates of components from the injection site. In addition, the possible occurrence of side effects related to nonantigen components (e.g., carriers, adjuvants, vehicle) must be monitored.

Interpretation of Results

Although a phase I trial is aimed primarily at safety assessment, it is necessary that the measurement of one or more parameters of the immune response to the vaccine antigen give at least an indirect indication of potential efficacy. For the hCG vaccine this relied upon a theoretical calculation of the amount of circulating antibody required to neutralize effectively the early phase of the luteotrophic action of the target hormone. This level and its duration are central to the construction of a protocol for phase II (efficacy and safety) studies.

With regard to safety, it is important to differentiate, if possible, any potentially adverse findings related to the vaccine itself from those occurring, either incidentally during the trial or as inconsequential phenomena related to vaccination in general. This may be difficult when, as in the phase I hCG trial, no group of human trial subjects had been so intensively investigated particularly with regard to immunological parameters. In addition there are no baseline data on the transient serological perturbations that may follow any form of vaccination. Thus a wide variety of mostly low titer autoantibodies may be demonstrated in trial subjects that must be categorized variously as baseline serological epiphenomena, transient consequences of polyclonal activation, or reactions to specific vaccine components with implications for potential harmful cross-reactive autoimmunity.

Clinical abnormalities unrelated to the vaccine may occur in any group of trial subjects. For example, in the phase I trial five significant unrelated medical disorders were diagnosed during the period of follow-up observation. They were acute cholecystitis, Wolf-Parkinson-White syndrome, iron deficiency anemia, acute pyelonephritis, and colonic diverticulitis.

Trial-Related Research

With appropriate ethical approval, it is important to utilize the unique opportunities offered by phase I trials of novel contraceptive vaccines to pursue relavent trial-related research. This may aim to address basic questions in immunology, to determine possible modes of action, or to accrue information of value in future vaccine development.

REFERENCES

Ada GL, Basten A, Jones WR (1985): Prospects for developing vaccines to control fertility. Nature 317:288–289.

Griffin PD (1986): A fertility regulating vaccine based on the carboxyl-terminal peptide of the beta subunit of human chorionic gonadotrophin. In Talwar GP (ed): Immunological Approaches to Contraceptive and Promoting Fertility. New York: Plenum, pp 43–59.

Griffin PD (1988): Vaccines for fertility regulation in WHO Special Programme of Research, Development, and Research Training in Human Reproduction. Annu Rep p 177–198.

Hearn JB (1976): Immunisation against pregnancy. Proc R Soc Med 195:149–160.

Jones WR (1982): Immunological Fertility Regulation. Melbourne: Blackwell, pp 38–70.

Jones WR, Bradley J, Judd SJ, Denholm EH, Ing RMY, Mueller UW, Powell J, Griffin PD, Stevens VC (1988): Phase 1 clinical trial of a World Health Organisation birth control vaccine. Lancet 1:1295–1298.

Stevens VC (1976): Perspective of development of a fertility control vaccine from hormonal antigens of trophoblast. In Development of Vaccines for Fertility Regulation. (WHO Symposium). Copenhagen: Scriptor, pp 93–110.

Stevens VC, Jones WR (1983): Pre-clinical safety studies on a HCG vaccine. In Isojima S, Billington WD (eds): Reproductive Immunology 1983. Amsterdam: Elsevier pp 233–237.

Stevens VC, Powell JE, Lee AC, Griffin PD (1982): Antifertility effects of immunisation of female baboons with C-terminal peptides of human chorionic gonadotrophin. Fertil Steril 35:98–105.

DISCUSSION

DR. GUPTA: I was concerned when you commented that in all five groups you got the contraceptive antibody titers using a cut-off point of 0.25 to 0.5 nmole hCG. The antibody titers are not very high, keeping in mind that the hCG levels vary a lot in the initial stages of pregnancy. We do not known how long the hCG should be neutralized by these antibodies to bring about a contraceptive effect. Another issue that is of relevance that has not be discussed is the avidity of these antibodies. Thus I feel that it is an overstatement to say that you have achieved the contraceptive levels of the anti-hCG antibodies in all five groups.

DR. JONES: We won't know whether it is contraceptive until we do the phase II trial, but I understand your point. No one will know whether their vaccine is contraceptive until they do an efficacy study.

DR. SWERDLOFF: How did you deal with the issue of costs, for instance, for those women who got pregnant? That's an important issue in these type of studies.

DR. JONES: We didn't have to address that for the phase I trial. The hospital was actually prepared to indemnify the cost of hospitalization for any trial-related side effects. We really haven't, as yet, specifically addressed who is going to be responsible for the management of any pregnancies that arise. Clearly, part of the responsibility for the care will be clinically and financially absorbed by the hospital. But as for the liability for any compensation, we do not yet know who will absorb that.

DR. MAZZOLLI: Are you planning to inject your vaccine at a special time into the menstrual cycle?

DR. JONES: No. That is not necessary or practical in relation to a phase II trial in which we plan to recruit women who are using intrauterine contraception, and possibly barrier methods, and who will be immunized. The current method will then be withdrawn when they reach a contraceptive level of antibodies that will be set higher than the one that we have set here. Thus it will not be necessary to time it into the cycle, but to get the most mileage out of the cycles, and to look at progesterone levels and so forth, there is a need to control the immunization schedule.

39

Lessons Learned and Future Needs

N.A. Mitchison

It is a pleasure to have been asked to give my opinion on the possibilities for immunocontraception. Let me begin by saying that it is now generally accepted that vaccines will come to be used for the control of fertility. There is general agreement concerning their potential value in terms of acceptability, safety, and easy availability (see Chapter 33, this volume). At present, the vaccines that are most advanced for this purpose are directed against the hormone human chorionic gonadotropin (hCG), but recently interest in a second type of vaccine, directed against gamete antigens, has grown. That interest has been fostered by the Contraceptive Research and Development CONRAD Program and by the WHO Special Programme in Human Reproduction, and accordingly it was appropriate that this meeting should be sponsored by these two agencies, with the help of colleagues in Argentina. The aims of the meeting have been to survey the stage that has been reached in the development of this type of vaccine and to identify optimal strategies for future development.

One might ask why a new type of vaccine is needed if the antihormone vaccines are making such good progress, as is described in Chapters 37 and 38 (this volume). The fact is that efficacy has yet to be demonstrated for these vaccines, and accordingly it seems prudent to prepare an alternative. More importantly, it is likely that gamete-based vaccines would be applied in other ways (for example, in males as well as in females) or in countries that might forbid the use an antihormone vaccine.

Gamete-based vaccines are still at an early stage of development, and thus the scope of this workshop was fairly far-ranging. It examined the functional biology of sperm in some detail, paying particular

Gamete Interaction: Prospects for Immunocontraception, pages 607–613
© 1990 Wiley-Liss, Inc.

attention to the later stages of development that are likely to be the principal targets of immunological intervention, in the belief that this will help in choosing the best antigens. It examined naturally occurring antibodies to sperm and also, in passing, the iatrogenic antibodies that appear after vasectomy. It tried to relate these to naturally occurring infertility and found this a difficult task, as has been the experience with other conditions supposedly resulting from autoimmunity. Here again the aim was to obtain guidance in the choice of antigens. It paid close attention to recent progress with the hCG-based antifertility vaccines, because these are further along the road that the new vaccines must travel, and that experience is, therefore, very valuable. As Chapter 33 (this volume) emphasizes, that experience shows that the creative ideas and exciting discoveries at the start of a vaccine development program provide but a prelude to the lengthy, laborious, and expensive later stages.

It seems to me that two major messages emerge. One is that we are beginning to acquire a full understanding of the developmental program that mammalian gametes follow. Among these, the most important apply to the later stages of sperm development. This refers to the process of maturation that takes place in the epididymis that enables sperm to swim up the female reproductive tract, to bind to and penetrate through the zona pellucida and finally to bind to and penetrate the ovum, all understood in full molecular detail. Most of the descriptive biology has been known for some time, and recent progress with sea urchin sperm has opened the way into molecular biology. Another important developmental program is executed during maturation of the ovarian follicle.

The second message is that gamete-based vaccines fully merit development. The conclusion of this workshop can be formulated in the following way: We do not yet know for certain whether such a vaccine will work, but we are sure that not to find out would be to take a serious and unnecessary risk. Furthermore, we have identified enough candidate vaccine molecules, and we know enough about their molecular biology, to begin to ask sharp questions about future strategy.

GAMETE DEVELOPMENTAL PROGRAMS

Sperm Maturation in the Epididymis

Chapters 9, 10, and 11 (this volume) outline the chronology of sperm maturation in the epididymis, which varies greatly from one mammalian species to another. During the process many glycoproteins already present on the sperm surface undergo redistribution, and others are acquired from the epithelium of the epididymis. In addition to those acquired by human sperm as described in Chapter 10 (this volume), fibronectin is also acquired (Abstract 6, this volume), as also is a glycoprotein in the rat (Abstract 15, this volume). The physiological counterparts of these surface changes include gradual acquisition of full motility and the specialized metabolism of mature sperm.

The extent to which this sequence of events is controlled by a clock internal to sperm, or, alternatively, by signals transmitted from epididymal epithelium, is unclear. A program of this complexity is likely to need at least some extrinsic biological control. Any such signals that may emanate from the epithelium clearly offer a tempting target for intervention, whether by immunological or by pharmacological means.

In terms of research strategy, an important lesson from recent research on other comparable developmental programs is the value of establishing in vitro systems. Parallels to the problem of the interaction between sperm and epididymal epithelium can be found in the cell interactions involved in hemopoiesis, lymphopoiesis, and glial differentiation; in each case, progress became possible only when the cells concerned could be grown in vitro, preferably in the form of long-term cell lines. In studying epididymal epithelium, and perhaps in other current technologies for transformation, a substantial investment in the transfection of temperature-sensitive oncogenes is called for. For instance, the glycoproteins secreted by the epithelium will no doubt be cloned and their upstream control sequences identified: If those sequences prove unique, it would be worth hooking them up to transforming genes and making transgenic animals.

The question of the value as vaccine candidates of epididymal proteins taken up by sperm was touched on in discussion. They might seem unattractive, because residual unattached protein would be likely to block access by antibodies and because loosely attached protein would seem unlikely to exercise a major physiological function. However, at the present time we do not know enough about these proteins to exclude them from consideration.

Follicle Development

Chapters 19 and 20 (this volume) describe follicle development, which involves a sequence of events at least as complex as that of sperm maturation. As Chapter 22 (this volume) points out, it can best be understood in terms of control of expression of the genes encoding the three major zona pellucida proteins ZP1, ZP2, and ZP3. Thus far only the latter two have been cloned. Abstract 1 describes how the formation of a mature zona can be understood in terms of self-assembly of these proteins.

The considerations outlined for sperm maturation apply equally to the follicle: the importance of cell–cell signals as potential targets for intervention and the potential value of in vitro systems and cell lines for any full analysis. Control by the classic endocrine system is of course a conspicuous feature of follicle development. Because many of the crucial interactions take place between cells that are adjacent to one another within tissue, it is likely that cytokines will also be involved. Here, again, there is a lesson to be drawn from other cell interactions: The total repertoire of cytokines seems to be fairly restricted, and the same molecules tend to function in a variety of systems. A systematic search for expression of the major cytokines within follicles is therefore called for.

Do epitopes exist on the zona pellucida that develop so late that antibodies against them would not damage immature follicles? If such structures could be identified, much of the fear about the zona as the basis of a vaccine would dissipate. Chapter 20 (this volume) argues that this possibility remains open as a valid target of research.

The Acrosome Reaction

The acrosome reaction lends itself well to molecular analysis, and remarkable progress has been made. Chapter 1 (this volume) describes the mobilization of glycoproteins that occurs on the surface of guinea pig sperm and raises the question of why a glycoprotein such as PH-20 should have a phosphatidylinositol anchor. Does the mobility that this permits facilitate adhesion, or does cleavage of the anchor transduce a signal? The acrosome reaction emerges as a miniprogram, with its own trigger(s) and a well-defined sequence of events. Chapters 17 and 22 (this volume) single out binding of ZP3 as the trigger, and the former describes a monoclonal antibody that identifies a 95 Kd transmembrane protein with a binding site for ZP3 on the outer side and tyrosine phosphokinase activity on the inner side. This important molecule may or may not be identical to a protein of similar size defined by a monoclonal antibody described in Chapter 4 (this volume); that antibody has a definite antifertility effect. Other receptors in the form of lectins able to bind zona carbohydrates have been identified (see Chapter 16, this volume), and these raise the question of whether a meaningful distinction can be made between adhesion and signalling molecules on the sperm surface. If experience with the CD glycoproteins of the lymphocyte surface is anything to go by, such a distinction is unlikely.

As judged from what is known about sea urchin sperm and from the latest information about mammalian sperm discussed at this meeting, human sperm are likely to carry a subset of the standard transmembrane signalling machinery and to use this principally for triggering the acrosome reaction. The hunt is on, for instance, for G proteins and other components of the inositol triphosphate pathway. One imagines that for such a simple program not all the standard pathways will be required; sperm with their formidable packaging problem are unlikely to carry unnecessary luggage. For the purpose of fertility control, it is important to identify just what sperm do carry in order to design inhibitors (including antibodies and pharmacological methods). Another equally exciting possibility would be to design agents able to trigger a premature acrosome reaction, which might be brought about in the lower female reproductive tract or even within the male. Tentative essays in that direction can be found in Abstract 11 (this volume), concerning a factor from follicular fluid that induces the reaction. *Roblero* (Abstract 8, this volume) identifies high potassium concentration as another favorable factor.

Following the initial triggering event(s), the release of acrosin with its tripartite proteolytic site and its zona-binding site is a major component of the reaction. This is traced in elegant and extensive molecular detail by Topfer-Peterson (see Chapter 15, this volume).

Binding of Sperm to the Oolemmal Surface

Binding of sperm to the oolemmal surface has been less amenable to molecular analysis, but real progress has been achieved. Chapter 1 (this volume) describes cleavage of PH-30 on the surface of guinea pig sperm so as to reveal an oolemma-binding site. The surprise is the involvement of molecules hitherto known only in the immune system. Bronson (Abstract 18, this volume) defines an oolemmal Fc receptor and by implication an immunoglobulin-type structure on sperm. Anderson (in collaboration with Johnson; see general discussion following Chapter 13, this volume) identifies a complement receptor (for C3b) on the inner acrosome membrane that is exposed after the acrosome reaction; for this purpose, she used a monoclonal antibody to the CD-46 receptor on human lymphocytes. The corresponding C3b-like activity was found on the oolemmal surface. All this is encouraging, and progress with known molecules should be rapid, although the surfaces involved may be too cryptic to be much use for vaccination.

ISSUES OF VACCINE STRATEGY

During the course of this meeting at least five proteins of the sperm surface merged as serious vaccine candidates, as defined in this volume by Blaquier (Chapter 10), Goldberg (Chapter 5), Herr (Chapter 2), Moore (Chapter 4), and Primakoff (Chapter 7). Shaha (Chapter 6) has another candidate, and several participants, including Aitken (Chapter 21), have candidate zona molecules. Thus the most urgent question is whether the time has come to press ahead with what we have or to keep the net open in the hope of trapping something better.

In this connection, I want to re-emphasize that finding good candidates is relatively cheap compared with the enormous cost of developing and testing a vaccine. This argues against going for broke at too early a stage. But, on the other hand, funding is competitive, and the sooner we have something to show for our efforts, the more likely we are to secure further support. In this sense a prototype vaccine is needed, even though we know that it may not be the optimal choice and may never enter widespread use.

What can be learned from other vaccine development programs? The message is pretty confusing, as the WHO Special Programme in Human Reproduction has hitherto singled out just one vaccine for development (here described in Chapters 33, 35, and 38) in contrast to the WHO Tropical Disease Research Programme, which currently has about 20 candidate malaria vaccine molecules but has not yet singled one out. There are of course good reasons for this difference, but that does not help us with our immediate problem.

The guidance that might have been expected from natural and iatrogenic antisperm immunity has on the whole not been forthcoming. This is a topic dealt with here by Hjort (Chapter 23) and by Jones (Chapter 30). The effort put forth by WHO in sperm workshops is amply justified by the wide acceptance of standarized antibody assays, which have proved their worth in the clinical study of infertility. However, as pointers to useful antigens these antibodies turn out to be too weak and to bind to too many components of sperm.

Several voices were heard during the meeting expressing the view that simply to accumulate more monoclonal antibodies cannot be the right route. Can molecular genetics, as outlined here in Chapters 28 and 29 offer an alternative? The latter chapter described a strategy potentially able to identify all membrane-integral proteins expressed on the surface of sperm. The importance of this approach is obvious; the question is whether it will work!

Related to this issue is the question of how much importance should be attributed to functional assays. If we single out a test such as the adherence of sperm to zona (Chapter 31, this volume) and use it to identify good antibodies and therefore good antigens, may we thereby neglect other perfectly good antibodies able, say, to cause sperm to adhere to cervical mucus? Taken to its logical conclusion, this line of argument implies that we should simply collect surface antigens one by one and then test them only for their antifertility effect in an appropriate animal model. It might be argued that functional assays at least help us to assign priorities within our collection; but one needs to remember that an assay is of limited value unless failure would constitute an exclusion criterion.

This workshop summary reflects only my opinion, and I apologize to authors of chapters or abstracts that I did not mention. Their work and presentations were both interesting and relevant. My own opinion for, what it is worth, is that a gamete-based vaccine is entirely feasible and that such a vaccine would fulfill a valuable role in family planning and in population control. Support for research to that end deserves high priority. I doubt if we are yet in a position to identify the best vaccine antigen(s); the net cast for new antigens should therefore remain open. This stance should be maintained until we have obtained 1) a valid estimate of the total number of usable antigens on the surface of spermatozoa and 2) acceptable criteria that would allow us to exclude ineffective antigens. In the meantime, the implementation of one or more prototype vaccines should go ahead, and I wish the enterprise luck. As long as we know what we are doing and do not take an exaggerated view of the value of a prototype, implementation of a prototype should benefit the program as a whole.

General Discussion

MR. SPIELER: The floor is now open for general discussion. This is an opportunity for anyone who has something to contribute to speak.

DR. BLAQUIER: I would like to raise the issue of candidates for vaccine development. Dr. Mitchison mentioned that he feels that the tide is in favor of integral proteins versus acquired proteins, because antigens in seminal fluid might be a disadvantage for neutralization. I disagree. We foresee neutralization of sperm biological action in women, but it would not be at the site of deposition of sperm. It would be in the uterine cavity or the fallopian tube, where there would be a very reduced number of sperm and no free antigens from seminal fluid. Also, I think that if we ever developed a vaccine that could be used by men, it might be an advantage to have an antigen that is entirely foreign to the testes and, therefore, avoid orchitis.

DR. MITCHISON: I don't have an opinion on that subject myself. I was reminding the group about an earlier discussion when I repeatedly heard that the place to look for sperm was in the caput epididymis, before they have acquired the proteins that they acquire as they move down through the epididymis. I appeal to those who spoke up for focusing on caput sperm to take up the discussion with Dr. Blaquier.

MR. GRIFFIN: I think that the acquired antigens, such as the one that Dr. Cuasnicu talked about, are very good candidates.

DR. HAMILTON: We heard during the meeting that zona pellucida antigens cause atrophy of the ovary, to say it in simple terms. And in the male, even immunization with very sperm-specific surface antigens caused orchitis. Yet, now it has been suggested that we should define more and more epitopes to get more specific antigens. But doesn't the inherent problem remain—that we are immunizing against body constituents and that this may cause autoimmunity? Although you may say we have examples already from human chorionic gonadotropin (hCG) immunization, I think that these cases have not been followed properly. What do we known about those women who were immunized? Do you know what sort of delayed autoimmune disease is possible? I am very skeptical that immunization against body constituents would ever work without side effects.

Gamete Interaction: Prospects for Immunocontraception, pages 615–617
© 1990 Wiley-Liss, Inc.

Are there any other examples in medicine in which, in clinical terms, immunization against body constituents has been performed without side effects?

MR. GRIFFIN: You are absolutely right, but you are showing your prejudice as a member of the WHO Task Force on Male Methods of Fertility Regulation. I think that there is a tremendous application for antisperm research for women, although your points about the potential cross reactivity of an antisperm vaccine in men is valid.

DR. TALWAR: One cannot group the sperm and the zona antigens in the same category as a hCG; there is a marked difference in the two cases. Most of the antigens that you see on the sperm leading to orchitis are common antigens. They are intrinsically foreign to the immune system. On the other hand, a woman "bathes" in hCG and she is normally tolerant to that, and it requires a lot of administration for many years to make her even react against hCG. A negative reaction to hCG usually occurs in certain rare cases of clinical gonadotropic deficiencies or resistence caused by repeated administration of hCG. The antibodies are again of a type that are directed against the whole hormone and not subunits. This is the contrast that we should keep in mind. Also, over the years, clinicians have observed these cases of natural infertility in which there has been reaction against a common antigen; what sort of price do we pay clinically?

DR. HANDELSMANN: I wanted to respond to a question raised by Dr. Mitchison. He seemed to attach a rather low priority to the use of functional assays. In the WHO Sperm Antigen Workshop, they include functional assays in order to know where an antigen is blocking and if it is going to be functional. I was rather surprised to hear this suggestion to try and de-emphasize these assays. I was more impressed with the opposite view to focus on functional assays rather early and then attempt to find things that clearly had functional significance. The intellectual value of cataloging all the antigens is quite useful in its own right, but for now I would rather give high priority to antigens that perform well in functional assays.

DR. MITCHISON: Data to date add up to a whole list of cautions. Concerning functional tests, there is logic in saying that something that is active in a functional test is a good vaccine candidate, but while the net is still open, the question is, what's an exclusion factor? Do you want to exclude molecules because you don't know their function? There are probably many functions that we don't yet understand, although we may in a hundred years. Would you regard failure to perform in a functional test as a valid exclusion criterion at this stage?

DR. SWERDLOFF: I am not saying that I would not continue this approach. It is a question of how one considers the future. But I don't see that the clinical application of sperm antigens is close. So, it seems that we only disagree on the assessment of the future and the availability of contraceptive vaccines in the near future.

MR. GRIFFIN: Apart from the question of discarding candidates that may not prove to be active in some in vitro or in vivo test of functional significance, there is the question of discarding candidates that, in initial screening, appear to be potentially hazardous. This brings us back to the question of seminal plasma antigens. Some of the earlier work that was done in this area with much cruder preparations indicated that although seminal plasma antigens were highly immunogenic, and in many cases didn't affect fertility, they did stimulate an IgE response. That is not to say that all such antigens are going to react in this manner, but would an event like that exclude a candidate from consideration?

DR. SWERDLOFF: It is hard to argue with the concept that you want to find out as much as you can about the possible repertoire of sperm antigens. But, unless you apply some type of functional testing, how will you know when the net is full? And, how will you know when it is time to begin to apply what we have? It may be that we don't have all the appropriate functional tests that we would like to have, but, at some point, we are going to have to decide on some means to select one or two products and move forward.

Abstracts of Poster Presentations

1. Dissolution and Reconstitution of Zona Pellucida Filaments In Vitro

M.H. Vazquez and P.M. Wassarman

Department of Cell and Developmental Biology, Roche Institute of Molecular Biology, Roche Research Center, Nutley, NJ 07110

Mammalian fertilization is initiated by binding of sperm to the egg extracellular coat, or zona pellucida (ZP). The mouse ZP consists of three glycoproteins, called ZP1, ZP2, and ZP3, that interact with one another via noncovalent bonds to form the coat. ZP2–ZP3 dimers ($\sim$1800,000 M_r) serve as repeating subunits (every 15 nm) of filaments (several μm in length) that make up the ZP. Filaments are cross-linked by ZP1, giving rise to a thick ($\sim$7 μm) three-dimensional matrix that completely surrounds unfertilized eggs. To gain insight into the assembly and structure of the mouse ZP, dissolution and reconstitution of ZP filaments were studied under a variety of conditions in vitro. In each case, the status of ZP filaments was assessed by using transmission EM of rotary shadowed specimens sprayed and dried onto mica sheets. Kinetics of dissolution (i.e., decrease in length) and reconstitution (i.e., increase in length) of ZP filaments are affected by several parameters, including pH, temperature, and ionic strength. For example, at 37°C filaments are unstable in 10 mM ammonium acetate, dissociating to predominantly ZP2–ZP3 dimers in less than 5 hr. On the other hand, at the same temperature, but in 100 mM ammonium acetate, filaments remain essentially intact for up to about 30 hr. The stabilizing effect of ionic strength is also observed under conditions of high temperature (42–50°C) and low pH (3.5–5.5), as well as in the presence of reducing agents (e.g., dithiothreitol, 10–100 mM) and proteinases (e.g., elastase). Results of such experiments suggest that interactions between ZP2 and ZP3 in dimers are significantly more stable than interations between ZP2–ZP3 dimers that constitute ZP filaments. Reconstitution of dissociated ZP filaments also was studied under a variety of conditions and

Gamete Interaction: Prospects for Immunocontraception, pages 619–633
© 1990 Wiley-Liss, Inc.

found to be affected by the method used to dissociate filaments, as well as by reconstitution conditions. For example, the extent of reconstitution of filaments from ZP2–ZP3 dimers was enhanced at low temperatures and high ionic strengths. Dialysis of ZP2–ZP3 dimers (prepared at 37°C in 10 mM ammonium acetate, pH 7.5) at 4°C in 200 mM ammonium acetate, pH 7.5, yielded filaments up to 1,500 nm in length (ave. 487 ± 26 nm; N = 300). Thus, under certain conditions, filaments can be reconstituted in vitro from solubilized ZP glycoproteins. On the other hand, ZP2–ZP3 dimers prepared at 50°C or at low pH exhibited a significantly decreased capacity to be reconstituted into filaments. Results of such experiments suggest that the ZP is an example of a self-assembly system. Apparently, all of the structural information required to produce ZP filaments is present in ZP2 and ZP3. These and other experimental approaches are providing insight into the mechanism of assembly of the ZP during oocyte growth.

2. Domains of Different N-Linked Oligosaccharides on the Surface of the Human Spermatozoon

Alberto S. Cerezo and Josefina M.S. de Cerezo

Centro de Investigaciones en Reproduccion, Facultad de Medidina and Departmento de Quimica Organica, Facultad de Ciencias Exactas y Naturales, UBA, Buenos Aires, Argentina

In previous work we demonstrated the domains of high mannose-type asparagine-linked oligosaccharides in the membrane of the normal human spermatozoon. Desialication does not change the results, but these domains were altered in some cases of infertility. We compared these domains with those of N-linked complex–type oligosaccharides in spermatozoa from fertile and infertile men. Spermatozoa obtained by centrifugation or swim-up were treated with FITC-Con A for the detection of oligomannosidic type structures and FITC-1-PHA and FITC-e-PHA for complex type N-linked oligosaccharides, in limited concentrations, i.e., the highest concentration at which one can discern between different oligosaccharide densities. The smears were incubated 15 min at room temperature and observed by fluorescence microscopy using a BG 12 filter at 530 nm. The highest densities of oligomannosidic structures were found (visual estimation) in most spermatozoa to be in the equatorial zone of the acrosome (55–80%), the postnuclear cap (79–99%), the neck (70–90%), and the intermediate segment (20–40%), and an even smaller percentage of spermatozoa showed fluorescence over the entire head.

No structures of this type were found in the tail. In greater than 90% of the spermatozoa, the lactosaminic oligosaccharides covered the entire head of the sperm, slightly less dense in the postnuclear cap (80–90%), and significantly lower in the anterior part of the acrosome (15%). Both types of oligosaccharides share domains that are of great importance in the sperm–egg interaction. High mannose structures are precursors of the complex molecules, but it is also known that both structures may have different biological purposes. On that basis it is not known at the moment whether our results reflect a point in the synthesis of a system of a complex type of N-linked oligosaccharides, an equilibrium, or a peculiar state producing both structures as a result of restricted glycosylation.

3. An Aanalysis of the Oocyte Surface After Cortical Granule Release

S.H. Lee, K.K. Ahuja, and D.G. Whittingham

MRC Experimental Embryology and Teratology Unit, St. George's Hospital Medical School, Crammer Terrace, London SW17 ORE, England

The release of cortical granules (CG) and the completion of meiosis are two of the earliest responses observed during the process of mammalian oocyte activation induced either by the entry of a fertilizing spermatozoon or by artificial activating agents. The newly released CG contents modify the properties of the oocyte plasma membrane and the overlying zona pellucida to prevent the entry of further spermatozoa into the oocyte, the so-called block to polyspermy. An immunocytochemical method has been established in the mouse model to study the kinetics of the release of CG glycoconjugates and their fate during the early stages of development. We extended these studies involving UEA-I to rat, golden hamster, and human oocytes. FITC-UEA I binding to the plasma membranes of rat, hamster, and human oocytes showed a punctate distribution over the entire surface except the microvilli-free area overlying the meiotic spindle, which is known to lack CG. The CG-free area of the rat oocytes was identical to that of the mouse, but it was smaller in the hamster and rather insignificant in the human fertilized oocytes. It is tempting to suggest that the fucosyl glycoconjugates may be universally present in the CG of mammalian oocytes and that a simple staining method involving FITC-UEA I could provide a powerful tool for the study of fertilization-associated changes in mammalian oocytes.

4. Effect of Diffusible Glycoproteins From the Vitelline Envelope on Sperm Fertility in *Bufo Arenarum* (Amphibia, Anura)

M.O. Cabada, J.N. Valz-Gianinot, and E.J. del Pine

Departmento de Ciencias Biologicae, Facultad de Ciencias Bioquimicas y Farmaceuticas, Universidad Nacional de Rosario, Suipacha 531, Rosario (2000), R. Argentina (M.O.C.): Departmento de Biologia del Desarrello (INSIBIO), CONICET-Universidad Nacional de Tucuman, S.M. Tucuman (4000), R. Argentina (J.N.V.G., E.J.D.P.)

The vitelline envelope (VE), the acellular coat of amphibian oocytes, and its role on polyspermy prevention have been well studied. The VE also seems to have a role in gamete interactions during fertilization. The VE of deposed, dejellied, oocytes can be isolated and substantially freed of oocyte cytoplasm or fertilization envelopes (FE; VE modified by oocyte activation) by sieving oocyte's homogenate obtained in calcium-free Ringer's solution supplemented with EDTA through a nylon mesh. Isolated VEs release glycoproteins upon incubation in saline solutions. Spermatozoa incubated in the presence of these molecules lose their fertilizing capacity. Glycoproteins extracted from FE do not have this property. Affinity chromatography with Sepharose–concanavalin A indicate that glycoproteins bearing α-D-methylmannoside or α-D-methylglucoside residues are responsible for this activity, whereas glycoproteins retained by either Sepharose–soybean agglutinin or Sepharose–phytohemagglutinin do not eliminate sperm fertility. Enzymatic digestion of the protein fraction of the glycoprotein does not affect its activity, while elimination of the glycosidic moiety results in activity loss. Preliminary experiments labeling the glycoproteins with ^{125}I indicate that spermatozoa bind these molecules. These results suggest a direct interaction between the components of the VE and spermatozoa that could regulate the number of sperm passing through the VE and could explain the low number of spermatozoa found in the perivitelline space.

5. Epididymal Maturation of Spermatozoa in Guinea Pig and Galea Musteloides

M.H. Burgos, J.C. Cavicchia, L.S. Gutierrez, A. Vincenti, M. Montorzi, and M.W. Fornes

Instituto de Histologia y Embriologia, Universidad Nacional de Cuyo, Mendoza, Argentina

Spermatozoa obtained from caput epididymis in both cavidae when compared with those obtained from cauda epididymis show significant changes in the head shape, acrosome density, localization of polysaccharides (methenamine-silver), cholesterol reaction (digitonin and pilipin), and freeze-fracture characteristics of plasma membrane in the acrosomal region (hexagonal pattern) and in the postacrosomal region (increase in the concentration of intramembrane particles). In the guinea pig, localization of a monoclonal antibody PH-30 (gift of D. Myles) appears gradually in the postacrosomal region of spermatozoa obtained from proximal cauda epididymis that is in close contact with the apical surface of the epididymal epithelium. Reaction was negative in the rest of the spermatozoa as well as in the epithelium. All spermatozoa become positive only in the postacrosomal region at the distal cauda epididymis. An interaction of the epithelial surface and spermatozoa is the postulated mechanism for revealing PH-30 antigen.

6. Equatorial Segment Fibronectin is a Marker for Sperm Maturation in Humans

Patricia V. Miranda and Jorge G. Tezon

Instituto de Biologia y Medicina Experimental, Obligado 2490, 1428 Buenos Aires, Argentina

Fibronectin, a protein that mediates cell–cell interactions in many biological systems, localizes over the equatorial segment of human ejaculated spermatozoa. When fibronectin immunostaining was analyzed on spermatozoa from different regions of the epididymis (N = 6), 80% of spermatozoa from the caput exhibited a diffuse distribution over the entire head, while the equatorial segment was stained in 10% of the cells. This distribution changed gradually along the epididymis. The equatorial segment was immunoreactive in 80% of spermatozoa from the cauda. A main immunoreactive band with a molecular weight of 200 kd was detected by Western blot on extracts from ejaculated spermatozoa. Soluble fibronectin was detected in the epididymal secretions. De novo synthesis of proteins by cultured epidiymal tubules was studied by ^{35}S-methionine incorporation and analyzed by SDS-PAGE and fluorography. Active synthesis of fibronectin and its release into the medium were detected in cultures from caput, proximal, and distal corpus epididymis. An antiserum raised against secretions of the cauda epididymis immunoprecipitated radioactive fibronectin. These results suggest that equatorial segment fibronectin of ejaculated spermatozoa appears during epididymal transit probably as a result of incorporation of epididymal secretions.

7. Expression of Human LDH-C$_4$ Toward Development of an Immunocontraceptive Vaccine

Kay M. LeVan and Erwin Goldberg

Department of Biological Sciences, Northwestern University, Evanston, IL 60208

Immunization of female baboons with the mouse sperm-specific antigen LDH-C$_4$ reduces fertility by 70%. Immunization with the human LDH-C$_4$ would be expected to generate an immune response with greater specificity more effective in neutralizing primate sperm function. Because human sperm enzyme is not readily available in large quantities, recombinant DNA methodologies were used for production of human LDH-C$_4$. Antibodies to mouse LDH-C$_4$ were used to screen a λgtll human testis cDNA expression library, and a full-length human Ldh-c clone was identified and sequenced. A "cassette" was engineered consisting of only the human Ldh-c open reading frame bounded by synthetic linkers. The modified cDNA was subcloned into the prokaryotic expression vector pKK223-3 and introduced into *Escherichia coli*. Cells were grown to midlog phase and induced with isopropyl-D-B-thiogalactopyranosive (IPTG) for positive regulation of the strong hybrid tac promoter. Induced cells overexpressed the 35 kd subunit that spontaneously associated into the enzymatically active 140 kd tetramer. Human LDH-C$_4$ was purified 196-fold from liter cultures of cells by two-step affinity chromatography to a specific activity of 90 I.U./mg. Amino acid sequencing and composition and immunochemical and kinetic studies proved authenticity of the human LDH-C$_4$ produced in *E. coli*; Milligram quantities of purified human LDH-C$_4$ are now available for immunogenicity and fertility studies. Also, an Ldh-c recombinant vaccinia was engineered for development of a viral contraceptive vaccine. The cassette was subcloned within flanking vaccinia thymidine kinase (tk) sequences in the plasmid transfer vector pSCll. Human tk cells were cotransfected with the plasmid and wild-type vaccinia to allow homologous recombination between the tk sequences, and the Ldh-c recombinant vaccinia was selected in the presence of bromodeoxyuridine. Monkey and human tissue cultured cells infected with the purified recombinant vaccinia expressed the human sperm-specific enzymatically active tetramer. Immunization of rabbits with the recombinant vaccinia generated antibodies that recognized human LDH-C$_4$. A viral delivery system is highly immunogenic without the use of adjuvant and may prove to be a more convenient and effective birth control vaccine.

This work was supported by NIH grants HD05863 and HD23771.

8. High Potassium Concentration and the Cumulus Corona Oocyte Complex Stimulate the Fertilizing Capacity of Human Spermatozoa

L. Roblero, A. Guadarrama, M.E. Ortiz, E. Fernandez, and F. Zegers-Hochschild

Departmento de Obstetricia y Ginecologia, Clinica Las Condes, Instituto Chileno de Medicina Reproductiva, Santiago, Chile

This poster shows the influence of high (25 mM) potassium (K) concentration and the presence of hamster cumulus oophorus on ability of human spermatozoa to undergo the acrosome reaction (AR) and to penetrate zona-free hamster oocytes. Progressively motile spermatozoa recovered from fertile men were incubated for 24 hr in culture media containing either 4.7 or 25 mM K with or without hamster cumulus corona oocyte complexes (CCO). Aliquots of medium from each culture condition were obtained at various intervals up to 24 hr of incubation for assessment of viability, progressive motility, AR, and sperm penetration into zona free hamster oocytes. The percentage of spermatozoa with progressive motility was significantly higher at 24 hr ($P = 0.01$) in the presence of CCO, irrespective of K concentration. A significant decrease in sperm mortality ($P = 0.0001$) was observed in the association of 25 mM K and CCO. A higher percentage of AR was observed with spermatozoa incubated in 25 mM K than in 4.7 mM K, irrespective of the time and the presence or absence of CCO ($P = 0.0001$). The percentage of penetrated oocytes in 25 mM K was higher at 2 and 5 hr of incubation than in 4.7 mM K ($P = 0.0001$). The presence of CCO in the culture medium provoked an additional significant increase in the percentage of penetrated oocytes ($P = 0.0001$). Although at 24 hr of incubation the percentage of AR was higher than that found at 2 and 5 hr, the percentage of penetrated zona-free hamster oocytes did not increase proportionally. The data show that incubation in culture medium prepared with 25 mM K and in the presence of hamster CCO significantly increased the percentage of sperm with progressive motility, viability, AR, and the percentage of penetrated zona-free hamster oocytes.

9. Immune Response and Infertility: Oral Immunization With 24 kd Sperm Antigens in Rats

A. Suri, G.P. Talwar, and Chandrima Shaha

Sperm Biotechnology Laboratory, National Institute of Immunology, New Delhi, India

A group of 24 kd antigens from rat testicular cytosol was previously identified, and antibodies to this antigen were found to reduce fertility significantly by the systemic route. To improve upon efficacy, studies on a different route of immunization were initiated. Rats were immunized orally with the 24 kd antigens. Immune responses in the reproductive tract washings and serum titers were measured by estimating IgA and IgG antibodies and also by localization of IgA and IgG isotype plasma cells in the reproductive tract. All the rats showed both IgG and IgA antibody response in vaginal washings and in serum. The IgA antibody response was observed to be higher in vaginal washings of the immunized animal after mating. However, IgG antibodies were also higher, which could be of serum origin. Specific plasma cells of the IgA and IgG isotypes were present in higher numbers in the uterine horn of representative rats on day 1 and day 3 following mating as compared with control animals on the same days after copulation. The results provide data on the effectiveness of oral immunization in producing humoral immune response in the reproductive tract as well as in serum against 24 kd antigens.

10. Induction of Cell-Mediated Immunity to Sperm in the Female Reproductive Tract: An Alternate Approach to Intercept Gamete Interaction

Shaki N. Upadhyay, Charu Kaushic, and Gursanan P. Talwar

National Institute of Immunology, New Delhi, India

Female wistar rats were immunized against homologous sperm using vaccinia as an immunopotentiating agent through the intrauterine (IU) route. The immune response to sperm in the genital tract was evaluated. Animals were put on continuous mating for 6 weeks; antisperm antibody titers in serum (IgG) and vaginal fluid (IgG and

IgA) were checked at regular intervals. All animals in the experimental group were rendered infertile, while the animals of the control group receiving only vaccinia through the IU route were unaffected. No antisperm antibodies could be detected in serum or vaginal fluid. The regional lymph nodes in the experimental group showed significantly higher lymphocytic proliferative activity in response to antigenic challenge; supernatants from lymphocytic cultures of this group were found to have spermicidal effects. Immunohistological study of the uterus also showed greater leukocytic infiltration in the experimental group. The results of this study indicate that a local cell-mediated immunity to sperm in the genital tract can be induced through intrauterine immunization using vaccinia as immunopotentiating agent and that such an immune response does affect fertility.

11. Inhibition of Sperm Binding to Zona Pellucida Upon Treatment With Follicular Fluid

David L. Fulgham, Deborah Johnson, Chalres C. Coddington, Pius Adoyo, Douglas Danforth, Stephen Beebe, and Nancy J. Alexander

The Jones Institute for Reproductive Medicine, Eastern Virginia Medical School, Norfolk, VA 23510

Ninety percent of human sperm treated with human follicular fluid (hFF; 1:2, v:v) for 40 min were confirmed by electron microscopy to be acrosome reacted (AR) within 3–15 min. The sperm had been previously prepared using a swim-up into an overlayer of Biggers, Whitten, and Whittingham (BWW) medium and then allowed to undergo capacitation for 18 hr ($37°C$, 5% CO_2 and air). Because AR sperm are impaired in their ability to bind tightly to the zona pellucida, we investigated the effect of hFF on sperm–zona interaction with bisected salt-stored human eggs. One hemizona (HZ) was incubated with the capacitated sperm and the other with similar sperm that had been pretreated for 40 min with hFF prior to incubation with the zona. After 4 hr of sperm–HZ coincubation, there was a range of 88% to 100% reduction in sperm binding to zona pellucida (N = 4). The average number of sperm bound (no hFF) was 43 ± 31 compared with 5.5 ± 4.4 for those sperm exposed to hFF. To clarify the effect of the 18 hr incubation on sperm acrosome changes, fresh sperm were prepared using a swim-up into BWW and immediately treated with hFF prior to performance of the HZ assay. Again there was a marked reduction in sperm binding to the zona pellucida (N = 4): 49.8 ± 16 versus 1.7 ± 1.5. This reduction was in a range of 92% to

99%. Additionally, there was no difference in sperm binding ability of non-hFF–exposed sperm whether the sperm were fresh or capacitated for 18 hr (40 vs. 32 tightly bound sperm). Thus it is our impression that the reduction in binding ability was due to the effect of hFF treatment on the sperm.

12. Isolation of a Protein From Human Follicular Fluid That Induces the Acrosomal Reaction in Human Sperm

Patricia Saragueta, Jorge G. Tezon, and J. Lino Barañao

Instituto de Biologia y Medicina Experimental, Obligado 2490, 1428 Buenos Aires, Argentina

The stimulatory effect of follicular fluid on the acrosome reaction (AR) in sperm from homologous or heterologous species has been documented by several groups. We have isolated a protein factor from human follicular fluid (hFF) that was able to induce the AR in human sperm. This protein was purified by affinity chromatography with blue Dextran/agarose (Affi-gel Blue) followed by Mono Q^{TM} HR5/5 anionic interaction chromatography and Superose^{TM} 12 HR 10/30 gel filtration HPLC. The active fraction thus isolated eluted as a single peak of apparent molecular weight of 272,000 when analyzed on the superose column under nondenaturing conditions and as a single band of apparent molecular weight of 46,000 on EDε gel electrophoresis under denaturing conditions using silver stain. Dose–response studies indicated that an optimal concentration existed for both crude hFE and the purified protein. Maximal effects were observed with concentrations of 0.4 and 5×10^{-4} mg/ml, respectively. These results indicate that this protein might be the factor responsible for the AR-inducing activity in hFF. The highly purified preparation obtained will allow a further characterization of its mechanism of action and physiological role.

13. Monoclonal Antibodies Against Pig Zona Pellucida and Their Contraceptive Potential

M. Betancourt, H. Serrano, R. Fierro, E. Bonilla, and E. Casas

Departmento de Ciencias de la Salud, Universidad Autonoma Metropolitana-Iztapalapa, Mexico, D.F. CP.09340 Mexico

Porcine zona pellucida (ZP) is composed of three glycoprotein families, a 90 K family and two 55 K families denoted 55Kβ and 55Kα, which have polypeptide backbones of 40 K and 37K, respectively. To produce monoclonal antibodies (mAbs), the 55 K glycoproteins and the whole heat-solubilized pig ZP were used as immunogens. Using Western Blots those mAbs prepared using 55 K as the immunogen reacted only with the reduced 37K polypeptide. The mAbs obtained by using the whole ZP as the immunogen reacted with the 37K polypeptide on Western blots only when the disulfide bonds were not reduced. Thus the ZP immunogen mAbs are conformational dependent. The mAbs were tissue specific and did not recognize heart, lung, muscle, or kidney antigens. They cross-reacted with rabbit oocyte ZP but did not recognize the ZP of rat or mouse oocytes. Of nine mAbs against the 55K family, eight inhibited boar sperm binding to pig oocytes in vitro. These results indicate that the 37K polypeptide moiety appears to be highly immunogenic, a property that may be useful in the formulation of immunocontraceptive agents.

This work was supported in part by CONACyT (Mexico), grant PCSACNA-050314.

14. Partial Characterization of Human Sperm Antigens With a Role in Gamete Interaction

Adriana Dawidowski and Jorge A. Blaquier

Instituto de Biologia y Medicina Experimental, Obligado 2490, 1428 Buenos Aires, Argentina

A polyclonal antiserum (anti-KCl) against sperm surface antigens of epididymal origin disrupts the function of normal ejaculated human spermatozoa. Exposure to serum significantly decreased hamster oocyte penetration without altering movement characteristics or the occurrence of the acrosome reaction and also blocked the union of capacitated spermatozoa to human zonae pellucidae, suggesting that the antigens recognized are important for gamete interaction. We report on the preliminary characterization of the antigens recognized by anti-KCl. Western blots of SDS gels in which epididymal fluid or sperm extract were analyzed revealed the presence of two moieties, 18.7 ± 0.7 kd and 17.6 ± 0.6 kd, that were the main antigens specifically recognized by anti-KCl (N = 9). When analyzed under nondenaturing conditions, immunological activity was associated with a fraction with molecular weight $>1,000$ kd. Using an ELISA assay, the amount of antigens (U/100 ng protein) present in fluid obtained from the caput, proximal corpus, distal corpus, and cauda regions from five human epididymides was determined. The values were 0.30, 2.08, 4.89, and 10.94, respectively. In one instance, the amount of antigens present in spermatozoa recovered from the different segments was also determined. The values (U/10^4 spermatozoa) were caput, 2.23; corpus, 7.1; and cauda, 17.87. These data suggest that antigens are secreted into epididymal plasma, where they accumulate and interact with maturing spermatozoa.

This work was supported by NIH grant HD 15920 and by the National Research Council (Argentina).

15. Participation of a Rat Sperm Epididymal Glycoprotein in the Acquisition of Sperm–Egg Fusion Ability During Maturation

L. Rochwerger, P.S. Cuasnicú, and D. Conesa

Instituto de Biologia y Medicina Experimental, Obligado 2490, 1428 Buenos Aires, Argentina

Rat epididymal glycoprotein DE (molecular weight of 37,000) is associated with the dorsal region of the sperm (SP) acrosome during epididymal transit. Indirect immunofluorescence assays showed that, during in vivo and in vitro capacitation, DE redistributes to the equatorial segment, a region likely involved in fusion with the oolemma. Previous results showed that incubation of capacitated SP with anti-DE in vitro completely inhibited their ability to penetrate zona-free (ZF) eggs, suggesting a role for DE in the sperm–egg fusion event. The purpose of this study was to examine the participation of DE in the development of egg fusion ability by maturing SP. We observed that incubation of capacitated SP with the CA^{2+} ionophore A23187 (5 μM) for 1 hr raised the percentage of cells showing redistribution (R) from 50% to 92%, suggesting that this phenomenon might occur as a consequence of the acrosome reaction (AR). Because the ability of SP to undergo AR and fertilize eggs increases during maturation, SP recovered from successive segments of the epididymis (caput, H; proximal corpus, B1; distal corpus, B2; and cauda, T) were incubated under in vitro capacitating conditions and either tested for R of exposed to ZP eggs. The results indicate a gradual increase in the percentage of R (H:6, B1:38, B2:49, T:51) parallel to the increase in the percentage of ZF egg penetration (H:5, B1:16, B2:28, T:72). Finally, preincubation of B2 SP with purified protein DE (2 μg) significantly increased ($P < 0.05$) the percentage of ZF egg penetration (59 vs. 28) compared with control. Taken together, these results strongly favor the participation of protein DE in the development of sperm–egg fusion ability that occurs during maturation.

This work was supported by WHO grant 87094.

16. Percoll Separation and Functional Study of Semen Round Cells From Asthenozoospermic Men With Infection History

Alicia Mazzolli, Clydes Barrera, E. Salama, and Graciela Kortebani

Centro de Investigaciones en Reproduccion, Facultad de Medicina, Universidad de Buenos Aires, Paraguay 2155, Argentina

Sterile men with a history of infection in accessory glands or of orchiepididymitis frequently show a high number of round cells in semen simultaneously with asthenozoospermia. In this work we selected 20 asthenozoospermic men who had suffered infection 2 to 8 years prior to the time of this study but presently are uninfected, as shown by negative cultures and less than 10% semen neutrophils. Semen samples were submitted to gradients of 40, 50, 60, and 70% Percoll in RPMI-1640 medium. After centrifugation, the cells recovered from the different interphases were shown to be enriched populations of macrophages (Mac) and lymphocytes (Ly), 69% and 65%, respectively. The bottom contained mostly spermatozoa devoid of round cells. Ly subsets were studied by monoclonal antibodies (mAbs) and activated lymphocytes: anti-CD3, anti-CD4, anti-CD8, anti-IL-2 receptors, and anti-B. Mac were identified by mAbs (M5) and phagocytosis tests and functionally analyzed by immunobead tests for surface–specific immunoglobulins and by the antisperm cytophilic antibody test. Enriched Ly populations consisted mainly of T-Ly (80.5%), and within them T helper prevailed over suppressor/cytotoxic T subset (46.9 ± 5.7 vs. $33.6 \pm 4\%$). Within the total Ly population, 60% of the cells expressed the IL-2 receptor, indicating the activated state of these cells. Immature germinal cells were negative in all cases to mAbs used. Enriched populations of Mac exhibited antisperm immunoglobulins $40 \pm 6\%$ as determined by the antisperm cytophilic antibody test with a characteristic complex of sperm cells attached to Mac surfaces. In summary, our data suggest that the asthenozoospermic sterile men with leukocytospermia studied here possessed mainly activated T-helper lymphocytes. Simultaneously, Mac showed an activated state committed toward specific immunoglobulins. These findings reinforce the hypothesis that monokines and lymphokines may play a role in sperm motility and therefore in male fertility.

17. Protein Kinase Activity During Human Sperm Capacitation

Dora C. Miceli, Dolores Lamb, and Norka Ruiz Bravo

Department of Developmental Biology, CONICET—University Nac. de Tucuman (D.C.M.) and Department of Urology, Baylor College of Medicine (D.L., N.R.B.), Houston, TX 77030

Protein phosphorylation by protein kinases is associated with signal transduction in a number of cellular events important in reproduction. These events include egg activation and sperm motility. We therefore explored the possibility that protein phosphorylation by sperm cell surface protein kinases correlates with sperm capacitation and/or the induction of the acrosome reaction. Protein kinase activity was assessed by measuring the transfer of the terminal phosphate from ^{32}P-ATP to exogenous protein. We confirmed that intact, washed sperm from human ejaculates have cyclic AMP–dependent and cyclic AMP–independent cell surface protein kinase activities. The location of the enzymes was shown to be at the cell surface by their ability to be inhibited by p-chlorophenyl sulfonic acid, a thiol reagent that does not enter cells. The cyclic AMP–dependent and –independent kinase activities of freshly ejaculated sperm were not significantly different from the activities of sperm capacitated in vitro. Likewise, no significant difference was found between the kinase activities of sperm before and after treatment with calcium ionophore to induce the acrosome reaction. During in vitro capacitation, however, the cyclic AMP–independent protein kinase phosphorylated endogenous proteins on the sperm surface. Proteins phosphorylated by the cyclic AMP–dependent actokinase[´] have not yet been identified. Our results indicate that an active sperm cell surface kinase phosphorylates proteins on the sperm cell surface and proteins from capacitating media during in vitro capacitation. Whether an analogous phosphorylation of sperm cell surface proteins occurs during in vivo capacitation and whether a modulation of the phorphorylation state of these proteins is required for sperm capacitation are not yet known.

18. The Mechanism of Enhanced Fertilization of Zona-Free Hamster Eggs by Antibody-Labeled Human Spermatozoa

R.A. Bronson and G.W. Cooper

Division of Reproductive Endocrinology, Health Sciences Center, State University of New York, Stony Brook, NY 11794 (R.A.B.); Laboratory of Human Reproduction,

North Shore Hospital—Cornell University Medical Center, Manhasset, NY 11030
(G.W.C.)

Antisperm antibodies (ASAs) may promote as well as inhibit the penetration of zona-free hamster eggs by human spermatozoa. Following coincubation of gametes, a greater number of spermatozoa labeled with ASAs were found adherent to the oolemma when compared with antibody-free sperm, in association with increased egg penetration frequencies. To determine whether ASA-promoted fertilization is mediated by an enhanced ability of antibody-labeled sperm to fuse with the oolemma or solely through an increased binding of more sperm to the egg surface, zona-free hamster eggs were exposed to sperm suspensions for short periods of time, then washed out of sperm. In this manner, those sperm adherent to the oolemma could be observed serially, without the interference of continued binding by additional motile sperm. Antibody labeled spermatozoa were found to bind to the oolemma earlier than antibody-negative spermatozoa. During coincubation with eggs, greater numbers of the former sperm were found despite their exposure to equal concentrations of motile sperm in both groups. The chance of penetration of an egg by ASA-labeled versus ASA-free sperm, however, once the spermatozoan was adherent to the oolemma, was the same for both groups. We propose that certain ASAs promote fertilization by increasing the likelihood of adherence of antibody-labeled sperm to the oolemma either through a common epitope present on both gametes (Fab mediated) or through binding of antibodies to oolemmal Fc receptors.

Workshop Participants

Pius A. Adoyo
Eastern Virginia Medical School
Norfolk, Virginia

Kamal K. Ahuja
Cromwell Hospital
London, England

R.J. Aitken
Centre for Reproductive Biology
Edinburgh, Scotland

Javier Alahiz
Group of Interdisciplinary Studies
  of Fertility
Bariloche, Argentina

Isabel Albental
School of Biochemistry & Pharmacy
Rosario, Argentina

Nancy J. Alexander
Eastern Virginia Medical School
Norfolk, Virginia

Deborah J. Anderson
Harvard Medical School
Boston, Massachusetts

Enia Comini Andrada
Institute of Medical Investigations
Buenos Aires, Argentina

John A. Andrada
Institute of Medical Investigations
Buenos Aires, Argentina

Lydia T. Antolin
Eastern Virginia Medical School
Norfolk, Virginia

Miguel Bentacourt
Metropolitan University
  Autonoma-Iztapalapa
Mexico D.F., Mexico

Gabriel Bialy
National Institute of Child Health &
  Human Development
Bethesda, Maryland

Jorge A. Blaquier
FERTILAB
Buenos Aires, Argentina

Ricardo M. Borda
Pontificia University
Bogota, Colombia

Rose-Marie Bradley Jones
Eastern Virginia Medical School
Norfolk, Virginia

Alfonso Briones
Tajamar Echography Medical
  Building
Santiago, Chile

Richard A. Bronson
State University of New York
Stony Brook, New York

Cosima Brucker
Eastern Virginia Medical School
Norfolk, Virginia

Maria E. Bruzzone
University of Chile
Santiago, Chile

Mario H. Burgos
Institute of Histology and Embryology
Mendoza, Argentina

Eduardo Bustos-Obregon
University of Chile
Santiago, Chile

Marcelo O. Cabada
National University of Rosario
Rosario, Argentina

Mónica A. Cameo
FERTILAB
Buenos Aires, Argentina

Robert Capetola
R.W. Johnson Pharmaceutical Research
  Institute
Raritan, New Jersey

Christopher P. Carron
Duke University Medical Center
Durham, North Carolina

Maria V. Castagnino
School of Biochemistry & Pharmacy
Rosario, Argentina

Enrique A. Castellon
University of Chile
Santiago, Chile

Alberto S. Cerezo
University of Buenos Aires
Buenos Aires, Argentina

William W. Chin
Brigham and Women's Hospital
Boston, Massachusetts

Lee E. Claypool
U.S. Agency for International
Development
Washington, DC

Daniela Cone
Institute of Biology and Experimental
Medicine
Buenos Aires, Argentina

Patricia S. Cuasnicú
Institute of Biology and Experimental
Medicine
Buenos Aires, Argentina

Victor Cussac
Group of Interdisciplinary Studies of
Fertility
Bariloche, Argentina

J.L. Dacheux
Laboratory of Physiology of Reproduction
Nouzilly, France

Francoise Dacheux
National Institute of Scientific Research
Monnaie, France

Jurrien Dean
National Institute of Diabetes & Digestive
& Kidney Diseases
Bethesda, Maryland

A.E. De Ioannes
Pontifical Catholic University of Chile
Santiago, Chile

Luigi C. Devoto
University of Chile
Santiago, Chile

Gustavo F. Doncel
University of Buenos Aires
Buenos Aires, Argentina

Bonnie S. Dunbar
Baylor College of Medicine
Houston, Texas

Raina Fichorova
Brigham and Women's Hospital
Boston, Massachusetts

Vilma F. Fleites
Institute of Endocrinology & Metabolic
Disease
Havana, Cuba

David L. Fulgham
Eastern Virginia Medical School
Norfolk, Virginia

Henry L. Gabelnick
Eastern Virginia Medical School
Arlington, Virginia

Erwin Goldberg
Northwestern University
Evanston, Illinois

Gustavo Gonzales
Height Investigations Institute
Lima, Peru

David Griffin
World Health Organization
Geneva, Switzerland

Johan Anton Grootegoed
Erasmus University Rotterdam
Rotterdam, The Netherlands

Liu Guo-zhen
Peking Union Medical College Hospital
Beijing, China

Satish K. Gupta
National Institute of Immunology
New Delhi, India

David W. Hamilton
University of Minnesota
Minneapolis, Minnesota

David J. Handelsmann
University of Sydney
Sydney, Australia

Norman B. Hecht
Tufts University
Medford, Massachusetts

Marcelo las Heras
Centro de Investigaciones Reproductivas
Perez Companc
Buenos Aires, Argentina

John C. Herr
University of Virginia
Charlottesville, Virginia

Tage Hjort
University of Aarhus
Aarhus, Denmark

Carolyn L. Hudgens
Eastern Virginia Medical School
Norfolk, Virginia

Christian A. Huidobro
Las Condes Clinic
Santiago, Chile

M.A. Isahakia
Institute of Primate Research
Nairobi, Kenya

Shinzo Isojima
Hyogo Medical College
Nishinomiya, Japan

Deborah E. Johnson
Eastern Virginia Medical School
Norfolk, Virginia

Peter M. Johnson
University of Liverpool
Liverpool, England

Warren R. Jones
University of South Australia
Adelaide, S.A., Australia

Archil Khomassuridze
Human Reproduction Institute
Tbilisi, USSR

Maciej Kurpisz
Polish Academy of Sciences
Poznan, Poland

Estrella Lay-Diaz
Center of Investigation in Human
  Reproduction
Ministerio de Salud
Panama City, Panama

Chi-Yu Gregory Lee
University of British Columbia
Vancouver, Canada

Kay M. LeVan
Northwestern University
Evanston, Illinois

Livia Lustig
University of Buenos Aires
Buenos Aires, Argentina

Lorenzo E. Mallea
Institute of Endocrinology & Metabolic
  Disease
Havana, Cuba

Bernadette M. Mannaerts
Organon International bv
Oss, The Netherlands

Bonina J. Manuel
Group of Interdisciplinary Studies of
  Fertility
Bariloche, Argentina

Daniel de Matos
Centro de Investigaciones Reproductivas
  Perez Companc
Buenos Aires, Argentina

Alicia B. Mazzolli
University of Buenos Aires
Buenos Aires, Argentina

Michael E. McClure
National Institute of Child Health &
  Human Development
Bethesda, Maryland

Teodoro Mendez-Barria
Reproductive Medicine Unit
Santiago, Chile

Dora C. Miceli
Conicet University
Tucuman, Argentina

Patricia Miranda
Institute of Biology and Experimental
  Medicine
Buenos Aires, Argentina

N.A. Mitchison
University College London
London, England

Harry D.M. Moore
Zoological Society of London
London, England

Patricio J. Morales
Catholic University of Chile
Santiago, Chile

Diana G. Myles
University of Connecticut Health Center
Farmington, Connecticut

Eberhard Nieschlag
Max Planck Clinical Research Unit
Muenster, West Germany

Michael G. O'Rand
University of North Carolina
Chapel Hill, North Carolina

Lynda Pasini
World Health Organization
Geneva, Switzerland

Mario Perichon
Center of Biology of Reproduction
Rosario, Argentina

Maria Margarita Porta
Center of Medical Education and Clinical
  Investigations
Buenos Aires, Argentina

Paul Primakoff
University of Connecticut Health Center
Farmington, Connecticut

Vichai Reutrakul
Mahidol University
Bangkok, Thailand

Alexandro Ridley
Humana Hospital
Rosario, Argentina

Leonora Rochwerger
Institute of Biology and Experimental
  Medicine
Buenos Aires, Argentina

Mario A. Rubio
University of Chile
Santiago, Chile

Anthony G. Sacco
Wayne State University
Detroit, Michigan

Patricia M. Saling
Duke University Medical Center
Durham, North Carolina

Patricia E. Saragueta
Institute of Biology and Experimental
  Medicine
Buenos Aires, Argentina

Luis Schwaustein
School of Biochemistry & Pharmacy
Rosario, Argentina

Shobha Sehgal
Postgraduate Institute of Medical
  Education and Research
Chandigarh, India

Chandrima Shaha
National Institute of Immunology
New Delhi, India

Glenn F. Spaulding
Cytogam, Inc.
Chandler, Arizona

Jeffrey M. Spieler
U.S. Agency for International
  Development
Washington, DC

V.C. Stevens
Ohio State University
Columbus, Ohio

Anil Suri
National Institute of Immunology
New Delhi, India

R.G. Sutcliffe
University of Glasgow
Glasgow, Scotland

Ronald S. Swerdloff
Harbor-UCLA Medical Center
Torrence, California

G.P. Talwar
National Institute of Immunology
New Delhi, India

Jorge G. Tezon
Institute of Biology and Experimental
  Medicine
Buenos Aires, Argentina

Rosemarie B. Thau
The Population Council
New York, New York

Ivani Tokunaga
Sao Paulo Medical School
Sao Paulo-SP, Brazil

Claudia N. Tomes
School of Natural & Exact Sciences
Buenos Aires, Argentina

E. Töpfer-Petersen
University of Munich
Munich, West Germany

Shakti N. Upadhyay
National Institute of Immunology
New Delhi, India

David Vantman
University of Chile
Santiago, Chile

Fernando J. Vasquez
University of Chile
Santiago, Chile

Monica H. Vazquez
Mount Sinai School of Medicine
New York, New York

Geoffrey M.H. Waites
World Health Organization
Geneva, Switzerland

Christina Wang
University of Hong Kong
Hong Kong

Yi-Fei Wang
Shanghai Second Medical University
Shanghai, China

David G. Whittingham
St. George's Hospital Medical
    School
London, England

Chong Xu
Family Planning Research Institute of
    Sichuan
Chengdu, China

Index